MOLD CONTROLLED
by John C. Banta

Published by John C. Banta Publishing
contact: johncbanta@gmail.com
https://johncbanta.com

ISBN: 978-1-62660-177-2

Book design: Michael Campbell, MC Writing Services, mcwriting.com
Illustrations: Atik Sugiwara, fiverr.com/atiksugiwara

Printed in the United States of America

MOLD
CONTROLLED

A Guide to Finding, Fixing, Preventing, and Getting Help with Mold Problems in Homes

JOHN C. BANTA

Disclaimer

The information contained in this book, *Mold Controlled,* is provided for informational and educational purposes only. The author and publisher make no representations, warranties, or guarantees, express or implied, regarding the accuracy, applicability, fitness, or completeness of the contents of this book. The methods and materials described herein are based on the author's expertise and experience but may not be suitable for every situation or individual.

Readers are strongly advised to consult with qualified professionals, including medical practitioners, Indoor Environmental Professionals (IEPs), and remediation specialists, before applying any information, methods, or materials discussed in this book to their circumstances. The author and publisher expressly disclaim all liability for any damages, losses, or adverse outcomes arising from the use of, or reliance on, the information provided in this book.

This book is not intended to replace professional advice, medical diagnosis, or treatment. It is the reader's sole responsibility to ensure that any actions taken based on this book are appropriate for their specific needs and circumstances. The reader acknowledges that the author and publisher are not liable for any injuries, health complications, or damages resulting from the use or misuse of the information or materials provided.

By using this book, the reader agrees to the terms of this disclaimer and accepts full responsibility for any risks associated with its use.

Praise for
Mold Controlled

I have had the privilege of working with John Banta for the past 15 years, and am delighted that his new book *Mold Controlled* is now available. This will expand upon his previous book *Prescriptions for a Healthy House,* and will be invaluable for those countless patients and their families who are wrestling with mold toxicity. Mold toxicity is not rare, but thought to impact 10 million Americans, and those suffering with it are in desperate need for clear advice about how to minimize their exposures at home and work so that they can heal. In *Mold Controlled,* John has brought together a wealth of information that will enable these patients to learn how to do this properly. This is a "must read" for all who are struggling with mold toxicity.

NEIL NATHAN MD, AUTHOR OF *TOXIC: HEAL YOUR BODY* AND *THE SENSITIVE PATIENT'S HEALING GUIDE*

John's advice helped me through some of the most challenging times in my life. I attribute much of my healing and comfort in my home to him. This book is a must for anyone dealing with toxic mold.

MELANIE YUNK, HEALTHY HAVEN CONSULTING

WOW! This book brings clarity to mold in a way that is simple, comprehensive, and masterful. Whether you need quick wins or step-by-step actions, it delivers the tools to diagnose, remediate, and manage mold effectively. A must-have resource that places the power to change your home and health back in your hands.

LYNNE WHITE, BBEC, BBNC, EMRS, STABLE ENVIRONMENT CONSULTING, INC.

To Trisha, my wife and my greatest love for the past 50 years. Your unwavering support, patience, and strength have carried me through every challenge. I am forever grateful for you.
To my daughters, Tiffany and Jamie. Jamie, your sharp editorial eye, organization, computer skills, and encouragement kept me going when I struggled. Tiffany, your practical wisdom and reminders to lighten up helped me find clarity and balance.

Without the three of you, this book—and so much more— would not have been possible. Thank you for your love, your guidance, and for always keeping me grounded.

Contents

Acknowledgements

I WANT TO EXPRESS PROFOUND GRATITUDE to those who have supported and influenced my journey to create healthier homes.

I am grateful to have met Helmut Ziehe, founder of IBE, early in my career. Helmut's translation of Dr. Anton Schneider's teachings from German into English reinforced my belief in the principles of building biology, 'do no harm' and 'simple is better.' Early collaborations with Peter Sierck and David Bierman helped expand my knowledge through shared teaching and discussions.

Special thanks to my co-authors Paula Baker-Laporte and Dr. Erica Elliott for inviting me over 25 years ago to join their collaboration, which has resulted in four editions of *Prescriptions for a Healthy House*. My work with them inspired and gave me the confidence to write this book, with *Mold Controlled* becoming a companion guide to *Prescriptions for a Healthy House*. Paula's expertise in building science and occupant health is genuinely exceptional.

I joined RestCon Environmental in 1997 and was fortunate to work under Jim and Pam Holland, the company's owners, until 2020. Jim mentored me in water damage restoration, guiding me to train with top experts. His generosity in sharing his knowledge has profoundly influenced my approach to balancing science and empathy in restoration.

In 2020, Peter and Shara Lyons became the new owners of RestCon Environmental. Their encouragement in developing Pathways™ Testing and support in shaping *Mold Controlled* have been invaluable. I also want to acknowledge the dedicated team at RestCon Environmental—Jennifer Germond, Amy Cluck McCalister, and Danielle Minitti—whose support has been essential in keeping operations running smoothly and making this work possible.

I am grateful to the microbiologists who helped me understand microbiological laboratory procedures, notably Chin Yang, PhD, Sean Abbott, PhD, and Boni Passmore, PhD. My ongoing collaboration with Boni Passmore has been essential to my work at RestCon Environmental and the development of this book.

Special thanks also to the team at Roots and Branches. Dr. Eric Dorninger recognized that I was developing an uncontrolled tremor and insisted I get checked. Healthcare providers Dr. Dana Bjerke, ND, LAc, and Genevieve Lamancusa, FNP-C, oversaw and managed my care. CIRS took away my ability to write. At first, I thought it was just writer's block, but as my condition worsened, I went into denial. Eric's intervention and Dana and Genevieve's care led to a complete recovery and a new perspective. Over the last eight months, the book has been entirely rewritten with many new additions beyond what I had initially planned. I once feared this book would never be finished. Thanks to their expert care and hard work, it has come together and, in the process, given me firsthand insight into what my wife and clients have endured. Experiencing CIRS from the inside out has deepened my understanding in ways I never anticipated.

I also want to thank Dr. Ritchie Shoemaker, whom I was introduced to by my friend and colleague Will Spates shortly before his passing. Looking back, I see how a series of unexpected events guided me to Dr. Shoemaker and his extensive work. His groundbreaking research and dedication to training physicians have been instrumental in advancing the understanding of CIRS. His willingness to review sections of this book, provide clarifications, and offer encouragement was invaluable. His insights into chronic inflammatory response syndrome (CIRS) have provided a scientific framework that underpins much of the guidance in this book. This book might never have taken shape without his pioneering research and leadership.

I am also grateful to many others whose guidance, expertise, and support have been essential in shaping this book. Specifically, Mary Brooker, and Willie and Elaine Swenson. I want to thank contributors Jennifer Schrantz, Jane Prescot, Laurie Rossi, Jenny Johnson, Ken Larsen, Dr. Ryan Holsapple, Alex Kessler, Ramona Gallagher, Scott Forsgren, Cindy Edwards, and Atik Sugiwara for their invaluable contributions. Their insights, research, and encouragement have been instrumental in the development of this work. Special thanks to distinguished environmental consultant contributors Bill Weber, Michael Schrantz, Marilee Nelson, Greg Weatherman, and Mary Cordaro, whose professional expertise and friendships I deeply value.

Lastly, I want to thank my wife, Trisha, and daughters, Tiffany and Jamie, for their unwavering trust and support. My goal has always been to protect them and help turn the tide on their health struggles by understanding and improving our living environments.

Foreword

by Doctor Eric Dorninger

MOLD IS A BEAST. I've had patients describe it as "an entity" and a family-wrecking, relationship-stealing, mind-numbing, exhausting thief that overwhelms, confuses, depletes, and wipes out patients, healthcare providers, and environmental professionals despite their best efforts to understand and conquer it.

Although these are all accurate descriptions, mold is ultimately a biotoxin that can trigger non-sensical, over-zealous innate cytokine storms of inflammation that need no passport to cross every 'body' border into every 'body' system and drive multi-system, multi-symptom illness. The fancy term for this multi-symptom, multi-system illness is CIRS or Chronic Inflammatory Response Syndrome.

Peer-reviewed, published sources of biotoxins that can trigger CIRS include seafood toxins (e.g., *Pfiesteria,* ciguatera); cyanobacteria from algae blooms; Lyme disease from tick bites and tick-related co-infections; recluse spider venom; molds and bacteria from water-damaged buildings (e.g., actinobacteria); and bacterial endotoxins (e.g., sewer gas, fecal matter).

Biotoxins, or "nature toxins," are special substances called ionophores or amphipaths/amphiphiles that have both water-soluble (hydrophilic) and fat-soluble (hydrophobic) properties. This dual nature allows biotoxins to move easily from one cell to another, almost like they can "walk through walls," due to their tiny size (as small as 1.4 angstroms) and ability to share electrons. These toxins tend to be stored in fat and nerve tissues, where they interact with cellular receptors, such as Toll-like receptors (specifically TLR2 and TLR4), mannose receptors, dectin receptors, and C-type lectin receptors, which can trigger ongoing immune system activation. (Shoemaker R. C., 2010), (Berry, 2014)

Hence, biotoxin illness is not so much a disease of toxicity but more a disease caused by overactive, unregulated, self-made cytokine storms. Chronic, unchecked, and uncoordinated innate immune responses are the leading cause of CIRS. The result of CIRS includes MHM or molecular hypometabolism, which means the body's energy production slows down, leading to chronic fatigue, along with neuroendocrine dysregulation (failure of the body's hormone systems) and brain atrophy (shrinkage of the brain). Molecular hypometabolism (MHM) is just a scientific term for the chronic fatigue that comes from CIRS.

Consequently, urinary mycotoxins cannot be used to diagnose CIRS. We all have urinary mycotoxins, and mycotoxins in the urine are simply a measure of exposure, not a measure of immune reactivity, and not a measure to confirm illness. Elevated urinary mycotoxins could come from a moldy building, a moldy blueberry, or a peanut.

The awakening of chronic innate immune responses to biotoxins is what "turns on" the illness and why a husband and wife could be living in the same moldy house, and one spouse is feeling relatively well while the other feels deathly ill.

Often, one spouse and the kids feel ill while the other spouse is thriving. This familial discrepancy is most often due to genetic predisposition (Mom and kids have the gene, but Dad doesn't, or vice versa). HLA (Human Leukocyte Antigen), or our "Immune Response Genetics" from our biological Mom and Dad, exists on Chromosome 6.

Chromosome 6 is where the majority of immune response genes for all the inflammatory diseases exist. There is most likely an HLA for every inflammatory disease known to humans, and we are bound only by our current knowledge. Crohn's, Ulcerative Colitis, Psoriatic Arthritis, ankylosing spondylosis, Type 1 Diabetes, Celiac, Rheumatoid Arthritis, and Hashimoto's are just some of the illnesses that we have discovered HLA (genetic predisposition). CIRS has the greatest HLA genetic predisposition for any inflammatory illness I have ever worked with.

Having an HLA genetic predisposition does not guarantee that you will get this illness, but it dramatically increases the statistical likelihood of getting that particular illness. This is why we often see that the grandma, mom, daughter, and granddaughter all have Hashimoto's thyroid antibodies.

"Genetics loads the Gun; environment pulls the trigger." Hence, the goal with CIRS is to ensure the environment (a water-damaged building) doesn't get introduced to those with CIRS genetics (that would be dreamy). Unfortunately, the EPA estimates that over 50% of American buildings are water-damaged... Sigh.

For those overloaded with understanding the "threshold" of expression of an inflammatory illness, celiac disease is an easy example. People born with the HLA DQ 2 or 8 have a higher statistical likelihood of getting Celiac (an autoimmune or self-attack on your intestinal lining partially driven by environmental exposure to gluten). Yet, many people who "wake up" celiac have been eating gluten for years, even decades. Modern Celiac research shows a multi-factorial trigger approach (i.e., low Vitamin D, gluten ingestion, and finally, a cold or the flu) to be the multi-factorial environment that finally woke up the genetic expression of the illness.

Nevertheless, if someone with the HLA for Celiac never had Gluten exposure, they would never express or "wake up" Celiac disease.

The same is true for CIRS. Many patients who have one of the multiple HLA genetic predisposition genes for biotoxin illness have been living/working/recreating in water-damaged buildings for years (home, school, work, relatives, church, yoga studio, gym, etc.) but felt fine. Then, one day, they get a cold or the flu, and although they didn't die from the flu, they never fully recovered, and a new triggered paradigm of brain fog, fatigue, and multi-symptom illness is their "new norm."

During COVID, Richie Shoemaker, MD, published a pilot study of 19 patients (5 were from our clinic, including yours truly). (Shoemaker R. C., 2022) This small study demonstrated that in these 19 patients, COVID Long hauling is a CIRS. Yet unlike previous CIRS cases where Mold was the biotoxin culprit, Actinobacteria and/or bacterial endotoxin was the biotoxin exposure this time.

To say this clearly, 19 people were in Actinobacteria and/or bacterial Endotoxin and doing relatively fine (despite the fact that sewer gas is good for no one). They got COVID, then they made it through COVID, but now specific inflammatory genes that were sitting dormant turned on to "manufacture" or express chronic inflammatory proteins, making the patient sick with all the symptoms of CIRS. To our relief, strict, earnest adherence and execution of the Shoemaker protocol restored these patients and turned off those genes, including my very own inflammatory responses.

Fortunately, *Mold Controlled* covers the topics and approach of endotoxin and actinobacteria and many other non-CIRS environmental inflammatory phenomena (e.g., allergies, MCS, aspergillosis, hypersensitive pneumonitis). Unfortunately, most people needing this book will have CIRS as their primary diagnosis. Nevertheless, CIRS is a vicious *yet treatable* illness, but it all starts with the buildings.

In his book *Mold Controlled*, John Banta shows you meticulous, clear, effective steps to get to "Healthcare Clean." Many of his approaches in this book are the same as those taught in the CIRSx Institute "Medically Important Remediation" (MIR) Course that John helped author. The inspiration for that course was my plea for our best environmental professionals to write a course to teach well-intentioned remediation companies to get buildings to "healthcare clean." Tragically, without Step 1 of the Shoemaker Protocol, "Remove Patient from Biotoxin Exposure," the patient's improvements remain mediocre instead of miraculous.

When working with patients who can't get proper inspection, remediation, and home maintenance in place ("Remove patient from biotoxin exposure"), I feel like a doctor giving antibiotics to someone whose water supply is contaminated. To treat the village, you need water engineers more than doctors to solve and resolve the situation. A proper remediation company is the "water engineer" for those with CIRS. In *Mold Controlled,* John empowers the patient with the knowledge, questions, and nudging necessary to ensure service companies understand healthcare clean.

Imagine a world where building architecture, engineering, and construction practices prioritized "healthcare clean." John Banta and Paula Baker-Laporte meticulously served this world in their first book *"Prescriptions for a Healthy House"* (4th Edition). Although this book is more of a reference book for everything from home design to building materials, wall systems, and plumbing, it is a staple and mainstay for anyone designing a home and evaluating best practices for construction projects, including reconstruction and remodeling after mold remediation. *Mold Controlled* addresses an even bigger looming problem in society: our current buildings and how to fix them and maintain them.

In a recent medical paper that several colleagues and I published with Dr. Shoemaker, we discovered a specific genetic expression pattern or "fingerprint" for Parkinson's disease in patients with chronic inflammatory response syndrome. (Shoemaker R. R., 2024) Although the data sets were small, this paper suggests CIRS as one potential underlying cause of Parkinson's Disease (PD). PD patients showed substantial improvement when this pattern was present, and the Shoemaker protocol was implemented. Moreover, people without any symptoms of PD who evidenced the same gene expression turned off the expressed gene fingerprint with the implementation of the Shoemaker protocol, potentially rewriting the genetic destiny of Parkinson's.

So, the stakes are high, and the buildings are low-quality and in very bad shape. We need trusted human beings with scientific integrity and a desire to serve, teach, organize, and standardize best practices to help CIRS patients and all humans access "healthcare clean" buildings. John Banta is one of those human beings.

When I try to explain who John Banta is, I tell people if "Einstein and Santa Claus" had a child, his name would be John Banta. He is jocund, benevolent, gritty, and brilliant. He is a man of the people, for the people. He has been informed by high-brow academia, tech lab work, relentless building experience, and the challenging camaraderie of honest peers. Yet, the most important influence in John's work is his family's suffering and the trials and tribulations they undertook to attain their health and wellness.

No one has all the answers, but John has many. This book actualizes the best of building science. It includes practical approaches to remediation and maintenance, guidance on professional versus DIY moments, and practical step-by-step advice accessible to those experiencing CIRS. Moreover, it has phenomenally practical tips for patients navigating their healthcare. John does not claim to be a doctor but a witness to all the pitfalls the CIRS community endures and has set up practical explanations on building and environmental illness with checklists and guideposts for navigating your way back to health.

John is one of the best teachers I know. He is a scientist and an educator. Over the years, his Mold Congress, Surviving Mold, and CIRSx conference talks are always "not to be missed," and attendees walk away with literal applications to improve building and healthcare outcomes for themselves and their community. Many of John's impactful talks can be seen on CIRSx.com under the curated videos tab: "Indoor Environmental Professionals & Buildings." As you'll see in John's lecture style, he doesn't talk over people; he talks into people, generously pouring all the knowledge and experience necessary to WIN building health.

As a Naturopathic Doctor who has been in healthcare for 30 years and private practice for 20 years, it's only been the last 12 years that I fully realized for CIRS patients Building Health IS Human Health. Once I surrendered to the painful and joyous truth of Step 1 of the Shoemaker Protocol, "Remove Patient from Biotoxin Exposure," I realized the true Heroes and Healers of this Healthcare crisis are the environmental professionals who do their job in earnest with pride, grit, integrity and the latest in building ecology knowledge. As a cherished senior counsel member of the CIRS community and a selfless leader in building science, John Banta leaves it all on the page in *Mold Controlled: A Guide to Finding, Fixing, Preventing, and Getting Help with Mold Problems in Homes*. This is an essential companion for graduating those afflicted with CIRS.

May this book bless your journey back to wellness.

In health and graduation to restored wellness,
Eric Dorninger ND, LAc

References

Berry, Y. (2014). *Physicians' guide to understanding and treating biotoxin illness: Based on the work of Ritchie Shoemaker, MD.*

Shoemaker, R. C. (2010). *Surviving mold: Life in the era of dangerous buildings.* Otter Bay Books.

Shoemaker, R. C. (2022). Treatable metabolic and inflammatory abnormalities in Post COVID Syndrome (PCS) define the transcriptomic basis for persistent symptoms: Lessons from CIRS. *Surviving Mold.* Retrieved from https://www.survivingmold.com/Publications/2493-Treatable_metabolic_and_inflammatory_abnormalities_in_Post_COVID(2).pdf

Shoemaker, R. R. (2024). A transcriptomic fingerprint for Parkinson's disease found in patients with chronic inflammatory response syndrome: Implications for diagnosis, treatment, and prevention. *Medical Research Archives, 12*(10). Retrieved from https://doi.org/10.18103/mra.v12i10.5788

Introduction

This book is about protecting two of our most valuable assets: Our home and our health. We spend as much as 90% of our time indoors. (USEPA, 2008) Our homes should protect and keep us healthy, but modern materials, design, maintenance, and construction practices often result in a healthy home rapidly deteriorating and attacking our health and well-being.

Why Water-damage Organisms Matter

Homes are continually becoming more expensive and are often built with cheaper composite materials that do not stand up to the test of time. It was standard for crafted homes built in the 1800s to last a century without major deterioration. They tended to be cold and drafty and require a higher energy input to make them comfortable—but they were sound. If they got wet, the materials used for construction tended to be more resilient, holding up well to the frequent wetting and drying cycles without rapidly falling apart. Contrast that with today's buildings, which cannot dry by themselves rapidly. This results in a greater vulnerability when water intrusion occurs. When materials get wet, they have a limited time to dry before that moisture begins to result in deterioration.

Our modern homes need ongoing maintenance to keep the water out. We need to perform the maintenance in ways that promote the health and longevity of the structure and the people living inside. Unfortunately, one of our teachers, the television, often sacrifices quality information for entertainment value and is not providing us with the information we need to do a safe and healthy job. Television reality shows focusing on flipping houses or do-it-yourself home renovation frequently skip over the more foundational aspects of home repair and maintenance and often concentrate on cosmetics.

Our homes are typically one of our most expensive purchases ever. Our monthly housing expenditure commonly exceeds our food budget, even when renting or leasing. (U.S. DOL, 2022) We expect the places where we live to be resilient, low maintenance, and to increase in value. Regrettably, today's construction materials and practices almost guarantee they will deteriorate—in many cases, this begins before the construction is complete. EPA guidance tells us that newly constructed buildings often start their lives with water damage from:

1. Use of building materials that are repeatedly or deeply wetted before the building is fully enclosed.
2. Poor control of rain and snow resulting from roof, window, siding, and flashing leaks
3. Wet or damp construction cavities
4. Moisture-laden outdoor air entering the building.
5. Condensation on cool surfaces. (IOM, 2004)

Construction defects, accidents, and routine wear and tear can lead to mold growth. Much of the deterioration in our homes is directly related to water. Excess moisture accelerates building deterioration. (USEPA, 1989)

Buildings are constructed of various materials with varying degrees of mold resistance. Stones, cement, and masonry are generally resistant to mold growth, with some buildings made exclusively from these materials surviving centuries. The rot resistance of wood lumber varies according to the type of wood and what part of the tree was milled for the lumber. Various sticks, stones, and other chunks of materials are typically assembled into the features we use to build our shelter. When we start with dry organic materials for constructing our buildings, we must prevent them from getting and staying wet with excess moisture to arrest the natural decay that would typically happen.

When sensitive construction materials remain wet for too long, the structure experiences the same processes as compost piles. It decays and begins to fall apart. Some parts degrade faster than others, but decay happens without proper care. Understanding how to care for our homes is necessary to be good stewards of our environment. Modern construction requires continuous maintenance to keep our buildings dry, healthy, and habitable.

PURPOSE OF THIS BOOK

In *Mold Controlled: Understanding, Finding, Fixing, and Preventing Problems Associated with Water Damage in Homes,* my goal is to equip you with the knowledge and skills to establish and maintain a clean, dry, healthy living environment. By applying the principles laid out in this book, you'll learn how to recognize a healthy home and take proactive measures to prevent the development of elevated levels of water-related microorganisms.

You'll acquire techniques for applying quality control measures during construction or remodeling to help avoid water entry and subsequent microorganism growth. If water damage does occur, this book will help you understand the thorough, rapid, non-toxic, professional restoration techniques necessary to bring your home back to a healthy state.

Moreover, you'll understand how to manage risks and control expenses effectively, preventing the costs and complications often associated with chronic water damage. This includes professional remediation methods for existing mold and the prevention of unwanted spores spreading into unaffected areas of your home.

WHAT YOU WILL LEARN: A SUMMARY OF CONTENTS

This book is a practical guide to help individuals navigate the complexities of renting, buying, evaluating, or fixing an already damaged home and personal possessions. With a particular focus beyond mere safety in favor of healthfulness, it is specially tailored for those with environmental sensitivities, offering guidance to help ensure the spaces they choose promote well-being. This book is divided into Four Parts:

Part One: Understanding Mold and Water Damage

Part one of this book sets the foundation for what you, as a homeowner or renter, need to know about managing water damage and controlling mold. This book is designed to empower you with the essential knowledge and tools to take charge of your home's health. By understanding how to identify, address, and prevent mold and water damage, you can confidently manage the remediation process and distinguish true expertise when hiring contractors. This is particularly crucial if you or someone in your household has hypersensitivities to mold, chemicals, perfumes, or typical remediation practices. Many so-called solutions will frequently worsen the problem for those with these sensitivities, which is why this book emphasizes a thoughtful, health-first approach.

You'll learn the importance of physically removing mold, controlling moisture, and cleaning contamination without relying on harmful chemicals, biocides, or deodorizers. The key to mold control isn't killing it but preventing and eliminating the conditions that allow it to grow. Maintaining a dry environment is essential. Mold remediation isn't the only step—keeping your home *Mold Controlled* means cleaning up and managing mold spores and fragments over time. Once you understand this process, you can implement immediate and lasting measures to protect your home's structural integrity and safeguard the health of its occupants.

This book isn't just for homeowners—renters will also find valuable insights on how to identify mold and water-related issues in their living spaces. Whether you're dealing with a minor leak or major flooding, this knowledge will equip you to take control of the situation before it escalates into a more significant issue.

Part Two: Navigating the Mold-Controlled Plan

This section guides managing water damage emergencies, navigating the process of owning or renting a home, and following my Five Stage, 25 Step Process for addressing water damage and mold. It combines expert insights with practical steps to help you recognize and respond to emergencies, make informed home selections, and oversee remediation and restoration for a healthier living space. Whether you own the property or not, the approach to investigating and resolving issues remains the same. For spaces you don't own—like rentals, workplaces, or temporary housing—this section helps you understand the situation, advocate for a healthier environment, and assess how your goals can be achieved or address complications that may arise.

Emergency Water Damage and Response

The first section of Part Two begins with guidelines on what to do when unexpected water damage occurs. While we hope these situations never happen, the reality is that they often do, and they can pose significant challenges, particularly for individuals with sensitivities. Swift action is always crucial. This section is dedicated to preparing for and responding to such emergencies. It offers practical advice on how to plan and equip yourself with strategies to mitigate damage yourself or immediately determine when professional help will be essential to ensuring a safe, healthy environment is restored after unforeseen events.

Preparedness is key. By familiarizing yourself with these procedures in advance, you can respond promptly when faced with water damage, minimizing its impact and maintaining a healthier living space.

Home Evaluation Guide: Things to Know When Buying, Renting, or Maintaining a Home

This second section serves as a comprehensive guide for anyone assessing a potential living space, whether you are considering renting or purchasing. Parts of this section are also important for reviewing a property you already occupy. It provides insights into evaluating both new and older homes across different climate zones, aiding in assessing the current condition of a structure and identifying potential issues before they manifest. Additionally, it helps recognize weak points or areas for consideration or concern once you have already occupied the space.

- With strategies for spotting visible problems, subtler signs, available information, and coverups, this section is designed to help you detect or foresee water damage and related issues in homes. Understanding your living space, especially if you are mold-sensitive, is crucial for making appropriate decisions for planning and adjusting your life and actions. The objective is to enhance your ability to identify risks associated with any living space, ensuring you are well-prepared to understand how to select, restore, and maintain a home that promotes the health and well-being of its occupants. This proactive approach minimizes surprises and adverse conditions, providing you with the knowledge to make informed decisions about your living environment.

The Five Stage, 25 Steps for Problem Identification, Remediation and Restoration

- The third section is the heart of the book. It delves into a Five Stage detailed 25 Step process, especially for those with mold and water-damage hypersensitivities. This Section of the book helps with the process of diagnosing and addressing past and present water damage and microbial issues within a home. My goal is to turn you into your own best expert regarding your home, helping address your needs regarding water damage and the organisms that can develop when a building gets wet and stays wet too long. It is not specifically a do-it-yourself manual but will help you evaluate if you and the professionals you may need to hire have the know-how, compassion, and ability to provide the assistance you will need. Mold work is always full of surprises, but my desire is to help minimize these issues and help you approach them with eyes wide open! These include methods for uncovering hidden problems when there are no obvious visual signs or odors, tailored remediation approaches for those with environmental

sensitivities, and rigorous quality control measures to confirm the success of remediation efforts. It also emphasizes the importance of rectifying the source of water intrusion and provides considerations for the reconstruction phase to ensure the long-term health of the home environment.

- **Stage One: Determine if Your Home Has a Problem** with water damage and the associated microorganisms. Here, you will focus on identifying potential water damage and the related organisms in your home. In this initial phase, you'll leverage your knowledge, accessible resources, and expert assistance to gather information through the property's non-destructive 'surface survey.' This stage is dedicated to collecting as much data as possible via visual inspections, historical research, and professional investigations to ascertain if any underlying issues may exist.

- **Stage Two: Tracking down clues of hidden water damage**, where it may have spread, and how to more closely examine the potential issues with associated microorganisms in your home. In this phase, you will apply both your own knowledge and that of professionals, utilizing available resources to zero in on areas of concern. The objective is to formulate a detailed remediation plan, potentially including the need for invasive investigations in areas suspected of concealing problems. By employing advanced testing methods and comprehensive inspections, you aim to locate and determine how to address these concealed issues precisely.

- **Stage Three: Commence Needed Remediation.** Here, we move forward with remediation and further investigation of suspected issues using destructive investigation techniques. Landlords may not allow tenants to commission destructive investigations or remediation. If we own the property, we can generally authorize and oversee destructive investigation and remediation. However, if others own or have specific legal controls over the property, such as with a Homeowners Association (HOA), we must obtain appropriate permissions. This phase addresses and corrects the identified problems. As the mysteries and secrets are exposed and remediated, we can move to the next stage and determine if the work has successfully returned the home to an acceptable state or if further exploration and remediation is needed.

- **Stage Four is all about 'Quality Control and Monitoring.'** This phase is the post-remediation review, where decisions are scrutinized, and laboratory confirmations are sought. We want to ensure we have collected enough information to provide accurate answers about the site. In this stage, we prioritize quality control methods such as visual inspection and testing to confirm the successful removal of issues associated with water damage. It's about thorough evaluation to avoid premature reconstruction that could cover up or hide additional bacteria, mold, and biotoxins, ensuring the effectiveness and safety of the remediation process to provide healthful results.

- **Stage Five: The Preservation and Reconstruction Phase.** Here, we evaluate the repair and reconstruction needs based on the findings collected during remediation. We conducted post-remediation testing in Stage Four to confirm that the problem conditions have been effectively addressed. In Stage Five, we also implement a strategy to help the building recuperate from any residual building memory, take preventive measures, and implement safeguards against future issues.

By working through the 25 Steps found in these Five Stages, we can help ensure that the reconstruction not only restores your indoor environment but also promotes its long-term health.

Part Three: Contents and Personal Possessions

Thus far, *Mold Controlled* has focused on the structural aspects of buildings. Yet, the significance of your possessions and contents should not be overlooked. Part Three provides the information to make informed decisions about the belongings within your home.

A frequent concern, especially among those hypersensitive to mold who turn to internet forums for advice, revolves around whether it's necessary to discard all personal items, including antiques, valuables, and memorabilia. It's heartbreaking to meet clients who, in a state of despair, have already disposed of all their belongings, only to realize their mold problem persists, leading them to consider another complete replacement. Unfortunately, much online advice overlooks the fact that each situation is unique.

The contents and personal possessions information aims to demystify the process, offering effective strategies for cleaning, moving, and storing your possessions. It's crucial to distinguish between items damaged by water, where water and microbial growth have physically damaged the item, versus those merely affected by contamination that consists of superficial settled spores. While not everything can be cost-effectively saved, a significant majority of items can be. Recognizing that there's no one-size-fits-all solution is key. By the conclusion of this section, you'll be prepared to devise a strategy tailored to your unique needs and situation.

Part Four: Epilog

The afterword includes additional information that may not integrate into the main flow of the preceding material, combined with my reflections on my personal journey in this field and additional background information that has directed much of my philosophy. It explains why I reject some aspects of the mold investigation and remediation industries' current direction and the confusion that has resulted.

Together, the sections of this book form a comprehensive guide, blending expert insights with my personal experiences, leading to practical actions to empower you. Whether you are preparing for life in a new home, recovering from an emergency, or striving to enhance the healthfulness of your current residence, this book is structured to support you at each juncture. With the help of this resource, you can approach each phase of home selection, emergency response, and ongoing maintenance with greater assurance and insight, ensuring a safer and healthier living space for you and your family.

Essentials Information Boxes

The "Essentials"—Information Boxes provide quick, practical guidance for important information with minimal technical explanations. By summarizing key points, it facilitates quick decision-making and evaluation of options. The summaries distill crucial information and dispel common myths. The book aims to empower readers to make informed decisions, whether handling issues themselves or hiring professionals. It's particularly beneficial for those sensitive to mold and water damage, providing actionable insights for prevention and remediation.

||||||||||||||||||||||||||||||||||||||||||||||||||||||||||||||||||||||||||||||||||||||||||||||||||||||||||||||||||||||||||||||||||||||||||||||||||

Essentials: Quick Wins

Here is your first Essentials Information

Before delving into the extensive guidance provided in this book, you may wish to implement some immediate measures. This can help to prevent and recognize mold and water damage risks. That's why I've compiled a list of 'Quick Wins'— simple, actionable steps you can take right now to minimize mold and water damage risks. However, it's crucial to note that some actions could destroy evidence or make it more challenging for professionals to diagnose your mold or water damage issues later. Always balance the urgency to act with the need for proper assessment and remediation, especially if you suspect a severe problem has already developed.

- Ventilation Boost: Use exhaust fans in bathrooms and kitchens to reduce humidity, a simple step that can help prevent additional mold growth.

- Air Circulation: It is even better to use open windows to improve air circulation in damp areas, reducing the chance of mold settling in.

- Dehumidifier Deployment: Putting your home on temporary life-support with a dehumidifier may be necessary. I would rather have a healthy house that is able to maintain proper relative humidity levels without mechanical invention. Still, emergency moisture control may sometimes be required, such as emergency water damage or in especially damp areas of the home, like the basement. According to the EPA, in most cases, the Ideal humidity level will be maintained between 30–50% and never over 60%. (USEPA, 2008)

- Do a Quick Leak Check: Check for leaks regularly. By identifying water leaks early, significant damage can be avoided. Routinely check under sinks and areas with water fixtures. During rainy periods, Search for wet areas around windows. If you see or feel moisture—it needs attention.

- Buy a Moisture Meter and Learn to Use It: Your hand can tell if it is very wet, but a moisture meter is necessary to tell when it is dry.

- Daily Wipe Down: perform a daily wipe-down of surfaces where moisture accumulates, like bathroom tiles, kitchen counters, and windows with condensation. Use an absorbent towel or sponge to remove excess moisture.

- Spot-Check for Mold: Learn the difference between mold and dirt.

- Remove Clutter: Removing items that block airflow and can reduce the risk of moisture accumulation, such as furniture or mattresses touching exterior walls or stacks of magazines on floors preventing air circulation.

- Gutter Check: Check and clean gutters regularly, as blocked gutters can lead to water seeping into the home.

- HEPA Vacuum Regularly: Regular vacuum cleaners don't capture mold spores and fragments. They spew them out into the room. Always use properly functioning HEPA vacuum cleaners, especially when cleaning carpets and upholstery.

Previous Work and New Focus

Drawing on my 25-year collaboration with architect Paula Baker-Laporte and medical doctor Erica Elliott, I co-authored *Prescriptions for a Healthy House: A Practical Guide for Architects, Builders, and Homeowners.* Now in its 4th edition, this comprehensive guide offers insights into designing, constructing, and remodeling homes to be healthy, sustainable, and durable. It aims to guide readers toward creating spaces that not only avoid harm but actively promote health and well-being from the ground up. (Baker-Laporte, 2022)

While "Prescriptions" lays the groundwork for elevating your home to a healthy standard through sustainable practices and materials, *Mold Controlled* zeroes in on the challenges of water damage, mold, and other related organisms within the home. It provides a detailed roadmap for recognizing, addressing, and preferably preventing these specific issues, emphasizing the importance of moisture control as a cornerstone of maintaining a healthy indoor environment.

The two books are complementary: *Mold Controlled* aims to help you choose a new place to rent or own, then identify and rectify water-related deficiencies and contamination to make your living space supportive of your health through moisture management. At the same time, "Prescriptions" guides you through construction, remodeling, and reconstruction with a focus on indoor environmental quality to create a truly healthy living space or sanctuary. Together, these books offer a holistic view of how to approach the creation and restoration of living spaces that are not only structurally sound but also supportive of occupants' health.

Prescriptions for a Healthy House serves as an essential reference for those looking to build or renovate with health in mind, laying the foundation for a healing home. *Mold Controlled* builds on this foundation, offering targeted remedial strategies for recognizing and dealing with the pervasive issue of mold and moisture for mold-aware and mold-sensitive individuals. Before any mold problem resolution is complete, the cause of the mold growth must be identified and remedied. This almost always necessitates discovering and addressing the source(s) of moisture, which involves remodeling and reconstruction. By integrating the guidance from both works, homeowners, builders, and architects can tackle the complex challenge of water damage and indoor air quality, ensuring homes are not just repaired but transformed into the healthiest environments possible.

It is exceedingly uncommon for a home to be irreparable; almost every home can indeed recover from water damage and be transformed into healthy living spaces. However, it's crucial to acknowledge that full restoration, tailored to everyone's health requirements, may not always be achievable, and outcomes cannot be guaranteed.

Conflict of Interest Statement

Early in my career, I sold air purifiers, specialty paints, sealants, coatings, and other miscellaneous products as part of my consulting work. These were the days when such products were not widely available. When I began collaborating with Paula Baker-Laporte and Dr. Erica Elliott on the first edition of *Prescriptions for a Healthy House: A Practical Guide for Architects, Builders, and Homeowners,* I stopped selling or accepting a commission on product sales. Since then, all my income has been based on my salary as a consultant and instructor, honorariums for public speaking, teaching online and in-person courses, and income from book sales. I have performed expert witness work as a consultant working on behalf of my employer, RestCon Environmental, without any additional salary. When I began writing this book, I realized that there were areas where I had questions that I did not believe had been adequately answered by independent scientific research publications. I started a crowdfunding site to provide financial resources for researching some of these topics and cover book production expenses. My crowdfunding efforts have raised over $16,300, mostly from $25 donations, and the findings have been included throughout this book. I am the developer of the Pathways™ Testing method; as I approach my retirement from full-time consulting, I anticipate l will begin receiving a commission for developing Pathways™ Testing. I have no other conflicts of interest.

References

U.S. Environmental Protection Agency. (2008). *Mold remediation in schools and commercial buildings* (EPA 402-K-01-001). Retrieved from https://www.epa.gov/mold

U.S. Department of Labor, Bureau of Labor Statistics. (2022). *Consumer expenditures – 2021* (USDL-21-1804). Washington, DC.

Institute of Medicine (U.S.) Committee on Damp Indoor Spaces and Health. (2004). *Damp indoor spaces and health.* Washington, DC: National Academies Press. Retrieved from https://www.ncbi.nlm.nih.gov/books/NBK215649/

U.S. Environmental Protection Agency. (1989). *Report to Congress on indoor air quality: Volume 2* (EPA/400/1-89/001C). Washington, DC.

Baker-Laporte, P., & Banta, J. (2022). *Prescriptions for a healthy house: A practical guide for architects, builders, and homeowners* (4th ed.). BLB Publications.

Part One: Understanding Mold and Water Damage

Chapter One: Save Your Home and Health

Mold Controlled is your comprehensive guide for understanding, finding, fixing, and preventing water damage and mold-related home issues. Our homes are as individual as we are, and so are the challenges they present. Your health, family, and personal preferences are unique. This book helps you to become the best judge of what is acceptable in your home. I aim to empower you to take control of your project, whether you're handling tasks personally or enlisting the help of professionals. This book is designed to equip you with the knowledge necessary to recognize genuine expertise in the field of water damage and mold remediation. This is crucial, especially for households where members have hypersensitivities to organisms resulting from water damage and chemicals, perfumes, fragrances, and common remediation practices that might not support occupant's health post-remediation. My goal is to ensure you can confidently steer the recovery process, prioritizing the health and safety of all occupants.

Renters will find value by learning to identify mold and water-related issues in their living spaces. Even though renters may not have the authority to make construction changes, they can use the book's practical tips for ongoing maintenance, non-toxic cleaning, and various mitigation control techniques. It also empowers renters to make informed decisions and discuss substandard living conditions, necessary repairs, and improvements that can lead to a healthier living environment. As with all sections of this book, there is a strong emphasis on people with hypersensitivities or other medical conditions triggered or worsened by mold and other water-damage organisms.

Correcting a Misconception

The good news is that the path to mold control is not through chemical warfare but through diligent and careful cleaning combined with maintaining a dry environment. The organisms that create these infestations are prevented by controlling and eliminating moisture. Growth in our homes can be physically removed, and excess spores and fragments can be cleaned to safeguard both the structural integrity of the building and the health of its inhabitants. This book advocates for a pacifist approach to remediating water damage problems in homes—an approach that provides benefits for all yet is particularly crucial for individuals with hypersensitivity to mold and chemical exposures.

||||||||||||||||||||||||||||||||||||||||||||||||||||||||||||||||||||||||||||||||||||||||||||||||||||||||||||||||||||||||||||||||||||||||||||||||||||||||||||||||||||||||||||||

Essentials: Why Biocides and Antimicrobials Create Problems

In most cases, it doesn't matter if problem organisms are alive, dormant, or dead since adverse reactions to mold and biotoxins can still occur from exposure to both viable (living or able to grow) and non-viable (dead) organisms. The U.S. Environmental Protection Agency says, "The purpose of mold remediation is to remove the mold to prevent human exposure and damage to building materials and furnishings. It is necessary to clean up mold contamination, not just to kill the mold. Dead mold is still allergenic, and some dead molds are potentially toxic." (USEPA, 2008)

My recommendation is against using biocides, antimicrobials, and similar compounds, often marketed for mold elimination. Here is why:

- **Ineffectiveness in Removing Mold:** Successful mold remediation requires physically removing organisms. Dead mold can still cause allergic reactions and potentially be toxic. Killing agents fail to eliminate the biological remnants like spores, fragments, and biotoxins, which are the real culprits in associated health-related issues. (ACGIH, 1999)

- **Fragmentation:** Killing mold can break it into tiny nanoparticles, which are easily inhaled and more readily absorbed via the air sacs in the lungs to enter the bloodstream. (Harding, 2019)

- **Practical Limitations and Health Concerns:** In real-world scenarios, even the most toxic of chemicals are frequently unable to kill mold. One reason is that many molds produce hydrophobic water-repelling spores and fragments resistant to chemicals. (Krasowska, 2014)

- **Toxic Chemical Residues:** Antimicrobials, biocides, and other agents for killing microorganisms can leave behind toxic residues, contaminating the indoor environment and interfering with the goal of creating a healthy home. Many of the chemicals advertised as "non-toxic" or "natural" are especially problematic for people with multiple chemical sensitivities. Additionally, the chemical residue left behind can react with environmental factors like moisture or heat and other forms of oxidation, leading to even more potentially harmful exposures. (Pall, 2009)

- **Problems With Using Essential Oils to Kill:** The use of products that kill or claim to kill mold is unnecessary and often counterproductive in water damage remediation. The term "natural" does not automatically imply healthfulness, effectiveness, or absence of side effects. Thyme oil, oregano oil, basil oil, citrus oil, and other essential oils are commonly used in small quantities for culinary purposes, enhancing flavor, and promoting and enhancing therapeutic effects. Similarly, tea tree oil and others may offer medicinal benefits when properly utilized in appropriate doses and can be effective in treating various physical ailments. However, employing these products in the home in the amounts necessary for mold eradication by spraying or fogging a structure frequently results in adverse reactions in sensitive people and may severely impact people, especially children, and individuals with chemical sensitivities. (Smith, 2016) Dogs, Cats, and birds have been found to be particularly at risk from exposures, resulting in warnings from veterinarians. (ASPCA, 2023) (Kahn, 2014)

- **Interfere with Laboratory PCR Analysis:** The natural phenol biocides contained in essential oils can disrupt DNA testing methods, such as Mold Specific Quantitative Polymerase Chain Reaction (MSQPCR), used for identifying mold issues in homes. This interference can lead to the presence of mold and bacteria going undetected and resulting in claims that the product was effective when, in fact, they have rendered laboratory results ineffective by inhibiting the detection of the organisms. (Schrader, 2010)

- **Risk of Creating More Harmful Conditions:** Some chemicals may stimulate actively growing molds to produce additional and more toxic secondary metabolites as a defense mechanism. (Murtoniemi, 2003)

- **Resistance:** Moreover, the use of certain antimicrobials has already led to the development of resistant fungal strains, similar to antibiotic resistance in bacteria. (Shoemaker R. C., 2010)

- **Emphasis on Physical Removal:** The most effective strategy for addressing mold is physical removal from surfaces. This includes discarding affected porous materials and maintaining hard surfaces in clean and dry conditions to avoid introducing potentially harmful chemicals and their residues into the living environment. (USEPA, 2008) (ACGIH, 1999) (IICRC, 2024)

- **Avoidance of Sensory Masking:** Avoiding products that mask odors or induce olfactory fatigue (inability to smell odors, even when they are present) is important. Buildings that are dry will not have these odors, and the removal of actively growing mold biomass and residues eliminates their odors because they are gone and not because fragrances or deodorizers hide the odors. (Kioumourtzoglou, 2024) (Hickey, 2008) (Steinemann, 2019)

- **Misting and Fogging Misapplications:** While misting can be used for dust suppression during cleanup, its uncontrolled or inappropriate use can result in additional mold growth. Additionally, science does not support the use of fogging or misting as a method for eliminating, 'killing' or 'destroying' mold. Inappropriate applications can cause extreme problems for people with sensitivities. (Hinds, 1999)

- **Perhaps the best reason for not using these products** is that they are not necessary or helpful! Physical removal and cleaning of contaminants work great! (CIRSx Academy, 2024)

THE COST OF IGNORING EARLY WARNINGS: A CAUTIONARY TALE

I will never forget the lesson of one family's vacation home I inspected over 30 years ago. The cottage was located in a popular resort community. It had been inherited by a family of brothers and sisters when their parents passed. I was hired by one of the adult children. He reported becoming very ill whenever they were vacationing in the home. I began my inspection with my customary initial walk-through. I immediately noted the overpowering stench of room deodorizers. It immediately became apparent that my sense of smell was overpowered, and I could not use it to help me track musty odors. The chemical deodorizers had become a problem themselves.

I quickly exited the home and met my client outside to learn more about the house's history.

I asked about the strong fragrance from the deodorizers. I was told a problem with a musty odor had developed about five years earlier. The family's solution to the smell was to place 17 room deodorizers or air fresheners throughout the home. I donned an organic vapor carbon-filtered respirator to complete my initial inspection.

When I inspected the crawlspace under the home, I discovered water was draining from a nearby hillside and accumulating under the house. The resulting dampness had resulted in multiple wood portions of the foundation and understructure developing severe rot and mold. The malodor had provided an early warning of a problem starting five years earlier. The addition of appropriate drainage to correct the odor was estimated to cost about five thousand dollars. However, damage caused by the delay would cost them ten times more to repair. Had the smell been addressed when it was first noticed instead of covering it up, over fifty thousand dollars in damage could have been avoided.

The Downfall of Quick Fixes: Deodorizers and Beyond

When dealing with mold issues, quick fixes like deodorizers or chemical treatments are often tempting. However, these solutions can be deceptive. They may temporarily mask the problem but rarely tackle the root cause, and for those with chemical hypersensitivities, persistent lingering odors can be devastating.

Complicating matters further, many individuals hypersensitive to mold also suffer from multiple chemical sensitivities (MCS), making chemical-based quick fixes a "double whammy" that exacerbates health problems. Given these complexities, a comprehensive, multi-disciplinary approach involving healthcare providers and environmental consultants is often the most effective way to address the environmental and health-related aspects of mold and chemical sensitivities.

Financial Ramifications: The Unseen Costs

The financial implications of mold and water damage are often underestimated and misunderstood. Many homes undergo cosmetic fixes that address the visible damage but neglect the underlying water source that led to mold growth in the first place. Even when the water source is corrected, lingering mold can still pose health risks, particularly for those who are hypersensitive. Mold needs to be physically removed to fully address these health concerns.

Insurance policies for water damage typically focus on returning the home to a pre-loss condition, often ignoring the health ramifications. This leaves a significant gap, passing the burden of healthcare costs onto the Medical Health Care System. However, the medical system also has its limitations, often not covering the chronic impacts of health issues caused by water damage, which ultimately passes the financial burden onto the consumer.

Navigating the insurance landscape becomes significantly more complex when dealing with Chronic Inflammatory Response Syndrome (CIRS) symptoms, impacting both medical and financial aspects of mold-related issues. The insurance sector, with its nuances and the evident gap between standard coverage and the needs of those with environmental sensitivities, presents a formidable challenge. It's crucial to understand the strategies and limitations that insurance companies operate within, including policy limits, vague language, and coverage caps, which often do not fully meet the requirements of hypersensitive individuals. Additionally, the practice of reporting claims to the Comprehensive Loss Underwriters Exchange (CLUE), even denied ones, can affect policy renewals and increase difficulties in obtaining affordable insurance coverage. This book will later delve into strategies for navigating these insurance complexities, suggesting that a proactive approach could have mitigated many of these challenges long ago. For the moment, acknowledging how CIRS symptoms can complicate insurance claims is vital. Seeking out resources that offer guidance on effectively handling these challenges is key to ensuring restoration efforts are aligned with the health needs of sensitive individuals.

Limitations of Simply Killing Mold

The notion that killing mold alone can resolve health issues is a misconception, one that's contradicted by authoritative references and my own extensive experience with water damage. Individuals hypersensitive to mold don't experience relief when exposed to dead mold structures; the key to improvement is physical removal and thorough cleaning.

Understanding the scope of water damage and its resulting organisms is crucial. Various inspection and testing methods can pinpoint the location of mold growth and guide its effective elimination, along with other water damage-related organisms. While most environmental consultants concur that physical removal is an essential and best course of action, some allow for killing mold, leading to confusion and misinformation. (USEPA, 2008) (ACGIH, 1999)

Be wary of manufacturers claiming their products, often touted as plant-based or non-toxic, can safely kill or inactivate mold. Such claims should be met with skepticism. Substances potent enough to kill mold are unlikely to contribute to a healthful home environment. Even if they can kill, dead mold bodies are not conducive to hypersensitive individuals' health. Exercise caution and equip yourself with the right knowledge to make informed decisions. (USEPA, 2008)

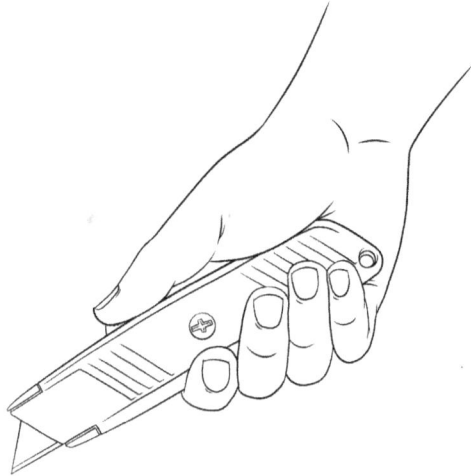

Figure 1-1 Razor Knife in Hand: A handheld razor knife is an affordable and versatile tool commonly used to cut tape and plastic and remove small gypsum wallboard sections with visible mold growth. However, it must remain within the containment zone or be bagged once it contacts contaminated materials to prevent cross-contamination. Mishandling tools like this is a frequent cause of spreading contamination.

Other Routes of Exposure: More than Just Inhalation

While inhalation is the most prevalent way people are exposed to mold, several other routes of exposure are equally important to consider. Direct skin contact with moldy surfaces can result in irritation or allergic reactions, especially when handling contaminated materials without appropriate protective gear. Ingestion is another route, where moldy food or water can lead to gastrointestinal issues. Some molds can even produce mycotoxins or biotoxins that are most commonly harmful when ingested. Inhalation and contact with mucous membranes, such as the eyes, nose, and mouth, can also serve as entry points, particularly if one rubs their eyes after contact with mold. Additionally, mold spores can adhere to clothing, pets, or objects, which can then be transferred to other areas, including skin and mucous membranes. Although extremely rare, mold can also enter the body through puncture wounds or skin breaches, typically in immunocompromised individuals. (ACGIH, 1999)

||||||||||||||||||||||||||||||||||||||||||||||||||||||||||||||||||||||||||||||||||||||||||||||||||||||||||||||||||||||||||||||||||||

Essay: Trading One Contaminant for Another: Why Ingredients Matter

by Marilee Nelson, Founder of Branch Basics All Purpose Cleaner

My experience over the last forty years has revealed that a significant hindrance to our health and ability to heal and reach our potential is the elephant in the American home, the ever-present chemical soup created from products with harmful ingredients scattered throughout the house.

I have worked predominantly with susceptible people (the chemically sensitive, mold-sensitive, and EMF-sensitive), whom I propose—serve as our modern-day canaries. The term "canary" originated from using canaries in coal mines to detect unsafe levels of carbon monoxide. A sudden halt to their singing would warn workers to turn around and not to go any further to avoid exposure. Today's canaries identify and warn us of hazardous products in our homes that contribute to health issues.

In the 1990s, I began receiving calls for help from people exposed to mold, who had their homes remediated yet were sicker than ever. They had become so ill that some had to abandon their homes and belongings because they kept reacting. They commented, "We got clearance after mold remediation, but I feel like I'm losing my mind. I am reacting so much, and no one believes me. They think I am crazy!" Their doctors and families had a hard time understanding what was wrong as it appeared there was no reason they should be reacting. Many were prescribed sedatives and other medications for depression or paranoia.

From the recovery of my son and other chemically sensitive canaries, I learned that toxic building materials and cleaning products such as those with toxic surfactants, aromatic hydrocarbons, quats (quaternary ammonium compounds), phenolics—essential oils like thymol, chlorine bleach, and other disinfecting agents, enzymes, masking and fragrance chemicals were especially inflammatory. So, I would first get a list of all materials and products used in the mold cleaning process.

Upon investigation, I discovered that in every case, much of the problem was in the materials and products used for remediation. Therefore, I recommended a deep cleaning procedure of all surfaces using a fragrance-free soap and water or a human-safe surfactant-based soap to remove remaining live or dead mold, MVOCs, mycotoxins, and chemical residues (harmful VOCs and SVOCs) left from toxic cleaning products. I would also recommend the systematic removal of all products with toxic chemicals from their homes based on a process I developed when recovering my son from a chemical injury. His miraculous recovery uncovered how essential it is for our homes to be a haven as products with harmful ingredients, even when not in use and sitting under a sink, create a chemical soup in the home that is inflammatory, exacerbates symptoms, and undermines the ability to heal.

The result was a radical reduction of inflammation and symptoms of other chronic conditions in the mold injured.

Improvement of other family members (such as increased well-being, more energy, improved sleep, brain fog lifted, headaches and migraines gone, mood elevated, hormone disruption, and allergies resolved) substantiated that these chemicals impact everyone. Continued deep cleaning was unnecessary, provided the source of biotoxins had been controlled. If they still reacted, I would have them do another deep clean and further testing (if necessary). I recommended deep cleaning as needed or once or twice a year for maintenance.

Studies verify that building materials, cleaning products, and other products used in the home may contaminate a home's air with chemicals that are neurotoxins, asthmagens, carcinogens, obesogens, hormone disruptors, and more. In other words, it's crucial to consider the potential health impacts of the materials used in remediation, as using these products trades one contaminant (moldy materials and biotoxins) for another (harmful chemicals in replacement building materials and cleaning products).

Before attempting mold remediation, it's crucial to understand the process of effective remediation. This means removal (not killing) of mold and associated biotoxins. This understanding can provide a sense of confidence in decision-making and help avoid the temptation to believe in quick-fix claims that involve spraying or fogging a chemical to kill mold.

Antimicrobials, biocides, fungicides, quats, bleach, and other EPA-registered pesticides (disinfectants and phenols like thymol) that kill mold create unintended consequences. They may kill the mold, but dead mold is inflammatory. Dead mold releases spores and toxic secondary metabolites or mycotoxins, and killing mold may create microscopic fragments that are so light that they linger in the breathing air space and are not captured by standard cleaning practices. Disinfectants also may not kill all the mold as resistant fungal strains that are even more virulent may emerge just as antibiotic-resistant superbugs have become an issue. In addition, endotoxins (lipopolysaccharides) are released from gram-negative bacteria when killed, and exotoxins from actinomycetes, which are gram-positive bacteria, are other inflammogens that may be a part of the biotoxin chemical soup that can cause inflammation. Cleaning initially to remove mold with soap and water can avoid the unnecessary creation of some of these biotoxins. Thankfully, deep cleaning all surfaces with simple soap and water REMOVES the mold and biotoxin chemical soup.

Disinfectants are not the only products that hinder effective remediation. Enzyme-containing cleaning products may leave behind residues of peptides and proteins that can interfere with the ability to tell if a surface is truly clean. The trend of using products containing thymol to kill mold is especially concerning. Understanding the dangers of using thymol or any essential oil to remediate mold can empower you to make informed decisions and take proactive steps, ensuring that you control your home's safety.

1. Thymol and other essential oils permeate porous materials and are difficult to remove. Thymol is an EPA-registered pesticide. As long as the VOCs are still present in the air, the thymol also acts as a pesticide that impacts people.

2. Many essential oil products are contaminated by processing methods or by materials the oils come into contact with, such as plastic tubing, which contaminates the oil with phthalates and other plasticizers that are neurotoxic, carcinogenic, asthmagens, obesogens, allergens, and hormone disruptors.

3. It has been discovered that inhibition can occur when essential oils are used to kill mold, making DNA-based clearance testing unreliable. This is very important, especially for people who assume essential oils don't bother them. Based on these points, I have had people unable to continue living in their homes.

Repercussions from aggressive mold killing can be avoided with deep cleaning practices using plain soap and water or surfactant-based cleaners that are fragrance-free and contain no essential oils, enzymes, masking chemicals, or other harmful substances. The great news is that obtaining clearance from the entire mold and biotoxin chemical soup can be fully accomplished via the simple power of removal, not killing.

One question we have to ask is: How can products with harmful ingredients be sold for use in our homes? The conventional and non-toxic cleaning industry uses the "Dose Makes the Poison Toxicology Model" to determine safe levels of product ingredients. The explanation is, "Our products contain only a small amount of harmful chemicals based on laboratory studies on animals and the LD50, the dose at which the ingredient is lethal for 50% of the test animals. Our products are safe, and such small amounts of these ingredients don't matter".

Our canaries are warning everyone that our homes should be our haven—*free of products with harmful ingredients*. Scientific research, in study after study, validates my contention, based on experience with the canaries and their families, that the "Dose Makes the Poison Toxicology Model" is not a viable benchmark for what is safe for the human body. Exposure to even small amounts of harmful chemicals DOES, in fact, MATTER.

We now know, from the science of epigenetics, that even a tiny amount of one chemical can turn off and on gene expression, initiate disease, inhibit recovery, and impact the ability of the body to heal. Scientific studies directly link the exponential rise of degenerative disease to our exposure to these harmful chemicals in our food, products, water, air, and homes. The power of removal of products with harmful ingredients from our homes is an unrecognized and underutilized weapon against chronic disease. We don't know how much they impact us until they are removed.

The good news is that you don't have to be a chemist or have a scientific background to read labels and evaluate products. You can quickly vet the ingredients and feel confident about your decisions because we have great tools at our fingertips.

- Use EWG Skin Deep to rate cleaning and personal care products. To Create a Healthy Home, use products with all ingredients rated a one or two on EWG Skin Deep with some exceptions (Products such as toothpaste and makeup may be difficult to find with all ingredients rated a one to two. Exceptions have to be made until better products are discovered or introduced into the market). Go to EWG Skin Deep's website and type in the last ingredient listed in the product you want to evaluate. The ingredients are rated one to ten, with one being the safest and ten being the most toxic. Avoid products with any ingredient rated three or more. Hint: Start with the last ingredient on the list to save time. Typically, you will find preservatives here and may only have to look at one ingredient to find a three or above rating. Once you find an ingredient rated three or more, look no more and remove that product from your home.

- Think Dirty is a great app to rate cleaning and personal care products; scan your product's barcode, and Think Dirty will rate it on the spot. We recommend products rated "o" on this app. Get the Think Dirty app at thinkdirtyapp.com.

Note: People trying to heal inflammatory skin conditions, hormone disruption, CIRS, or chronic illness should also avoid products used on the skin with the following ingredients that can be inflammatory (citric acid, sodium coco sulfate, sodium benzoate, potassium sorbate, phenoxyethanol, SLS, SLES, and any ingredient with a quaternary ammonium component like polyquaternium-11) even though they are rated a one or two on EWG Skin Deep.

In conclusion, CIRS canaries have taught us how using products with harmful chemicals to remediate mold is inflammatory. They have also demonstrated how having these products in the home under sinks and in cabinets continually emits VOCs and SVOCs that undermine our health and inhibit healing. The canaries also opened our eyes to the inflammatory biotoxin chemical soup created by the unforeseen consequences of using products that kill instead of remove!

THE EVOLVING VIEW ON MOLD AND WATER-DAMAGE HEALTH IMPACTS

The Evolving View on Mold and Water-damage Health Impacts captures the shift in understanding and addressing health issues related to mold and water damage. Historically, individuals reporting sensitivity to mold or health problems due to water damage were often not taken seriously and sometimes labeled as having psychosomatic disorders. This skepticism was partly because mold and water damage are not always visibly apparent, and their health effects were poorly understood. However, current medical and environmental health research is changing this perspective, showing that mold and water damage can profoundly affect health, causing respiratory problems, allergies, inflammatory conditions, and neurological impacts. This growing body of knowledge increases recognition of these health issues as genuine concerns.

The variability in individual reactions to mold and water damage—with some people becoming severely ill from minimal exposure while others remain unaffected—was a source of confusion. It is understood as a reflection of genetic differences in how bodies react to environmental stressors. The stigma of being labeled 'crazy' for experiencing these health issues has been challenging, leading to feelings of isolation and reluctance to seek help. Fortunately, health professionals and affected individuals are making strides in educating the public and healthcare providers about the realities of mold and water damage sensitivities. Their efforts are fostering a more empathetic and informed approach to these issues.

Effective assistance for those reporting mold and water-damage sensitivities involves a comprehensive evaluation, including environmental assessments, medical testing, and understanding individual health histories. By validating the experiences of those affected, it provides a pathway to appropriate treatment and management. While some skepticism remains, ongoing education, research, and advocacy steadily increase understanding and support for those affected.

Essay: A Journey of Recovery

by Ryan J. Holsapple, Ph.D.

If you are anything like my wife Victoria, you have scoured the medical world, searching tirelessly for a solution to your debilitating illness. Even though she saw an ensemble of decidedly competent healthcare providers, including some of the most reputable doctors and hospitals in the nation, Victoria was bereft of answers for over a decade. During that time, her ability to exert energy slowly diminished to the point where she became bedbound. By the time we found the right medical and professional help, Victoria had suffered long under a medical system that had failed her and millions of other Americans. I have a story to tell about our journey of dealing with CIRS (Chronic Inflammatory Response Syndrome), which I hope readers will resonate with and find encouraging.

A Long and Tired Path

Much of Victoria's 20s were a struggle with her health. The road to what would eventually become complete disability was long and wearisome. Along the way, she had little choice but to become her own lead physician. She spent countless hours researching, trying to piece together the often puzzling and contradictory course of treatment coming from varying medical experts and practitioners. We shuttled ourselves to countless doctor's appointments and tried many protocols and treatment plans, only to have her health and quality of life continue to descend.

The Descending Illness

Victoria's struggles eventually culminated in a complete physical breakdown. To put it succinctly, her mitochondria were not making energy for her cells, which caused profound disability and fatigue; her immune system was in total dysfunction, and her brain was inflamed. A small fraction of her symptoms included chronic and debilitating fatigue, acute nerve pain, migraines, tachycardia, complete light and noise intolerance, exertional intolerance—e.g., difficulty even rolling around in bed –, inability tolerate mild stimulation and post-exertional malaise—that is, her symptoms would significantly worsen after exerting energy and would increase her state of disability for weeks.

Finding a Solution

It was not until she was completely bedbound for 10 months, with me as her primary caregiver and medical manager, that Victoria became a patient at Roots and Branches Integrative Healthcare. They are a clinic in Colorado that understood the complex immunological and mitochondrial dysfunction she was facing and knew how to properly treat it. Dr. Dorninger, Dr. Bjerke, and others at Roots and Branches patiently walked us through the complex reality that is CIRS treatment. I learned about the process involved in getting a home up to standards for CIRS patients. Eventually, Dr. Dorninger referred me to John Banta,—the author of this book—who became our environmental consultant.

Embracing the Process

In reflecting on what drove me to be receptive to John's advisements and the general CIRS protocols, I discovered that it was initially desperation; I was losing my wife. That desperation was slowly replaced by hope as I listened to the doctors and to John, acquainted myself with anecdotal stories of recovery, and researched the biological mechanisms underlying the disease and its treatment. After many months of enduring hope came belief; I saw positive changes occurring in Victoria's

symptoms, abilities, and blood work as we diligently continued the treatment process. Belief rooted itself in me and became unshakable. Still, after more time, something more powerful than belief began to grow, I knew. Knowing that this process of getting out of biotoxin exposure and undergoing treatment works came directly from seeing Victoria's progress and my continued research on the science of CIRS recovery.

Our Healing Journey: *Addressing our Home*

The beginning of Victoria's healing progress was after we did the work required to get our home safe. Initial Actino Panel and MSQPCR testing revealed that we had significant issues with actinomycetes, and moderately high mold levels. I brought these results to John for further direction. Because of the severity of Victoria's situation, John helped us create an expedited plan of action. We removed Victoria from the home, performed detailed inspections, underwent several iterations of deep cleaning, resealed and cleaned the crawlspace under John's guidelines, and referred to part 3 of this book to address items and cleaning items. We were on a tight timeline as we had no way of knowing whether the other home Victoria was staying in was safe or if it, too, was compromised. We wanted her in a safe environment immediately. Our urgency was well-founded; we were engaged in painful discussions about whether she needed a feeding tube, given how much she was struggling to eat. Fortunately, the feeding tube never came to pass, in large part thanks to the home being properly addressed.

Adapting our Approach

After completing the major efforts of addressing our home and the items therein, we were able to settle into a sustainable routine. The house was cleaned regularly according to John's suggested methods. We took—and continue to take—an aggressive and consistent approach to cleaning our house because we want to keep the environment safe for Victoria. Collecting Pathways™ samples 24 hours after having cleaned gave us the knowledge that there was a low level of peptide bonds and proteins in the home, which means the cleaning worked.

While we did our best to ensure a safe home, we did not have the luxury of deep cleaning and then waiting a couple of weeks without cleaning to further assess the Pathways™ results and see if there was a concerning increase in peptide bonds and proteins. Such a thorough investigation may suggest an unseen issue with actinomycetes or mold. However, Victoria was too sick, and I was not willing to risk any further biotoxin exposure by foregoing cleaning if I could help it. John taught me that cleaning could "bail the boat," meaning there may very well be mold issues in the house that have not been caught, but by regular cleaning and assessing pathways results within 24 hours after a cleaning, we were able to assess a strong probability that she is breathing clean air. Her subsequent healing supports our conclusion.

Later, when Victoria is even more functional than she is now, we will be working with John and use Pathways™ testing to see if our home has lurking issues with mold. Fortunately, none of the species or levels of mold or actinomycetes we have had come back in our testing suggest water damage. In essence, we have converging lines of evidence that allow us to be comfortable with the decision to handle our home this way in the short term.

Healing

Having the home adequately addressed allowed Victoria to undergo the next phases of the Shoemaker Protocol. It took many months, yet as Victoria went through the various steps of treatment needed, we saw continuous improvement in her abilities. She began laughing, speaking more, eating more, and moving more. Her legs, which had atrophied—a sight I would not wish on any husband—began to develop muscle again. Her blood markers improved, and her light and sound tolerance expanded. She was healing.

As I write this, Victoria is presently in the middle of that healing journey. We still closely monitor our home through various methods of the sort laid out in this book. We make adjustments as necessary. I have come to accept that this is an ongoing process, and it is a process that works. We now celebrate that it is not a matter of "if" she gets back to a full, enjoyable life; it is only a matter of "when." Considering how incapacitated she was, what we have been a part of is a medical miracle. The treatment process and getting out of biotoxin exposure have pulled her back from the clutches of death and given her a new lease on life.

References

U.S. Environmental Protection Agency. (2008). *Mold remediation in schools and commercial buildings* (EPA 402-K-01-001). Retrieved from https://www.epa.gov/mold

American Conference of Governmental Industrial Hygienists. (1999). *Bioaerosols: Assessment and control*. ACGIH.

Harding, C. F., Pytte, C. L., Page, K. G., Ryberg, K. J., Normand, E., Remigio, G. J., DeStefano, R. A., Morris, D. B., Voronina, J., Lopez, A., Stalbow, L. A., Williams, E. P., & Abreu, O. (2019). Mold inhalation causes innate immune activation, neural, cognitive, and emotional dysfunction. *Brain, Behavior, and Immunity*. https://doi.org/10.1016/j.bbi.2019.11.006

Krasowska, A., & Sigler, K. (2014). How microorganisms use hydrophobicity and what does this mean for human needs? *Frontiers in Cellular and Infection Microbiology, 4*. https://doi.org/10.3389/fcimb.2014.00112

Pall, M. L. (2009). Multiple chemical sensitivity: Toxicological questions and mechanisms. In *General and applied toxicology* (Online). John Wiley & Sons, Ltd. https://doi.org/10.1002/9780470744307.gat091

Smith, C. (2016, May 11). Poison Center warns of toxicity of essential oils. *Clarksville Now*. Retrieved from https://clarksvillenow.com/local/poison-center-warns-toxicity-essential-oils/9

ASPCA. (2022, June 23). The essentials of essential oils around pets. *ASPCA*. Retrieved from https://www.aspca.org/news/essentials-essential-oils-around-pets

Kahn, C. M., McLean, M. K., & Slater, M. (2014). Concentrated tea tree oil toxicosis in dogs and cats: 443 cases (2002–2012). *Journal of the American Veterinary Medical Association, 244*(1), 95–100. https://doi.org/10.2460/javma.244.1.95

Schrader, C., Schielke, A., Ellerbroek, L., & Johne, R. (2010). PCR inhibitors—Occurrence, properties, and removal. *Analytical and Bioanalytical Chemistry, 396*(6), 1977–1990. https://doi.org/10.1007/s00216-009-3150-9

Murtoniemi, T., Nevalainen, A., & Hirvonen, M.-R. (2003). Effect of plasterboard composition on *Stachybotrys chartarum* growth and biological activity of spores. *Applied and Environmental Microbiology, 69*(7), 3751–3757. https://doi.org/10.1128/AEM.69.7.3751-3757.2003

Shoemaker, R. (2010). *Surviving mold: Life in the era of dangerous buildings*. Otter Bay Books. Retrieved from https://www.survivingmold.com/

Institute of Inspection, Cleaning and Restoration Certification. (2024). *ANSI/IICRC S520 standard for professional mold remediation* (4th ed.). IICRC.

Kioumourtzoglou, M.-A. (2024, February 5). Do air fresheners impact our health? *Columbia Doctors*. Retrieved from https://www.columbiadoctors.org/news/do-air-fresheners-impact-our-health

Hickey, H. (2008, July 23). Toxic chemicals found in common scented laundry products and air fresheners. *UW News*. Retrieved from https://www.washington.edu/news/2008/07/23/toxic-chemicals-found-in-common-scented-laundry-products-air-fresheners/

Steinemann, A. (2019). The fragranced products phenomenon: Air quality and health, science, and policy. *Air Quality, Atmosphere & Health, 12*(11), 1197–1204. https://doi.org/10.1007/s11869-019-00729-9

Hinds, W. (1999). 12.3 Kinematic coagulation. In *Aerosol technology: Properties, behavior, and measurement of airborne particles* (pp. 274 and 288). Wiley.

Hinds, W. (1999). 13.9 Evaporation. In *Aerosol technology: Properties, behavior, and measurement of airborne particles*. Wiley.

CIRSx Training Institute. (2024). *Fundamentals of medically important remediation—101*. Developed by a team of seasoned industry experts assisted and reviewed by medical professionals, MIR101 provides 16 hours of self-paced, comprehensive training. Retrieved from https://institute.cirsx.com/p/medically-important-remediation-101

Chapter Two: The Health Consequences of Uncontrolled Water Damage

Hypersensitivity due to mold and other water-damage organisms extends beyond mere allergic reactions and asthma. Scientific research indicates that the issue can be far more complex, affecting multiple bodily organs and systems, including the skin, digestive, nervous, respiratory, and immune systems. Also, Lyme disease and other confounding diseases can further complicate the situation and hinder progress.

When mold particles, whether alive or dead, are inhaled, they interact with the immune system, triggering various responses that can vary from person to person. Live, viable mold spores are metabolically active. Not only can they produce biotoxins, but they can also lead to rare fungal infections (more common during the initial HIV crisis, before quality antiretrovirals became available). But this doesn't mean that killing mold is the answer! Not only can dead mold particles and fragments cause allergic reactions, but they also contain the already produced biotoxins. Although biotoxins are chemicals and are not alive, they can still elicit an innate immune response. This immune system response recognizes the molecular patterns on these substances and may react by initiating inflammatory responses. Over time, chronic exposure to biotoxins, microbial volatile organic compounds (MVOCs) gases, and living or dead particles can lead to persistent inflammation. This chronic inflammatory response syndrome (CIRS) can have long-term health implications.

Myth: Dead Mold Doesn't Cause Health Problems:
Fact: Even when mold is dead, the spores and byproducts can still cause health issues for certain individuals. Proper removal and remediation are necessary to address these risks.

THE MULTIFACETED CONSEQUENCES OF WATER DAMAGE

When it comes to water damage in your home, the stakes are more than just structural. The organisms that thrive in damp environments are varied and not limited to mold. Many bacteria, insects, and rodents thrive in damp areas; these invaders can lead to a range of health issues that are as diverse as the organisms themselves. Much remains unknown about the potential health consequences of many types of organisms associated with water-damaged buildings, but what is clear is that merely drying a building and addressing the aesthetics or structural integrity is not enough—keeping buildings dry, quickly discovering and addressing water intrusion, remediation, and restoration lead to lower recovery costs and healthier living spaces.

Allergic Reactions

Allergic reactions occur when the immune system overreacts to a substance perceived as harmful, even when it isn't. Exposures to certain foods, seasonal pollens, insect bites or stings, and molds can cause symptoms like sneezing, itchy eyes, or skin rashes. It's worth noting that the severity of allergic reactions can vary greatly among individuals, ranging from mild discomfort that can be relieved by over-the-counter medications and herbal or other remedies to the treatment of more severe, even life-threatening, responses such as anaphylaxis that may require emergency treatment and hospitalization. (Kurup V. P., 2000)

Aspergillosis and Other Mold-Related Infections

Aspergillosis is a fungal infection primarily caused by *Aspergillus fumigatus* and sometimes *Aspergillus flavus, A. terreus, A. parasiticus*, and others. These species can amplify in water-damaged buildings and lead to infections in immune-compromised people by colonizing the lungs, most commonly, but sometimes spreading to the heart and brain. Once established, they are difficult to treat and frequently lethal. Of particular concern, aspergillosis is a leading cause of death among individuals whose immune systems are compromised by chemotherapy or anti-rejection drugs used after organ transplants. (Tischler, 2019)

In the early HIV/AIDS epidemic, aspergillosis posed a significant risk to those with HIV, primarily due to their compromised immune systems. Thanks to advancements in HIV treatment, notably the use of effective antiretroviral therapy and better overall management of the condition, the risk of aspergillosis has dramatically diminished. Improved treatments, alongside heightened awareness and preventive strategies against mold exposure, have significantly lowered these aspergillosis cases in countries where treatments are available.

Myth: A Little Mold Isn't a Big Deal.
Fact: Even small amounts of mold can be a health hazard, particularly for individuals with biotoxin illness, allergies, asthma, or other respiratory conditions. It's also a sign of a larger moisture problem that can lead to more significant mold growth over time.

Asthma Trigger

Asthma is a chronic respiratory condition characterized by inflammation and narrowing of the airways, leading to symptoms like wheezing, shortness of breath, and coughing. Exposure to water-damaged buildings and the associated organisms, even after drying, can act as an asthma trigger, exacerbating symptoms in those who are sensitive or have pre-existing asthma. (Dales, 2000)

Chronic Inflammatory Response Syndrome (CIRS)

Chronic Inflammatory Response Syndrome (CIRS) is a complex, multi-system, multi-symptom illness primarily triggered by exposure to biotoxins, such as mold, certain bacteria, and toxic algae. It occurs when the body's immune system fails to effectively clear these toxins, leading to an ongoing inflammatory response. CIRS requires a comprehensive approach to diagnosis and management, focusing on removing the source of biotoxin exposure and addressing the body's inflammatory and other reactions. (Shoemaker R. J., 2018)

Hypersensitivity pneumonitis

Hypersensitivity pneumonitis (HP) is a complex lung condition triggered by an immune response to inhaling very tiny particles of substances, such as soils (farmer's lung), flour (baker's lung and miller's lung), and often including mold spores or fragments from mold cured foods (cheese washers' lung, salami washers' lung). This condition can manifest in acute, subacute, or chronic forms, each with varying symptoms and severities. It is noteworthy that unresolved water damage results in mold growth in the home, as these settings can be a potent source of the offending particles. Given its potential to cause irreversible lung damage if not addressed, early diagnosis and intervention are crucial. (Gomes, 2021)

Skin Disorders

Mold-related skin disorders can manifest as symptoms, from mild irritations like itchiness and redness to more severe conditions like dermatitis. These skin issues arise when there's direct contact with mold growth or an accumulation of settled spores or fragments, often in environments with water damage or elevated humidity. Given the potential for escalation and secondary infections, prompt attention to mold-related skin disorders is vital for effective management and recovery. (CIRS Academy, 2021)

Toxicosis

Toxicosis is the term used for the harmful effects of exposure to biotoxins. Certain molds, bacteria, and algae produce these toxic substances. The symptoms of toxicosis can vary widely, ranging from mild issues like stomach discomfort to more severe effects, including neurological problems and weakened immune response. The risk of experiencing toxicosis increases in places with water damage because these environments tend to have higher levels of toxins. (Shoemaker R., 2005)

Vagal Nerve System Responses

The vagal nerve system, centered around the vagus nerve, is essential to the body's "rest and digest" functions as part of the parasympathetic nervous system. Musty odors, such as those from mold and bacteria, can trigger the olfactory system, which is closely linked to emotional and physiological response centers in the brain. This activation can lead to a stress response, as the brain interprets these odors as potential threats, causing various reactions, including changes in breathing patterns, nausea, and even emotional distress in some individuals. The vagus nerve plays a pivotal role in managing these responses by helping to calm the body after stress has been perceived, regulating heart rate, digestion, and respiratory rate, among other functions. (Waxenbaum JA, 2024)

Water Damage & Sensitivities: Late is Not Too Late

Coping with sensitivities to organisms associated with water damage, such as mold, often means confronting a silent yet significant burden. Many people don't realize the impact of these sensitivities until serious health issues arise. However, recognizing the problem even later is an important step forward. Acknowledging these sensitivities can lead to meaningful actions to reduce their impact on the home's and its occupants' health.

You can't ask a pet, a young child, or a building to explain where it hurts—each can suffer from hidden issues that can't be verbalized and may go unnoticed until the problem worsens. Just as a pediatrician or veterinarian must poke and prod to find the source of discomfort in a child or pet, homeowners must also investigate hidden areas in their home. A house doesn't cry, but it offers clues—like subtle signs of water damage or changes in air quality. Sometimes, these clues come from the health of the occupants themselves. The most sensitive person in the home often acts as an early warning system. Recognizing when our homes are "hurting" is key to optimizing both the home and the occupants' health and longevity. The following section will explore the conditions and symptoms commonly experienced by individuals with mold and water-damage sensitivities. These symptoms can often be the first indication that something is wrong with the building itself. It is a vital diagnostic tool for identifying underlying structural issues that may go unnoticed.

Chronic Inflammatory Response Syndromes (CIRS)

It is estimated that 52 million people in the U.S. population, have a genetic predisposition to Chronic Inflammatory Response Syndrome (CIRS), Mold Sensitivity, or Biotoxin Illness. Approximately 25% of the U.S. population carries this genetic predisposition, making them susceptible to inflammatory responses from exposure to mold, bacteria, and other biotoxins commonly found in water-damaged environments. (McMahon S. , 2019)

The concern is more significant for the 25% who are genetically predisposed but may not yet be symptomatic. Significant health events, such as "Long Covid" or excessive chemical exposures, can trigger latent sensitivities in this group. This activation could increase their reactivity to various organisms in water-damaged settings, potentially expanding the number of individuals affected beyond the current levels already showing symptoms. (Shoemaker R. M., 2021)

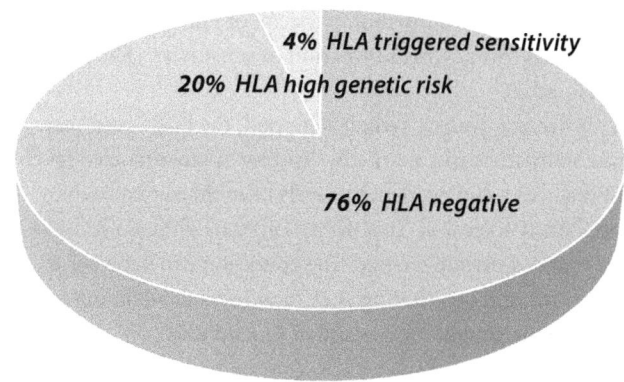

Figure 1-2: This pie chart illustrates the approximate distribution of genetic predisposition to hypersensitivities related to mold and other water damage contaminants in the U.S. population, based on HLA genotypes. Approximately 76% of the population does not carry alleles associated with increased susceptibility to mold, endotoxins, exotoxins, or multiple chemical sensitivities. Among the remaining 24% with genetic predispositions, environmental exposures play a significant role in determining whether these sensitivities are expressed. Current estimates suggest that 1–4% of the population actively expresses hypersensitivities, though this percentage could increase with greater exposure to environmental triggers.

Chronic Inflammatory Response Syndrome (CIRS) can coexist with other medical conditions triggered by mold or organisms found in water-damaged environments, presenting a complex challenge for diagnosis and treatment. While CIRS requires a specific approach focused on managing the systemic inflammatory response and addressing biotoxin exposure, other concurrent conditions, such as asthma, allergies, or infections, demand treatments tailored to relieve symptoms or target the infection directly. This complexity often necessitates collaboration among various medical specialties, each bringing expertise to address the patient's health issues. Effective treatment, therefore, involves a personalized and comprehensive approach that considers the unique aspects of each condition and a coordinated effort among specialists, working together to ensure that all aspects of the patient's health are addressed. Bridging the gaps between these specialties is crucial for developing an integrated treatment plan that tackles both CIRS and any coexisting conditions, acknowledging that the path to healing is multifaceted and requires a unified approach. (McMahon, 2017)

Many individuals may not realize they are predisposed to mold sensitivity until a significant triggering event occurs, such as encountering severe water damage or acquiring a building with mold issues that trigger their condition. The genetic predisposition is not being expressed, so the genetic factor is not recognized until specific conditions activate it. Elevated exposure to problematic types of mold, combined with a stressor—environmental, physical, or emotional—can switch on this genetic expression of sensitivity. (Shoemaker R. N., 2021)

Once this genetic switch is flipped, the body's immune reactivity increases markedly, leading to an enhanced level of reactivity and even lower levels of mold exposure than previously tolerable. This transition to heightened sensitivity marks a pivotal change. The condition can evolve into a chronic and debilitating state, making it challenging to reverse the genetic expression of sensitivities.

Consequently, the remediation process in a building for individuals with such sensitivities demands far more than a standard cleanup. It requires an approach to not only eliminating mold but also lowering spore counts and biotoxins to levels that do not trigger this now persistent sensitivity. This meticulous remediation is vital to creating an environment that accommodates those affected by mold sensitivities, reflecting the complex interplay between genetic predisposition, exposure levels, and stressors that contribute to the condition's development.

Who is Dr. Ritchie Shoemaker?

Dr. Ritchie Shoemaker, a pioneering physician in biotoxin-related illnesses, began his practice in a small fishing town in rural Maryland. He first identified the connection between exposure to toxins produced by *Pfiesteria piscicida*—an organism associated with harmful algal blooms—and a multi-symptom, multi-system illness in humans, often stemming from water-damage organisms rather than contaminated seafood. He later recognized similarities between ciguatera poisoning, resulting from the consumption of fish contaminated by *Gambierdiscus toxicus* (another toxic algal species), and mold-related biotoxin illnesses, thereby advancing the understanding of chronic inflammatory responses to environmental toxins. Though now retired from active medical practice, Dr. Shoemaker remains deeply involved in research and education. He is regarded as the foremost expert regarding Chronic Inflammatory Response Syndrome (CIRS). He has developed groundbreaking diagnostic protocols and treatment methods, significantly advancing the understanding and treatment of biotoxin-related illnesses, particularly those associated with water-damage organisms, including mold, endotoxins from gram-negative bacteria, and exotoxins from actinobacteria. Dr. Shoemaker continues to share his expertise and the latest research through his website, SurvivingMold.com. In addition, the site, CIRSx.com, provides valuable resources and insights for physicians, professionals in functional and integrative medicine, and others dedicated to improving patient care in this field.

Chronic Inflammatory Response Syndrome (CIRS) Symptoms

Chronic Inflammatory Response Syndrome (CIRS) presents a bewildering array of challenges, primarily because it is a syndrome that is multi-symptom, multi-system. That is, CIRS creates many healthcare symptoms in many body systems. Triggered by exposure to biotoxins from sources like mold, gram-negative bacteria, actinobacteria, and toxic algae, CIRS can be particularly severe in individuals with certain genetic predispositions. This susceptibility is often related to specific variations in the Human Leukocyte Antigen (HLA) genes on chromosome six. CIRS manifests as a persistent inflammatory response that the body struggles to resolve, even after removing the biotoxin source. The syndrome encompasses a broad spectrum of symptoms, including but not limited to fatigue, headaches, respiratory complications, and cognitive difficulties. These symptoms' wide-ranging and variable nature and commonality with other conditions currently make mainstream CIRS diagnoses challenging to recognize and treat. Addressing CIRS effectively requires a multifaceted approach, encompassing the removal of affected people from the exposure sources, treatment to help remove biotoxin deposited in the body, management of symptoms, and ongoing monitoring to manage this complex condition. To further illustrate the complexities of understanding HLA research, it has connected mold sensitivity in children with moderate to severe asthma. (Knutsen AP, 2010)

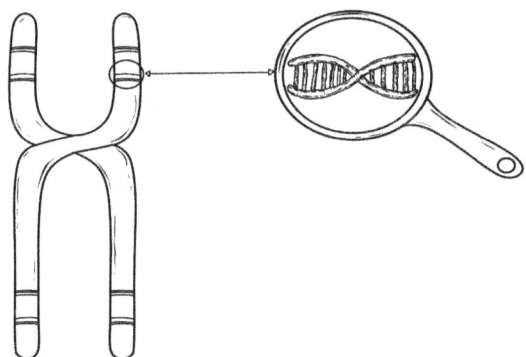

Figure 1-3: Chromosome 6, highlighting the approximate location of the HLA-DR gene segment, which is associated with genetic predispositions to sensitivities involving mold, water-damage organisms, multiple chemical sensitivities, and other environmental exposures.

Symptoms of CIRS

Individuals hypersensitive to water damage-related organisms may experience a wide range of symptoms that can be subtle or, in many cases, profoundly disruptive. Chronic Inflammatory Response Syndrome (CIRS) presents through a complex set of symptoms, reflecting its impact on multiple bodily systems. (CIRS Academy, 2021)

Chronic fatigue and sleep disorders

Chronic fatigue and sleep disorders are often exacerbated in the context of Chronic Inflammatory Response Syndrome (CIRS), a condition triggered by exposure to biotoxins like mold. In CIRS, the immune system's prolonged inflammatory response can lead to a cascade of symptoms, including debilitating fatigue and disrupted sleep patterns. This creates a vicious cycle: exhaustion makes it difficult to manage CIRS, while sleep disorders further compromise the body's ability to heal, reinforcing both conditions.

Difficulties with memory, focus, and concentration (Brain fog)

Brain fog is a particularly insidious symptom. It manifests as a clouding of consciousness, affecting cognitive functions such as memory, focus, and decision-making. This mental haze is not merely an inconvenience; it's indicative of the systemic inflammation that CIRS triggers, which can have a profound impact on neural pathways and neurotransmitter activity.

Understanding the role of brain fog in CIRS is essential, as it affects the quality of life and complicates the management of the syndrome. It's like navigating through a maze while wearing a blindfold; you know you need to find a way out, but the condition you're trying to manage makes it challenging to see the path.

Aches, pain, and weakness

Aches, pain, and weakness are more than just physical discomforts; they are tangible markers of the body's ongoing struggle with systemic inflammation. These symptoms are often the result of cytokine release, small proteins that play a key role in cell signaling during immune responses. Elevated levels of cytokines can lead to muscle and joint pain, as well as generalized weakness.

The presence of these symptoms in CIRS complicates both diagnosis and treatment. They can easily be mistaken for other conditions, such as fibromyalgia or chronic fatigue syndrome, leading to potential misdiagnosis. Moreover, physical discomfort often exacerbates other CIRS symptoms, like fatigue and brain fog, creating a challenging cycle of symptoms that feed into each other.

In essence, aches, pains, and weakness are not just symptoms but signals alerting us to the deeper, systemic issues at play in CIRS. Understanding their role can help devise more targeted treatment strategies, offering a glimmer of light in what can often feel like a never-ending tunnel of discomfort.

Muscle cramps and morning stiffness

Muscle cramps and morning stiffness indicate the body's underlying systemic inflammation. Muscle cramps, often sudden and painful, may be linked to electrolyte imbalances worsened by the inflammatory state induced by CIRS. Morning stiffness, experienced upon waking, can be attributed to overnight inflammatory processes that lead to fluid accumulation in joints and muscle tissues.

Headaches and light sensitivity

Headaches and light sensitivity are more than mere discomforts; they are symptomatic of the neurological impact of systemic inflammation. Headaches, often ranging from dull aches to debilitating migraines, can directly result from the inflammatory cytokines affecting the nervous system. Light sensitivity, or photophobia, is another neurological symptom that can be particularly distressing. It often manifests itself as an intolerance to varying light conditions, making even simple tasks like reading or driving challenging.

Red Eyes, Blurred vision, and tearing.

Symptoms like red eyes, blurred vision, and tearing are not merely ocular annoyances but indicative of the syndrome's systemic reach. These eye-related symptoms can be attributed to the body's inflammatory response to biotoxins, which affects the ocular tissues and leads to irritation, visual disturbances, and excessive tearing. While they may seem less severe than other CIRS symptoms, their presence can significantly impact daily activities and quality of life.

Sinus congestion, coughing.

Sinus congestion and coughing are more than just respiratory irritations; they are key indicators of the body's inflammatory response to environmental biotoxins. These symptoms often manifest as the respiratory system's attempt to expel or neutralize irritants, leading to inflamed sinus passages and persistent coughing. While they may appear to be common ailments, in the setting of CIRS, they provide valuable diagnostic insights and can significantly affect one's quality of life.

Shortness of breath

Shortness of breath is a particularly concerning symptom, indicative of the syndrome's impact on respiratory function. Often experienced as a sensation of being unable to draw a full breath, this symptom can sometimes be attributed to the inflammatory processes affecting the lungs and airways. While it may not be immediately life-threatening, shortness of breath can significantly impair physical activity and quality of life.

Painful joints and morning stiffness

Painful joints and morning stiffness are not merely discomforts; they are significant indicators of systemic inflammation. These symptoms often manifest because of elevated cytokine levels, which lead to inflammation in the joints and surrounding tissues. Upon waking, individuals may experience stiffness, making even simple movements challenging.

Word-finding difficulties.

Word-finding difficulties are more than just frustrating lapses; they are a telling sign of the neurological effects of systemic inflammation. Often manifesting as the inability to quickly recall specific words or names, this symptom can be attributed to the impact of inflammatory cytokines on cognitive function and neural communication.

Problems Assimilating New Knowledge

Difficulties in assimilating new knowledge are not just educational hurdles but indicative of the neurological toll of systemic inflammation. This cognitive impairment can be attributed to the disruption of neural pathways and neurotransmitter activity, making the acquisition and retention of new information challenging.

Confusion, Disorientation

Confusion and disorientation in CIRS are more than momentary lapses; they are significant indicators of the syndrome's neurological impact. These symptoms can manifest as a lack of mental clarity or even a temporary loss of spatial awareness, often attributed to the inflammatory processes affecting the brain.

Skin Sensitivity, Rashes, Eczema, Hives

Skin issues like sensitivity, rashes, eczema, and hives are not merely dermatological concerns but manifestations of systemic inflammation. The body's heightened immune response to environmental biotoxins can trigger these conditions, leading to various forms of skin irritation.

Unusual Sweating (Especially at Night)

Unusual sweating, particularly at night, is a symptom that can be particularly telling in the context of CIRS. This can be attributed to the body's attempt to regulate temperature and eliminate toxins through perspiration, exacerbated by systemic inflammation.

Mood Swings

Mood swings in CIRS are not just emotional fluctuations; they indicate the neurological and hormonal imbalances caused by systemic inflammation. These mood changes can be sudden and extreme, affecting one's emotional well-being and interpersonal relationships.

Excessive Thirst

Excessive thirst in CIRS can be attributed to inflammatory conditions resulting in the body's inability to regulate fluids.

Static Shocks

Static shocks in CIRS may seem trivial but can indicate an imbalance in the body's electrical system, possibly exacerbated by systemic inflammation. While not life-threatening, they serve as an unusual but telling symptom.

Numbness or Tingling

Numbness or tingling sensations are often neurological and can be attributed to the inflammatory processes affecting nerve function in CIRS. These symptoms provide valuable diagnostic insights into the syndrome's neurological impact.

Vertigo or Dizziness

Vertigo and dizziness in CIRS are significant indicators of the syndrome's impact on the vestibular system. These symptoms can be disorienting and debilitating, affecting one's ability to perform daily tasks.

Metallic Tastes

A metallic taste in the mouth can be a peculiar but telling symptom in CIRS. It possibly indicates the body's response to toxin exposure and provides a diagnostic clue.

Abdominal Pain, Diarrhea

Gastrointestinal symptoms like abdominal pain and diarrhea in CIRS can be attributed to the systemic inflammation affecting the digestive tract, providing diagnostic insights.

Exercise Intolerance

Exercise intolerance in CIRS can be attributed to the body's compromised metabolic and respiratory systems, exacerbated by systemic inflammation, and serves as an important diagnostic marker.

Tremors

Tremors in CIRS are often neurological, indicative of the syndrome's impact on motor function and coordination, as crucial diagnostic symptoms.

Unusual Pain, Especially Migraines or Facial Pain

Unusual pain, particularly migraines or facial pain, can be debilitating and often indicates the neurological and inflammatory aspects of CIRS.

Appetite Swings, Gastrointestinal Disorders

Fluctuations in appetite and gastrointestinal disorders in CIRS can be linked to systemic inflammation affecting the digestive system, serving as diagnostic clues.

Increased Urination (Especially at Night)

Increased urination, particularly at night, can be a symptom of the body's attempt to eliminate toxins, providing valuable insights into the body's physiological state in CIRS.

Depression and Anxiety

Mental health symptoms like depression and anxiety in CIRS are often linked to the neurological impact of systemic inflammation and serve as diagnostic symptoms.

Infertility/Miscarriage

Infertility in CIRS can be a devastating symptom, often linked to hormonal imbalances caused by systemic inflammation. Moreover, CIRS patients have been observed to have a higher incidence of miscarriage.

Multiple Chemical Sensitivities

Multiple chemical sensitivities in CIRS indicate a heightened immune response to various environmental factors, serving as a significant diagnostic clue.

Each of these symptoms, while varying in severity and impact, contributes to the complex diagnostic and treatment landscape of CIRS. Is it any wonder that navigating this condition can feel like a maze with shifting walls? The multifaceted nature of CIRS symptoms not only complicates diagnosis but also makes treatment a challenging endeavor. It requires a multi-disciplinary approach involving healthcare providers, environmental consultants, and legal advisors to navigate insurance complexities. The symptoms of CIRS are more than just a list of ailments; they represent a web of interconnected challenges that extend into various aspects of life, from health to finances to emotional well-being. (McMahon, 2017)

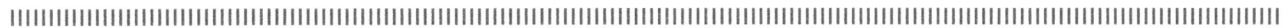

Essay: Children and Mold; Pediatric Considerations
by Scott McMahon, MD

"Our nation's children are our greatest asset and our most precious treasure." These words, quoted from Christopher Dodd, echo the sentiments of many, if not all, devoted parents. Our children are not just our future; they need to be our "now."

As a pediatrician for over 30 years, I have watched epidemics of obesity, Type 2 diabetes, hypertension, autism, etc., torment our children. One cannot discount at least a portion of the causation of these plagues from environmental changes experienced over recent generations. GMO foods, an adulterated food pyramid, a panoply of vaccines, removing physical education at school, and the development of over 300,000 new chemicals in the last century are likely contributors. However, as a kids' doctor, my greatest concern for our current and future generations is chronic exposure to increased microbial growth in water-damaged buildings.

The medical literature reports that 17% of children aged 4–18 years have chronic headaches. (Lateef, 2009) That constitutes 10 million U.S. children! Additionally, 13.5% of all children aged 0–18 have chronic stomach issues, which often cannot be easily traced to a specific cause. (Reust, 2018) That is another

10,000,000 kids, though many youngsters will suffer from both. What causes these headaches and stomach issues? Modern medicine does not know. Pediatricians are taught at the finest temples of medical learning that recurrent head and stomach pains are usually stress-related and do not have an organic cause. These are "functional" symptoms. (Wessely S, 1999) "Functional" is a nice way of saying, "It's all in your head." The same thing happens in adult patients, too. These are medically unexplained symptoms (MUS).

Well-meaning doctors run all the relevant tests *they know* and find nothing. There are only a few conclusions to which they can arrive.

1. The patient is faking illness or hiding information.
2. The patient has mental illness.
3. The patient has a disorder of which the physician is not aware and does not know the confirmatory tests to run. As one who knows hundreds of physicians, I believe this is the least likely deduction a medical professional will make.

As such, children with chronic headaches and/or abdominal pains are told that there is really nothing physically wrong with them. The patient is healthy, but their pains are a manifestation of psychological issues. If the child truly has an organic illness of which the physician is unaware, this is abusive doctoring, and many of my patients have experienced this medical malpractice before transferring to my care.

Enter chronic inflammatory response syndrome (CIRS). CIRS is a chronic, progressive, and debilitating disease if left undiagnosed and untreated. CIRS has been found in at least 7% of evaluated children. One-quarter of the population is genetically predisposed, and 50–85% of buildings have some degree of water damage, per the U.S. EPA. Up to 11.4 million American children (15.8%) are both exposed and predisposed. Most patients with CIRS have a predisposition, and ALL have an environmental exposure, most commonly water-damaged buildings. (McMahon S. W., 2023)

I have evaluated ~800 children for CIRS over 15 years. When these children have one or more MUS, such as headaches, IBS-like stomach issues, atypical chest pains, chronic fatigue, persisting growing pains, prolonged bed wetting, and more, I perform the standard workup for these symptoms—and I assess them for CIRS. Patients with CIRS will have several abnormal lab tests related to their immune and endocrine systems; however, the diagnostic lab tests are unfamiliar to many doctors. If you do not know about CIRS, you will not see it. Once you know about CIRS, you will see it in patients every day. (McMahon, 2017)

Around 90% of my children with chronic headaches will have multiple abnormal tests confirming CIRS. Of those with "functional" abdominal pain, just less than 90% have numerous positive CIRS tests. My research demonstrates similar numbers for children with growing pains lasting longer than 2 months, children not toilet-trained by 6 years old, and kids with chronic fatigue. Maybe these MUS have an explanation after all! Psychiatrist NOT required!!!

Treatment is simple, effective, and, in small children, often completely restorative. If mold exposure is the cause, removing them from the exposure and treating for 2–4 weeks with a binder like cholestyramine is very effective in younger children. Older children sometimes require additional short-term therapies, but resolution or reduction of symptoms is still the expectation. Recurrence of symptoms does not usually occur unless the kids are re-exposed to water-damaged buildings. CIRS is an extremely rewarding illness to treat.

Missing the CIRS diagnosis and misdiagnosing an incorrect malady leads to incorrect treatment, unnecessary side effects, excessive costs, and delays in proper therapy. If the wrong diagnosis also warrants a trip to the psychiatrist, it harms patient trust and is abusive. Is there any wonder why patients are flocking to the internet and alternative medicine constructs to bring relief?

Summarizing, there are a number of MUS that lead to misdiagnosis and wrong therapies, even in children. CIRS explains all of these MUS, but many physicians are unaware of this extremely common environmental illness. The most popular symptoms in children are chronic fatigue, recurrent headaches, frequent abdominal pains, persisting growing pains, inattention (often misdiagnosed as ADHD), and failure to toilet train by 6 years old. Small children with CIRS can exhibit one or all six symptoms. By 11 years old, typically, these children manifest symptoms in at least four different body systems involving their eyes, lungs, muscles, joints, urinary frequency, exercise tolerance, GI tract, energy level, cognition/behavior, and much more. CIRS is more easily treatable at younger ages of discovery, has better outcomes in the young, and becomes preventable after initial therapy. Diagnosis is made by a few blood tests, and screening at birth or shortly after is possible.

It is time we looked at Pediatric CIRS, not only for its terrible toll on our youth but also for the possible preventative potential this illness affords. It is time for Pediatricians, Family Practitioners, and Internists to learn about CIRS.

UNDERSTANDING ALLERGENS AND ALLERGIES

Normal quantities of mold spores are everywhere outdoors and, over time, will migrate into our homes. With continued exposure, allergic sensitivities to mold may worsen, resulting in increased reactivity with normal outdoor mold accumulation.

The National Allergy Bureau (NAB), a section of the American Academy of Allergy, Asthma & Immunology (AAAAI), has been monitoring outdoor allergen levels for decades. News outlets, weather services, and health organizations frequently use NAB's pollen and mold spore counts to inform the public about current allergen conditions in various cities. (Levetin, 2023)

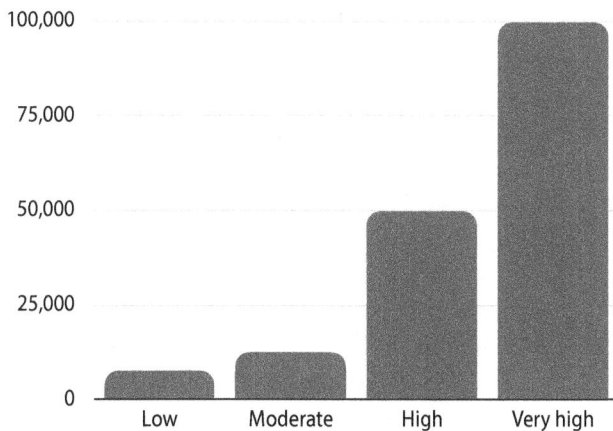

Figure 1-4: Spore Counts per Cubic Meter across Four Categories of Concentration (Low, Moderate, High, and Very High).

In understanding the impact of mold on health, it's important to note that mold allergies have been identified in about 6% of people who have recognized a genetic tendency to develop allergic reactions such as asthma, eczema, and hay fever. These individuals often have heightened immune responses to common allergens like pollen, dust mites, and certain foods. This predisposition is associated with the production of elevated levels of Immunoglobulin E (IgE) antibodies, which play a key role in allergic reactions. Recognizing this link can help guide effective strategies for managing mold exposure and mitigating its impact on those susceptible to such allergies. (Kurup V. P., 2000)

ALLERGENS: BEYOND MOLD

While mold is a significant concern for many, it's crucial to remember that various other environmental factors can trigger allergies and asthma reactions. If you don't find relief from mold mitigation, you may need to look to other common allergen sources, including dog and cat dander. These can cause symptoms ranging from mild sneezing and itching to more severe respiratory issues. Rodent urine is another less discussed but potent allergen, especially in urban environments or older buildings. Dust mites are ubiquitous in homes and can trigger symptoms like pollen allergies, such as sneezing, runny or stuffy nose, itchy or watery eyes, and scratchy throat or skin. These symptoms are often grouped under the term "allergic rhinitis." Cockroach frass (feces) is another indoor allergen that can cause significant health problems, particularly in densely populated areas where cockroach infestations are more common.

Outdoor allergens like pollens from trees, grasses, and weeds can also wreak havoc. These allergens are often seasonal but can cause perennial issues for those particularly sensitive. Symptoms can range from mild discomfort, such as itchy eyes and sneezing, to more severe conditions like allergic rhinitis or even anaphylaxis in extreme cases.

Importantly, moisture control also plays a role in mitigating allergens like Dust mites and roaches, which tend to thrive in damp conditions. Maintaining a dry environment can effectively help control more than just mold. Similar moisture control techniques used for mold prevention offer a practical approach to reducing exposure to other allergens and improving indoor environmental quality.

IMPACTS AND SIDE EFFECTS OF WATER DAMAGE

The adverse health effects of water damage involve more than mold. Water-damaged homes can harbor amplified bacteria, which can be harmful to everyone and especially problematic for those with inflammatory responses. Additionally, many chemicals used to treat these problems are, at best, unnecessary or useless and, at worst, can harm people and pets. Chemical treatments can interfere with the successful restoration of homes occupied by people with multiple chemical sensitivities (MCS), making the house uninhabitable for them. Killing organisms instead of physically removing them can interfere with the investigation and remediation process by creating false negative results. Physical removal and cleaning are necessary to eliminate the exotoxins and endotoxins left behind when organisms die.

The good news is that bacterial issues in the home can be resolved by discarding unrestorable damaged materials, cleaning the remaining structure, and restoration using many of the same techniques used for mold without harmful chemicals. By understanding the different threats to our indoor environment, you can take steps to protect your health and your home.

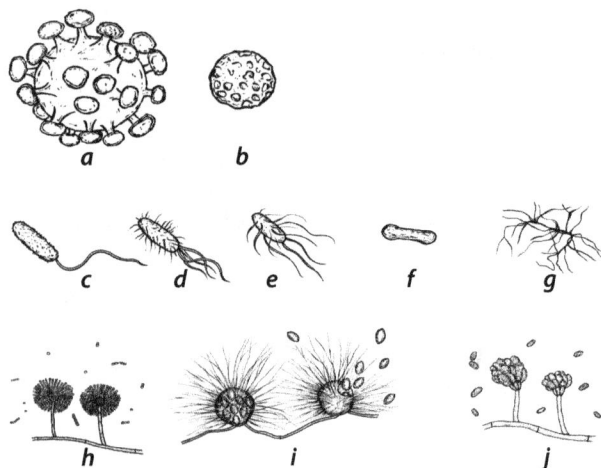

*Figure 1-5: Relative sizes of different microorganisms. Top line, viruses: COVID-19 60 to 140 nm in diameter (**a**). Hepatitis A virus ~27 nm (**b**). Middle line, bacteria: whole bacteria are slightly smaller than mold spores. Cholera bacteria 1 to 3 μm in length, 0.5 to 0.8 μm in diameter (**c**). Escherichia coli (E. coli) 1 to 2 μm in length and 0.5 μm in diameter (**d**). Salmonella 1 to 3 μm in length and 0.5 to 1 μm in diameter (**e**). Corynebacterium acnes (Cutibacterium acnes) 1.0 to 1.5 μm in length and 0.5 to 0.8 μm in diameter (**f**). Water-damage Actinobacteria (e.g., Streptomyces species) 0.5 to 2.0 μm in diameter for filaments, which can be many micrometers long (**g**). Bottom line, mold: Hyphae are typically 2 to 4 μm wide. And long. Aspergillus 2 to 4 μm diameter for spores (**h**). Chaetomium 6 to 12 μm in diameter for spores (**i**). Stachybotrys 5 μm width, 10 μm in length for spores (**j**).*

GRAM-NEGATIVE BACTERIA AND ENDOTOXINS

Gram-negative bacteria present significant indoor health risks. They can thrive in diverse environments such as drinking water, swimming pools, and natural bodies of water. They are most commonly present in homes affected by sewage backflow but also can be the result of a dried P-trap, failed toilet wax ring, Studor vent (air admittance valve), unkept cat litter box, or animal fecal buildup, rodent or other animal infestations, manure, and septic line failures. These can introduce high concentrations of endotoxins from fecal organisms like E. coli and Salmonella, leading to widespread health issues, from gastrointestinal disturbances to infections impacting the skin, ears, eyes, and respiratory system. These bacteria and their endotoxins demand prompt and trained professional cleanup to mitigate exposure risks and prevent infections.

The primary strategy for addressing these contaminants emphasizes thorough cleaning with soap and water. Soap, detergent, or appropriate surfactant is practical by emulsifying the hydrophobic, lipid, or fatty membranes found in gram-negative bacteria, mold, and viruses. The surfactant action emulsifies these fatty membranes, enabling the physical removal of these organisms and helping minimize the risk of the endotoxins they produce and the related health problems. Avoid harsh chemicals that can leave harmful residues and exacerbate health issues by prioritizing soap and water for cleaning. Endotoxins from sewage and the associated pathogenic organisms do not dissipate on their own and require removal and disposal of porous, contaminated materials such as gypsum wallboard and insulation, followed by thorough cleaning to mitigate their health risks. You can't kill a biotoxin. Addressing fresh sewage intrusion is critical, as discussed in the emergency water-damage section. (IICRC, 2021)

ACTINOBACTERIA AND EXOTOXINS

Actinobacteria, known for their crucial role in soil ecology, are a diverse group of filamentous bacteria that contribute significantly to the decomposition of organic matter. In the natural environment, they are predominantly found in soil, where they help break down complex compounds, including cellulose and chitin, thus playing a vital role in the carbon cycle. Their presence is not limited to soil; actinobacteria can also thrive in aquatic ecosystems and areas where organic material is abundant. Soil-related actinobacteria can be tracked into a home but are not currently believed to be organisms of concern for home environments.

Water-damage actinomycetes generally refers to the filamentous, spore-forming bacteria that are a part of the phylum actinobacteria and are typically found at low levels in indoor environments but can proliferate, especially in damp or water-damaged spaces. They flourish in many of the same moist conditions as water-damage-associated molds, making flooded or wet areas of buildings ideal for their growth. Due to their filamentous structure, actinomycetes colonies can closely resemble mold, leading to potential confusion during visual inspections. This similarity is not just superficial; like mold, actinomycetes can release spores (conidia) infused with exotoxins into the air and onto surfaces, contributing to indoor environmental quality problems and potentially causing health issues, especially for hypersensitive building occupants.

The confusion between actinomycetes and mold goes beyond identification; it has practical implications for diagnosis and remediation. Traditional mold testing typically relies on spore counts and species identification via microscopic examination or culture techniques but generally does not detect any actinobacteria. Identifying bacteria requires specific testing procedures distinct from mold testing, which can be part of a laboratory's bacterial identification services. This disconnect between environmental consultants and laboratories can easily lead to confusion and ineffective remediation strategies—especially when filamentous growth results from actinomycetes, yet mold testing of those surfaces yields negative results. The ecological requirements and growth characteristics of actinomycetes differ somewhat from molds; actinomycetes are more commonly found on wood or soil-related substrates, while non-filamentous actinobacteria are often associated with human or animal skin flora. Consequently, what appears to be mold in water-damaged buildings may be filamentous actinomycetes, necessitating tailored approaches for accurate testing and identification. Remediation methods for mold, however, may still be effective for actinomycetes.

Given the potential overlap in appearance and habitat between Actinomycetes and mold, environmental health professionals must consider the presence of Actinomycetes in their assessments of water-damaged environments. This awareness can ensure that testing and remediation efforts are appropriately directed, addressing the actual contaminants present and mitigating their impact on indoor air quality and occupant health.

For decades, it has been understood that Actinobacteria can develop indoors, especially within water-damaged buildings. Advancements such as Next-Generation Sequencing (NGS) and transcriptomic assays have significantly enhanced our understanding, revealing how these bacteria, when present in unacceptably high levels, can cause the innate immune system to overreact, causing Chronic Inflammatory Response Syndrome (CIRS) in genetically predisposed people. This overreaction is particularly prevalent in individuals exposed to water-damaged environments, underscoring the need to identify actinobacteria and not misinterpret them as being the same as mold. (Shoemaker R. e., 2021)

Recognizing the sources of actinobacteria and their identification in buildings has paved the way for more focused treatment and remediation strategies. Crucial steps include identifying these bacteria, understanding their origins, and recognizing their health impacts. The methods for remediation and cleaning of Actinomycetes that result from water-damaged environments are generally the same as those for mold remediation and involve physical removal of non-restorable affected materials like gypsum board and insulation to provide access to wall cavities and otherwise inaccessible spaces as well as cleaning to remove the organisms and exotoxins. (IICRC, 2021)

Skin-related actinobacteria conditions often require cooperation between patients, environmental consultants, cleaning specialists, and medical practitioners. Typically, harmless when residing on our skin, under poorly understood circumstances, some individuals become carriers of unusually high levels of these bacteria, which can be shed along with skin cells into their living spaces.

This is necessary to break the cycle of contamination where the infected person sheds bacteria into the home and can then become exposed to the shared organisms if they are not cleaned and physically removed to normal levels within the home. When shed by others within the house, these organisms may affect people afflicted with CIRS symptoms. However, they face a special predicament when they have infected skin and CIRS directly impacts them. (Dorninger, 2022)

A comprehensive approach involves:

- The medical practitioner diagnoses and prescribes the appropriate treatments for the affected person to help reestablish a normal skin microflora.

- The environmental consultant's role includes identifying actinobacteria contamination in indoor environments and distinguishing between those caused by water damage, those affecting the skin, and the normal flora that may be tracked into the home by people and pets but are unlikely to result in adverse effects.

  › Water Damage: When Actinomycetes result from water damage, remediation involves removing water-damaged porous materials, such as gypsum wallboard and affected insulation, and aggressive abrasive cleaning of affected wood followed by thorough cleaning of the rest of the affected environment.
  › Skin Conditions: For skin conditions, effective cleaning methods are required for the building, furnishings, and personal possessions. The cleaning methods outlined in this book's 25 Steps and Contents sections can effectively remove Actinobacteria from homes, undergarments, clothing, bedding, pillow covers, and other personal items.
  › Normal routine effective housekeeping should be able to control soil-related actinobacteria.

A notable distinction is that actinobacteria associated with skin-related conditions are not caused by water damage and, therefore, do not require destructive remediation efforts, only effective structural cleaning. Successfully cleaning a home removes these organisms and their exotoxins, so, as with mold, killing the microorganisms directly is unnecessary and may even be counterproductive. For skin-related conditions, where the person is the source of the contamination, medical treatment is essential to address the person(s) that is the infection source and prevent reinfection. In cases where exposure is building-related, the focus should be locating and remediating the water damage. (Shoemaker R. e., 2021)

This area of research continues to develop, with advancements in identifying, evaluating, and treating actinobacteria-related issues. For effective management, it is recommended that one stay informed on the latest research and work with professionals who understand the most current findings.

MULTIPLE CHEMICAL SENSITIVITIES

Multiple Chemical Sensitivities (MCS) is a condition that makes people unusually sensitive to everyday substances. By understanding the intricacies, you'll be better equipped to create an environment that minimizes exposure, enhances well-being, and addresses issues from mold and other organisms and exposures associated with water damage.

MCS can arise from a variety of factors. One potential cause is genetic predisposition, where individuals may have a natural inclination toward developing sensitivities. Environmental exposures, such as long-term interaction with pollutants or toxic chemicals, can also contribute. Additionally, initial sensitizing events, like acute exposure to organisms associated with water damage, chemical exposure, or a series of exposures, can act as a catalyst for the onset of MCS. Understanding these root causes is crucial for effectively diagnosing and managing the condition. (Molot, 2023)

Physical Symptoms

The physical symptoms of MCS can vary widely, making early recognition crucial for effective management. Individuals may initially experience mild symptoms like headaches and fatigue but, over time, can face more severe manifestations such as difficulty breathing, skin rashes, and digestive issues. These physical symptoms can significantly interfere with daily activities and impact the quality of life. The challenge lies in the fact that these symptoms often overlap with other medical conditions, complicating the timely diagnosis and intervention process. Chemical exposure can accentuate the physical symptoms associated with MCS. Understanding the range and severity of these physical manifestations is essential for healthcare providers and individuals to manage MCS effectively. (Bell IR H. E., 1995)

Psychological Impact

The psychological toll of Multiple Chemical Sensitivities (MCS) is often as challenging as the physical symptoms. Anxiety and depression are everyday experiences for those affected, further intensified by the lifestyle restrictions necessary to avoid potential chemical irritants. Exposure to triggers like mold can remarkably heighten these psychological aspects, making individuals more susceptible to cycles of mental distress. The presence of these psychological symptoms complicates the diagnostic process significantly. They can mimic or exacerbate the physical symptoms, making it challenging for healthcare providers to accurately identify MCS as the underlying cause. Understanding this interplay between psychological and physical symptoms is vital for comprehensive diagnosis and effective management. (Kilburn, 2009)

Multi-System Involvement and Common Chemical Triggers

Multiple Chemical Sensitivities (MCS) is a complex condition involving symptoms that affect multiple bodily systems, including respiratory, dermatological, and neurological systems. This multi-system involvement can complicate diagnosis and treatment, often leading clinicians to incorrect or incomplete treatment plans. Common household chemicals such as cleaning agents, perfumes, and laundry detergents are among the most prevalent triggers for MCS symptoms, often making routine activities challenging for those affected. Individuals can take an essential first step in managing their condition by raising their awareness of these chemical triggers and eliminating them. Secondary triggers like pollen, pet dander, mold, actinobacteria, endotoxins from gram-negative bacteria, and other factors associated with water damage can further aggravate MCS symptoms, especially when an individual is already sensitized to different substances. Therefore, it's crucial to consider the immediate chemical environment and the broader setting, such as the home or workplace, when managing MCS. Occupational environments often contain chemicals, from industrial solvents to office supplies like printer ink, which can exacerbate symptoms. Workplace adaptations like enhanced ventilation and safer materials can significantly improve the quality of life for individuals with MCS. Indoor air quality also plays a pivotal role, as poorly ventilated areas can trap pollutants and intensify symptoms, especially in buildings with water damage or mold issues. Enhancing ventilation and regularly assessing air quality is key in any comprehensive MCS management strategy. Outdoor air quality also impacts those with MCS; even areas distant from direct pollution sources are increasingly affected by intermittent wildfire smoke due to climate change, posing a substantial challenge for individuals with chemical sensitivities. (Molot, 2023)

Mold exposure uniquely impacts individuals with MCS, often acting as a trigger and an amplifying factor for other symptoms. Molds release compounds like mycotoxins and volatile organic compounds (VOCs), which can be highly irritating or toxic. For those with MCS, mold exposure can trigger immediate symptoms and increase sensitivity to other chemicals, expanding their vulnerability to various triggers. The immune response to mold exposure can be complex and more intense in MCS patients, often heightening overall chemical sensitivity. This response necessitates a multi-faceted approach to MCS management that includes mold remediation and attention to materials and methods used for repair, reconstruction, and remodeling as a foundational component. (Baker-Laporte, 2022)

Mold Remediation as a Component of MCS Management

Given the significant impact that mold can have on MCS, mold remediation becomes a part of an effective management strategy. This involves identifying and eliminating mold sources, improving ventilation, and possibly using air purification methods to improve indoor air quality. It is crucial to address mold problems comprehensively to achieve a significant reduction in symptoms associated with mold, other organisms associated with water damage, and MCS. Understanding the intricacies of how water damage-related exposure interacts with MCS allows for more effective symptom management and contributes to creating healthier living spaces. (CIRSx Academy, 2024)

|||||||||||||||||||||||||||||||||||||||||||||||||||||||||||||||||||||||||||||||||||||||||||||||||||||||||||||||||||||||||||||||||

Essay: Addressing the Emotional Aspects of Hypersensitivities
by Jane Prescot, FMCHC. Shoemaker Proficiency Partner Diplomate, CIRS Coach and Consultant

Historically, individuals with environmental sensitivities have been misunderstood or dismissed by the medical profession. Most have been sick for some time with a progressively debilitating, often multi-system unexplained illness. Navigating the health care system with a medically unexplained illness can be a traumatizing process. These individuals have wasted time, money, and energy trying to get a diagnosis for their bewildering symptoms. They may have been referred to multiple specialists, been given multiple misdiagnoses and prescribed ineffective treatments. Ultimately, they are given a neuropsychiatric or somatization explanation for their symptoms.

But there is more recently a growing awareness that medically unexplained symptoms and environmental sensitivities may have a common underlying etiology.

The biological, psychological, and social aspects of environmental sensitivity are inseparable. The brain is a target organ in this condition. Alterations in brain structure and function affect mood and emotional responses, cognitive function, attention, and strategic thinking. There is a loss of motivation and the ability to feel pleasure. Symptoms of anxiety and depression are often part of the broader constellation of neuro-immune symptoms, with the main aspect of anxiety being the anticipation of danger. Those who are severely affected are often unable to function normally in their personal, social and professional lives.

Environmental hypersensitivities take a toll on the individual with the condition and their whole family. Relationships can be challenging. For some, there is very limited spousal support. For others, the partner is supportive but can feel helpless and overwhelmed by the unpredictability of symptoms and the financial & practical considerations surrounding the illness. Suffering with this chronic, bewildering illness is often a traumatic and grievous process. There can be the loss of significant relationships, impaired family roles, loss of employment or underemployment, and social isolation. Impacted individuals and their families feel powerless. The environmentally sensitive individual may have been misunderstood and stigmatized by employers, friends, and family. They may have illegitimately been denied accommodation in the workplace or housing and are often denied disability benefits. Stress caused by isolation, social and occupational losses, stigmatization, a lack of health care, and physician gaslighting takes its toll.

Finally, the environmentally sensitive individual is relieved to find a health care practitioner who understands their condition, but then there is grief and loss associated with getting a diagnosis. There is fear and anxiety over the complexity and cost of the illness and remediation of their living space. They can be overwhelmed by the challenges of finding knowledgeable environmental professionals. There may be trauma over wasted time, money and effort with a previous failed remediation. For many of these individuals the prospect of having life-long susceptibility to re-acquiring biotoxin illness can seem daunting.

Dysregulation of the nervous system and the stress response in the environmentally sensitive individual can manifest in a number of ways. Some individuals get their diagnosis and run with it. Others flounder in overwhelm or struggle to move ahead and experience frustration and shame at not being able to do everything needed to support their recovery. The overwhelmed individual is likely to interact with health care providers and environmental professionals who may not understand overwhelm and may stigmatize this individual as non-compliant or difficult.

An individual in an activated sympathetic state may appear aggressive, angry, or belligerent. The medical provider and environmental team may perceive this as a patient or client lacking confidence in their clinical or professional management.

Discovering the *Biotoxin Pathway* (Shoemaker R. C., 2011) can be an aha moment for many environmentally hypersensitive individuals. They are now able to understand how exposure to mold and biotoxins made them sick with so many seemingly disparate symptoms and how ongoing environmental exposure is also keeping them sick.

Poor psychological health can accompany environmental sensitivity simply as a consequence of inflammation. But we don't want to discount the effects that are secondary to the trauma, grief and loss that accompanies this diagnosis. Ultimately, this individual needs to navigate the stages of grief to fully regain their health.

The Stages of Grief

Denial: Initially, individuals may find it hard to accept that their symptoms are related to mold exposure. This denial can delay necessary actions, such as consulting a healthcare professional or an environmental consultant.

Anger: Once reality sets in, anger often follows. Individuals may feel frustrated with their living conditions, their inability to get immediate relief, or even with themselves for not recognizing the signs earlier.

Bargaining: At this stage, people may try to make "deals" with themselves or others, thinking that minor changes in lifestyle or quick fixes could solve the problem. This is often a misguided attempt to regain control.

Depression: As the gravity of the situation sinks in, individuals may experience depression. The ongoing physical symptoms, emotional stress, and lifestyle changes can be overwhelming.

Acceptance: This is the turning point where individuals fully acknowledge the issue and take proactive steps to address it. Acceptance doesn't mean resignation; it means understanding the reality and working collaboratively with healthcare providers and environmental consultants to improve conditions.

Action and Hope: While not traditionally a stage of grief, this is an essential step in this context. With acceptance comes the ability to take informed action. This is where the collaborative efforts between the patient, their health care team, the environmental consultant, and other supporting trades come into play. It's also the stage where individuals often find hope, realizing that their condition can improve and they can regain a sense of normalcy.

Understanding and navigating these emotional stages can be as crucial as treating the physical symptoms. The emotional and physical experiences are deeply interconnected, and addressing both is key to holistic well-being. By recognizing these emotional stages, individuals can better manage their symptoms and take more effective steps toward both emotional and physical healing.

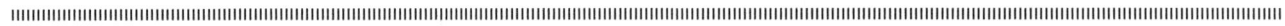

TAKING ACTION: A COLLABORATIVE EFFORT

Addressing mold sensitivities, especially when they are more severe or discovered after a significant amount of time has passed, requires a higher standard of care and a multidisciplinary approach. A combined collaborative effort between the patient, their medical practitioner, the environmental consultant, the water damage restorer, the mold remediator, supporting trades, family, friends, and others may be needed to regain the ability to function more appropriately. The cause of the problem must be identified and corrected, remediation must be successfully performed, and the maintenance and cleaning plan must be updated to prevent future issues.

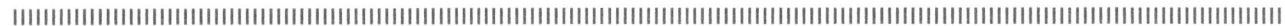

Essay: Mold Illness: Surviving and Thriving
by Paula Vetter, RN, MSN, FNP-C; Laurie Rossi, RN; Cindy Edwards, CBA

Mold Illness: Surviving and Thriving is an essential guide for individuals & families seeking recovery from Chronic Inflammatory Response Syndrome (CIRS). It provides a comprehensive guide to the personal journey required for healing. While *Mold Controlled* focuses on the environmental aspects—primarily how to create a safe, mold-controlled home—*Surviving and Thriving* goes beyond this by offering a detailed roadmap of the personal actions necessary for full recovery. This unique recovery manual is written by a nurse practitioner, a Shoemaker-certified CIRS Practitioner, an environmental contractor and specialist in building science, and an RN case manager who has spent more than 14 years navigating CIRS recovery for herself and then for scores of CIRS practitioners and their patients. The book's focus on health, including managing the detailed practical aspects of recovery, gives CIRS patients a more holistic view of what specific personal actions they need to take for long-term success. (Vetter, 2018)

The book strongly emphasizes the step-by-step actions a person must take to recover from CIRS. This includes navigating medical treatments, managing lifestyle changes, and ensuring that the physical environment supports healing. It delves deeply into the personal aspects of recovery—what patients need to do on a physical, emotional, and psychological level—making it a vital resource for those facing this challenging condition.

One of the standout features of *Surviving and Thriving* is the inclusion of multiple practical tools, such as sample letters to employers, landlords, sellers, and schools. These letters offer templates that patients can adapt when seeking help, advocating for their needs, or making requests for accommodations. These resources help empower individuals who may otherwise feel overwhelmed by the complexity of navigating their illness. Additionally, there are detailed lists of specific actions and checklists that patients, caregivers, and environmental professionals can utilize to create a supportive and effective recovery environment.

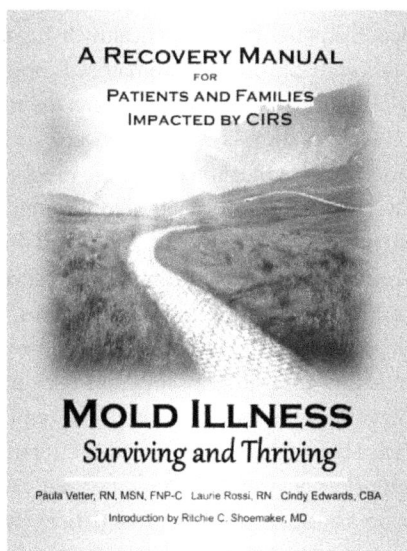

Figure 1-6: Mold Illness: Surviving and Thriving

The book's unique strength lies in its blend of personal and practical actionable advice. The authors' deep understanding of CIRS recovery reflects a balance between the physical actions needed to clean and detoxify one's living space and the personal strategies required for a sustainable healing process. Readers are guided through detoxification challenges, the importance and personal tracking of mold avoidance, and strategies for maintaining long-term health once the worst illness has passed.

Surviving and Thriving serves as a compassionate and empowering companion for anyone on the journey of CIRS recovery. It provides the necessary information and practical tools to navigate each process stage. Including personal letters, checklists, and actionable steps ensures that this book will be an invaluable guide for patients, caregivers, and environmental professionals in helping patients take control of their health and move toward a brighter future.

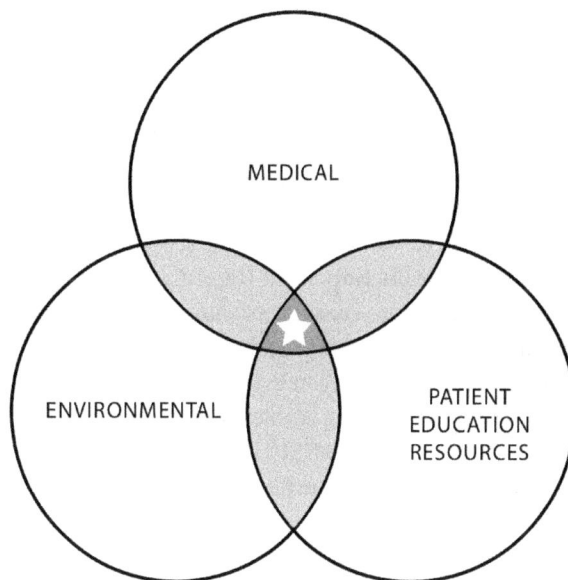

Figure 1-7: *This diagram illustrates the three interdependent professional disciplines essential for effective Chronic Inflammatory Response Syndrome (CIRS) management: medical (health care providers and their adjuncts), patient education (trusted resources), and environmental (Medically Important trained Indoor Environmental Professionals and Remediators). Each discipline is patient-centered and science-based and must complete its specific, practical steps in the correct sequence, with validation of efficacy. When all disciplines collaborate effectively, they achieve the "sweet spot" at the center—representing a recovered CIRS patient. Proper project management bridges gaps, fosters teamwork and supports recovery while minimizing setbacks, emotional strain, and wasted resources.*

BEYOND MEDICAL CARE: THE ROLE OF ENVIRONMENTAL CONSULTANTS

While doctors today rarely make house calls, someone needs to recognize when health problems stem from the buildings we occupy. That's where a qualified Environmental Consultant or Building Scientist becomes essential. These professionals conduct medically necessary investigations and recommend effective remediation strategies, especially for clients with extreme sensitivities to mold, water-damage-related organisms, and environmental contaminants. Their role requires an understanding beyond the vested interests of insurance companies,

real estate agents, landlords, or other parties who may not fully appreciate the unique needs of hypersensitive clients. Selecting an empathetic Environmental Consultant with specialized expertise is crucial for individuals adversely affected by mold and related organisms.

Specialized Qualifications for Medically Important Work

An Indoor Environmental Professional (IEP) working with hypersensitive clients must possess qualifications beyond the standard Industrial Hygienist training. Typical industrial hygiene programs emphasize assessments aligned with general occupational health and safety standards, often catering to insurance or real estate needs. However, environmental consultants working with medically sensitive populations should pursue specialized training for these complex cases.

CIRSx is developing training to address the medical practitioner/patient needs for medically important investigations. While this training is in progress, it is recommended that environmental consultants become familiar with the knowledge and skills required of remediation contractors. Foundational training in water damage and remediation from the **Institute for Inspection, Cleaning, and Restoration Certification (IICRC)** provides essential insights into the science of drying and remediation. This background is also for IEPs and can be supplemented with the **CIRSx Medically Important Remediation 101** online training, which equips consultants with skills to adjust work processes to understand and specify remediation methods suited to sensitive individuals.

This additional training enables IEPs to bridge the existing gap between the **ANSI/IICRC S500 Standard for Professional Water Damage Restoration** and the **ANSI/IICRC S520 Standard for Professional Mold Remediation** to align these industry standards with the specialized needs of mold-injured or hypersensitive patients. Equipped with this expertise, IEPs can create practical specifications and protocols tailored to medically sensitive individuals.

In this context, **specifications** outline the materials, methods, and standards necessary for effective remediation, while **protocols** are step-by-step instructions for implementing these specifications. Specifications set the overall plan, defining goals and best practices, whereas protocols provide the exact actions required to meet these standards. Together, they guide safe and comprehensive remediation work, creating an environment supportive of health and recovery for hypersensitive individuals. (CIRSx Institute, 2024)

THE REMEDIATION CONTRACTOR, AS A MEMBER OF THE TEAM

For households with individuals sensitive to mold, bacteria, or multiple chemical sensitivities (MCS), working with remediation companies that understand and address these needs is essential. Unlike general contractors who often aim to minimize costs and time by using unacceptable harsh chemicals to kill microorganisms, health-focused remediation contractors prioritize physical removal, detailed cleaning, and non-toxic methods that safeguard the well-being of occupants. These specialized companies recognize the complexities of sensitivities. They are committed to restoring safe environments for those whose health can be easily triggered by exposure to

contaminants and chemicals inappropriate for use in medically important cases.

Given the unique requirements of health-focused restoration, it is increasingly important for sensitive individuals to seek out remediation contractors who adhere to these principles. Though this dedication to health-centered quality may come at a higher cost, the investment is essential for those impacted by sensitivities to create a healthy living space.

For patients with Chronic Inflammatory Response Syndrome (CIRS) caused by mold exposure, the role of the Remediation Contractor is crucial to recovery. As the "boots on the ground," these professionals execute precise mold removal and structural repairs. Without thorough, expert remediation, healthcare practitioners often find that patients struggle to recover fully, as ongoing mold exposure within the home continues to trigger immune responses. Effective remediation goes beyond visible cleanup; it addresses hidden mold, controls moisture, and employs non-toxic methods to support healing genuinely. In many cases, Remediation Contractors are the bridge between medical treatment and a health-supportive environment, making their expertise and dedication a basic consideration for patients with mold sensitivities to reclaim their health.

Despite over 6,000 certified water and mold remediation firms and countless trained technicians, a shortage exists of contractors qualified to work with mold-sensitive patients. This shortage is partly due to market forces prioritizing satisfying insurance interests over addressing the health needs of hypersensitive individuals. Many companies focus on quick, low-cost solutions, with an industry mindset that "cheap is good" rather than emphasizing meticulous, health-centered remediation.

Compounding this issue, the antimicrobial manufacturing sector has heavily influenced the remediation industry, leading many technicians to believe that killing mold with chemicals is the only solution. However, this approach can be unnecessary and even harmful for patients with mold and chemical sensitivities. Applying antimicrobials in sensitive environments frequently exacerbates symptoms, making conditions worse rather than facilitating recovery.

There are several steps in the restoration process that restorers should perform or facilitate, which can return the structure to a sanitary condition without using antimicrobials (biocides). These steps should include ensuring the water intrusion has been stopped, removing un-restorable contaminated materials, followed by remediation, drying, and final cleaning of affected materials, systems, and contents. —ANSI/IICRC S500–2015

The lack of expertise in medically conscious remediation highlights the importance of organizations like CIRSx, founded on the belief that successful mold remediation requires a knowledgeable, collaborative team. CIRSx sponsors continuing education designed to help Remediation Technicians and their companies develop the specialized skills needed to bridge the gap between standard practices and the medical needs of hypersensitive populations. Through CIRSx training, contractors learn effective, non-toxic techniques for creating a health-supportive environment, enabling them to meet the unique requirements of patients affected by mold and water-damage organisms.

Medically Important Remediation (MIR101) – Advanced Training

For individuals suffering from Chronic Inflammatory Response Syndrome (CIRS) and other illnesses related to water damage, selecting a qualified remediation company is essential. Industry experts and medical professionals have developed the CIRSx "Medically Important Remediation" (MIR101) course program to bridge the gap between standard remediation practices and the critical needs of medically sensitive individuals.

CIRSx was founded by physicians who recognized that the only way for their patients to recover from mold illness is to remove harmful molds from their living environments or remove harmful mold exposures altogether. CIRSx empowers medical, environmental, and remediation professionals with the knowledge and skills to address CIRS and other mold-related illnesses, providing patients with safe, health-focused remediation solutions. This organization envisions a future where individuals impacted by mold and water damage illnesses can live in spaces that support healing, with the highest standards of environmental care in place.

MIR101 Training

The MIR101 course elevates traditional remediation skills to meet the needs of patients affected by mold-related illnesses. This intensive, 16-hour self-paced program offers science-based training on creating a health-supportive home environment where harmful molds and other water-damage organisms are physically removed instead of chemically treated and hidden conditions allowed to fester. The course teaches technicians how to work alongside healthcare providers to support patient recovery, as CIRSx understands that only after removing inflammatory exposures can medical care help reverse and repair the damage that has been done.

Course Highlights

Advanced Techniques: Training focuses on cutting-edge microbial remediation for sensitive environments.

Medical Collaboration: Emphasis on supporting healthcare practitioners' work through proper environmental care.

Expert Instruction: Delivered by leaders in environmental and medical fields.

Continuing Education Credit: Earn a digital badge to certify understanding of Medically Important Remediation. This course has earned two days of Continuing Education Credit from the IICRC.

My Endorsement

As one of the instructors, I can personally vouch for the quality and depth of information in MIR101. This course is vital for any remediation company looking to support mold-sensitive individuals with expertise and care.

For *Mold Controlled* readers: I encourage you to select companies with MIR101 training to ensure they meet the highest standards in medically focused remediation care. If no certified companies are available in your area, consider recommending CIRSx training to local firms to help develop access to these specialized services so they will be available when you or your community needs them.

General audiences wanting only informational content should take the "Medically Important Remediation—MIR100." MIR100 has the same content as MIR101 but without the navigation controls, quiz requirements, and digital badge.

Medically Important Remediation MIR100 & MIR101 are offered by the CIRSx Institute at:

https://institute.cirsx.com/p/medically-important-remediation-101

https://institute.cirsx.com/p/medically-important-remediation-1012

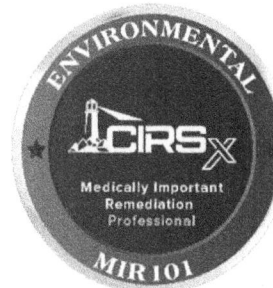

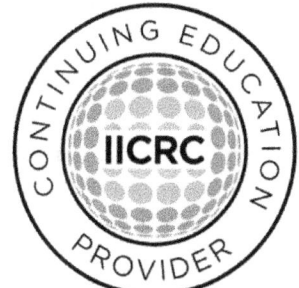

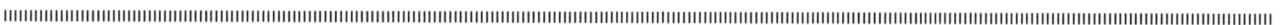

THE IMPORTANCE OF A SUPPORT NETWORK

Never underestimate the power of a strong support network. Whether it's family, friends, or online communities, shared experiences and advice can make a world of difference.

Discovering you are being affected by mold sensitivities may seem like an isolating experience; However, it can also be the beginning of a journey toward a healthier life. With the right information, professional guidance, and emotional support, you can navigate this challenging period and come out stronger on the other side. Your home should be a healthful, nurturing refuge—a place of comfort and well-being. And that's entirely achievable with the right approach and resources.

||||||||||||||||||||||||||||||||||||||||||||||||||||||||||||||||||||||||||||||||||||||||||||||||||||||||||||||||||||||||||||||||||||||||||

Essay: Health Support Networks

by Jenny Johnson, MSPT, FMCHC, NBC-HWC

The US Surgeon General declared an epidemic of loneliness in America in 2023 after participating in a "listening tour" across the country. In his subsequent Advisory, he shared the daunting research that subjective social disconnection is not only harmful to our mental health but significantly increases the risk of heart disease, stroke, dementia, and premature death. (U.S. HHS, 2023). In fact, perceived loneliness is comparable to smoking 15 cigarettes per day when it comes to all-cause mortality. (Murthy, 2023) If the average American suffers from loneliness, then the risk for those experiencing environmental sensitivities is exponentially greater. Why? For starters, many are isolated in a very literal sense due to the nature of their health condition. Successful health outcomes often necessitate that they avoid exposure to buildings of unknown air quality. This means that restaurants, churches, grocery stores, shopping malls, friends' homes, office buildings, hotels, and public transportation may be unavailable to them—limiting access to natural avenues of social gatherings and community support. In addition, many people with environmental illnesses have symptoms and disabilities that are not visible or easily identified on standard laboratory testing. This leaves them feeling misunderstood, invalidated, poorly supported, or even gaslighted by their friends, family members, colleagues, and under-trained medical professionals. Public awareness and compassion about environmental sensitivities are still lacking, leading to additional suffering and isolation for those experiencing them.

Knowing that loneliness and disconnection can perpetuate chronic illness and serve as an obstacle to recovery, it is valuable for individuals suffering from environmental illness to assess their own experiences and potential risks. While not everyone will need support outside of their existing community, many find very meaningful connections and healing within "external" support networks.

Health support networks can offer a range of benefits for individuals dealing with health issues, particularly those related to environmental sensitivities. One of the key advantages is the emotional support and understanding that comes from interacting with peers facing similar challenges. This sense of community can significantly reduce feelings of isolation. Additionally, these groups serve as platforms for sharing valuable information about treatments, coping strategies, and resources, which is especially helpful in navigating the complexities of environmental health issues. Being part of a support network can also motivate and empower individuals to actively manage their health, drawing inspiration from others' success stories and varied approaches to similar problems. Engaging in discussions about personal challenges and achievements within the group can provide emotional and mental health benefits, alleviating stress, anxiety, and depression often associated with chronic health issues.

However, there are risks associated with some health support networks, particularly those that are free and easily accessible on social media platforms. Such groups may be facilitated by volunteers who are not proficient in the content area or who don't have adequate time, energy, training, or personal well-being to effectively moderate the quality of the information and sensitive group dynamics. This can sometimes result in conflicts or a negative atmosphere, which can be counterproductive for individuals seeking safety and support.

The role of a qualified professional in leading a safe and effective support network is critical. A professional leader can provide necessary guidance, structure, and moderation, ensuring that the group's activities and discussions are constructive and aligned with health and safety principles. They can also ensure that the information shared is accurate and reliable, reducing the risk of misinformation. By tailoring discussions and activities to address the specific needs of group members, professionals can offer more personalized support. They are also better equipped to manage situations where members may experience severe emotional or physical distress, providing appropriate assistance or referrals. Moreover, a professional leader can help integrate the support network's activities with members' overall care plans, ensuring that the group's support complements professional medical advice.

The nature of **Health Support Networks** varies, providing something for everyone. Below are three types that are most common:

- **Group Therapy**: Individuals experiencing clinical depression, anxiety, panic, trauma, PTSD, or grief may be best served by licensed counselors or therapists who are highly skilled in group therapy facilitation. Sometimes, these mental health conditions were present before the individual became chronically ill and have been exacerbated or triggered by aspects of their medical condition. In other cases, they were brought on by the illness itself and/or surrounding stressors. An illness-based group therapy program can be incredibly validating and healing, as members are provided a safe space to share experiences and explore evidence-based healing modalities with a professional guide who can collaborate with other members of their care team as needed.

- **Educational Communities:** Many people have a strong desire to better understand their chronic illness to improve their personal agency and confidence with their treatment. While they may experience stress, overwhelm, and other challenging emotions, they do not necessarily need to be under the care of a mental health specialist. These individuals may be best served by a support group that is intentionally oriented around their specific illness and professionally facilitated by an expert in the field who is also skilled in group coaching. This way, the educational content and dialogue can be carefully curated and monitored to prevent misinformation, and favorable group dynamics can be ensured. Members "speak the same language," share evidence-based tips and resources, celebrate one another's successes, and encourage each other when the road gets particularly tough. Mutual support, from a place of shared experience and common humanity, can greatly enhance the sense of being seen and known and of having purpose and meaning—antidotes to loneliness.

- The **CIRS Healing Collective** is one example of an illness-based, professionally-facilitated, educational support network. It was created in 2019 by Jenny Johnson, Shoemaker Proficiency Partner and Certified Health Coach of Simplified Wellness Designs, who continues to curate the content and group dynamics. This virtual community is maintained on a private platform with a user-friendly phone app; members can participate from any country and from the safety and convenience of their own home (or tent!). There is a monitored "activity feed" where members ask questions and share experiences and helpful resources. A professional facilitator provides protocol updates, wellness tips, member polls, recipes, live group coaching sessions, live group discussions with expert guests, and patient-oriented educational programs (**Equipped to Overcome CIRS** and **Salugenex™ for CIRS**).

- **Support Groups**: Some individuals don't have serious mental health concerns and are not looking for information but are simply seeking meaningful connections with others who have similar experiences and may benefit from a support group. Support groups can vary quite a bit in nature and quality. Some are professionally facilitated, and others are peer-led. They may or may not be in-person, faith-based, or illness-based. Successful support groups typically offer group members a safe space to share experiences and mutual encouragement, which can greatly reduce perceived loneliness and social disconnection.

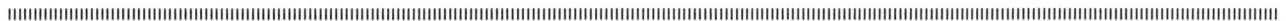

HEALTH SUPPORT GROUPS

Health support groups can offer a range of benefits for individuals dealing with health issues, particularly those related to environmental sensitivities. One of the key advantages is the emotional support and understanding that comes from interacting with peers facing similar challenges. This sense of community can significantly reduce feelings of isolation. Additionally, these groups serve as platforms for sharing valuable information about treatments, coping strategies, and resources, which is especially helpful in navigating the complexities of environmental health issues. Being part of a support group can also motivate and empower individuals to actively manage their health, drawing inspiration from others' success stories and varied approaches to similar problems. Engaging in discussions about personal challenges and achievements within the group can provide emotional and mental health benefits, alleviating stress, anxiety, and depression often associated with chronic health issues.

|||||||||||||||||||||||||||||||||||||||||||||||||||||||||||||||||||||||||||||||||||||||||||||||||||||||||||||||||||||||||||||||||||

Essay: The Use of Limbic System Retraining and Vagal Tonification: Moving the Needle Towards Health in Complex, Chronic Illness Patients

by Scott Forsgren, FDN-P, HHP

The role of **limbic system retraining** and **vagus nerve tonification** in optimizing health, including for those dealing with mold and biotoxin-associated illnesses, cannot be overstated. Together, they offer a powerful approach to support recovery from complex, chronic illness.

The **limbic system**, which includes the hypothalamus, hippocampus, amygdala, and cingulate cortex, is often called the "feeling and reacting brain." This system processes sensory information, such as touch, light, sound, smell, and taste, to assess safety. When impaired, the limbic system can become like an overly sensitive alarm system, overreacting to minor stimuli.

The limbic system impacts the functioning of the immune system, endocrine system, and autonomic nervous system (ANS); the ANS, in turn, controls blood pressure, heart rate, breathing, digestion, and more.

Limbic system impairment can result from various triggers, including mold or biotoxin exposure in water-damaged buildings, chemical or pesticide exposures, microbial overgrowths, and trauma, whether physical, mental, or emotional. This ongoing, inappropriate response can lead to a cascade of symptoms as the body continually overreacts to perceived threats.

When a serious threat, like significant mold exposure or Lyme disease, is reduced from a roaring tiger to a gentle kitten purring outside the window, the limbic system needs to recognize this change and not continue to react as though the tiger is still prowling nearby.

There is almost certainly a limbic component at play for individuals with multiple sensitivities, such as light, sound, food, fragrances, and even supplements. You might recognize this by avoiding places like the detergent aisle at the store or may react to someone wearing perfume or may be tolerating only five foods.

Limbic system retraining can help to "recalibrate" or "reboot" the system, adjusting the perceived threat level to be more aligned with the actual threat level.

Even if the tiger is still present, limbic system retraining often increases tolerance to supplements, medications, foods, and even some environments that a sensitive patient may otherwise react to. Thus, limbic system retraining is a foundational component of the healing process and would ideally be implemented as early as possible.

Limbic system retraining approaches may be categorized as either **"driver's seat" tools**, which are more active retraining programs, or **"passenger seat" tools**, which are more passive and may serve as beneficial adjunct therapies. Generally, "driver's seat" methods provide the primary foundation for limbic system retraining, while "passenger seat" therapies offer additional support. These tools collectively aid in recalibrating the limbic system's perception of threat and enabling greater resilience to numerous triggers. Additionally, while tools like yoga and meditation may have many benefits, they are not directly aimed at supporting the limbic system and thus do not replace a focus in this realm.

Neil Nathan, MD, emphasizes the importance of creating a sense of "safer" in both the mind and body to achieve effective healing. This approach often includes addressing emotional traumas and other personal triggers that may contribute to a heightened sense of threat.

Working in this realm does not mean your condition is all "in your head." The limbic system is part of the "brain," and so technically, the problem can be in the "head," but that does not mean it is in the "mind." As Dr. Nathan says, "It's not psychological; it's neurological." (Nathan, 2024)

Driver's Seat Limbic System Tools Resources:

- **DNRS (Dynamic Neural Retraining System™)** by Annie Hopper; RetrainingTheBrain.com

- **Gupta Program** by Ashok Gupta, MA (Cantab), MSc; GuptaProgram.com

- **Primal Trust™** by Cathleen King, DPT; PrimalTrust.org

- **Passenger Seat Limbic System Tools Resources**:

- **Frequency Specific Microcurrent** by Carolyn McMakin, MA, DC; FrequencySpecific.com

- Some herbs, homeopathics, essential oils, thiamine, as well as mast cell stabilizers and antihistamines

The vagus nerve acts as a two-way communication channel between the brain and gut, regulating essential functions like digestion, heart rate, and respiration. Techniques for **vagus nerve tonification**, which help to calm the nervous system, may include humming, gargling, and vagal exercises detailed in Stanley Rosenberg's *Accessing the Healing Power of the Vagus Nerve*. Stephen Porges, PhD's "Safe and Sound Protocol" is often beneficial for adults and children alike. Other supportive modalities may include cranial osteopathy, EFT (Emotional Freedom Technique), and vagus nerve stimulators such as gammaCore and others, as well as devices such as the Apollo Neuro and the NIKKI, which may help promote a shift from a sympathetic-dominant (fight or flight) state to a more parasympathetic (calm and relaxed) state supportive of healing.

Vagus Nerve Tonification Resources:

- **Stanley Rosenberg's Book**: *Accessing the Healing Power of the Vagus Nerve*; Amazon.com

- **Safe and Sound Protocol** by Stephen Porges, PhD; IntegratedListening.com

- **Apollo Neuro**: wearable device supporting the vagus nerve and parasympathetic nervous system; ApolloNeuro.com

- **NIKKI**: wearable device supporting the parasympathetic nervous system; WeAreNIKKI.com

- **gammaCore**: vagus nerve stimulator; gammaCore.com

Robert Naviaux, MD, has coined the term **"Cell Danger Response"** to describe a cellular protective response or survival response that occurs when the body is under threat. Limbic system retraining and vagus nerve tonification may promote a shift from a survival mode to a healing state, essential for the body to "rest, digest, detoxify, and repair" effectively.

The combination of limbic system retraining and vagus nerve tonification is powerful—it's not simply 1+1=2, but the benefits are often exponentially greater. Neil Nathan, MD, underscores the importance of working on both the limbic system and vagus nerve simultaneously to optimize outcomes.

While limbic system retraining and vagal tonification tools are foundational, it's crucial to note that they do not replace environmental mitigation. If someone is significantly mold-exposed, implementing these tools does not mean the external environment can be ignored. Eliminating significant mold growth is essential, but if one reacts to small amounts of mold in their environment, recalibrating the perceived threat level with the actual threat level may help to reduce hypersensitivity to minor exposures.

As Sandeep Gupta, MD, explains, "The limbic brain and nervous system have a certain type of intelligence. Their role is to protect us from what these brain areas perceive as dangerous experiences, including severe environmental exposures, such as mold, chemicals, or tick bites. Our job is to bring a level of subtlety and discernment into this response so as not to continue to be caught in the limbic loop of stress, anxiety, and inflammation".

In the context of complex and chronic illnesses such as Chronic Inflammatory Response Syndrome (CIRS), Lyme disease, Chronic Fatigue Syndrome/Myalgic Encephalomyelitis (CFS/ME), Fibromyalgia, Long COVID, Small Intestinal Bacterial Overgrowth (SIBO), Postural Orthostatic Tachycardia Syndrome (POTS), Mast Cell Activation Syndrome (MCAS), Multiple Chemical Sensitivity (MCS), Electromagnetic Hypersensitivity Syndrome (EHS), and others, limbic system retraining and vagus nerve tonification hold great promise for improving quality of life and fostering healing.

Explore Scott's Resources:

- Interview: Neil Nathan, MD, on *The Sensitive Patient's Healing Guide*; BetterHealthGuy.com/episode200

- Book: *The Sensitive Patient's Healing Guide: Top Experts Offer New Insights and Treatments for Environmental Toxins, Lyme Disease, and EMFs* by Neil Nathan, MD

- Interview: IEP Radio Episode #34: Chronic Illness, Environmental Exposures, and the Limbic System; Interview with Scott Forsgren, FDN-P; IEPRadio.com

- Interview: Annie Hopper, creator of DNRS; BetterHealthGuy.com/episode42

- Interview: Ashok Gupta, MA, (Cantab), MSc, creator of Gupta Program; BetterHealthGuy.com/episode133

- Interview: Cathleen King, DPT, creator of Primal Trust™; BetterHealthGuy.com/episode201

- Interview: Carolyn McMakin, MA, DC, creator of Frequency Specific Microcurrent; BetterHealthGuy.com/episode102

- Interview: Eva Detko, PhD on the Vagus Nerve; BetterHealthGuy.com/episode135

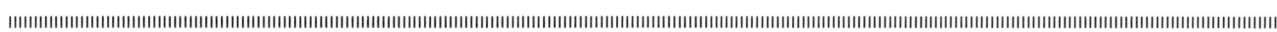

LIMBIC SYSTEM INVOLVEMENT

The limbic system, a complex network of brain structures, plays a decisive role in our emotional and physical responses, especially concerning environmental factors like mold and water damage. This system integrates emotions, behavior, motivation, long-term memory, and olfaction, acting as an emotional nervous system trigger. A key part of this system, the amygdala, prepares the body for fight-or-flight reactions in emotional situations, impacting both heart and breathing rates and influencing the consolidation of emotionally charged memories. The limbic system also affects physiological aspects like blood pressure and heart rate through hormonal responses, with chronic stress leading to long-term health issues. Individual differences in limbic system reactivity contribute to sensitivities to environmental stimuli, as seen in conditions like multiple chemical sensitivity (MCS), linking limbic function with environmental sensitivity. The dynamic nature of the limbic system, changing with environmental input, shows that psychological and physiological experiences can be modified, offering potential pathways for improving indoor environmental health. (Bell IR H. E., 1995)

||||||||||||||||||||||||||||||||||||||||||||||||||||||||||||||||||||||||||||||||||||||||||||||||||||

Essentials: Mold, Water Damage and Health

- Genetic factors often reveal individual sensitivities to mold and water damage only after a sensitizing event has occurred.

- Rapid, heightened standard of care is essential for water-damaged homes, especially for those already sensitized to mold.

- Effective remediation requires a multi-disciplinary approach involving healthcare providers, environmental consultants, and remediators.

- Ignoring early signs like musty smells can worsen problems and increase costs. Masking odors is counterproductive.

- Outdoor mold is generally less concerning than spores from man-made sources, particularly for those with heightened sensitivities.

- Even if mold growth from water damage has been addressed by remediation, regular, effective cleaning is essential for managing mold risks and preventing the migration of accumulations of settled spores due to building memory. Building memory is caused by mold spores, fragments, and particles that migrate from inaccessible nooks and crannies into the living space. Examples of hidden areas inaccessible for routine cleaning include electrical outlets, areas under baseboards, sill plates, and carpets.

- Mold exposure can occur through inhalation, direct skin contact, and occasionally ingestion, making it particularly risky for hypersensitive individuals.

- Sensitivities can also stem from other allergens like pet dander and pollen.

- Remediation aims for overall health, not just mold elimination. Substitution of one problem for another is not acceptable. Chemical agents used to kill, even if natural, such as essential oils, are not recommended.

- Physical removal and effective cleaning are the best methods for mold remediation.

- Multiple Chemical Sensitivities (MCS) are complex and linked to genetic and environmental factors, including mold exposure.

- Mold's role in MCS is dual: it acts as both a trigger and a sensitizer, emphasizing the need for effective indoor air quality management.

- HLA genotypes may indicate genetic predispositions for sensitivities to mold, chemicals, and other stressors.

- The goal is to create safe homes that actively contribute to occupants' health.

- Remediation effectiveness varies; not all homes can be healthy for everyone.

||||||||||||||||||||||||||||||||||||||||||||||||||||||||||||||||||||||||||||||||||||||||||||||||||||

Essay: The Learning Process and Key Psychological Takeaways
by Ryan Holsapple, PhD

Introduction: A Psychologist's Journey with CIRS

As a psychologist, this journey has led me to a unique understanding of individuals with chronic illnesses and the intense issues they face. It inspired me to specialize in working with individuals, caregivers, and families facing illness. My wife, Victoria, faced a profound journey of illness and recovery, standing as a testament to what it means to confront CIRS with strength and purpose. Her experience of being bedbound and then gradually regaining her health was driven not only by medical treatment but also by her removal from exposure and the remediation of her environment. She also focused on understanding how her psychological healing could support her physical healing.

Now, with my own recent CIRS diagnosis and beginning treatment, though my condition is less severe than Victoria's, has offered me insights into the resilience required to heal. As I embark on my own recovery, I hope to share practical psychological tools that, while not a replacement for addressing environmental issues related to water damage

or medical intervention, can provide real support for anyone affected by this illness.

Understanding the Barriers

As I can attest, properly dealing with mold and biotoxin illness can be downright challenging and stressful. Many committed to their home's cleanliness and healthfulness are also undergoing complex multi-step medical treatment. Despite overwhelming challenges, the fortunate fact is that while we cannot change our genetic susceptibility for CIRS, we can adjust our lifestyles and environments to increase our prosperity and health. Victoria and I have found the rewards of this process outweigh the challenges. Still, there is often much that is out of our control, and this makes the process more challenging and potentially stressful.

Challenges in creating a CIRS-friendly home range from financial constraints and chronic disability to caregiving responsibilities and limited resources. Putting all these issues aside and assuming someone has all the resources they need, properly addressing environmental issues for people with CIRS is still a demanding process. Covering a spectrum from those with ample resources to those with few, my intention is to empower readers to do what they can with what they have.

Tapping into tools for our inner resiliency allows us to address issues and heal more effectively. It also puts us in a more functional and relaxed psychological state. Our psychology and our bodies are inextricably connected; in fact, they are not separate realities. Environmental adjustments alone remain demanding, even for those who can afford complete remediation. Yet, regardless of individual circumstances, improvements can be made that empower our physical and psychological well-being. The most important guiding principle is to focus on where we have the power to act and letting go of what we cannot control. People like John—the author of this book—are expert at showing individuals what can be done to improve environmental circumstances, providing them with a more measurable manner to assess for themselves what can or cannot be controlled.

The Mind-Body Connection

CIRS affects more than the body; it deeply impacts the mind. The symptoms and stresses of CIRS can affect our emotions, thinking, and outlook. This is true with any illness; stress and negative emotions simply aggravate the body more. Victoria and I found that managing our psychological states positively impacted our physical responses. The illness still demands treatment, and yet we work within those boundaries to do everything we can to feel better. Our perceptions, emotions, and attitudes are the lens through which we experience symptoms, setbacks, and progress.

Each individual's personality affects how they experience and respond to CIRS. People are born with specific personality traits, which, combined with other complex developmental factors and prior life experiences, lead to how they interpret the illness. This is why no two people handle CIRS the same way—one person may feel optimistic, while another may struggle with ongoing fear or worry. Recognizing this diversity without judgment helps create space for self-compassion, allowing each person to honor their own journey.

The placebo effect powerfully illustrates this connection, where beliefs and expectations can condition our body's responses. Many studies show that belief alone can impact different levels of our physiology. Expecting improvements can trigger the brain and body to produce real, positive responses. The placebo effect reveals how interconnected our minds and bodies are; it shows how we think and what we expect, changes our experience of symptoms, and empowers our body's healing potential. For someone with CIRS, managing beliefs and outlook can help alleviate stress and boost resilience. Yet, studies also confirm that the placebo response is not an unlimited cure for disease. The ability for us to change our own bodily response depends on the context and the level of the body's complexity and ailments. While improving beliefs, attitudes, and expectations undoubtedly helps the process of CIRS treatment—as it would with many diseases—it is crucial

that physical sources of mold and other biotoxins are removed to create a truly healthful environment for recovery.

The human brain is among the most complex entities in the known universe. Perhaps even more incredible is the fact that we can proactively direct the process of its change. Neuroplasticity is the brain's ability to reshape by forming and strengthening new connections, as well as pruning old connections. Our brains contain billions of neurons that link up through trillions of pathways. When we repeatedly use specific thoughts, emotions, or behaviors, these pathways become stronger, much like how a trail becomes clearer the more we walk on it. This ability allows us to change our perceptions, attitudes, behaviors, skills, and even emotional responses over time. However, it doesn't mean we can change everything in our brain—or that we'd want to. For example, essential functions like breathing or heartbeat are managed by self-regulating parts of the brain, which we wouldn't want to rewire, as they are deeply ingrained features that keep us alive without needing our constant attention. While these ancient parts of the brain function autonomously for survival, some of the more emotional and cognitive layers of our brain function can be proactively altered through neuroplasticity.

Neuroplasticity gives us the power to actively shape our experiences by choosing the thoughts, emotions, and behaviors we want to reinforce. There are three essential components to rewiring the brain for more psychological benefit. Those are: 1) stop mechanisms, 2) redirecting attention, and 3) proactively rewiring. Stop mechanisms are often not taught, and research shows they are a crucial part of the equation of change. They simply include finding ways to stop when going down an undesirable path of thought, emotion, or behavior. Through stop-mechanisms, long-term disuse of certain pathways can eventually lead to neural pruning, which allows it to become increasingly easier to disengage undesired pathways as they slowly weaken. Consider how we naturally stop ourselves all the time, whether it's pausing before saying something hurtful or stopping ourselves from overindulging at the dinner table—examples are countless. When we interrupt ourselves and stop a behavior, emotion, or thought that is not serving us, we are stopping those brain pathways from firing in full force. Stopping without redirecting simply leaves a vacuum that is often filled with more negative experiences. After stopping, it is equally important to immediately redirect our focus to what we want and then repeatedly use that focus to rewire. I provide some functional tools for redirecting and rewiring below.

The important issue is that if we do not find a way to stop and then use our full focus to redirect and rewire, the notion of using neuroplasticity for our benefit becomes much less functional. There is no room for bringing in the new state of being we want if we are still preoccupied with the old one. *"Stop, Redirect, and Rewire"* is a process that truly works. If any one component is missing, it will not be as effective; the brain will be working against itself. With my clients, I often say,

"It takes what it takes," meaning change often requires hard work consistently repeated over time.

Finally, rewiring does not have to be followed by stopping an unwanted experience. I encourage taking advantage of rewiring to enhance our positive experiences and enjoy life more at any time we choose. The process of rewiring the brain can take consistent and highly focused efforts over many months, and the results we can get over time are well worth the effort. Neuroplasticity is one of our greatest allies on the path to psychological wellness and physical healing when dealing with CIRS.

What We Do for Love

Sometimes, life presents difficult choices where protecting others or achieving a larger goal may come at our own expense. Imagine holding a pot of boiling water that begins to slip. For most, the reflex is to drop it to avoid getting burned. But if a baby is nearby, that reflex to drop the pot must be suppressed to prevent harm to the child. This is an extreme example, but it illustrates the loving sacrifices we sometimes make at our own expense. When it comes to Victoria and myself, I often handle issues with biotoxins that I wouldn't want her to go near. Even though I have CIRS, I understand that her sensitivity is much more extreme. I delegate handling biotoxins wherever I can, and yet, at the end of the day, I make sure she is not exposed, even if that means I have to risk exposure.

For those with CIRS, decisions like these come with an additional price because exposure to triggers can be extremely harmful. To the extent possible, it's helpful to structure one's life to minimize the need for these kinds of choices. By anticipating situations where exposure or stress might arise, one can make plans or modifications to avoid them. Building a support system, arranging for environmental safety, and adopting strong boundaries can empower us to avoid difficult self-harming decisions without also putting our loved ones at risk whenever possible.

The Importance of Reducing Stress

Reducing stress is one of the most powerful ways to support healing in CIRS, as stress can worsen inflammation, which is already a core issue in this illness. For CIRS patients, stress is not just an emotional experience; it can also intensify physical symptoms. Research shows that stress heightens the body's release of inflammatory compounds, such as cytokines, which can upregulate genetic expression, aggravate CIRS symptoms, and prolong recovery.

CIRS affects the limbic system, amplifying stress and negative emotions. Many CIRS patients have encountered cycles of depression and heightened anxiety, which reinforces stress and inflammation. It's not uncommon for individuals with CIRS to find themselves stuck in a feedback loop, where the illness drives negative emotions, which in turn exacerbate physical symptoms. Breaking this cycle isn't easy, but the effort to reduce stress pays off by allowing the body to focus on healing.

While stress most certainly does not explicitly cause CIRS, it can reinforce inflammatory issues, arguably making healing harder than it otherwise would be. I am outlining this to solidify the importance of finding ways to practice psychological self-regulation while also treating the physical disease. Those with personality tendencies toward stress will benefit significantly from incorporating stress-reducing practices, which can ease the body's inflammatory responses and contribute to improved outcomes. This knowledge that individuals can become major sources of inflammation may empower those of us dealing with CIRS to practice tools and techniques for stress regulation and relaxation.

Tools and Techniques for Recovery

Various practices can support the mind-body connection and improve resilience in the face of CIRS. Keeping in mind what I shared earlier about "Stop, Redirect, Rewire," these tools can be very effective for redirecting and rewiring portions of that process. While none of these tools replace proper medical treatment, they offer support for reducing stress and enhancing psychological strength.

- **Mindfulness and Meditation**: These practices foster a focused awareness of the present moment, free from judgment. For individuals with CIRS, this can provide a sense of calm amid uncertainty. Over time, mindfulness and meditation can reduce stress and even retrain the brain to respond differently to triggering situations, reducing inflammation and promoting relaxation.

- **Somatic Practices**: Gentle movements, such as yoga, tai chi, or walking meditation, help calm the mind and regulate the body. Physical movement can be particularly grounding and beneficial for CIRS patients, especially when undertaken at a comfortable pace and with approval from a healthcare provider.

- **Visualization and Affirmation**: Visualization exercises involve creating peaceful or uplifting images in the mind, which can help the brain develop positive connections and promote healing. Affirmations, meanwhile, use repeated positive statements to reinforce self-worth and well-being, allowing individuals to retrain their mental responses over time.

- **Therapy**: Working with a therapist who understands chronic illness can be invaluable. Therapy allows people to explore and work through their journey's psychological and emotional aspects. Additionally, a skilled therapist can support patients in building resilience, validating their experience, and uncovering strengths.

Ultimately, these tools can be powerful allies in recovery, but they can reach their full potential only in a healthful environment free of CIRS triggers.

Concluding Remarks

Going through this long journey of recovery with Victoria has enabled me to reflect on what helped us through the process and allowed us to find success. It has also given me much to reflect on as a psychologist. In considering the process, the general themes I hoped to portray here are that CIRS is a serious condition that needs medical treatment, that there is a vital connection between our psyche and our bodily processes, and that restoring our water-damaged indoor environments is a primary requirement for our path to healing. We can empower ourselves to heal and maximally enjoy life, given the fact that our consciousness affects our bodily states in important ways. While the CIRS disease process and its genetic components are complex, our understanding and available treatments continue to advance, opening up empowering steps we can take to support our physical and psychological well-being. (Kaptchuk, 2010)

References

Kurup, V. P., Shen, H. D., & Banerjee, B. (2000). Respiratory fungal allergy. *Microbes and Infection, 2,* 1101–1110.

Tischler, B. Y., & Hohl, T. M. (2019). Menacing mold: Recent advances in *Aspergillus* pathogenesis and host defense. *Journal of Molecular Biology, 431*(21), 4229–4246. https://doi.org/10.1016/j.jmb.2019.03.027

Dales, R. E., Cakmak, S., Burnett, R. T., Judek, S., Coates, F., & Brook, J. R. (2000). Influence of ambient fungal spores on emergency visits for asthma to a regional children's hospital. *American Journal of Respiratory and Critical Care Medicine, 162*(6). https://doi.org/10.1164/ajrccm.162.6.2001020

Shoemaker, R., Johnson, K., Jim, L., Berry, Y., Dooley, M., Ryan, J., & McMahon, S. (2018). Diagnostic process for chronic inflammatory response syndrome (CIRS): A consensus statement. *Internal Medicine Review, 4*(5), 1–47.

Gomes, M. L., Morais, A., & Cavaleiro Rufo, J. (2021). The association between fungi exposure and hypersensitivity pneumonitis: A systematic review. *Porto Biomedical Journal, 6*(1), e117. https://doi.org/10.1097/j.pbj.0000000000000117

Shoemaker, R. (2010). *Surviving mold: Life in the era of dangerous buildings.* Otter Bay Books. Retrieved from https://www.survivingmold.com

Shoemaker, R., & House, D. (2005). A time-series of sick building syndrome; chronic, biotoxin-associated illness from exposure to water-damaged buildings. *Neurotoxicology and Teratology, 27*(1), 29–46.

Waxenbaum, J. A., Reddy, V., & Varacallo, M. (2023, July 24). Anatomy, autonomic nervous system. In *StatPearls* [Internet]. Treasure Island, FL: StatPearls Publishing. Retrieved from https://www.ncbi.nlm.nih.gov/books/NBK539845/

Shoemaker, R., & Vukelic, A. (2023, February 28). The evolution of chronic inflammatory response syndrome and the biotoxin pathway. In *Nutrition and integrative medicine for clinicians.* CRC Press.

Shoemaker, R., McMahon, S., Heyman, A., Lark, D., van der Westhuizen, M., & Ryan, J. (2021). Treatable metabolic and inflammatory abnormalities in post-COVID syndrome (PCS) define the transcriptomic basis for persistent symptoms: Lessons from CIRS. *Medical Research Archives, 9*(7), 1–18.

McMahon, S. W. (2017, March). An evaluation of alternate means to diagnose chronic inflammatory response syndrome and determine prevalence. *Medical Research Archives, 5*(3). Available at https://esmed.org/MRA/mra/article/view/1125

Shoemaker, R., Neil, V., Heyman, A., van der Westhuizen, M., McMahon, S., & Lark, D. (2021). Newer molecular methods bring new insights into human- and building-health risk assessments from water-damaged buildings: Defining exposure and reactivity, the two sides of causation of CIRS-WDB illness. *Medical Research Archives, 9*(3), 1–36.

Lateef, T. M., Menkanagas, K. R., He, J., Kalaydjian, A., Khoromi, S., Knight, E., & Nelson, K. B. (2009). Headache in a national sample of American children: Prevalence and comorbidity. *Journal of Child Neurology, 24*(5), 536–543. https://doi.org/10.1177/0883073808327831

Knutsen, A. P., Vijay, H. M., Kumar, V., et al. (2010). Mold sensitivity in children with moderate-severe asthma is associated with HLA-DR and HLA-DQ. *Allergy, 65*(11), 1367–1375.

The CIRS Academy. (2021). Surviving mold indoor environmental professional panel consensus for microbial remediation 2020. *Medical Research Archives, 9*(1), 1–25. KEI Journals. Retrieved from https://www.survivingmold.com

McMahon, S. W. (2023, February 28). Pediatric chronic inflammatory response syndrome. In *Nutrition and integrative medicine for clinicians.* CRC Press.

Levetin, E., Pityn, P. J., Ramon, G. D., Pityn, E., Anderson, J., Bielory, L., Dalan, D., Codina, R., Rivera-Mariani, F. E., & Bolanos, B. (2023). Aeroallergen monitoring by the National Allergy Bureau: A review of the past and a look into the future. *The Journal of Allergy and Clinical Immunology: In Practice, 11*(5), 1394–1400. https://doi.org/10.1016/j.jaip.2022.11.026

Institute of Inspection, Cleaning and Restoration Certification. (2021). *ANSI/IICRC S500 standard for professional water damage restoration* (5th ed.). IICRC.

Shoemaker, R., et al. (2021). Exposure to *Actinobacteria* resident in water-damaged buildings and resultant immune injury in chronic inflammatory response syndrome. *Medical Research Archives, 9*(10). https://doi.org/10.18103/mra.v9i10.2585

Dorninger, E. (2022, October). *Actinomycetes: The problem is YOU. I Dream of GENIE—Volume 5 Webinar,* CIRSx.com, Salisbury, MD, United States.

Molot, J., Sears, M., & Anisman, H. (2023). Multiple chemical sensitivity: It's time to catch up to the science. *Neuroscience & Biobehavioral Reviews, 151,* 105227. https://doi.org/10.1016/j.neubiorev.2023.105227

Bell, I. R., Hardin, E. E., Baldwin, C. M., & Schwartz, G. E. (1995). Increased limbic system symptomatology and sensitizability of young adults with chemical and noise sensitivities. *Environmental Research, 70*(2), 84–97. https://doi.org/10.1006/enrs.1995.1052

Baker-Laporte, P., & Banta, J. (2022). *Prescriptions for a healthy house: A practical guide for architects, builders, and homeowners* (4th ed.).

CIRSx. (2024). *Medically important remediation general course MIR100, and medically important remediation professional course MIR101* [Online course]. CIRSx Institute.

Shoemaker, R. C. (2011). *Biotoxin pathway chart.* Surviving Mold. Retrieved from https://www.survivingmold.com

Kaptchuk, T. J., Friedlander, E., Kelley, J. M., Sanchez, M. N., Kokkotou, E., Singer, J. P., … & Lembo, A. J. (2010). Placebos without deception: A randomized controlled trial in irritable bowel syndrome. *PLOS ONE, 5*(12), e15591. https://doi.org/10.1371/journal.pone.0015591

Nathan, N. (2024). *The sensitive patient's healing guide: Top experts offer new insights and treatments for environmental toxins, Lyme disease, and EMFs.* [Self-published].

Reust, C. E., & Williams, A. (2018). Recurrent abdominal pain in children. *American Family Physician, 97*(12), 785–793.

Wessely, S., Nimnuan, C., & Sharpe, M. (1999). Functional somatic syndromes: One or many? *The Lancet, 354*(9182), 936–939.

U.S. Department of Health and Human Services. (2023, May). New Surgeon General advisory raises alarm about the devastating impact of the epidemic of loneliness and isolation in the United States. Retrieved from https://www.hhs.gov/about/news/2023/05/03/new-surgeon-general-advisory-raises-alarm-about-devastating-impact-epidemic-loneliness-isolation-united-states.html

Murthy, V. H. (2023). *Our epidemic of loneliness and isolation: The U.S. Surgeon General's advisory on the health effects of social connection and community.* U.S. Department of Health and Human Services. Retrieved from https://www.hhs.gov/sites/default/files/surgeon-general-social-connection-advisory.pdf

Chapter Three: Physiology, Particle Behavior, and Natural Ecology of Water-Damage Organisms

When we discuss mold, it's easy to lump it into a singular category, overlooking its vast diversity. Molds are microscopic fungi. The fungal kingdom is not limited to molds; it includes many visible organisms such as mushrooms, bracts, and puffballs. Unlike these larger fungi, molds distinguish themselves by their microscopic size.

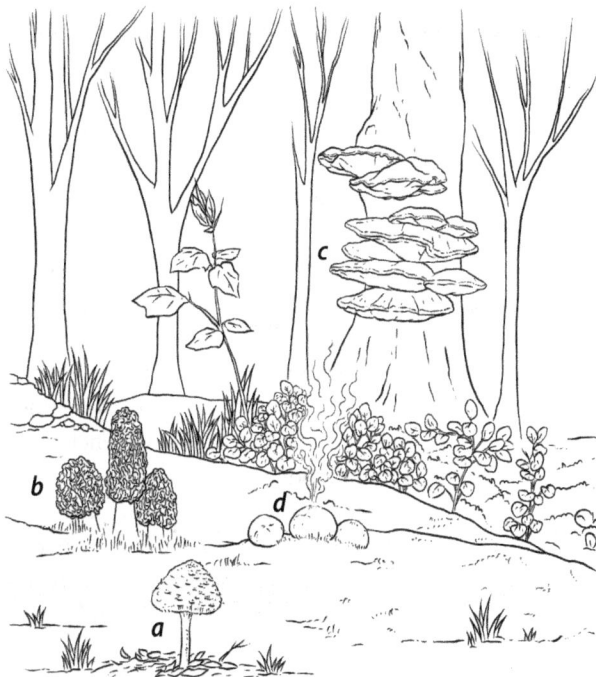

*Figure 1-9: Mushrooms (**a**), morels (**b**), bracts (**c**), and puffballs (**d**) are the fruiting bodies (spore-producing structures) of various types of macrofungi visible to the naked eye in nature. However, the spores they release are microscopic and typically reported as basidiospores on mold reports. Basidiospores are also produced by both dry rot and wet rot fungi, though they cannot be further identified by type under a microscope.*

As climate change impacts our world, shifts in microflora are expected. Harvard Medical School's Center for Health and the Global Environment reports that elevated CO_2 levels could stimulate faster growth and increase spore production in certain fungi. More research is needed, but climate change will likely continue to influence fungal ecology. (Epstein, 2005)

THE DIVERSE, ECOLOGICAL, AND BENEFICIAL ROLES OF MOLDS

Molds and yeasts distinguish themselves from other fungi as they are too small to see without a microscope. Each type of mold has its niche in nature, where it competes for survival, with estimates of the number of mold species existing in the hundreds of thousands, far surpassing the number of plant and animal species. New types of molds are continuously discovered and exhibit diverse relationships with their environments; some molds are parasitic, scavenging, and living on a host, while others are symbiotic, with one organism's survival dependent on another. Many molds are saprophytic, playing a crucial role in breaking down organic matter and recycling nutrients essential for maintaining soil health and ecosystem balance. However, the same organic materials that mold breaks down in nature are often used in constructing our homes, meaning that these beneficial organisms can turn our homes into self-composting structures simply by adding water. While molds are frequently perceived as agents of decay, they are indispensable in food preservation and pharmaceuticals. Molds and other fungi have been used for centuries in practices like fermentation, traditional medicine, and even art, underscoring their significance beyond health concerns. If it were not for mold, our planet would be thick with organic debris and waste. Antibiotics would not have been discovered to fight bacterial infections. Foods such as bread and beer would be flat. Many varieties of wine and cheese would be lost. *Aspergillus niger* is instrumental in the production of citric acid, a common food preservative.

Pharmaceuticals Based on Mold

Molds have found their way into our lives in other beneficial ways. There are different toxins produced by various types of molds that may, in the proper dose, be medicinal. In 1928, Alexander Fleming discovered penicillin, the world's first true antibiotic, when he observed something unexpected during his research. He noticed that a petri dish, accidentally contaminated with *Penicillium notatum* mold (now classified as *Penicillium chrysogenum*), had a clear area around it with no bacterial growth. This suggested that the mold produced a substance toxic to bacteria but harmless to humans at these effective levels. Fleming deduced that the mold was naturally defending its territory by releasing this antibacterial compound. This observation ultimately led to the development of penicillin, a revolutionary antibiotic that has since saved countless lives by effectively treating bacterial infections with high toxicity to bacteria but low toxicity to people. (Gaynes, 2017)

Various other medical treatments have their origins in the secondary metabolites produced by different molds. Indigenous cultures worldwide have been studied and contributed to the knowledge of many pharmaceuticals based on varieties of molds used for traditional treatments. Pharmaceutical firms have often begun their search for new drug formulations by looking at natural medicines produced by mold.

The LDL cholesterol-reducing statin drugs are another example of a pharmaceutical that was first naturally produced as a secondary metabolite of mold. The first statin discovered in the early 1970s was Mevastatin, which was produced by the mold *Penicillium citrinum*. The mold *Aspergillus terreus* is now being used commercially instead for making this widely used medicine. The cancer-fighting drug Paclitaxel™ has been manufactured using a strain of *Penicillium raistrickii*. *Aspergillus flavus* produces the potent carcinogen aflatoxin but can also produce an anticancer metabolite called solamargine. The anti-fungal treatment Griseofulvin is derived from the mold *Penicillium griseofulvum* but is currently being manufactured using a *Penicillium patulum* strain. *Penicillium stoloniferum* and *Stachybotrys subglutinans* have been used to produce immunosuppressants to help prevent the rejection of

transplanted organs. *Aspergillus sclerotiorin* has metabolites that are used to treat diabetes. (Frontiers Editorial, 2023)

Uses of Mold in Food Production

Often, molds are very specific about the nutrients required to grow. The mold *Botrytis cinerea* thrives on mature grapes. It is called the "Noble Rot" because it produces a fine, rich, sweet wine when made from grapes that are infected with this mold. To make this wine, the first part of the fermentation occurs by leaving the grapes in the field until they begin to ferment on the vine. When the juice is squeezed from the grapes, these molds transfer into the fermentation tank and continue the process. Alcohol is only one of the many compounds that are produced as mold grows. In the case of wine, beer, and other fermented beverages, molds can enhance the flavors and aroma of the grapes, grains, or other ingredients as they progress from a lush, fresh consumable into an intoxicating and delicious brew.

Penicillium nalgiovense is often used on the surface of salami to aid in the curing process. This mold helps to create a white coat on the surface of the salami, contributing to its flavor, texture, and safety by inhibiting the growth of undesirable microorganisms. *Penicillium camemberti* is another example of a mold used for food production; it's essential to produce soft, ripened cheeses like Camembert and Brie. However, it's crucial to differentiate between the beneficial role molds play in food production and the potential hazards they pose when inhaled. Occupations involving artisanal food production, for example, are at risk for conditions such as "Cheese Washers Lung" or "Sausage Workers Lung." These conditions are attributed to the inhalation of mold spores during the process of preparing the foods for market. While these molds are beneficial or essential when ingested in food, inhaling them can lead to a respiratory issue called hypersensitivity pneumonitis. Therefore, occupational safety measures, such as proper ventilation and protective gear, are imperative in these industries to mitigate the risk of mold-related health issues. (Juneja, 2018)

Physiology of Mold

Understanding how mold grows and spreads is essential before we can effectively tackle mold in our homes. The life cycle of a fungal organism, such as mold, typically involves several stages, including germination, growth, reproduction, and sporulation:

Spore Formation: Let's begin the life cycle with mature growth, releasing spores into the environment. These spores are tiny, lightweight structures easily dispersed by air, water, or other vectors. Spores serve as the

reproductive units of the fungus and can remain dormant until suitable conditions for growth are encountered.

Germination: The fungal spores germinate when favorable environmental conditions are met, such as adequate moisture and a suitable nutrient source. Germination involves spore swelling and developing into a germ tube structure.

Hyphal Growth: A network of thread-like structures called hyphae begins to grow from the germ tube. These hyphae extend and branch, forming a mycelium, which is the filament or rootlike body of the fungus. The mycelium consists of a vast network of hyphae that explore and colonize the substrate in search of nutrients.

Hyphal Structure and Formation: Fungal hyphae are composed of individual cells called hyphal cells. These cells are elongated and tubular, allowing for efficient nutrient uptake.

Absorption and Exploration of the Substrate: The formation of hyphal cells is a result of the fungal growth process. As the fungal spore germinates, it elongates to form a germ tube, which eventually develops into a mature hyphal cell. The elongation of the hyphal cell is a complex biochemical process involving the synthesis of cell wall components, including chitin. Fungal hyphae can branch and form a complex network called the mycelium. Branching occurs when new hyphal cells are generated at specific sites along the hyphae. These branches allow the fungus to explore a larger area and access more nutrients.

In addition to growth, fungal hyphae can differentiate into specialized structures for reproduction, such as sporangia or conidiophores. These structures produce spores that can be released to initiate new fungal colonies.

Nutrient Uptake: Fungi, including molds, employ a unique strategy known as extracellular digestion, which involves secreting enzymes outside their cells into the surrounding environment to decompose complex organic compounds into simpler forms. Unlike plants, molds cannot perform photosynthesis to produce their own food and instead rely on obtaining nutrients from their environment. The hyphae of these fungi secrete various enzymes, such as proteases, cellulases, and amylases, to break down complex substances like proteins, cellulose, and starch outside the fungal cells. The fungal cell wall, far from being a barrier, features channels and transport proteins that facilitate the movement of these nutrients. Once extracellular enzymes have broken down the organic matter, the resulting simpler molecules, such as amino acids and simple sugars, are absorbed by the hyphae through the cell walls and membranes, enabling the fungi to sustain and grow.

Metabolic Processes: Inside the fungal hyphal cell, these absorbed nutrients are subjected to various metabolic processes. For example, amino acids can be used for protein synthesis within the cell, providing the building blocks for the fungal cell's own proteins. Simple sugars, such as glucose, can enter glycolysis and other metabolic pathways to generate energy for the fungal cell.

Growth and Reproduction: Growth and Hyphal Extension: The hyphal extension and growth process involves the coordinated expansion of the hyphal cell. This expansion is facilitated by the incorporation of new cell wall material and the synthesis of additional cytoplasmic components. The growing tip of the hyphal cell, known as the apical tip, is particularly active in cell wall synthesis and extension.

As the fungus continues to obtain nutrients, the hyphae grow, and the mycelium expands. When the fungal colony reaches a sufficient size and conditions are favorable, it may enter the reproductive phase. Fungi reproduce both sexually and asexually, depending on the species.

Sporulation: In the reproductive phase, the fungus produces specialized spore-bearing structures. These structures can vary among different fungal species. For example, molds may produce sporangia that contain spores, while yeast-like fungi may produce budding cells. When these structures mature, they release new spores into the environment, completing the life cycle.

Fungi's ability to efficiently break down complex organic matter into simpler nutrients, combined with their rapid growth, makes them successful decomposers and colonizers of various substrates. This life cycle allows mold and other fungi to thrive in environments with organic materials, such as decaying organic matter, wood, paper, or damp building materials.

MOLDS ARE IMPORTANT FOR DECOMPOSITION AND SOIL PRODUCTION

Cladosporium cladosporioides and *Cladosporium herbarum* are usually the most common types of airborne outdoor mold spores found in North America. Both commonly grow on leaf litter at cold temperatures all the way down to freezing. They help begin the digestion process by utilizing the moisture that accumulates from early morning dew or frost to become one of the first colonizers of loose plant leaf litter throughout the colder fall and winter months. Recent research shows some molds spend a part of their life cycle living in a symbiotic relationship with the leaves of many types of trees. While the leaves on the tree are alive, essential nutrients are provided to the mold by the tree, but the mold also cooperates with the tree by providing nutrients to the tree, making this a mutually beneficial relationship. When cold autumn temperatures result in the leaves falling off the trees, the *Cladosporium* mold is ready to fill its new role by assisting in the digestion or natural composting of the leaves and assimilating them into nutrient-rich soil. (Sieber, 2007)

When the piles of leaves are thick, a variety of mold spores will be distributed throughout the pile. *Penicillium*,

Aspergillus, and other heat-loving molds thrive in the warm compost pile and will colonize the organic material. No one type of mold becomes the sole or dominant type of mold found in the pile. Instead, a balance of different organisms is achieved.

As mold grows, it uses certain available nutrients. Mildews growing on green leaves may begin the process of digestion and break down one nutrient into another, which becomes available for consumption by other microorganisms. The process of digestion continues with different successions of life forms, reproducing and dying, then replaced by other organisms that continue to feed on the spoils of previous inhabitants. As dried leaves fall to the ground, molds that thrive at cold temperatures use dampness from rain, melting snow, frost, or dew to provide moisture to colonize the leaf litter and continue growing.

HOW MOLD TRAVELS

Mold travels primarily by means of airborne spores. It is common for these seed-like structures to be present in the outdoor air. The concentration is usually lowest in winter, especially when snow covers the ground. They are also rare in the air over open ocean expanses that are devoid of floating organic matter. Yet, even in these settings, a few resilient spores can survive. Astonishingly, spores have been detected traveling between continents at altitudes as high as the jet stream. This is a testament to their durability and their potential for global distribution. (Shinn, 2003)

Every breath we take typically includes a few particles or spores produced by mold, even when outdoor levels are normal. However, in certain regions and seasons, the outdoor spore count can surge, leading us to inhale more than 50 spores per breath. During such periods, it's more common for people to experience eye, lung, and mucous membrane irritation—even for those without mold sensitivities. Saint Louis, Missouri, has earned notoriety for its elevated mold counts, often reaching levels between 20,000 and 50,000 spores per cubic meter of air, primarily during hot, humid summers. (SLCDPH, 2024)

Most molds encountered outdoors in the air are relatively harmless leaf molds. However, certain soil-producing molds present in outdoor air can pose greater health risks, especially when they find their way indoors, land on a moist surface, germinate, and begin to grow when they can digest and obtain nutrients from the materials we use to construct, furnish and occupy our homes. These problem spores are found at low levels mixed in with the more common outdoor types, making it nearly impossible to isolate our indoor living spaces from outdoor influences.

|||||||||||||||||||||||||||||||||||||||||||||||||||||||||||||||||||||||||||||||||||||||||||||||||||||||||||||||||||||||||||||||||||||||||||||||||||||||

Composting: Safer Approaches for People With Mold Sensitivities

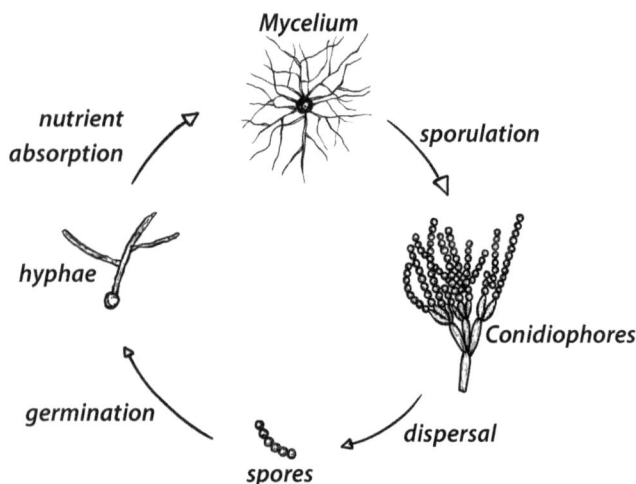

Figure 1-13: When mold grows, spores exposed to sufficient moisture germinate and form hyphae, which release digestive enzymes to absorb nutrients. Well-formed hyphae become denser mycelium, which matures, and sporulation leads to the formation of conidiophores.

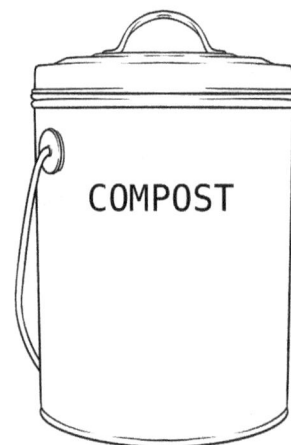

Figure 1-10: Many molds that cause contamination from water damage are the same as those that turn food scraps and organic waste into compost. When collecting organic waste for composting, it should be kept in a covered container and ideally emptied into your outdoor compost bin every day and the container cleaned. By the end of two days, bacteria will be out of control, and mold spores can begin to germinate and grow. Another option is to keep your scraps for composting in your refrigerator or freezer until you can take them to the compost bin.

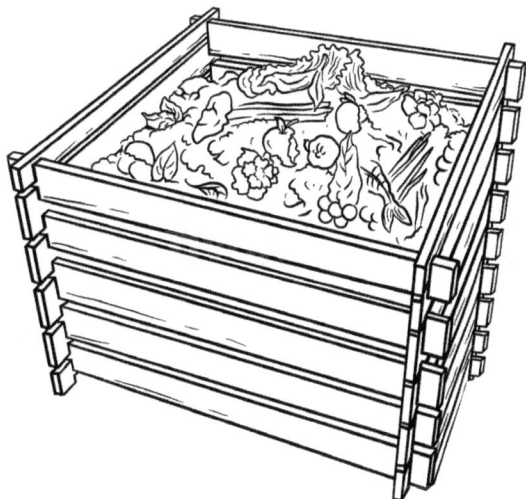

Figure 1-11: Open compost bins should be placed at least 50 feet away from homes or occupied buildings. Turning compost can release large quantities of mold spores, including those found in water-damaged buildings. Whenever possible, avoid open composting near living spaces to minimize exposure.

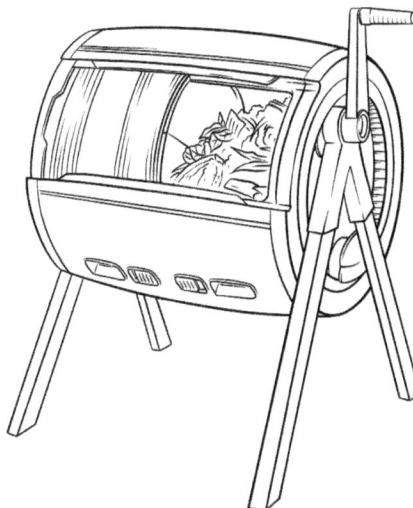

Figure 1-12: The best option is a closed compost bin with a sealable cover and built-in mixing capability. These bins contain mold spores during the composting process, allowing them to break down safely into nutrient-rich, well-rotted compost for the soil.

LIFE CYCLE AND SPORE DISPERSAL MECHANISMS

When conditions are optimal, a germinating mold spore grows a root-like structure known as a hypha. This hypha releases enzymes crucial for breaking down organic material and absorbing nutrients. The moisture level in the environment is pivotal for this enzymatic process; if too dry, the enzymes can't dissolve to work, and if too wet, they become dilute and ineffective. As the hypha metabolizes nutrients, it evolves into a complex network called "mycelium." When the mycelium matures, it undergoes sporulation, a key process in mold's life cycle and ability to colonize new environments. During sporulation, the mycelium produces tall, spore-bearing structures that lift the spores above the surface, allowing them to dry and develop a water-resistant coat. These mature spores are then released into the environment, where they can be carried by air, water, or other organisms to new locations. Upon finding a suitable environment with the right moisture and organic material, these spores can germinate and grow into new mycelium, thus continuing the life cycle of the mold.

Mold spores are both minuscule and incredibly resilient, capable of floating in the air for extended periods. Some have even been known to travel between continents, carried by jet streams or ocean breezes, although such intercontinental journeys are less common.

Some molds have specialized mechanisms that "shoot" their spores into the air, often propelled by the force of a raindrop. Outdoor air samples often reveal a mix of viable and non-viable spores, emphasizing the resilience of these organisms.

It's crucial to note that mold grows on surfaces, not in the air, and spores tend to settle in still air. If a spore lands on a dry surface, it remains dormant until conditions improve. On a wet surface, it typically soaks and remains wet for a couple of days before it can sprout or "germinate." The mold may remain dormant if conditions are less than ideal, such as insufficient food or a dry surface. Eventually, mold spores that fail to germinate and develop will die. Even dead, they can remain intact for extended periods and only decay slowly. The drier the conditions, the slower the decay.

Spores can also re-enter the air through disturbances like wind or interactions with insects and animals. This ensures they continue to move to new, potentially hospitable environments where they might find the right conditions to grow.

Mold is a natural part of our environment, thriving almost everywhere outdoors. It's important to recognize that mold spores will inevitably find their way into our homes, regardless of how well the house is constructed. These microscopic spores can travel through the tiniest of openings—cracks, electrical outlets, and other small gaps in walls, floors, and ceilings. To put it in perspective, a crack the size of a human hair is like a freeway for mold spores and fragments!

|||||||||||||||||||||||||||||||||||||||||||||||||||||||||||||||||||||||||||||||||||||||||||||||||||||||||||||

Essentials: Temporarily Sealing Pathways

Temporarily blocking the flow of air through pathway openings can be helpful in situations where contaminants such as spores, particles, or fragments are entering from hidden sources. This approach is not without risks but may provide temporary assistance if monitored carefully and used as a short-term measure.

Risks of Sealing Pathways:

Sealing wet materials can trap moisture, accelerating deterioration, promoting microbial growth, and worsening the problem over time. While sealing pathways containing dormant spores or particles may be acceptable if the source of moisture has been resolved, it carries the risk of intermittent moisture reappearing, especially during inclement weather, potentially leading to unrecognized issues. Additionally, sealing one pathway can alter airflow dynamics, potentially forcing contaminants to migrate through other, less prominent pathways, thereby exacerbating the problem in unexpected areas. Careful consideration and monitoring are essential when implementing such measures.

When Temporary Sealing Can Be Useful:

If the source of moisture has been effectively addressed and the risk of future moisture is minimal, sealing pathways may be an acceptable temporary measure to limit exposure to contaminants. In situations where options are limited, such as living in a property with a recalcitrant landlord unwilling to make permanent repairs, sealing can provide temporary relief when no better alternatives are available. Additionally, pathway sealing can be useful for creating temporary sanctuaries, such as during travel, relocation, or while your permanent residence—or portions of it—undergoes remediation. These measures, while temporary, can help reduce exposure and provide short-term solutions in challenging circumstances.

Key Considerations for Temporary Sealing:

It is essential to always monitor sealed pathways closely for any signs of new moisture or shifting airflow patterns, as these can indicate underlying issues that need immediate attention. Sealing should be used as a last resort or a temporary measure, with the goal of addressing the root cause of contamination or moisture as soon as possible. Temporary sealing is not a substitute for permanent and effective remediation but rather a short-term solution to reduce exposure while more comprehensive measures are planned or implemented.

Temporary sealing can provide short-term relief in challenging situations, but it must be approached with care and vigilance to avoid creating larger problems in the future.

Methods for Temporary Sealing

Temporary sealing can provide short-term relief in challenging situations, but it must be approached with care and vigilance to avoid creating larger problems in the future. Below are effective methods and considerations for temporary sealing, along with their advantages and limitations.

Quick-Release Tape

Using quick-release tape, such as painter's tape, blue tape, or green tape, can be a practical solution for covering long cracks (e.g., where the baseboard meets the floor) or sealing electrical outlets. Outlets can still be used by plugging through the tape, making this method versatile and easy to implement.

This approach is ideal when you do not have permission to make semi-permanent fixes, such as in rental properties or temporary living situations. However, there are precautions to consider. While designed to avoid damaging painted surfaces, quick-release tape should not remain in place for longer than two weeks, as it may cause surface damage. Additionally, tape will lose its adhesive properties if the materials become damp, failing to contain contaminants. It can also be visually unappealing, although brands like Shur-Tape offer white quick-release tape that is less obtrusive.

In hotels, bed and breakfasts, or other temporary accommodations, using tape may create misunderstandings with management, who might not realize it is being applied as an emergency measure. To mitigate this, consider informing management of your need for reasonable accommodation due to health concerns. Transparency can help avoid unnecessary conflicts while ensuring your temporary needs are met.

100% Silicone Aquarium Sealant

For a more semi-permanent seal, 100% silicone aquarium sealant is a safe option. This non-toxic product is suitable for hypersensitive individuals once cured, as it is specifically formulated to avoid releasing harmful substances (regular silicone is not appropriate and can be toxic to humans and aquatic life). Aquarium silicone is particularly effective for sealing cracks or gaps when permission for longer-lasting fixes is granted.

Tyvek Building Wrap for Damp Surfaces

When sealing wet or damp areas, Tyvek Building Wrap is preferable to polyethylene plastic. Tyvek allows some moisture permeability, reducing the likelihood of mold growth while still providing a temporary barrier to contaminants. However, it does not dry as effectively as leaving the area open to air circulation, which can release spores and fragments. In situations where dampness is present, creating a mini containment with negative air pressure may provide better drying and control than sealing alone.

Mini Containment for Wet Areas

For areas that are wet or likely to become wet, building a mini containment zone with negative air pressure is often more effective than sealing the surface itself. This method allows for proper drying while controlling the spread of contaminants.

Use in Temporary Living or Travel Situations

These methods can also be applied when creating a temporary sanctuary during travel or in situations where you must live elsewhere while your permanent residence or portions of it undergo remediation. This approach is discussed further (See below, Establishing a Mold and Chemical Controlled Safe Room).

Important Notes

Temporary measures will not prevent further deterioration of materials but can help reduce excessive exposure to contaminants. Monitor sealed areas closely for signs of moisture or airflow changes and prioritize permanent solutions as soon as possible to address the root cause of the problem. Using these methods responsibly and thoughtfully can achieve short-term relief while planning for more comprehensive remediation.

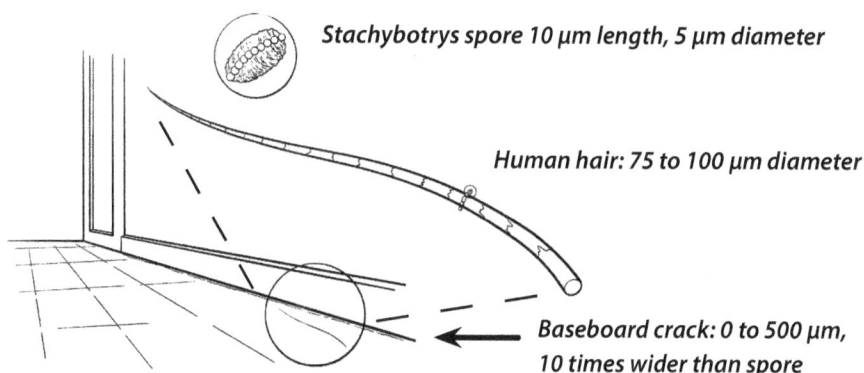

Stachybotrys spore 10 µm length, 5 µm diameter

Human hair: 75 to 100 µm diameter

Baseboard crack: 0 to 500 µm, 10 times wider than spore

Figure 1-14: A crack the size of a single human hair between the top of the floor and the bottom edge of the baseboard is like a freeway for mold spores and fragments to escape from a hidden location inside a wall cavity.

Essay: Establishing a Mold and Chemical Controlled Safe Room

by Marilee Nelson

Introduction: Mold Escape and Travel Plan

Creating a clean, safe sanctuary can be transformative, offering an away space for healing during home remediation, visiting others, or just vacationing. This "mold escape" plan removes you from contaminated belongings and places you in a nurturing environment, helping set the stage for recovery and a healthier future. With optimism and a sense of discovery, you may uncover unexpected insights about yourself and how your indoor environment may have influences on your well-being you have not yet identified.

Overview of the Decontamination Process

Decontamination involves isolating and thoroughly cleaning yourself and your belongings before entering the space set up as a healing sanctuary. When packing, you should leave behind items with even minor mold or contamination risks and products with inflammatory ingredients. Sensitive individuals often react to everyday items, like personal care products. This is a chance to strip away mold, water damage, and chemical problems and see how they may have affected you. Since sensitivities vary, not every recommendation will apply universally; adapt the process to best fit your situation.

Pre-Planning Preparation for Mold Escape and Travel

Deciding What to Bring

Organize items by importance and accessibility. Prioritize essentials—clean clothing, personal care items, and medical supplies—to make unpacking easier on arrival.

Safe Friend's Role

Ask a trusted friend in a mold-free home to store and double-bag essential items, keeping them in a clean space until transport. This avoids cross-contamination and helps ensure only clean items enter the sanctuary.

Packing Tips

Use food-safe zip bags made from virgin, non-recycled materials, which are less likely to leach chemicals. Bring only new, non-toxic, fragrance-free personal care products, reducing irritant exposure.

What to Take

Opt for organic cotton clothing, bedding, and towels without chemical treatments. Limit belongings to essentials for easy decontamination and a clean sanctuary space.

Preparation Assistance

Decontaminate essentials, like a driver's license and credit cards, with safe soap and sunlight to help them outgas. Then, store them in a zip-lock bag with desiccants to absorb moisture. This final step ensures items stay contaminant-free.

Finding Your Safe Haven

Selecting Accommodations

Choose accommodations free from recent remodeling, pesticides, or strong fragrances, ideally with non-carpeted floors. Openable windows and balconies are essential for natural ventilation, helping reduce odor and particles for a health-supportive environment.

Guidelines for Selecting Safe Accommodations

Hotels like Element by Westin and Home2Suites by Hilton often meet the above criteria.

The Carpenter Hotel in Austin, Texas, with its concrete walls and minimal carpet, is an example of a more mold-resistant accommodation. People with sensitivities have successfully used this hotel. However, upon check-in, inspect for prior leaks. The nearby Casa de Luz offers clean, organic meals, supporting a healthy stay.

Preplanning

Pre-vet accommodations using a checklist and online reviews. If possible, have a friend with a good sense of smell inspect the space. Staying organized and detail-focused will help avoid unnecessary stress.

Questions to Ask and Communicating Needs

When contacting accommodations, speak with someone in authority, not just front desk staff. Be clear about health needs, requesting pet-free, fragrance-free rooms without pesticides. Ask if they can accommodate fragrance-free cleaning and whether there are carpet-free rooms. These specific requests help ensure a low-toxin environment for a comfortable stay.

Hiring Staff Assistance for Room Preparation

Ask hotel staff if someone can follow your cleaning requirements, offering to compensate or tip for their extra effort. This additionally helps keep surfaces free of residual cleaning chemicals and allergens and reduces exposure since you are not personally stirring things up.

Backup Plans

Prepare a backup plan in case accommodations don't meet your needs, such as camping availability or where you can sleep in your vehicle with essentials like a portable air purifier, clean bedding, and protective sheets.

Preparation Steps: What to Bring and Ship

Items to Prepare and Ship

Gather new, mold-free items, like a wallet, body care products, bedding, and towels. Branch Basics offers fragrance-free options. Branch Basics Foaming Wash or Gel Soap serves multiple functions for a minimalist approach.

Organic Cotton Clothing and Bedding

Pack organic cotton clothing, pajamas, towels, and bedding. Ask your friend to pre-wash with fragrance-free detergent. Obtaining non-porous luggage that's easily cleaned is ideal.

Shoe Policy

Enforce a no-shoes policy in your sanctuary with a disposable walk-off mat at the entrance and indoor-only slippers stored in a zip-type bag with desiccant.

Optional Comforts

If desired, bring Epsom salts, a bath water purifier, and a cot with untreated fabric for sleeping outdoors or on an upstairs balcony. Reverse Osmosis water can be stored in glass containers to help ensure a clean water supply.

Essential Kits for Your Sanctuary

Prepare specific kits for cleanliness and comfort:

Cleaning Kit: Unscented Swiffer wipes or disposable microfiber cloths, Branch Basics All Purpose Cleaner, and irritant-free gloves for wiping down surfaces.

Protection Kit: Protective sheets, zip-type bags (assorted sizes—up to 5 gallons), and silica gel desiccant packets for storing personal items and controlling moisture.

Personal Care Kit: Branch Basics travel soap, body wash, and shampoo are gentle on sensitive skin.

Vehicle Preparation

Clean your vehicle to prevent cross-contamination. Use a HEPA vacuum to remove particles from seats and floors, ventilate by opening doors, and wipe surfaces with a safe soap like Branch Basics. Disposable microfiber cloths help avoid recontamination. These steps create a cleaner vehicle environment for sensitive travelers. For more information about vehicles, see the *Mold Controlled Contents* Chapter

Travel

Preparation Before Departure

Retrieve double-bagged, pre-packed items from your friend to ensure they remain contaminant-free until arrival at your sanctuary.

Changing Clothes at the Hotel

If the room has been prepared, change into clean organic cotton clothing in the hotel's public restroom before entering the sanctuary. Bag travel clothes securely to avoid contaminating the sanctuary. If uncertain about room conditions, inspect and get it cleaned first to avoid contaminating clean clothing.

Tyvek Suit for Entry

For added protection, wear a Tyvek suit anytime you can't go directly from the outdoors to your clean quarters. Remove the suit at the door, place it in a disposal bag, and step into house slippers to avoid tracking contaminants inside.

Arrival Procedure

Inspection

Inspect the room before bringing belongings, checking for musty odors or water damage. Request switching rooms if needed until you find a satisfactory one.

Hiring Assistance for Initial Cleaning

With management permission, consider tipping hotel staff to provide extra help. Brief them on safe cleaning practices and demonstrate using fragrance-free products like Branch Basics to clean specific areas. This partnership makes it easier to maintain a clean environment throughout your stay.

Initial Cleaning

It is best to avoid carpets and upholstered furnishings. If you must clean yourself, use a HEPA vacuum for soft surfaces, then wipe hard surfaces with microfiber cloths and safe, unscented cleaner. This deep cleaning prepares the room as a low-toxin sanctuary. When you have no choice but to clean a space yourself, the first time, you should clean it thoroughly. In that case, you may need personal protective equipment, which is unlikely to provide sufficient protection for someone with sensitivities but is better than nothing. Once the environment is clean, proactively clean often before contaminants can build up to levels that trigger your sensitivities.

Emergency Response Guidelines

Have a plan for unexpected contamination, such as ventilating the space, using an air purifier, or isolating contaminated items.

Setting Up Your Temporary Space

Air Out the Room

Open windows or doors to improve ventilation, dispersing any remaining odors or particles.

Bed Setup

Use personal organic cotton bedding and leave hotel linens untouched to ensure a toxin-free sleeping environment. See the Contents section for suggestions on mattress cleaning and wrapping.

Maid Service Restrictions

To prevent exposure to standard cleaning chemicals, avoid maid service by anyone you have not trained and approved. Use a "Do Not Disturb" sign and handle upkeep yourself, ensuring only safe products are used.

During Your Stay

Daily Maintenance

Monitor air quality and clean high-contact areas daily with unscented microfiber cloths. Periodically HEPA vacuum carpets, upholstery, and curtains to minimize irritants.

Regular Airing Out

When possible, open windows or doors for ventilation. A portable air quality monitor helps ensure fresh air flow is safe.

Protective Measures

Use a HEPA air purifier to capture airborne allergens, and wear a particulate mask when handling potentially contaminated items outside your quarters. These steps help sustain a low-allergen environment.

Food and Water

Safe Drinking Water

Bring RO water in glass bottles, as plastic can leach chemicals. Before bringing it into the sanctuary, wipe down containers with an unscented cleaner.

Food Options

Seek organic food sources or health-focused restaurants. Casa de Luz offers organic, plant-based meals in Austin, TX, near The Carpenter Hotel. Consider organic food delivery or accommodations with kitchens for meal preparation.

Daily Activities

Self-Care Practices

Take daily Epsom salt baths with filtered water for relaxation. To support a low-toxin routine, use non-toxic soaps like Branch Basics Foaming Wash.

Room and Personal Item Cleanliness

Clean surfaces and personal items daily, using safe cleaning products and disposable microfiber cloths to avoid contaminant buildup.

Monitor and Adapt

Stay attuned to changes in air quality or comfort. Adjust ventilation and track symptoms or triggers with a portable air quality monitor. A roll of safe quick-release tape can be a handy way to temporarily way to block offensive airflow pathways, such as electrical outlets, unsealed cracks between the baseboard and the flooring, and other openings you may discover.

Health Monitoring Tools

A portable air quality monitor can alert you to particle or humidity changes that affect comfort. A journal helps track symptoms and adjustments.

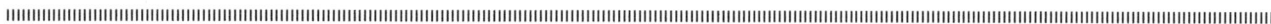

ABNORMAL LEVELS OF OUTDOOR MOLD: SOME UNINTENDED CONSEQUENCES

For many years, the prevailing wisdom among experts dealing with building-related mold issues was that *Stachybotrys chartarum* (formerly known as *Stachybotrys atra*) rarely existed in outdoor environments and posed no significant threat to indoor air quality—unless, of course, there was water damage within the home. However, I've encountered an increasing number of homes where *Stachybotrys* DNA persisted indoors, even after comprehensive remediation and cleaning efforts. At first glance, this would imply the need for further remediation. However, no new or different mold sources were evident or could be discovered inside these structures. A pattern was starting to emerge, and I found elevated levels of water-damage molds at the highest levels in areas of homes with significant ongoing natural ventilation, such as garages, attics, and crawlspaces. Intrigued, I began analyzing outdoor dust samples collected from smooth surfaces like glass patio tabletops, vinyl chair covers, and solar panel collectors. Astonishingly, the levels of *Stachybotrys* DNA in these outdoor samples surpassed those found throughout the occupied and unoccupied areas in the problem homes. This suggested the possible existence of one or more unidentified outdoor sources of problem molds customarily associated with indoor water damage infiltrating indoor spaces.

Myth: Black Mold Is the Only Dangerous Type.
Fact: While Stachybotrys, commonly known as "black mold," is toxigenic, other mold types can also pose similar health risks. Any mold growth indoors should be isolated with caution and addressed properly using appropriate physical removal methods.

Identified Problem Sources

Some mold species, especially *Stachybotrys*, have gained notoriety for thriving on the cardboard coatings of gypsum wallboard and the jute backings of carpets. Jute continues to be used for woven backings on carpets, especially those imported from Europe. It has become apparent that cardboard, paper, jute, and straw, when used for soil-related purposes, provide nutrients for supporting problem levels of mold growth in ways that have not traditionally been identified as problematic. When man-made materials like cardboard, jute-backed carpets, or certain types of insulation with kraft paper vapor retarders or ground-up cellulose typically from recycled newspapers are left outside, or in damp spaces, they can become breeding grounds for mold. When these materials remain chronically wet with sufficiently warm temperatures, the growth of *Stachybotrys chartarum* outdoors has been found to cover these materials.

The mold amplification on these types of materials poses a unique risk as these spores can migrate into living environments, adversely affecting individuals sensitive to mold exposure. Further investigations have shed light on several outdoor materials and practices that contribute to elevated levels of *Stachybotrys* mold. Using cardboard as a weed block on soil has gained popularity for its perceived environmental recycling benefits and cost-effectiveness. However, this trend has deeper roots in global trade dynamics, particularly with China. For years, the United States and other Western countries found it economically viable to ship recycled cardboard to China, where it was reprocessed into new materials with high recycled content. This symbiotic relationship was mutually beneficial: Western countries could offload their recyclable waste, and China could obtain inexpensive raw materials for manufacturing. However, the landscape changed dramatically when recycled paper and cardboard prices plummeted. The drop in prices made shipping these materials to China for reprocessing no longer profitable. As a result, an excess of recycled cardboard began to accumulate domestically. This surplus led to innovative, albeit not always safe, uses for cardboard, including its application as a weed block on the soil. While this practice may seem like a resourceful way to repurpose cardboard, it raises significant concerns, especially regarding the potential for mold growth, such as *Stachybotrys*, in outdoor environments. Therefore, while the practice emerged as a byproduct of shifting economic and trade realities, its long-term impact on soil health and indoor air quality is a subject that warrants scrutiny.

Most of the population in North America is not hypersensitive to mold and will not be aware of its presence; however, for people with mold sensitivities, the practice is proving to be devastating. Using cardboard as a weed block emerged with good intentions for helping use our excess cardboard that would otherwise end up in landfills as a byproduct of shifting economic and trade realities, but its unintended consequences may result in long-term impacts on soil health and indoor air quality, especially for hypersensitive people.

Other Issues from Cardboard and Paper Used in Construction and Repairs

An often overlooked issue affecting individuals with mold sensitivities is cardboard or paper left on the soil in crawlspaces beneath homes. While it might initially seem puzzling why such materials would be used this way, the answer often lies in practicality. Electricians, plumbers, and other professionals frequently work in these confined spaces and prefer to avoid direct contact with muddy or damp soil. Laying down cardboard provides a makeshift, yet effective, barrier that keeps them out of the mud, making their work environment more manageable. This would never become a problem if the cardboard and other debris were removed at the end of each day. Unfortunately, these materials are frequently left behind. This seemingly practical solution comes with unintended consequences. The confined nature of crawlspaces allows for the rapid amplification of problem types of mold growth, which can then infiltrate the living spaces above, posing a considerable risk to sensitive individuals. (Hayashi, 2014)

In construction, cardboard forms are commonly used for pouring concrete piers and foundations, particularly in areas with expansive clay soils or seismic activity, to accommodate ground movement. However, these forms share drawbacks with using cardboard and newspaper as weed blocks in landscaping. While economical and versatile, they readily absorb moisture, leading to mold growth as they decay. The resulting contaminants can pose health risks to sensitive occupants, entering living spaces through open windows, doors, foot traffic, or being drawn into the structure through cracks or expansion joints via the stack effect.

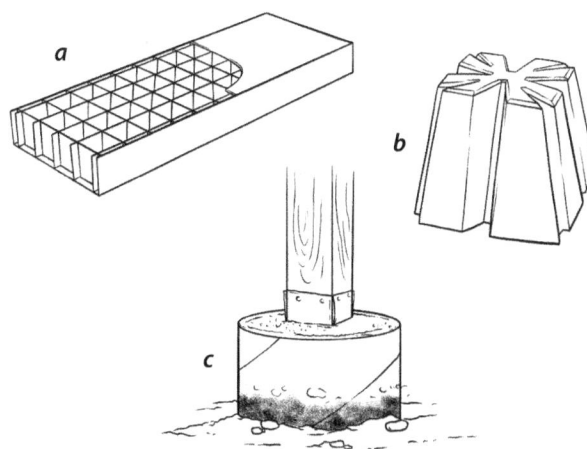

*Figure 1-15: Flat Ribbed Cardboard Form (**a**) is a ribbed cardboard form designed to create a flat concrete surface, often used as a base for the slab. The ribbing provides structural integrity to the form, reducing the risk of collapse during the pouring process while allowing for even distribution of the concrete. Cardboard Void Form (**b**) is commonly used in areas with expansive soils to create a void between the concrete and the soil. It allows the soil to expand and contract without exerting pressure on the concrete structure, preventing cracks or structural damage. Cardboard Pier Form (**c**) is used for pouring concrete piers or columns. It is designed to hold the shape of the concrete while it sets, creating a strong and stable vertical support for foundations or structural elements. Leaving the cardboard form in place can grow mold.*

Materials and Practices Requiring Further Consideration

Some materials and practices fall into a gray area and may require further investigation. For instance, compost piles could be a problem, depending on how they are managed. Entire books have been written on the correct balance of nutrients, moisture, and ventilation. Keep them balanced and healthy by understanding what they need, and the organisms that help break down the organic material into the soil will be balanced. Burlap, cardboard, and carpet should not be placed directly on soil because many of the organisms they produce when they begin to rot are the same type that cause problems in water-damaged buildings.

Adding to the concern, a technical report from the American Journal of Pediatrics has highlighted instances where moldy horticulture pots made of recycled paper had visible black masses of *Stachybotrys*. This led to symptoms among workers handling these pots. (Mazur, 2006)

Materials Not Proving Problematic

On the flip side, my research has also identified several outdoor materials that are not problematic regarding *Stachybotrys'* growth. I have tested over ten commercial decorative ground covers like bark and mulch and have not found *Stachybotrys* at elevated levels. Similarly, potting soils and other soil amendments have been non-problematic. Leaves in various stages of decay have been tested, but *Stachybotrys'* growth has not been identified.

While my research has identified several outdoor materials that have not been problematic regarding *Stachybotrys* growth, it's crucial to note that these findings are not exhaustive. The materials tested, such as commercial decorative ground covers like bark and mulch, as well as potting soils and other soil amendments, have shown no issues in the context of my studies but may not always be true.

Different environmental conditions, manufacturing processes, or even slight material composition variations could yield different outcomes. Therefore, additional testing should be conducted to confirm these findings in various settings and conditions. Always be aware that exceptions could exist, and what holds in one scenario may not necessarily apply in another.

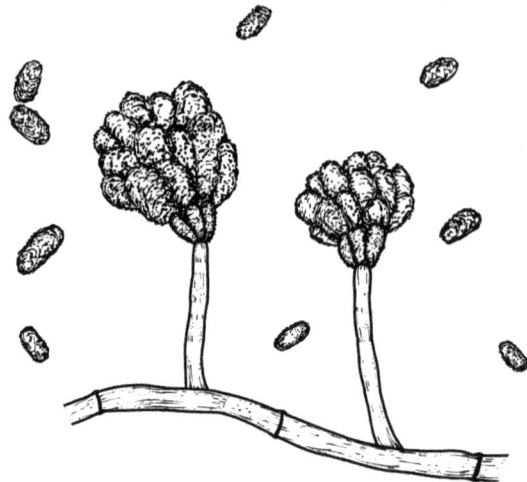

Figure 1-16: Stachybotrys chartarum (spore size 5 by 10μm).

Stachybotrys Chartarum: An Examination of Its Ecological Behavior

Stachybotrys chartarum is a mold species that predominantly colonizes wet stalks of rice and similar vegetation. This mold becomes problematic when it infiltrates corn silage stored with excessive moisture. Characterized by its slow growth rate, *Stachybotrys* necessitates near-saturated moisture conditions for a prolonged period, distinguishing it from other more rapidly growing molds.

When these conditions begin to change—specifically, when competing molds that thrive in less saturated conditions emerge—the biological stress on *Stachybotrys* triggers the production of secondary metabolites known as Biotoxins. These biotoxins serve a defensive role, essentially acting as a barrier to inhibit the establishment of competing molds, thereby preserving the *Stachybotrys* colony during its dormant phase.

Optimal conditions for *Stachybotrys chartarum* include a temperature range of 77 to 86°F and high moisture levels bordering on saturation. Under such conditions, it may still require seven to twelve days for germination and up to a month to achieve dense colonization. When the mold undergoes desiccation, its stress response can activate the production of biotoxins to impede the growth of other mold species, thereby securing its ecological niche.

Rapid desiccation minimizes the production of biotoxins as the mold transitions to a dormant state. However, if the *Stachybotrys* has been subjected to slow drying or cycles of wetting and partial drying, the biotoxins produced could effectively monopolize its environment, thwarting the encroachment of molds that require less moisture.

Should the moisture levels return to an optimal state, *Stachybotrys chartarum* can resume growth, having safeguarded its territory through biotoxin production. Regarding its life cycle, the half-life of *Stachybotrys* spores is approximately ten months. Therefore, significant spore death occurs over extended periods, with the majority expiring by the end of four years. If conditions turn favorable again—such as after significant rainfall—the mold can reactivate and proliferate, given that sufficient nutrients are available. (Dillon, 2005)

Stachybotrys is a mold that requires chronic moisture to thrive and continuous wetness to grow. If the moisture level drops below approximately 95% saturation at the surface, it goes dormant and ceases to grow. *Stachybotrys* is particularly finicky about its nutrients, preferring paper or cardboard. It is unlikely to grow on wood unless the wood comes in contact with paper or cardboard.

The growth of *Stachybotrys* in an attic, for example, depends on several factors. A leak must keep the nutrient source—such as gypsum board ceiling or cellulose insulation (ground-up recycled newspapers)—continuously wet for 7–12 days for *Stachybotrys* to germinate. The saturation must be maintained for a long enough period for this slow-growing mold to become well-established. The rainy season increases the likelihood of *Stachybotrys'* growth due to prolonged wetness. However, temperature is another factor. *Stachybotrys* thrives at around room temperature and stops growing when temperatures drop below approximately 60 degrees Fahrenheit, making it less likely to compete and grow in colder conditions.

When materials get wet, multiple organisms will compete to grow on them. Fast-growing molds can germinate in 2–3 days and become well-established within a week, using up space and nutrients to outcompete *Stachybotrys* before it has a chance to grow. If the material remains damp but not sufficiently saturated, other organisms requiring less moisture will dominate. Similarly, if the nutrient composition or temperature isn't ideal for *Stachybotrys*, other molds will prevail.

If the conditions change and become wetter to favor *Stachybotrys*, it may attempt to grow, but it must compete with other organisms that have already developed. This is when chemical warfare begins. *Stachybotrys* can produce over 200 different toxic compounds as a defense mechanism to secure its territory. These biotoxins are not specifically aimed at humans, but we and our homes become collateral damage.

Interestingly, fewer spores are released while *Stachybotrys* is actively growing. As it dries out, it becomes more friable, and spores, particles, and fragments are more likely to be released. Also, *Stachybotrys* spores are heavy and sticky; they do not travel much until we disturb them and spread them around.

Typically, *Stachybotrys* requires a slow but continuous leak that wets paper or cardboard for a long time without being discovered. It is more commonly found growing behind kitchen cabinets due to a slow drip than from roof leaks during the rainy season. Roof leaks are usually noticed quickly due to visible water stains, prompting immediate action.

Once discovered, spraying *Stachybotrys* with chemicals can exacerbate the situation by triggering biotoxin production. It is much safer and more effective to physically remove the affected area of a paper-covered gypsum board and dispose of it rather than using chemicals to kill the mold.

|||||||||||||||||||||||||||||||||||||||||||||||||||||||||||||||||||||||||||||||||||||||||||||||||||||||||||||||||||||||||||||||||||||||||

Essentials: Outdoor Molds

1. Mold is a normal part of our outdoor environment.

2. Unless you have a specific sensitivity to "normal outdoor molds," they will only occasionally be at levels that cause discomfort.

3. Outdoor air will generally provide healthier indoor conditions. Opening windows and having adequate ventilation are usually beneficial.

4. Certain outdoor activities and conditions can trigger higher levels of mold exposure.

   a. Avoid positioning open compost piles within 50 feet of homes. Compost piles are loaded with the same molds that commonly grow in water damage.

   b. If you are mold sensitive, avoid turning open compost piles yourself. Leave that to the 75% of the population that isn't mold sensitive.

   c. Once the compost has become soil and is completely digested, it's ready to use in your garden. The water-damage molds have been replaced with beneficial soil-type organisms that are found everywhere.

   d. Fruits and vegetables typically have enough internal moisture to support mold growth as they rot. Harvest fruit and garden vegetables when they are ripe, but before they drop to the ground and begin to rot or develop mold.

   e. Encourage the earthworm population. They will help by coming to the surface to aerate and turn the lawn and garden soil for you each night. Earthworms will also help turn compost piles without stirring up the molds in the hot interior parts of the piles until the molds have completed enough of the digestion process to cool to acceptable temperatures. The worms then pull the nutrient-rich compost downward into the soil and further digest the compost into a nutrient-rich loam that is perfect for growing plants.

5. Outdoor mold levels will usually be at their highest when it starts raining. Mold spores can be propelled into the air by the droplet hitting the moisture-repellant outer coating of the spore. Warm, moist, windy conditions are also more likely to result in high spores in the air.

6. Outdoor mold spore levels will usually be at their lowest when snowing or a layer of snow is on the ground.

7. Outdoor mold levels vary in different regions of the country. You will need to learn your sensitivities to mold and when to avoid outdoor conditions or activities that may cause flare-ups. An indoor sanctuary can be helpful during these times.

8. Outdoor mold levels are frequently published along with pollen levels by local news agencies. The American Academy of Allergy Asthma and Immunology publishes mold levels they monitor for many areas at AAAAI.org.

9. When left outdoors and exposed to moisture, materials like cardboard, paper, jute (burlap), hay bales, and high-density straw applications can become hotspots for the growth of *Stachybotrys* and other molds typically linked to indoor water damage. These materials are especially prone to mold proliferation when repeatedly or chronically wet, mainly when favorable temperatures are also present. Avoid using cardboard and newspaper as a weed block for gardens, pathways, or other areas where weeds grow. Instead, use synthetic weed-block materials that do not support growth.

References

Epstein, P. R., & Mills, E. (Eds.). (2005). *Climate change futures: Health, ecological and economic dimensions.* A project of the Center for Health and the Global Environment at Harvard Medical School.

Gaynes, R. (2017). The discovery of penicillin—New insights after more than 75 years of clinical use. *Emerging Infectious Diseases, 23*(5). https://doi.org/10.3201/eid2305.161556

Frontiers Editorial. (2023). Fungal bioactive metabolites of pharmacological relevance. *Frontiers in Pharmacology.* Retrieved from https://www.frontiersin.org

Juneja, V. K., Dwivedi, H. P., & Sofos, J. N. (Eds.). (2018). *Microbial control and food preservation: Theory and practice.* Springer. https://doi.org/10.1007/978-1-4939-7556-3

Sieber, T. N. (2007). Foliar endophytic fungi: Diversity in species and functions in forest trees. *Fungal Biology Reviews, 21*(2–3), 75–89.

Shinn, E. A., Griffin, D. W., & Seba, D. B. (2003). Atmospheric transport of mold spores in clouds of desert dust. *Archives of Environmental Health, 58*(8), 498–504.

St. Louis County Department of Public Health. (2024). *Pollen and mold center: Mold spore counts.* Retrieved from https://pollenandmold.stlouisco.com/Summary.aspx?Item=Mold

Hayashi, M., Osawa, H., Hasegawa, K., Honma, Y., & Yamada, H. (2014). Infiltration of mould from crawl space under the prefabricated bathroom. *Journal of Environmental Protection, 5*(10), 914–921. https://doi.org/10.4236/jep.2014.510093

Mazur, L. J., & Kim, J. (2006). Spectrum of noninfectious health effects from molds. *American Journal of Pediatrics, 118*(6).

Dillon, H. K., Heinsohn, P. A., & Miller, J. D. (2005). *Field guide for the determination of biological contaminants in environmental samples.* American Industrial Hygiene Association.

Chapter Four: Normal and Abnormal Indoor Environments

In typical homes without water damage, mold spore levels can vary widely due to outdoor mold spores entering our homes in several ways: through open windows and doors or by hitching a ride on our clothes and shoes. Once inside, many of these spores settle on surfaces where they can be removed by cleaning. Some become stirred up and removed by the furnace filter, or they might simply float outside.

This means the amount of mold spores inside a home always changes. Though it's hard to keep it constant, most homes have a usual range of mold levels. We can help keep our homes within this normal range by doing a few things: not bringing in as many spores from outside and keeping our homes clean and well-ventilated. If we let up on these efforts, mold levels can rise.

The "Pigpen Effect" and Its Relevance to Indoor Air Quality

Remember "Pigpen" from the Peanuts comics? He always walked around with a cloud of dust following him. This isn't just a funny cartoon idea—it's a real thing scientists have called the "Pigpen Effect." A study in 2005 even proved it happens. When we move around, we stir up a mini storm of tiny particles around us, including mold spores. The more active we are, the bigger this cloud gets. These particles don't just float aimlessly; they seem to cling to us and even move with us. (Penn State, 2019)

When we clean our homes by conventional sweeping or dusting, we spread tiny particles of molds and bacteria around. Some will find their way outside, some will be removed by HEPA vacuuming and effective cleaning techniques or caught by air filters, and others will settle down until we stir them up again. (Fugler, 2002)

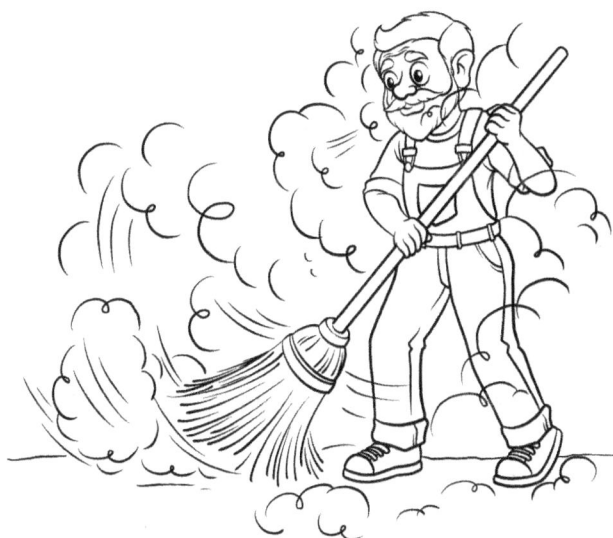

Figure 1.17: Ban the Broom. It does not clean mold spores or small particles and can scatter them, making cleaning more time-consuming.

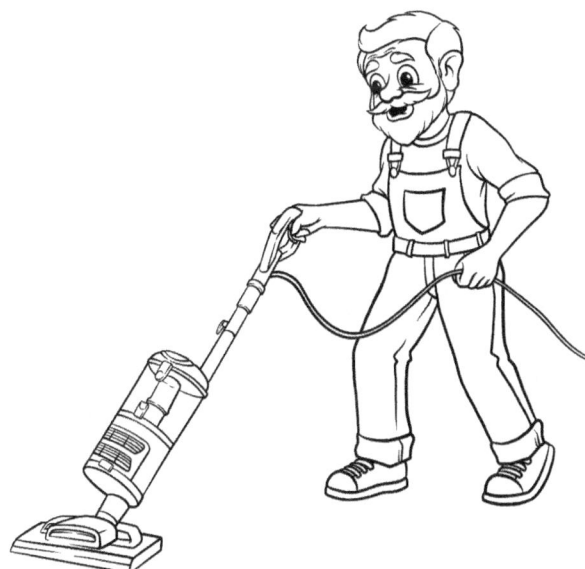

Figure 1-18: Always use a HEPA vacuum instead of an unfiltered vacuum. Only a properly functioning HEPA vacuum cleaner contains the small and fine particles.

HOW INDOOR MOLD TRAVELS

Understanding how mold and other water-damage organisms behave as particles in our homes can significantly affect remediation efforts. In 2005, our research team at RestCon Environmental contributed to the scientific literature with a publication entitled "Modeling the Equilibrium Spore Load for a Building." This computational model, albeit rudimentary, served as an invaluable tool for comprehending spore behavior in indoor settings. It accounted for many variables, including but not limited to infiltration, exfiltration, and surface settling. By manipulating these variables, the model could predict their individual and collective impact on indoor mold levels. Notably, the model corroborated certain intuitive assumptions while unveiling some counterintuitive phenomena. For instance, smaller spores such as *Penicillium* and *Aspergillus* are more likely to be expelled from the building, whereas larger spores have a higher propensity for surface settling. (Banta J., 2005)

Spore settling speed, as defined by Stokes' formula, reveals that mold spores with the same density settle at a rate proportional to the square of the mean aerodynamic radius of the particle. As we move around and perform various activities, we will re-aerosolize settled spores and elevate the indoor airborne mold concentration. Cleaning activities like using a regular vacuum cleaner can exacerbate mold challenges. HEPA vacuuming helps remove settled spores, whereas poorly filtered vacuum cleaners will spew contaminates back into the air.

Our shoes and clothing move mold spores between areas and assist in cross-contaminating indoor areas. The quantity of spores brought indoors is contingent upon the number of occupants, frequency of ingress and egress, external fungal load, and individual habits. The HVAC system also influences the mixing and distribution of contaminants. The study's model, developed to understand and predict indoor mold spore concentration, incorporates parameters such as air exchange rate, filtration efficiency, and spore size. While the model provided significant insights, it operated under specific assumptions, including the hypothesis that the air within a structure is homogeneously mixed, yielding uniform spore concentrations throughout. This is not the way particles behave. Instead, the closer one gets to a source, the higher the concentration. However, the model did assist with a greater understanding of why larger, heavier spores such as *Stachybotrys* tend to accumulate at higher concentrations near their growth site. In contrast, smaller, lighter-weight mold spores tend to spread further within a home but are also more likely to exit a home through exfiltration when doors and windows are left open for ventilation purposes.

Water damage can be likened to a slow-acting fire, acting as a catalyst for structural decay. The initial stages involve bacterial colonization, swiftly followed by mold proliferation. As custodians of our living spaces, rapid discovery and effective drying of wet areas are imperative for preventing microbial escalation.

GROWTH OF MOLD IS ASSOCIATED WITH WATER DAMAGE

When our home or personal belongings become moldy with growth, it is always due to a moisture problem. If materials contain nutrients, or if dust containing digestible ingredients is present and remains damp for a sufficient period, then mold will grow. Wet or damp wood, paper, cardboard, natural fiber cloth, and stuffed upholstered furniture are examples of materials that usually are nutrient-rich and will be invaded by the root-like structures. These structures, called hyphae, develop if the surface of the material remains wet or damp for a few days. The hyphae transport nutrients that support the development of mold growth, much like plant roots function by absorbing nutrients. In addition, mold aids the digestion of nutrients by releasing enzymes into the moisture layer to digest the material. This results in the nutrient becoming soluble in water and makes it available to nourish the development of growth. Digestion stops when the material dries out. The mold goes dormant and can rapidly begin again if damp condition returns. Mold growth can be caused by either liquid water or water vapor.

- Liquid water from rain, floods, pipe breaks, or other water-damage emergencies can saturate the structure and personal belongings. They all must be dried quickly and thoroughly to prevent mold from growing. In addition to mold growth, liquid water damage may cause cracking, swelling, buckling, cupping, warping, and staining beyond repair before mold growth can develop.

- High levels of water vapor in the form of excess humidity can support certain types of mold growth without any liquid water present. A few types of mold can germinate and begin to grow when the relative humidity at the surface of an item or construction material is sustained at higher than 61%. At a sustained 70% relative humidity at a surface, multiple types of mold readily germinate and begin to grow.

- Books and papers may develop a musty odor from excess humidity long before visible damage is apparent. The odor is frequently the first sign that something has become too damp. Immediate drying can arrest further deterioration, and detailed cleaning can often return the books or papers to a serviceable condition.

- When the dew point temperature of a surface is reached, condensation moisture forms. When sustained condensation wets the surface continuously for 2–3 days, some types of mold will germinate and initially result in a light layer of mold growing on the damp surface. If this is recognized and addressed early, it is frequently possible to restore these items by drying and cleaning the surface before the hyphae can cause permanent damage by penetrating into the item. If the condensation forms repeatedly on surfaces or maintains items in a continuously damp condition, cumulative damage from mold growth may mean the object is permanently damaged.

- Wet plastic, glass, metals, stone, ceramics, and tile only develop mold growth if there's a layer of nutrient-rich dirt or dust to nurture them. These hard-surfaced items can usually be cleaned to remove mold growth by removing the nutrient-rich filth. Moisture is always a critical component. If materials remain dry or are quickly dried, mold growth cannot germinate and begin growing.

- Wood rot, caused by Basidiomycetes class fungi (which includes mushrooms), takes months of wetness to develop and can have serious structural implications. Unchecked wet rot or dry rot can eventually lead to buildings collapsing. Despite its name, dry rot requires more moisture than faster-growing surface molds need. This means that any time dry rot or wet rot is present in a building, it is likely that surface mold will already have developed in nearby materials by the time the rot becomes apparent.

WHY IS WATER MORE DAMAGING TO OUR HOMES NOW?

Prior to the mid-1900s, construction was much more resilient to moisture. Buildings would get wet, but they could dry quickly by themselves because of significant amounts of air leakage. Since many homes were heated with wood or peat, the extra airflow allowed the necessary ventilation for efficient and safe fireplace operation. The smoke was carried up the chimney, while lots of moisture was able to exhaust from the home simultaneously.

When we exhale, our breath has moisture that was not present when we inhaled those same molecules of air. Every twenty-four hours, the average adult exhales about a quart of liquid water in the form of a vapor. Bathing or showering, cooking, and cleaning also release water vapor into the home. By the time it is all added up, the typical adult generates the equivalent of over a gallon of liquid water each day.

The typical home also has a certain amount of water vapor that passes from the soil under the house into the living space. An acceptable amount is generally considered three pounds per thousand square feet of soil exposure daily. This means a 2000-square-foot ranch-style home commonly takes on three-quarters of a gallon of daily water from the soil. The drafty air that passed through the pre-energy crisis structure easily managed these amounts of water. In the 1970s, energy conservation began to enter our consciousness. As energy costs rose, construction methods adapted to the changing conditions. Our homes became tighter and better insulated to reduce energy consumption, but this had the unintended consequence of reducing the amount of water vapor that would be swept from the home based on the inherent air leakage that had been present.

- According to the National Flood Insurance Program, "More than 20% of flood insurance claims come from people outside the mapped high-risk areas." High-risk areas have a 25% chance of flooding in a 30-year period.

- According to the Insurance Bureau of Canada, "One of every two dollars paid by home insurers is for damage caused by water." Examples of conditions leading to water damage include plumbing breaks, toilets, sinks, and washer overflows. Tree limbs can fall on our homes during a rainstorm, and a variety of other accidents, like broken pipes and water heaters, can release major amounts of water into our homes.

- According to the US Environmental Protection Agency's pamphlet, *Mold Remediation in Schools and Commercial Buildings*, it is necessary to respond to water damage within 24 to 48 hours and dry the building rapidly to eliminate the risk of mold growth developing.

The moisture capacity of our buildings has also changed. At one time, most buildings were constructed of heavy materials such as solid wood and masonry. These materials can absorb a lot of water vapor during damp periods and then moderate the indoor humidity levels by releasing that moisture when the weather creates drier conditions. The nature of the materials was such that it would be rare for water vapor to cause the material to become wet enough to support the organisms that cause decay. Over the years, resource conservation and modern construction techniques have resulted in construction materials with less capacity to absorb and release moisture. We have gone from using heavy timbers to using dimensional lumber. A two-by-four no longer measures 2 inches by 4 inches. It is now 1.5 by 3.5 inches. Losing half an inch on each side may not seem like much, but there is a third less wood. This also corresponds to a third less moisture buffering capacity. Some construction companies take this lost frame moisture buffering capacity to an extreme by eliminating it with the use of metal framing. The average moisture content of cured wood framing lumber in North America is 10%. Suppose the moisture content can vary during wet and dry times by ±2%. This means a typical wood-framed home can buffer about 200 gallons more water than a similar metal-framed home.

When it comes to mold growing in buildings, it is all about the water getting into places where it can contact nutritive materials to nurture mold growth. Without moisture and food, mold can't grow. Because water flows or migrates via capillary action, it can travel some distance from where it enters the building. So even if it entered at a point where non-nutritive materials were used for the construction, it may travel a long way and potentially cause damage to other nutritive materials along the path it followed. Water resulting in mold growth usually comes in one or more of the following forms:

1. Plumbing and fixture issues.
2. Falling rain or melting snow entering openings in the building envelope.
3. Flowing water, such as in floods and drainage issues.
4. Condensation from excess water vapor entering the home from earth, air, or fire
5. Liquid water, humidity, or condensation from occupant-generated activities like showering, bathing, cooking, cleaning, and breathing.

Humidity

The types of mold that can grow under humid conditions are fewer than the types that will germinate when conditions are wet, but some types of mold never require any liquid water, only elevated humidity.

- When humidity levels are high, permeable furnishings will take on the excess moisture, causing the moisture content to rise until the moisture in the item reaches an equilibrium with the home.
- The surface permeability acts as the gatekeeper for allowing moisture to enter the item. When there is more moisture trying to enter the item than can be absorbed, the surface moisture (also known as water activity or A_w) will increase. It is the excess moisture on the surface of our items that allows mold to grow.
- When conditions are dry, the moisture exits the item, and the moisture content will reduce until it is once again in equilibrium with the home.

- Correspondingly, if more moisture is trying to exit the item than can be carried away by the surrounding air through evaporation, then the A_w will again increase.
- Each type of mold has a different minimum water activity that permits mold growth to occur.

It is possible for indoor humidity levels to cause mold to grow on our furnishings without allowing it to grow on the structural materials. Gypsum wallboard with highly permeable, flat latex paint will quickly allow excess humidity to pass through the paint into the highly absorbent paper coating and interior gypsum material. Since mold growth can only begin growing at the surface of a material with enough moisture on that surface, it will not support mold growth until the A_w at the surface rises to the point needed by a particular mold for germination and growth. Furniture with a finish may have a lower permeability than unfinished wood. The finish on the surface causes a bottleneck that prevents moisture from passing as quickly into the wood. The A_w at the surface increases faster because the sealed wood under the finish is unable to absorb and buffer the excess moisture.

Condensation

In addition to the permeability of an object, another influence is changing temperature. Relative humidity varies quite dramatically based on a change in temperature. The relative humidity in the air may be low, but a nearby cold surface may be wet with condensation. We see this whenever condensation moisture forms on the outside of a can of cold soda sitting on a table.

A rapid 20° F (11° C) temperature drop will cause a doubling of the relative humidity at the surface of a material. At 50% relative humidity, lowering the temperature by this amount or more will cause condensation moisture to form.

I was contacted by an insurance company for a young lady who had lived in Australia for several years. While there, she purchased several pieces of furniture that had been hand-made from hardwood lumber collected from the indigenous trees found in Australia. When it came time for her to move back to the United States, a shipping company was hired to pack and transport all her furnishings from Sydney to San Francisco in a shipboard cargo container. When her cargo container was unloaded at the docks in San Francisco, her things were damp and completely covered with mold growth. It was fortunate that she had purchased mold insurance as a rider to her coverage for the shipment. I was hired to investigate the conditions that caused mold to grow so that the insurance company could pay her claim. Once the facts of the case became known, it was obvious to me what had gone wrong. On the day when the furnishings were loaded into the cargo container, the temperature in Sydney was recorded as being 97 °F (36 °C), and the relative humidity was 50%. The hold of the ship remained dry throughout the month-long transport, with a constant temperature of 57 °F (14 °C) for most of the trip.

Here's what happened—Relative humidity (RH) is relative to temperature. The cargo container was packed and sealed at the higher outdoor temperature. When the furnishings were lowered into the hold of the ship, the temperature inside the sealed cargo container began to cool to a temperature below the dew point. Condensation began to form on the furniture inside the air-tight storage box. In this case, the difference in temperature was 40°F (22°C), which resulted in a quadrupling of the RH. As the temperature dropped, condensation began to form, and it literally began to rain on the furnishings inside the storage container. The amount of moisture that had been present when the cargo container was loaded and sealed seemed to be in the ideal humidity range (30–50%), but it was more than enough for condensation to form and cause the mold to grow as the temperature dropped.

HOW QUICKLY MOLD GROWS IN OUR HOME

The Time Factor plays a pivotal role. Mold can germinate within 24 to 48 hours of moisture exposure, emphasizing the need for swift action in water-damaged areas. Once germination has occurred, you may still have time to finish the drying process to arrest the mold growth before it can develop to a point where amplification begins. If you can maintain a cycle of beginning drying within 24 hours of the initial wetting and have the surface or unbound moisture

dried by the time 48 hours have passed. In that case, you will likely successfully prevent mold growth from becoming established. Generally, the longer an item remains wet, the greater the likelihood of it developing damage in addition to mold growth.

During days three through seven, viable (able to germinate) mold spores infused with sufficient moisture can germinate and send out a single, small, root-like structure called a hypha. The germinated but not yet established mold growth is now quite vulnerable. If it can't digest and absorb sufficient nutrients to continue its life process, it will die and never reach a stage of exponential growth or sporulation.

Only when the proper amount of moisture, temperature, and nutrients are present can mold growth sustain itself until it reaches maturation. This is where the mold has produced sufficient growth and sporulated to a point where spores and growth structures exceed the normal background levels found in outdoor environments.

- In the landscape of mold growth within American homes, the hierarchy of influencing factors begins with Water Activity (Amount of Water). This is the most essential element, as all molds require moisture to thrive, but their needs vary. Water damage or high-humidity areas are prime locations for mold proliferation.

- Temperature follows with a twist: while most molds prefer warm, humid conditions typical of indoor environments, there are cold-loving molds usually found outdoors. Interestingly, these cold-tolerant molds are generally less toxic compared to the faster-growing, indoor water-damage-associated molds. The latter are often linked to health issues due to their ability to produce mycotoxins, potentially harmful substances.

- Nutrients (Food Sources) come next; molds feed on organic materials found in construction materials and household items, making our homes a buffet for them.

- Competition among various microbial species can influence mold growth. In environments where mold faces little competition, it can dominate and spread unchallenged.

||||||||||||||||||||||||||||||||||||||||||||||||||||||||||||||||||||||||||||||||||||||||||||||||||||||||||||||||||||||||||||||||||||||||||||||||||||||||

Essentials: The "Butter Test"

Most mycotoxins are water soluble, but a few are soluble in oils or fats. When fat-soluble mycotoxin-containing mold spores or fungal fragments land on a greasy surface, the bulk of the toxins remain in the settled particulates, but some of the mycotoxins diffuse into the surface film. Cleaning these fat-soluble residues is easy when you use methods to cut through and remove grease. A simple test can determine if a

household cleaning product will effectively clean fats, lipids, grease, or oils and the mycotoxins they contain from surfaces. Smear some butter or other cooking fat onto a dish or plate. Use the product you wish to test to clean the butter off the plate. Since dish detergent or dish soap is manufactured for this purpose, it passes the "butter test" and will work every time. Mycotoxins and oily residues will be removed.

||||||||||||||||||||||||||||||||||||||||||||||||||||||||||||||||||||||||||||||||||||||||||||||||||||||||||||||||||||||||||||||||||||||||||||||||||||||||

HOW SPORES SPREAD INDOORS

When mold growth matures, it produces seed-like structures called spores. Mold spores and their residual fragments have an inherent ability to spread throughout indoor environments. Spores can enter homes through ventilation systems, open windows, or by attaching to clothing and pets, accumulating on surfaces, and mixing with other dust particles. In moist and nutrient-rich conditions, viable spores may germinate and colonize surfaces. Conversely, in dry conditions, these particles can disperse into hidden areas like behind walls or within HVAC systems, contributing to "building memory," where spores and fragments can persist in concealed locations. Despite remediation efforts, completely eradicating all hidden spores and fragments is nearly impossible, leading to potential re-emergence and health implications over time. This building memory underscores the importance of comprehensive remediation to eliminate sources of contamination, followed by ongoing cleaning to maintain indoor environmental quality.

Managing mold involves keeping indoor environments balanced to prevent new growth and managing the spread of spores and fragments by cleaning. Complete eradication of mold residues is neither feasible, necessary, nor beneficial, as they are part of the natural environment. The objective is to maintain mold at levels that do not trigger health issues or structural damage, avoiding overly sterile conditions that disrupt the natural microbial ecosystem and could lead to other health risks. The overuse of antimicrobial agents, aiming solely at killing mold spores, can overlook underlying moisture problems, contribute to resistant microorganism strains, and interfere with accurate mold testing, emphasizing the need for sustainable mold control strategies.

How Mold Migrates from Hidden Locations into the Living Areas

A crack the size of a single human hair is like a freeway, allowing the much smaller mold spores to pass freely. For the mold spores to travel from the wall cavity through the crack and into the living space, there must be both a pathway and an airflow. Some common sources for airflow include the stack effect, the wind blowing on the outside of a wall, exhaust fans, the draw of air up a fireplace, clothes driers exhaust, and leaky ductwork. When these occur, small amounts of air are sucked through every available opening. If aerodynamic contaminated dust is in the direct path of airflow, it will be sucked into the indoor air in the building. Suppose you live in an apartment or condominium with a shared wall with your neighbor. In that case, there is a good chance you have experienced a demonstration of this air exchange from their unit into yours when you can smell them cooking dinner, smoking, or using air fresheners. These air flows occur in many ways that are not obvious, but if they pass by an area of contaminants with sufficient velocity, they can be picked up by the air currents and travel into the living space. Once the particles exit the crack or opening and enter the room, they either begin floating around and eventually settle onto a surface as dust or are attracted to and stick to nearby surfaces. Most particles will settle closer to their source. This proximity principle can help track down hidden sources and is one of the principles used with Pathways™ Testing.

> *Myth:* All Mold is Visible:
> *Fact:* Mold growth may not be dense enough to be visible. Also, mold growth can occur in places that are not immediately visible, such as inside ductwork, behind wallpaper, or within wall cavities. Just because mold isn't visible doesn't mean it's not present.

Essentials: Choosing and Using a HEPA Vacuum Cleaner

Despite marketing claims, I find an alarming number of consumer-grade HEPA vacuum clears do not properly filter at the HEPA standard of 99.97% effective at 0.3μm. I've tested several hundred HEPA vacuum cleaners in people's homes and found that over 50% of these "HEPA" vacuums failed a particle-counter test.

• Never use a non-HEPA vacuum in your home. Verify performance, not just labels. This is further confirmed based on independent research of HEPA-filtered air filtration equipment failure rates. (Brandys, 2012)

• **Reliable Choices:**

› *Inexpensive Options*: Shark Navigator and Shark Rotator Lift-Away models with "Complete Seal Technology" have performed well when I have tested them.

› *Premium Options*: Miele vacuum cleaners with True HEPA filters are excellent, but confirm the filter is present and properly labeled. Look for a pleated filter marked "HEPA" inside the vacuum. Some less expensive Miele's do not have a HEPA option.

- **Common Misrepresentations**:

  › A flat pad or activated carbon filter is not HEPA.

  › HEPA vacuum bags are not substitutes for a proper HEPA filter.

  › Salespeople can misrepresent models; verify specifications by inspecting inside the vacuum cleaner yourself.

- **Safe Bag Changes**:

  › Always empty your vacuum outdoors to avoid releasing fine particles and spores.

  › Wipe the vacuum exterior with a disposable microfiber cloth before bringing it back inside.

  › If mold-sensitive, delegate bag-changing and cleaning tasks to someone who is not.

- **Protect Your Home**:

  › Never allow housekeeping services to use their own vacuum cleaner in your home. Insist they use your properly functioning HEPA vacuum to avoid cross-contamination from other households.

  › The best way to confirm that a HEPA vacuum properly filters fine particles and prevents their release is to check your vacuum cleaner with a particle counter.

Do's When HEPA Vacuuming

- **DO follow the manufacturer's operating manual and owner instructions:** Most homeowner-grade HEPA vacuum cleaners are not heavy-duty and will burn out or break down quickly if used or anything more than minor remediation cleanups.

- **DO Inspect the Filter Regularly:** Check the HEPA filter before each use to ensure it is in good condition, securely seated, and free from visible damage or dirt buildup. Checking the exhaust from a HEPA vacuum cleaner with a particle counter can help determine whether it effectively removes particles.

- **DO Replace Filters as Recommended:** Follow the manufacturer's guidelines for replacing HEPA filters and pre-filters. Using filters beyond their recommended lifespan can compromise the vacuum's filtration effectiveness.

- **DO Empty the Vacuum Bag Carefully:** When the bag or dust container is full, empty it carefully outside, standing upwind, and double bag the waste to prevent releasing contaminants back into the environment.

- **DO Clean the Exterior Regularly:** Use a damp microfiber cloth to wipe down the vacuum's exterior, particularly around vents and attachments, to prevent dust accumulation. This is especially important after opening the vacuum cleaner to change the bag or service the equipment and filters. The interior of the vacuum cleaner is not clean! The HEPA filter has a clean side and a dirty side. The dirty side is the inside of the vacuum cleaner.

- **DO Use Attachments Properly:** Utilize the vacuum's various attachments, such as crevice tools and brushes, for effective cleaning of different surfaces. A crevice tool is designed to increase the air velocity where it is being used. An opening that is too small can overwork your vacuum cleaner and potentially burn it out. If an opening is too large, the vacuuming will provide less suction.

- **DO Store in a Clean, Dry Area:** Keep the vacuum in a designated storage area away from potential contamination sources, such as mold-prone spaces.

Don'ts When HEPA Vacuuming

- **DON'T Overfill the Bag or Container:** Do not let the dust bag or container reach full capacity, as this can reduce the vacuum's efficiency and strain the motor.

- **DON'T Use on Wet Surfaces Unless Specified:** Do not use the HEPA vacuum on wet surfaces unless specifically designed for wet/dry cleaning. Wet debris can clog the filter and damage internal components. Also, wet cleaning makes mud, which is more difficult to remove. Always dry vacuum to remove as much dust and debris as possible.

- **DON'T Use Without the HEPA Filter in Place:** Never operate the vacuum without the HEPA filter, as this will release contaminants back into the air and defeat its purpose.

- **DON'T Wash a Non-Washable HEPA Filter:** Most HEPA filters are not washable; refer to your vacuum's manual. Washing a non-washable filter can damage its structure and reduce filtration capacity.

- **DON'T Drag the Vacuum Across Contaminated Areas:** To prevent the transfer of mold or debris, do not allow the vacuum, hose, or power cord to come into direct contact with contaminated surfaces. The vacuum cleaner will need a detailed cleaning if it is going to be used in a clean environment after being used in a contaminated environment.

- **DON'T Use for Hazardous Materials Unless Approved:** HEPA vacuums should not be used for hazardous substances like asbestos or lead dust unless they are certified and equipped specifically for that use.

By following these steps, you can ensure your vacuum cleaner truly supports a healthy, mold-controlled home.

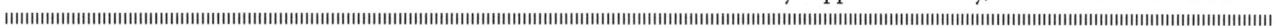

PRINCIPLES OF MOLD AND WATER DAMAGE ORGANISM BEHAVIOR

- The closer you are to an area or source of mold growth, the higher the concentrations of mold spores and fragments are likely to be. Visibly observable mold often contains concentrations ranging from 1 to 10 million colony-forming units per square inch, but hidden or inaccessible mold can also release spores and fragments into the environment. These contaminants can escape from hiding through tiny openings, cracks, or penetrations in walls, floors, or ceilings. Once released, they can migrate into occupied spaces, spreading through airflow and affecting indoor air quality. Identifying areas near potential sources allows for the tracking and planning of effective remediation of contamination.

- Spores, fragments, and particles bigger than one micron tend to settle downward onto horizontal surfaces due to gravity. Larger spores and particles, such as those from *Stachybotrys*, can settle from the ceiling to the floor in just a few minutes. Smaller spores, like those from *Penicillium* and *Aspergillus*, settle more slowly, typically requiring 4 to 8 hours to cover the same distance. These contaminants will be more concentrated in the room where the source is located, and their spread to adjacent areas in lesser amounts depends on factors like the size of doorways or openings between rooms.

- The pressure differential between rooms, driven by airflow, significantly influences how many contaminants spread and how far they travel into adjacent areas. Higher pressure differences create stronger airflows, which can carry more significant quantities of spores, fragments, and particles from one space to another, increasing the spread of contaminants throughout a home.

- Spores, fragments, and particles that exit hidden locations into occupiable spaces accumulate on clean surfaces near their release points due to electrostatic and molecular forces, which cause them to stick to nearby surfaces. These forces result in a denser concentration of particles at these release points, such as cracks under baseboards or where walls meet floors. Particles released from ceilings or upper wall areas similarly concentrate near the openings where they emerge. Once the surfaces near the release points become saturated—neutralizing the electrostatic and molecular forces—particles begin to settle. Larger particles typically fall mostly downward, while smaller particles disperse as they meander and settle more gradually over time.

- To observe electrostatic and molecular forces, try this simple demonstration: sprinkle a handful of bread flour on a smooth kitchen floor, then vacuum it up. This will illustrate how small particles, like mold spores, adhere to surfaces due to these forces. Although it may appear clean, running your finger over the area will reveal more sub-visible flour clinging to the surface, highlighting how small particles like mold spores can persist and adhere to surfaces, impacting efforts to remove contamination thoroughly. Bread flour particles, typically around the same size as mold spores (2–10 microns), behave similarly by adhering to surfaces at unseen levels due to electrostatic and molecular forces. This similarity demonstrates how both can persist on surfaces and require specific cleaning methods to remove them effectively. Your finger picks up these fine particles more effectively than a vacuum cleaner. For even better results at breaking the electrostatic and molecular forces, use a disposable dampened microfiber cloth, which acts as an excellent "particle magnet" for fine-settled contaminants. This demonstrates the importance of thorough cleaning techniques to overcome the electrostatic and molecular forces that make small particles, like mold spores, challenging to remove.

- Mold growth in an HVAC system will likely be distributed throughout the home via the ductwork. When the system operates, air movement carries spores, fragments, and other particles from contaminated areas into every space the system serves, significantly impacting indoor air quality. While a MERV or HEPA filter can help reduce the redistribution of contaminants from the house, it cannot prevent mold or particles that have grown inside or accumulated beyond the filter from spreading throughout the system and into the house.

- Mold growth in a specific segment of ductwork releases spores and particles carried by the HVAC duct system into the rooms served by that branch. The concentration of contaminants in each room will depend on the mold growth in that ductwork segment. Trunk lines with higher levels of development will distribute more contaminants into the corresponding rooms, while trunk lines without growth will distribute lower contamination levels. This variability can result in significantly higher contamination levels in some rooms.

THE DIFFERENCE BETWEEN SMALL PARTICLE AND FINE PARTICLE CLEANING

Small particle cleaning is necessary to maintain a healthful indoor environment, focusing on removing particles ranging from 1 to 10 microns in size. These particles exhibit behavior influenced by their size and weight: while gravity contributes to their settling on surfaces, settling rates vary significantly. For example, a 10-micron particle in still air will settle within a few minutes, whereas a 1-micron particle may take overnight to settle. Environmental factors such as airflow, turbulence, and mechanical agitation further influence their ability to remain airborne.

In contrast, fine particles—less than 1 micron in size—primarily exhibit Brownian motion, moving randomly and adhering to surfaces through mechanisms such as impaction, electrostatic attraction, or van der Waals forces.

Small particles are more predictable and can be addressed effectively using conventional cleaning techniques, making their removal an essential focus in maintaining indoor air quality.

Essentials: Effective Small Particle Cleaning

The following section addresses the essentials of small particle cleaning, emphasizing strategies that account for their dynamic behavior. Fine particle removal, with its distinct challenges and requirements, will be discussed in a dedicated text box.

- Preparation of Cleaning Solution: Combine five drops of Branch Basics all-purpose cleaner or a similarly acceptable detergent (no enzymes, essential oils, and will tolerated by hypersensitive people) with a quart of water.

- Place this diluted solution in a spritzer bottle for application. Dipping and wringing out microfiber cloths leaves them too wet and makes them less effective.

- Use gloves and other appropriate personal protective equipment (PPE) to avoid direct skin contact with surfaces.

- Cleaning Process—Dampening the Cloth: Use a disposable microfiber cleaning cloth dampened with the prepared solution. The microfiber material captures fine dust and particulates without leaving residues.

- Spritz the microfiber cloth with 3 to 4 sprays from the spritzer bottle. Do not spray the surface being cleaned with the cleaning solution. Be cautious not to saturate surfaces, particularly porous materials, to prevent secondary water damage. This dampening should be minimal to avoid over-wetting, which could lead to less efficient cleaning by the microfiber cloth and, in extreme situations, water damage or mold growth.

- Wiping the Surfaces with a dampened disposable microfiber cloth. The microfiber cloth's texture lets it pick up and hold fine particulates more effectively than paper, terry cloth, or other types of wipe towels. The cleaning is performed using an S-cleaning pattern, where the leading edge of the cloth is always moving in the same direction, as opposed to a back-and-forth scrubbing motion. If scrubbing is needed to get a surface free of crud and caked-on dirt, spot-clean those areas using your regular cleaning methods, followed by Effective Cleaning.

- Edge cleaning helps remove contaminants that build up next to the walls, which S-cleaning misses.

- After cleaning, each surface should be visually inspected to ensure it is visibly clean and free of debris and dust.

- You should be able to wipe 40 square feet of surface with a single wipe towel and not have it pick up any more visible residue. The wipe cloth should also be clean and free of stains. This is akin to performing a 'white glove test' using the disposable microfiber wipe and is an essential step to confirm that all particulates have been effectively removed.

- Properly Dispose of Used Cleaning Materials after use to prevent cross-contamination.

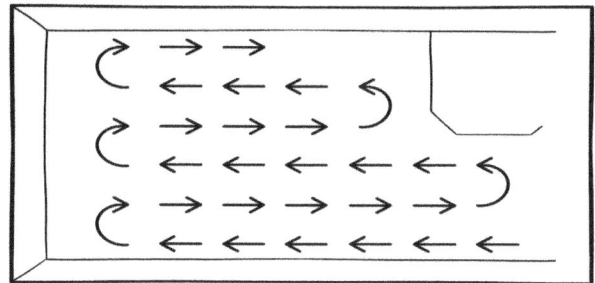

Figure 1-19: An S-Cleaning Pattern cleans large flat surfaces quickly and efficiently. When performed with a swivel-type mop head, the wipe pattern allows the leading edge of the wipe to collect the dirt because it is always moving forward.

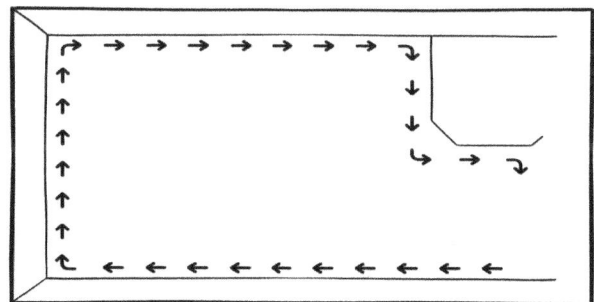

Figure 1-20: An Edge-Cleaning Pattern picks up the dirt and contamination close to the wall where they exit hidden locations, such as the space between the bottom edge of the baseboard and the top of the floor. It also collects the dirt that was missed around the edges by the S-Cleaning method.

These Effective Cleaning methods help ensure that surfaces are meticulously cleaned while minimizing the risk of damage or moisture issues from wet mopping and helping the overall remediation process by providing a surface ready-for cleanliness testing.

Why I Favor Disposable Microfiber Wipes Over Reusables

Disposable microfiber wipes are my preferred choice for cleaning because they provide superior hygiene and eliminate the complexities associated with maintaining reusable microfiber. To effectively clean reusable microfiber, it must be washed at temperatures exceeding 165°F, held at that temperature for over 45 minutes, and subjected to multiple wash and rinse cycles using a special detergent without bleach, softening agents, or other additives that could damage the fibers. Additionally, reusable microfiber cloths must be washed separately from other types of laundry to avoid cross-contamination and maintain their cleaning effectiveness. This rigorous process ensures that the fibers untwist and release trapped contaminants, but it is time-consuming and resource-intensive. Disposable microfiber wipes bypass these challenges entirely, reducing the risk of cross-contamination and ensuring that every cleaning pass uses a fresh, uncontaminated surface. For environments requiring meticulous cleaning, such as those impacted by mold or water damage, disposable wipes offer a practical and reliable solution.

THE CHALLENGES OF FINE PARTICLE CLEANING

Fine particles, defined as less than 1 micron in size, present significant challenges due to their unique behavior and physical characteristics. These particles are not effectively removed by conventional air purifiers or HEPA vacuums, as they often adhere to surfaces through mechanisms like impaction, electrostatic attraction, or van der Waals forces. Additionally, fine particles are dominated by Brownian motion, which keeps them suspended in the air for extended periods rather than traveling directly into capture zones or settling efficiently under gravity.

Essentials: Principles for Effective Fine Particle Removal

Effective fine particle cleaning requires specialized strategies. Disposable Electrostatic Microfiber Wipes are particularly effective for removing fine particles from surfaces because they attract and hold particles securely, minimizing re-aerosolization.

- **Agglomeration for Easier Removal:** Fine particles can be made to clump together into larger clusters through appropriate misting techniques, allowing them to behave like small particles and settle predictably onto surfaces.

- **Enhanced Surface Accessibility:** Once fine particles are agglomerated, they settle onto horizontal surfaces, where they can be effectively removed using proper cleaning methods, such as disposable electrostatic microfiber wipes.

- **Controlled Particle Removal Through Artificial Raindrops:** Effective misting promotes the formation of artificial raindrops, using fine particles as nuclei. These raindrops bring the particles down to surfaces, making them accessible for thorough cleanup.

- **Avoidance of Chemical Hazards:** Effective removal techniques should avoid misting agents that introduce petrochemical residues (such as those used in dry fogging), biocides, or antimicrobials. Since fine particles are not alive, using toxic chemicals to "kill" them is both unnecessary and counterproductive. These chemicals can pose significant risks to sensitive individuals and compromise environmental safety.

- **Reversible, Non-Damaging Approaches:** Particle removal methods should avoid irreversible solutions, such as sealing cracks or pathways, which can trap moisture and lead to long-term degradation. Appropriate strategies focus on eliminating particles without causing additional issues.

- **AeroSolver as a Method for Effective Removal:** AeroSolver aligns with these principles by safely agglomerating fine particles, facilitating their removal without introducing harmful chemicals or using damaging methods, and ensuring a practical, health-conscious approach to fine particle removal.

Detailed information about AeroSolver and its application can be found immediately following Exercise 14.3: Removing Ultra-Fine Particles from the Air. Combining complementary tools like AeroSolver with effective surface cleaning techniques makes fine particle cleaning a practical and achievable process.

THE NEED FOR CONTINUING POST-REMEDIATION CLEANUP

After a building has been thoroughly remediated to remove water-damage organisms, sources, and affected materials, followed by a detailed cleanup to eliminate elevated mold spores and water-damage organism residues, the indoor environment begins normalizing. Remediation tackles the root causes and removes the mold growth, while cleanup focuses on clearing away the bacteria, spores, toxins, and residues that are present. Research, such as the

RestCon equilibrium model, suggests it takes about four to six weeks for mold and bacterial levels to stabilize at a new equilibrium after successful remediation. Right after cleaning, the surfaces are free of contaminants. However, over time, the new equilibrium may reestablish with excess contamination levels due to building memory. The new equilibrium may stabilize at an unacceptable level, especially for people with mold sensitivities. Routine cleaning performed using effective cleaning techniques can help maintain controlled levels until the building "forgets" the trouble it experienced. (Banta J., 2005)

Essentials: Choosing Mold Cleaning Agents

1. Soap and Detergents: The Proven Choice

Why They Work for Mold: Most water-damage-related molds produce spores and fragments with hydrophobic outer layers composed of tough polysaccharides like chitin and glucans, combined with proteins that contribute to their water-repellent nature. Additionally, the plasma membrane of fungal cells, which lies beneath the spore wall, consists of a phospholipid bilayer that plays a role in cellular functions. Soaps and detergents are effective because they act as surfactants, breaking down the hydrophobic barriers on spore surfaces and emulsifying residues.

Additional Benefit: The action of soap or detergent allows for physically removing spores, fragments, and associated mycotoxins from surfaces. These cleaning agents can also target fatty residues where fat-soluble mycotoxins may accumulate, ensuring thorough decontamination. Mycotoxins, which can be fat- or water-soluble, are also emulsified and removed using a soap or detergent in water.

When to Use: Always use these as the primary cleaning agent for mold. Detergent or soap-based solutions are sufficient for effective cleaning and do not introduce harmful residues.

Other Considerations: Soaps, detergents, and other cleaning agents with enzymes can interfere with Pathways™ Testing (Enzymes are Proteins and will provide false positive Pathways™ results). Essential oil and chemical-based phenols can cause inhibition of DNA-based testing such as MSQPCR, (ERMI, HERTSMI, and Next Gen Sequencing). They should be avoided to prevent false negative results. Branch Basics All Purpose Cleaner has been formulated without these problem compounds, oils, or enzymes.

2. Vinegar

Why It's Promoted: Vinegar (acetic acid) is often marketed as a natural cleaning agent, effective for removing calcium and other mineral deposits. Its mild acidity dissolves mineral buildup and water spots, making it a popular household cleaner. However, claims that vinegar can effectively eliminate mold or solve mold problems are often exaggerated and unsupported by evidence.

Why It Doesn't Work for Mold: Vinegar is not effective for removing mold spores, fragments, or residues. Its acidity provides only mild antifungal effects on non-porous surfaces, insufficient for comprehensive mold remediation. Vinegar does not effectively break down the hydrophobic outer layers of mold spores. Additionally, mixing vinegar with anionic detergents can neutralize their cleaning power by altering the pH, reducing their ability to emulsify and remove fat-soluble residues and biotoxins from surfaces.

Be cautious when following internet advice for mold remediation and cleaning. Many cleaning agents contain Antimicrobials, biocides, and other substances that are ineffective in returning the home to an acceptable condition for people with environmental sensitivities to mold or chemicals. The following explains some of these intricacies further.

When Not to Use: Avoid using vinegar as a mold cleaning agent, alone or in combination with soaps or detergents. It offers no significant benefit in removing mold or mycotoxins and may create a false sense of security. Instead, use cleaning products specifically designed for mold remediation.

3. Baking Soda

- **Why It's Promoted:** Baking soda (sodium bicarbonate) is often recommended for its odor-neutralizing properties and as a mild abrasive for cleaning surfaces.

- **Why It Doesn't Work for Mold:** Baking soda does not break down the hydrophobic outer layers of mold spores or fragments. It is not a surfactant and cannot emulsify fats or residues where fat-soluble mycotoxins may accumulate. While its alkalinity may temporarily raise surface pH, this effect is insufficient to meaningfully inhibit mold growth or remove spores.

44444444

- **When Not to Use:** Avoid using baking soda as a cleaning agent for mold. While it can help with odors, it provides no effective benefit for removing mold spores, fragments, or mycotoxins and should not be relied on for mold remediation.

4. Hydrogen Peroxide

- **Why It's Promoted**: Hydrogen peroxide is widely marketed as a mold killer and oxidizer because it releases reactive oxygen species that break down organic materials.

- **Why It Doesn't Work for Mold**: While hydrogen peroxide has been shown in the laboratory to kill surface hyphae and degrade some structures, it does not penetrate porous materials effectively or remove mold spores, fragments, or mycotoxins. Mold spores are protected by their tough outer wall, composed of polysaccharides and proteins, which limits hydrogen peroxide's ability to eliminate mold. Additionally, hydrogen peroxide does not address the root cause of mold problems, such as moisture or contamination, leaving conditions for regrowth.

- **When Not to Use**: As a standalone cleaning agent. It is ineffective for comprehensive mold remediation and may damage surfaces. Mixing hydrogen peroxide with certain cleaning agents, including soaps, detergents, and other household products, can lead to potentially adverse chemical reactions. For example, hydrogen peroxide may react with certain surfactants, stabilizers, or enzymes commonly found in detergents, leading to excessive foaming, destabilization of the hydrogen peroxide, and reduced cleaning efficacy.

5. Bleach

- **Why It's Promoted**: Chlorine bleach (sodium hypochlorite) is widely marketed as a disinfectant and mold killer, often used to clean hard, non-porous surfaces. Its oxidizing properties can kill surface mold and bacteria, making it a common but problematic recommendation for mold cleanup.

- **Why It Doesn't Work for Mold**: Bleach does not effectively penetrate porous materials like drywall or wood, leaving deeper mold contamination untouched. While it can kill surface mold, the water content in bleach may soak into porous surfaces, potentially encouraging further mold growth. Moreover, killing mold is insufficient—dead mold remains allergenic, and some dead molds are still toxic, as noted by the EPA. Chemically sensitive individuals often cannot tolerate chlorine bleach or other chlorine-based products, as the fumes and byproducts can trigger respiratory irritation, headaches, and other adverse reactions. Additionally, bleach can produce unintended and noxious chemical reactions, such as the release of chlorine gas when mixed with ammonia or other cleaning agents. Furthermore, bleach is a known PCR inhibitor that interferes

with DNA-based mold testing (e.g., ERMI or HERTSMI) and causes false negatives by damaging the genetic material used for analysis.

- **When Not to Use**: Avoid using bleach for mold remediation on porous surfaces, in areas with embedded mold contamination, or around individuals with chemical sensitivities. The EPA specifically advises against the use of biocides like chlorine bleach for mold cleanup, highlighting its limitations and the potential health risks of leaving dead mold and residues behind. Instead, focus on physically removing mold spores

6. Essential Oils

- **Why They're Promoted**: Essential oils, such as tea tree, thyme, orange, and basil oil, are widely marketed as natural antifungal agents due to their antimicrobial properties demonstrated in laboratory studies.

- **Why They Don't Work for Mold**: While essential oils may have antifungal properties, they are ineffective for comprehensive mold remediation. Essential oils cannot physically remove mold spores, fragments, or mycotoxins, which are key components of mold contamination. Additionally, compounds in essential oils, such as phenols, are known PCR inhibitors and can interfere with DNA-based mold testing (e.g., ERMI or HERTSMI), potentially leading to false negatives. The strong odors of essential oils can also trigger adverse reactions in chemically sensitive individuals without addressing the underlying mold problem, making them unsuitable for sensitive environments.

- **When Not to Use**: Do not use essential oils as a cleaning agent or "natural" mold killer. They provide no effective remediation benefit and may introduce additional challenges for sensitive populations. Instead, focus on proven cleaning methods that physically remove mold and address the root causes of contamination.

7. Commercial "Mold Killers"

- **Why They're Promoted**: Commercial mold-killing products are often marketed as quick and easy solutions to eliminate mold and prevent its return. Their claims emphasize antifungal or antimicrobial properties that appeal to consumers seeking immediate results.

- **Why They Don't Work for Mold**: While many of these products rely on synthetic phenols, quaternary ammonium compounds, or other biocides, they are not effective for comprehensive mold remediation. These chemicals may kill surface mold but cannot physically remove spores, fragments, or mycotoxins, which remain allergenic and potentially toxic. Moreover, many biocides leave behind harmful residues that can exacerbate health issues for sensitive individuals. Relying on such products can create a false sense of security, as killing mold does not address the root cause—excess moisture—or remove contamination from the environment.

- **When Not to Use**: Avoid using commercial mold-killing products for remediation cleaning. They are unnecessary and may introduce harmful residues that pose risks to the home environment and its occupants, especially those who are chemically sensitive. Instead, focus on proven methods that physically remove mold, address moisture issues, and restore a safe living environment.

Key Takeaways

- **Focus on Cleaning, Not Killing**: Effective mold remediation involves physically removing spores, fragments, and residues using soap or detergent solutions. Killing mold without removing it does not address the root problem and leaves behind allergenic and toxic materials.

- **Avoid Harmful Substances:** Biocides, phenols, and other marketed mold-killing products are unnecessary and can provide a false sense of security. These chemicals may leave harmful residues, make chemically sensitive individuals ill, and damage homes. Focus on safer, proven cleaning methods.

- **Keep It Simple:** Aqueous soap or detergent solutions are sufficient for mold remediation. They remove contamination effectively without introducing harmful residues or interfering with mold testing processes, making them ideal for sensitive environments.

HOW BUILDING MEMORY CAN AFFECT A REMEDIATED HOME

Despite successful remediation and initial cleanup, new molds and bacteria continue to enter the home through various means: carried by air currents, people, pets, and even contaminated items brought inside. Monitoring how quickly mold levels rise post-remediation can indicate the success of the intervention. Mold spores that have settled into hard-to-reach places, like electrical outlets or under baseboards, may shift and migrate into the living space. Regular, effective cleaning after the remediation of growth sites is complete can help maintain low to normal spore levels, contributing to a healthier indoor environment.

POST-REMEDIATION ASSESSMENTS

Assessments should be conducted as needed during and after this stabilization period to ensure the continuing effectiveness of the remediation and cleanup. MSQPCR results that include a calculation of the HERTSMI-2 score, developed by Dr. Ritchie Shoemaker, is a test method that can help confirm a normal fungal ecology and provide guidance to understand if the building is functioning appropriately. Testing a home immediately after it has just been remediated and cleaned can help establish if the remediation area has been adequately cleaned. However, a single passing test does not provide a complete picture. Many nuances may also need to be addressed. Other considerations may need to include:

- Monitoring endotoxins and gram-negative organisms found in sewage, septic water, and other sources.

- Determining if remaining Actinobacteria are from water-damage-associated organisms or being shed from the skin of one or more occupants or pets.

- How often is effective cleaning required to maintain successful remediation and re-establish a healthy indoor ecology?

- Are additional contamination levels emerging over time? Do these emerging elevated levels indicate additional areas that also require remediation, new developing issues that need to be addressed, or building memory that can be controlled by effective cleaning?

- How can you anticipate future problems to ensure they are adequately addressed in the building maintenance and repair process rather than developing as a surprise later on?

Pathways™ Testing (Step 17) at two-week intervals can be used to monitor the levels of peptide bonds and proteins in dust migrating back into the building. This can help guide the frequency of necessary cleaning to help establish the stabilization rate and ensure the building regains a normal controlled balance.

CHALLENGE TESTING

Sometimes, people are acutely sensitive to their surroundings and can tell rapidly if a building will negatively impact their health. These individuals rely on personal perception as an early warning system to "sense" when an environment may trigger symptoms. Not everyone with this sensitivity will know immediately; some may be unable to separate the meaning of their symptoms. This presents a dilemma: how does one break the exposure cycle when you cannot sense whether you're being exposed?

Relying solely on perception may become unreliable for people whose bodies have become hyper-reactive, especially if it is accompanied by a sense of unease or discomfort. In such cases, a structured and systematic method like challenge testing can provide clearer insights by combining medical observation with controlled environmental exposure, helping to determine whether a space contributes to symptoms.

SAIIE (SEQUENTIAL ACTIVATION OF INNATE IMMUNE EFFECTS)

Some biomarkers can respond to mold and other environmental toxins more rapidly than physical symptoms might appear or be discerned, offering a more objective way to monitor exposure. This is the basis of SAIIE (Sequential Activation of Innate Immune Effects), which uses biomarkers such as C4a and tools like Visual Contrast Sensitivity (VCS) testing to detect subtle changes in immune and inflammatory responses that may not yet be felt physically. It is important to note that not all people's biomarkers respond in the same way, underscoring the need for a qualified medical practitioner to oversee this process. (Shoemaker R. M., 2008b)

The SAIIE protocol, developed by Dr. Ritchie Shoemaker, tests whether a specific building or environment causes a physiological response in people with CIRS. It uses a carefully planned process under medical supervision to check if exposure to a suspected building causes rapid inflammatory changes, helping to confirm that the environment, not another factor, is the problem. Before starting the re-exposure trial, you must provide informed consent, acknowledging that you understand the process, potential risks, and your right to stop the trial at any time if needed.

Here's how it works:

First Phase—Establish Baseline: The patient moves to a known clean environment and stops taking their CIRS medications for a set period. While monitoring symptoms, their medical practitioner arranges testing to establish a baseline, including laboratory tests and other objective health status measures. This baseline reflects the patient's condition without exposure to contaminated environments.

Re-Exposure Phase: The patient provides informed consent and re-enters the suspected building for 4 to 8 hours under controlled conditions so the medical practitioner can observe changes in symptoms or biomarkers that align with exposure.

Final Step—Check for Patterns: Over three days, testing continues to identify patterns of worsening results or symptoms that suggest the suspected building is a significant factor in the patient's illness.

Dr. Shoemaker's SAIIE method was initially developed to help demonstrate causation—establishing a direct link between a specific exposure and resulting symptoms. Proving causation means showing that a particular environment, such as a mold-contaminated building, is directly responsible for triggering a patient's symptoms rather than merely being associated with them. This can be particularly useful in both medical and legal contexts.

"C4a is the most important short-lived marker we have for mold illness; It reflects ongoing activation."
—*Ritchie Shoemaker, M.D.*

The Sequential Activation of Innate Immune Effects (SAIIE) protocol demonstrates unique strengths that align with key elements of the Bradford Hill criteria for establishing causation. One strength is its focus on **temporal relationships**, as SAIIE's sequential design tracks how physiological effects develop after specific environmental exposures, clearly demonstrating that symptoms follow the trigger. Additionally, SAIIE relies on **biological plausibility** by incorporating biomarkers, which provide measurable, objective evidence of the body's inflammatory or immune responses. The protocol also emphasizes **reproducibility**, observing consistent patterns of symptom recurrence and biomarker changes across multiple re-exposure trials. Unlike population-based studies, SAIIE is highly individualized, tailoring its approach to the unique physiology of the person being tested, making it particularly useful for those with sensitivities like Chronic Inflammatory Response Syndrome (CIRS). By combining real-time observations with objective biomarker data, SAIIE offers a personalized, dynamic method for confirming causation in environmental health assessments, filling an essential gap in evaluating individual responses to potential exposures.

Beyond proving causation, SAIIE is a valuable tool for those unable to sense their body's reactions to an environment accurately. While testing the building itself can indicate general exposure levels, individuals may have unique sensitivities that fall outside typical expectations. For these cases, SAIIE offers a way to rely on objective biomarkers rather than subjective perception alone, enabling individuals to manage their health more confidently.

Practical Applications of SAIIE

SAIIE can be applied in several ways to support health and environmental decision-making, including:

- **Home Selection (Buying or Renting)**: SAIIE testing can help determine that a prospective home's environment supports health and clarify how the property might impact wellness over time.

- **Five Stages and 25 Steps to a Mold-Controlled Home:**

  › **Step 19: Confirmation of Remediation Success:** Pathways™ testing can confirm that remediation has effectively lowered peptide bond and protein-based contaminant levels on specific surfaces. SAIIE can further determine if the levels achieved are adequate to support healing.

  › **Step 23: Establishing a Maintenance Plan and Monitoring Schedule:** SAIIE can be incorporated into a proactive maintenance and monitoring plan by combining routine checks of your home with SAIIE-inspired monitoring by your healthcare practitioner. This helps preserve a healthful home, reduce the risk of future extensive water damage, and optimize the environment for healing and well-being.

||||||||||||||||||||||||||||||||||||||||||||||||||||||||||||||||||||||||||||||||||||||||||||||||||||||||||||||||||||||||||||||||||||||||||||

Essentials: Top Ten Actions for Preventing New Mold Growth

1. **Fix Water Leaks Promptly**

   a. **Repair leaks immediately:** Address any leaks in roofs, walls, or plumbing fixtures as soon as they are discovered.

   b. **Inspect regularly:** Regularly check for leaks under sinks, around appliances, and in the attic.

   c. **Learn to use a moisture meter:** Regularly check moisture levels in walls, floors, and other areas prone to dampness to detect potential mold problems early.

2. **Dry Wet Areas Immediately**

   a. **Dry spills and wet areas promptly:** Use towels, fans, and dehumidifiers to dry quickly.

   b. **Avoid leaving wet items:** Do not leave wet clothes, towels, or other items in a pile.

3. **Control Indoor Humidity and Condensation**

   a. **Keep humidity below 60%:** Aim for 30–50% to prevent mold growth.

   b. **Use dehumidifiers and air conditioners:** Treat these as a building life-support system when necessary to maintain the humidity.

   c. **Learn** to use and take advantage of materials' moisture capacity: Allow materials to buffer extra moisture when damp and release it when dry by increasing outdoor ventilation when it's dry outside and closing windows when it's wet outside.

   d. **Manage indoor temperatures:** Use heating and cooling to maintain consistent indoor temperatures and reduce condensation.

   e. **Address cold spots:** Use insulation and vapor barriers to manage and prevent condensation on cold surfaces.

4. **Properly Insulate and Seal (Preventative Maintenance)**

   a. **Insulate pipes and exterior walls:** This prevents condensation and maintains consistent temperatures.

   b. **Seal windows and doors:** Properly seal them to avoid moisture intrusion.

   c. **Learn to anticipate the failure of aging materials:** Regularly inspect and replace aging materials before they fail.

Ensure Proper Ventilation

5. **Use exhaust fans in high-moisture areas,** such as bathrooms, kitchens, and laundry rooms.

   a. **Be cautious about opening windows or using fans:** Avoid during high outdoor humidity, pollution, severe weather, or cold climates to prevent additional moisture or contaminants.

6. **Maintain HVAC Systems**

   a. **Clean and service HVAC systems regularly:** Ensure filters are changed and that systems are debris-free.

   b. **Use HVAC with humidity control:** Systems with humidity control features can help maintain optimal indoor humidity levels.

7. **Use Safe Cleaning Products**

   a. **Use non-toxic cleaners like Branch Basics**—Especially in high-moisture areas like bathrooms and basements.

   b. **Avoid toxic treatments and antimicrobials:** Focus on safe, non-toxic options.

8. **Don't Trap Moisture**

   a. **Avoid moisture-resistant materials that trap moisture:** Ensure building materials allow moisture to escape.

   b. **Properly ventilate enclosed spaces:** Use smart membranes or moisture-resistant barriers that allow moisture to escape.

9. **Improve Drainage**

   a. **Ensure proper grading:** The ground should slope away from your home's foundation to prevent water accumulation.

   b. **Maintain gutters and downspouts:** Clean regularly to prevent clogs and ensure water is directed away from the house.

Regular Physical Cleaning and Maintenance

10. **Clean regularly:** Use safe, non-toxic cleaning products.

    a. **Inspect for mold:** Regularly inspect your home for signs of mold and address any issues immediately.

    b. **Know who to call and when:** Seek professional help for issues you cannot address.

||||||||||||||||||||||||||||||||||||||||||||||||||||||||||||||||||||||||||||||||||||||||||||||||||||||||||||||||||||||||||||||||||||||||||||

||||||||||||||||||||||||||||||||||||||||||||||||||||||||||||||||||||||||||||||||||||||||||||||||||||||||||||||||||||||||||||||||||||||||||||

Essentials: Simplifying the Complexities

We are far from completely understanding the complexities of mold, and our knowledge base is continually changing and expanding. Even so, it is not necessary to understand every detail to manage mold effectively. Many decisions can be made based on general observations and following the most important principles:

- Keep it dry

- If it gets wet, dry it quickly.

- If it can't be dried quickly enough to prevent mold growth, use physical means to isolate and control the infestation while minimizing disturbances to contain the spread of spores and fragments.

- Physical removal is the primary means for remediating mold.

- Avoid attempts to kill the mold. This is more likely to spread the mold, increase toxicity, and have other unintended consequences, especially for people with hypersensitivity.

- Remediation by relocation is the best. Send the moldy debris to the landfill.

- Clean effectively.

- Use quality control and monitoring methods to ensure the mold has been effectively remediated and cleaned.

- Anticipate building memory that must be addressed after remediation is complete.

- Always use the least toxic and effective means available. This rarely involves trying to kill mold. Dead mold is almost as big a problem as live mold (and sometimes dead mold is a significantly more significant problem).

- If chemicals, even natural ones like essential oils, are used in ways toxic enough to kill mold spores, it is also toxic sufficient to affect hypersensitive people, kids, and pets adversely.

- Chemical methods for remediation and cleaning often interfere with the ability to test to determine if problems remain. It is extremely rare for a chemical approach to be necessary or effective.

- Before reconstructing, ensure the water source that caused the problem has been corrected and will not reoccur.

- Do Not Trap Moisture by trying to encapsulate mold in place on nutritive materials like wood or gypsum wallboard. Mold can still grow under and on top of antimicrobial coatings if moisture is present.

References

Penn State. (2019, June 28). Pig-Pen effect: Mixing skin oil and ozone can produce a personal pollution cloud. *ScienceDaily*. Retrieved October 13, 2024, from https://www.sciencedaily.com/releases/2019/06/190628120533.htm

Rabinovitch, N., Liu, A. H., Zhang, L., Dutton, S. J., Murphy, J. R., & Gelfand, E. W. (2005). Importance of the personal endotoxin cloud in school-age children with asthma. *Journal of Allergy and Clinical Immunology, 116*(5), 1053–1057. https://doi.org/10.1016/j.jaci.2005.08.046

Fugler, D., & Bowser, D. (2002). Reducing particulate levels in houses. In *Proceedings: Indoor Air 2002*. Canada Mortgage and Housing Corporation; Bowser Technical Inc.

Banta, J., Passmore, B., & Holland, J. (2005). Modeling the equilibrium spore load for a building. In E. Johanning (Ed.), *Bioaerosols, fungi, bacteria, mycotoxins and human health* (pp. 262–269). Fungal Research Group Foundation Inc.

Hodgson, M., & Scott, R. J. (1999). Prevalence of fungi in carpet dust samples. In E. Johanning (Ed.), *Bioaerosols, fungi, and mycotoxins: Health effects, assessment, prevention, and control* (pp. 268–274). Boyd Printing Company.

Shoemaker, R. (2008b). SAIIE meets ERMI: Correlation of indices of human health and building health. *AIHCE presentation*, Minneapolis, Minnesota, June 2008. Center for Research on Biotoxin Associated Illnesses. Retrieved from https://www.survivingmold.com

Mold Gallery: Illustrated Profiles of Important Fungi

TYPES OF MOLD

When viewed under a microscope, mold reveals a diverse world. These tiny fungi come in many shapes, sizes, and colors, making it easy to misidentify one type for another. The shapes seen under a microscope are affected by the collection and preparation methods used for the sample. The mold consists of long, delicate thread-like structures called hyphae, which form a network called mycelium, responsible for nutrient absorption and growth. Conidia are the spores responsible for fungal reproduction and dispersion. The arrangement of conidia on the hyphae can vary: some molds have aerial hyphae that lift spores into the air, like how a dandelion raises its seeds, while others create sticky masses of spores that cling to insects and animals, much like weed burrs on socks. Some spores are propelled through the air by a sling-shot-like distribution mechanism triggered by rain droplets.

This diversity in structure and dispersal mechanisms, combined with the microscopic size of the mold, makes distinguishing between different types based solely on appearance challenging. Molds may appear to mimic one another due to limitations in detection techniques when looking at them under a microscope. Scientists use a technique called MSQPCR (Mold-Specific Quantitative Polymerase Chain Reaction) for the genetic identification of molds, providing more precise information about the present types. This has led to the reclassification of some organisms, bringing further clarity. However, MSQPCR can also add confusion, as similar DNA segments can make it difficult to differentiate between molds that look alike but are quite different in behavior and habitat preferences.

To complicate matters, molds are constantly evolving, with some types becoming more common in certain areas and altering the biotoxins they emit. Mold adapts to its surroundings based on stresses or controls it encounters. Different nutritional sources can change mold's color, and water activity levels influence growth stages. The hyphae's appearance cannot distinguish mold types since they tend to look very alike. Differences between the appearance of conidia or spores are often the most important methods for determining the type of mold visually using a microscope.

The illustrations in this section are based on various microscopic examinations and aim to convey mold's tremendous diversity. They are artists' renditions created by examining photomicrographs of mold. The collection and preparation process usually involves scraping, flattening, and distorting the mold from how it would appear in its natural state. Think of this like the difference between a preserved flower that has been dried and pressed flat versus one growing in the garden. These depictions help to provide a clearer understanding of mold's diversity and complexity despite the inherent alterations caused by the sample preparation and microscopic examination process.

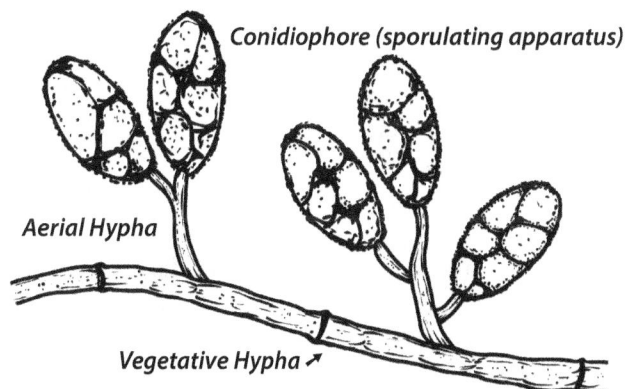

Figure 2-1: Alternaria (Ulocladium) chartarum is a mold that is frequently found growing on chronically wet gypsum board paper surfaces. It is an example of a mold associated with chronic water damage that is not included as one of the 36 mold species commonly offered by laboratories offering ERMI panel analysis. It should be noted that the genus Ulocladium has been reclassified to Alternaria based on genetic sequencing. Specialty laboratories may offer this organism upon request.

CLASSIFICATION AND NOMENCLATURE

Life forms are scientifically classified by their genus and species names. For example, house cats are known as *Felis catus*, while humans are *Homo sapiens*. Dogs and wolves, despite their different temperaments, belong to the same species, *Canis lupus*. The dog is a subspecies called *Canis lupus familiaris* to distinguish it from the wolf, *Canis lupus*. The coyote, *Canis latrans*, is a separate species but belongs to the same genus.

Molds vary by genus and species; their impacts can range from edible to toxic. For example:

- *Penicillium camembeti* is used to make Camembert and Brie cheese.

- *P. chrysogenum* is used for penicillin antibiotics.

- *P. roqueforti* is essential for Roquefort and blue cheese.

- *P. brevicompactum* can be harmful; it's often found in water-damaged buildings and produces a toxin called mycophenolic acid.

UNDERSTANDING KEY TERMS

Spore Equivalents: "Spore Equivalents" is a measure used to express total mold presence in a sample based on the amount of fungal DNA detected. This includes DNA from all fungal structures—spores, hyphae, and fragments—and is expressed as the equivalent number of spores. Rather than counting only intact spores, this method assesses the total DNA content to provide a fuller picture of mold exposure, capturing all cellular material that may impact indoor air quality.

Geometric Mean: The geometric mean is a statistical average used to understand typical mold concentrations in an indoor environment, especially when there is a wide range of values. It minimizes the impact of extremely high or low numbers, offering a clearer picture of normal mold levels expected in homes. This approach is particularly helpful when mold spore counts vary greatly across different samples, such as when some homes have abnormally high levels due to growth from water damage.

Opportunistic Pathogen: A microorganism (like certain bacteria, fungi, or viruses) that doesn't usually cause harm in healthy people but can lead to infections when someone's immune system is weakened. This can happen due to illness or medications that suppress the immune system, such as Prolonged or high-dose corticosteroid use (like prednisone), immunosuppressants used after organ transplants (such as tacrolimus or cyclosporine), or chemotherapy drugs for cancer treatment. These medications reduce the body's ability to fight off infections, allowing opportunistic pathogens to cause disease.

Water Activity: Water activity, or A_w, measures the moisture on a material's surface that is available for mold growth. It directly corresponds to the relative humidity at that surface (e.g., an A_w of 0.75 equals 75% surface humidity). Cooler surfaces can increase surface humidity and support mold growth, even if the surrounding air feels dry.

HUD/EPA BASE Study: The HUD/EPA Building Assessment and Survey Evaluation (BASE) Study was a comprehensive investigation of indoor air quality and building-related health effects in a representative sample of U.S. office buildings. It included an evaluation of mold by collecting data on visible mold growth, moisture problems, and air and surface sampling to assess microbial contamination. You will find information referenced multiple times from this important study in the following section. (Vesper, 2007)

THE GENUS ASPERGILLUS

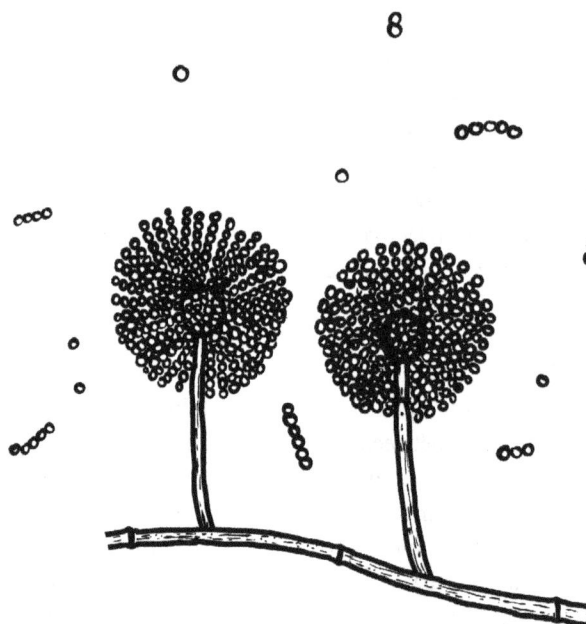

Figure 2-2: The genus Aspergillus has been estimated to consist of over 1000 species. New species continue to be discovered. All species of Aspergillus molds share several common characteristics that influence their behavior, growth, and potential impact on indoor environments.

Common characteristics of the genus *Aspergillus*

- **Spore Production**: All *Aspergillus* species produce spores (conidia), which are lightweight and easily dispersed by air currents. These spores are one of the primary ways mold spreads and can lead to indoor contamination.

- **Moisture Requirement**: While some species can tolerate drier conditions, all *Aspergillus* molds require some moisture for growth, whether from liquid water or high humidity levels. They are commonly found in environments with water damage, high humidity, or surface condensation.

- **Temperature Tolerance**: *Aspergillus* species generally thrive in warm environments, with many species capable of growing in a wide temperature range. Some can even tolerate extremely cold or hot temperatures, allowing them to colonize various indoor environments.

- **Organic Material Utilization**: These molds typically grow on organic materials as a food source. In buildings, they are often found on wood, drywall, carpet, and other cellulose-based substances. Many types of *Aspergillus* molds grow on food waste and are a major composter.

- **Health Risks**: Many *Aspergillus* species produce allergens and biotoxins, which can pose health risks, especially for individuals with CIRS, weakened immune systems, asthma, or allergies. Some species, like *Aspergillus fumigatus*, can cause more severe conditions, including infectious disease such as aspergillosis.

- **Survival in Diverse Conditions**: *Aspergillus* species are known for their resilience and ability to survive in a variety of environmental conditions, including lower nutrient levels, making them common in both indoor and outdoor settings.

Aspergillus flavus

The HUD/EPA BASE study found *Aspergillus flavus* in 36% of U.S. homes, typically at low background levels of around two spore equivalents per milligram of dust in homes without water damage. In water-damaged homes, levels can be significantly higher, with the highest recorded at 4,768 spore equivalents per milligram of dust. *Aspergillus flavus* requires a minimum water activity level of 0.74 to grow, with optimal growth at a water activity level of 0.98. (Pitt, 2009) (Flannigan, 2001) (Hung, 2005) (ACGIH, 1999) Under these conditions, it can thrive on cellulose-based materials such as wood, paper, cardboard, paper-faced gypsum board, and paper-backed insulation. *Aspergillus flavus* is an allergen that can also trigger respiratory issues like hypersensitivity pneumonitis and is an opportunistic pathogen capable of causing sinus infections, eye inflammation, skin infections, deep tissue infections, and bone infections. (Gravensen, 1994) (Kurup V. P., 2000) *A. flavus* is also a major producer of aflatoxin B1. This highly toxic and carcinogenic compound can contaminate peanut-based products, leading to FDA regulation in food. It can produce additional biotoxins, including sterigmatocystin, cyclopiazonic acid, kojic acid, β-nitropropionic acid, aspertoxin, aflatrem, gliotoxin, and aspergillic acid. (Gravensen, 1994) (Abbott, 2002) (Bennett, 2003)

Aspergillus montevidensis (Eurotium amstelodamii)

The HUD/EPA BASE Study found *Aspergillus amstelodami* in 98% of U.S. homes, typically at moderate levels of around 155 spore equivalents per milligram of dust in homes without water damage. Levels in damp or severely contaminated homes can be much higher, with the highest recorded at 1,100,000 spore equivalents per milligram of dust. Formerly known as *Eurotium amstelodami*, genetic studies have identified it as the sexual form of *Aspergillus*, leading to its reclassification as *Aspergillus montevidensis*. So, they are both the same organism. It tolerates drier conditions (0.70 at 25°C) compared to most other molds associated with water damage but but may grow at up to 0.96 water activity. (Pitt, 2009) (Flannigan, 2001) (Hung, 2005) (ACGIH, 1999) It can colonize cellulose-based construction materials and is commonly found outdoors in wheat chaff and other similar plant materials. While not known to produce biotoxins, *A. amstelodami* can cause allergic and asthmatic reactions and has been linked to respiratory health issues such as hypersensitivity pneumonitis. Proper ventilation and moisture management are essential to prevent its colonization in indoor environments.

Aspergillus fumigatus

The HUD/EPA BASE Study found *Aspergillus fumigatus* in 62% of U.S. homes, typically at low background levels of around three spore equivalents per milligram of dust in homes without water damage. In water-damaged homes, levels can be significantly higher, with the highest recorded at 5,800 spore equivalents per milligram of dust. Under elevated moisture conditions, *A. fumigatus* can colonize construction materials such as wood, drywall, and insulation. It requires moderate moisture, with water activity ranging from 0.80 to 0.95. This mold is known for its rapid growth, often forming visible colonies within days. (Pitt, 2009) (Flannigan, 2001) (Hung, 2005) (ACGIH, 1999) *A. fumigatus* is commonly found outdoors in soil, decaying organic matter, compost, and plant debris. It is an opportunistic pathogen, posing significant health risks to individuals with compromised immune systems or respiratory conditions. It is also a common allergen, known to trigger allergic reactions, especially in individuals with mold sensitivities, and has been linked to respiratory health issues such as hypersensitivity pneumonitis. Additionally, *A. fumigatus* produces gliotoxin, a potent biotoxin associated with immune suppression. (Gravensen, 1994) (Abbott, 2002) (Bennett, 2003)

Aspergillus niger

The HUD/EPA BASE Study found *Aspergillus niger* in 69% of U.S. homes, typically at moderate levels of around four spore equivalents per milligram of dust in homes without water damage. In water-damaged homes, levels can be much higher, with the highest recorded at 6,200 spore equivalents per milligram of dust. *A. niger* is known for its relatively fast growth, forming visible colonies on substrates like wood, drywall, insulation, and paper products, particularly in moisture-prone areas. It can grow across various moisture conditions, with a minimum water activity of 0.74 and optimal growth at 0.98. (Pitt, 2009) (Flannigan, 2001) (Hung, 2005) (ACGIH, 1999) Outdoors, *A. niger* is commonly found in soil and decaying plant material. It can cause allergic reactions in sensitive people, leading to hypersensitivity pneumonitis at high exposure levels. While primarily associated with less severe opportunistic infections, such as fungal ear infections (otomycosis), it has rarely been implicated in opportunistic invasive aspergillosis. *A. niger* is not typically known for producing significant biotoxins, but certain strains can produce low levels of ochratoxin A under specific conditions.

Aspergillus ochraceus

The HUD/EPA BASE Study found *Aspergillus ochraceus* in 27% of U.S. homes, typically at low levels of around two spore equivalents per milligram of dust in homes without water damage. In severely contaminated homes, levels can be much higher, with the highest recorded at 12,000 spore equivalents per milligram of dust. *A. ochraceus* can colonize various construction materials, including wood, drywall, insulation, cardboard, and wallpaper, particularly in areas with elevated moisture or water damage, such as HVAC system coil and condensate collection areas. It grows optimally in moderately humid environments, with water activity ranging from 0.80 to 0.90, though it can tolerate levels as low as 0.76. (Pitt, 2009) (Flannigan, 2001) (Hung, 2005) (ACGIH, 1999) Outdoors, it is commonly

found in soil and decaying plant matter and can contaminate damp agricultural products like grains, beans, and coffee. It can cause allergic reactions in sensitive people and lead to hypersensitivity pneumonitis at high exposure levels. *A. ochraceus* is known for producing ochratoxin A. This potent biotoxin is potentially carcinogenic in humans. (Gravensen, 1994) (Abbott, 2002) (Bennett, 2003)

Aspergillus penicillioides

The HUD/EPA BASE Study found *Aspergillus penicillioides* in 90% of U.S. homes, typically at moderate levels of around 91 spore equivalents per milligram of dust in homes without water damage. In severely contaminated, water-damaged homes, levels can reach as high as 6,000,000 spore equivalents per milligram of dust, indicating severe contamination. This mold species can rapidly grow, form visible colonies within days under suitable conditions, and thrive in areas with elevated humidity. It colonizes construction materials such as wood, drywall, insulation, and paper. *A. penicillioides* grows in environments with high humidity, requiring a water activity level as low as 0.585 (Stevenson, 2017), though its optimal growth occurs between 0.91 and 0.93. (Pitt, 2009) (Flannigan, 2001) (Hung, 2005) (ACGIH, 1999) It has been identified in ancient works of art, such as the brown spots found on the tomb paintings of the Egyptian Pharaoh Tutankhamun. It can even grow on materials containing lead with concentrations of 1000 ppm found in lead-containing paints. (Harvard Gazette). It is known to cause respiratory issues from hypersensitivity pneumonitis and allergies in sensitive individuals. Exposure to *A. penicillioides* has been linked to biotoxin-related inflammatory conditions like CIRS, although the specific biotoxins have not been identified. (Shoemaker R. &., 2006)

||||||||||||||||||||||||||||||||||||||||||||||||||||||||||||||||||||||||||||||||||||||||||||||||||||||||||||||||||||||||||||||||||||||||||||

King Tut's Tomb

King Tutankhamun's tomb, discovered in 1922, has fascinated the world not only for its treasures but also for the unusual microbial growth observed inside. Unlike other ancient tombs, King Tut's tomb exhibited significant mold growth on its walls and artifacts, prompting scientific investigation into the reasons behind this phenomenon. One theory suggests that the unusual mold growth may be linked to the fact that Tutankhamun died unexpectedly at a young age, around 18 or 19 years old. This sudden death may have rushed the completion of the tomb's interior, leaving insufficient time for plaster, paint, and other materials to properly dry before the tomb was sealed. The moisture trapped inside created ideal conditions for mold growth.

One of the key mold organisms found in the tomb is *Aspergillus penicillioides*, which is notable for its ability to grow at some of the lowest water activity (A_w) levels recorded. This characteristic allows it to thrive in environments with minimal moisture, making it a persistent issue in locations like ancient tombs, where the atmosphere becomes extremely dry after initial sealing. *A. penicillioides* is particularly adept at growing on organic materials such as paintings, wood, and textiles, which were abundant in the tomb. Even though the tomb eventually became dry, the initial dampness likely enabled this mold to establish itself on the delicate antiquities left in King Tut's burial chamber.

Additionally, *Aspergillus niger* and *Aspergillus flavus* were also found, contributing to the black and brown staining observed on the tomb walls. While these molds usually require higher moisture levels to thrive, their presence further supports the theory that the tomb's rushed preparation and sealing left a damp environment where mold could flourish. The growth of these fungi on the tomb's paintings, statues, and other organic materials underscores the preservation challenges, especially when mold species like *A. penicillins* can survive in even the most arid environments once established. (Harvard Gazette)

||||||||||||||||||||||||||||||||||||||||||||||||||||||||||||||||||||||||||||||||||||||||||||||||||||||||||||||||||||||||||||||||||||||||||||||||||

Aspergillus restrictus

The HUD/EPA BASE Study found *Aspergillus restrictus* in 12% of U.S. homes, typically at low levels of around two spore equivalents per milligram of dust in homes without water damage. However, levels reached 25,000 spore equivalents per milligram of dust in a severely contaminated home. *A. restrictus* can colonize construction materials such as wood, drywall, insulation, and paper products, particularly in areas with elevated moisture. It thrives in moderate humidity, with a minimum water activity reported between 0.70 and 0.76 and optimal growth between 0.82 and 0.93. (Pitt, 2009) (Flannigan, 2001) (Hung, 2005) (ACGIH, 1999) It can form visible colonies within days under suitable moisture conditions. Outdoors, *A. restrictus* is found in soil and decaying plant material. While not as extensively studied as other molds, exposure to *A. restrictus* and its potential biotoxins can cause respiratory issues and allergies, especially in mold-sensitive individuals. Its role in health issues is less documented compared to other molds.

Aspergillus sclerotiorum

The HUD/EPA BASE Study found *Aspergillus sclerotiorum* in 26% of U.S. homes, typically at low levels of around two spore equivalents per milligram of dust in homes without water damage. However, in one study home, levels reached 890 spore equivalents per milligram of dust. (Pitt, 2009) (Flannigan, 2001) (Hung, 2005) (ACGIH, 1999) *A. sclerotiorum* can grow rapidly under suitable moisture conditions, forming visible colonies within days. Although not typically associated with home environments, it can colonize organic materials if moisture is present. Outdoors, *A. sclerotiorum,* is commonly found in soil, plant debris, and marine or saline environments. (Ma, 2019) While not known for significant biotoxin production, exposure to its spores or secondary metabolites may cause respiratory or allergic reactions, particularly in individuals with mold sensitivities.

Aspergillus sydowii

The HUD/EPA BASE Study found *Aspergillus sydowii* in 29% of U.S. homes, typically at low levels of around three spore equivalents per milligram of dust in homes without water damage. In severely contaminated homes, levels can be much higher, with the highest recorded at 14,666 spore equivalents per milligram of dust. *A. sydowii* can colonize organic materials if sufficient moisture is present, particularly in environments with a water activity between 0.76 and 0.96, thriving at around 0.90 or higher. (Pitt, 2009) (Flannigan, 2001) (Hung, 2005) (ACGIH, 1999) It is commonly found outdoors in natural environments, such as soil, marine sediments, and coastal regions, where it often grows on decaying organic matter. Although *A. sydowii* is not typically linked to human health issues, exposure to its spores or secondary metabolites may cause respiratory or allergic reactions, particularly in mold-sensitive individuals. Unlike some other species, *A. sydowii* is not known for producing biotoxins.

Aspergillus unguis

The HUD/EPA BASE Study found *Aspergillus unguis* in 20% of U.S. homes, typically at low levels of around two spore equivalents per milligram of dust in homes without water damage. However, in cases of severe contamination, levels can reach as high as 5,588 spore equivalents per milligram of dust. *A. unguis* can colonize organic materials in indoor environments if sufficient moisture is present. It thrives in environments with moderately high water activity, typically around 0.90 or higher, and can form visible colonies relatively quickly under suitable conditions. (Pitt, 2009) (Flannigan, 2001) (Hung, 2005) (ACGIH, 1999) Outdoors, it is often found in soil, decaying plant material, and organic-rich substrates. While *A. unguis* is not typically linked to significant health issues, exposure to its spores may cause respiratory and allergic reactions in mold-sensitive individuals. It is not known for major toxin production, but it may produce secondary metabolites with various effects.

Aspergillus ustus

The HUD/EPA BASE Study found *Aspergillus ustus* in 40% of U.S. homes, typically at low levels of around two spore equivalents per milligram of dust in homes without water damage. In one home with higher contamination, the level reached 738 spore equivalents per milligram of dust. (Pitt, 2009) (Flannigan, 2001) (Hung, 2005) (ACGIH, 1999) While *A. ustus* is primarily an outdoor mold found in soil and decaying plant materials, it can travel indoors. This mold thrives in environments rich in organic matter, such as leaves, wood, and other plant debris. Though *A. ustus* is not commonly linked to significant health issues, exposure to its spores may cause respiratory or allergic reactions, especially in mold-sensitive individuals. It is not known for biotoxin production but may, under rare conditions, produce secondary metabolites with various effects.

Aspergillus versicolor

The HUD/EPA BASE Study found *Aspergillus versicolor* in 30% of U.S. homes, typically at low levels of around two spore equivalents per milligram of dust in homes without water damage. In severely contaminated homes, levels can reach up to 3,574 spore equivalents per milligram of dust. *A. versicolor* is commonly associated with water-damaged indoor environments, particularly on wetted or damp wallboard and materials like wood, drywall, insulation, and paper products. It can grow relatively quickly under moderate moisture conditions, with a water activity level between 0.80 and 0.90. (Pitt, 2009) (Flannigan, 2001) (Hung, 2005) (ACGIH, 1999) It has been frequently linked to subterranean termite infestations. Outdoors can be found in soil and plant debris. *A. versicolor* is known for producing the biotoxins sterigmatocystin and versicolorin. (Gravensen, 1994) (Abbott, 2002) (Bennett, 2003) It is also associated with health issues such as respiratory problems, hypersensitivity pneumonitis, allergies, and conditions like Chronic Inflammatory Response Syndrome (CIRS) and Sick Building Syndrome (SBS).

THE GENUS *CLADOSPORIUM*

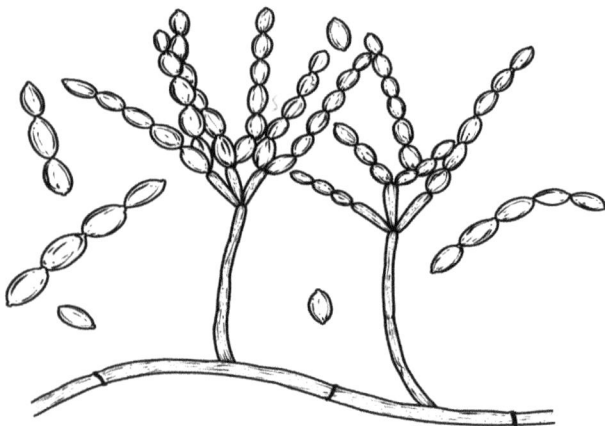

Figure 2-3: Cladosporium is one of the most common molds found in outdoor and indoor environments, with over 700 species identified. These molds thrive in various conditions and are known for their resilience. Species of Cladosporium share key characteristics that influence their growth and impact on indoor environments.

Common characteristics of the genus *Cladosporium*

- **Spore Production**: All *Cladosporium* species produce lightweight conidia (spores) that are easily dispersed through the air. They can travel long distances through air currents.

- **Moisture Requirement**: *Cladosporium* molds prefer environments with high humidity or moisture. While they can survive in lower moisture levels compared to other molds, they are typically found in areas with dampness, such as bathrooms, basements, and areas with water damage. They are also frequently found on damp building materials like wood and wallpaper.

- **Temperature Tolerance**: Many *Cladosporium* species thrive in moderate temperatures, but they can grow in a wide range of environments, from cold to warm conditions. Some species at temperatures found in refrigerators/freezers have even been documented growing (very slowly) on ice, making them common contaminants in food storage areas.

- **Organic Material Utilization**: *Cladosporium* molds typically grow on organic materials, utilizing them as a food source. Indoors, they can be found on a variety of surfaces, including wood, drywall, carpet, and insulation, particularly on colder surfaces where condensation moisture has formed. They can also grow on food products, painted surfaces, textiles, and household dust.

- **Health Risks**: Although *Cladosporium* is generally considered to be less harmful than some other mold genera, it can cause allergic reactions and respiratory issues, especially in individuals with mold sensitivities, asthma, or compromised immune systems. Exposure to large quantities of *Cladosporium* spores may lead to symptoms such as coughing, sneezing, and throat irritation.

- **Survival in Diverse Conditions**: *Cladosporium* species are known for their hardiness and ability to survive in a variety of environmental conditions. They can grow in areas with minimal nutrient availability and are found both indoors and outdoors. Outdoors, they are often found in decaying plant matter, soil, and on leaf surfaces, which makes them a frequent contributor to outdoor spore counts.

Cladosporium cladosporioides

The HUD/EPA BASE Study found *Cladosporium cladosporioides* (Type 1) in 99% of U.S. homes, reaching up to 140,000 spore equivalents per milligram of dust, indicating significant growth in some environments. Type 2 was present in 70% of homes, with levels as high as 4,100 spore equivalents per milligram of dust. Both types are primarily considered outdoor molds but can grow indoors under certain conditions, particularly in areas with condensation or high humidity. Type 1 typically shows moderate levels indoors, with a geometric mean of 331 spore equivalents per milligram, while Type 2 usually shows lower levels, with a geometric mean of 4 spore equivalents per milligram. These species grow on colder surfaces, such as poorly insulated walls or windows with condensation, and thrive in cooler temperatures, even down to freezing. Outdoors, both Type 1 and Type 2, exist in beneficial relationships with living tree leaves, each supporting the others beneficially; in fall, their role changes and becomes common in soil and decaying plant material, playing a beneficial role in breaking down the leaves where they formerly grew. Exposure to *Cladosporium* species may cause respiratory issues or allergies, especially in sensitive individuals. Still, these molds are not known to produce mycotoxins, but they gain a competitive advantage by thriving in cooler environments.

Cladosporium herbarum

The HUD/EPA BASE Study found *Cladosporium herbarum* in 84% of U.S. homes, with spore levels reaching up to 52,000 spore equivalents per milligram of dust in some environments, indicating severe contamination. Typically, *C. herbarum* grows at moderate levels indoors, with a geometric mean of 31 spore equivalents per milligram, but it can grow significantly under favorable conditions. While primarily an outdoor mold, it can colonize indoor environments, especially in areas with fluctuating moisture levels, ranging from damp to very wet. *C. herbarum* grows well at cooler temperatures, tolerating conditions as low as -10°C (14°F) and up to 32°C (90°F), allowing it to grow slowly even on frozen materials. It is one of the common forms of *Cladosporium* that grows on condensation films on painted window sills. Outdoors, it plays a beneficial role in plant decay and soil formation. *C. herbarum* is a major allergen known to exacerbate asthma and hay fever, causing symptoms like sneezing, coughing, and skin irritation. However, it is not known to produce biotoxins.

Cladosporium sphaerospermum

The HUD/EPA BASE Study found *Cladosporium sphaerospermum* in 82% of U.S. homes, typically at low levels of around 13 spore equivalents per milligram of dust. In some severely contaminated environments, levels can reach up to 23,000 spore equivalents per milligram of dust, indicating significant growth in the vicinity. *C. sphaerospermum* is often found indoors, particularly in condensation areas, such as on windows and even in mattresses, where perspiration provides moisture and salt, supporting its growth as a halotolerant microorganism. In the outdoors, it is commonly found in soil and decaying plant material. This species is known to cause allergic reactions and asthma in sensitive individuals and can occasionally lead to skin, nail, or sinus infections, with lung infections being rare. However, *C. sphaerospermum* is not known to produce significant toxins.

THE GENUS *PENICILLIUM*

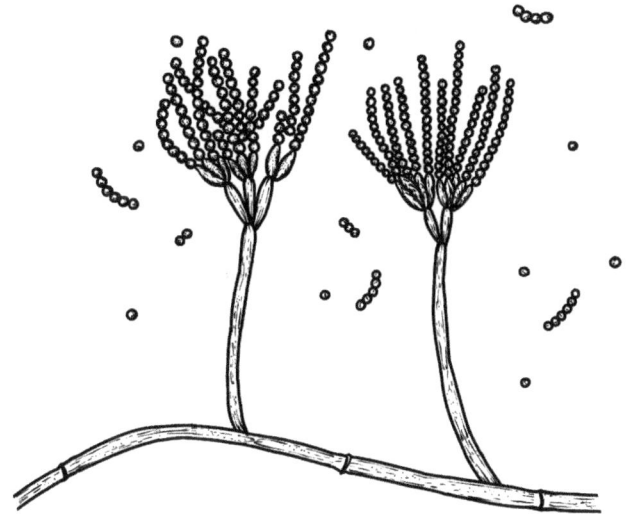

Figure 2-4: The genus Penicillium consists of over 300 species, with more being discovered regularly. These molds are widely distributed in various environments, including soil, decaying organic matter, and indoor settings. Penicillium molds share several common characteristics that influence their behavior, growth, and impact on indoor environments.

Common characteristics of the genus *Penicillium*

- **Spore Production**: All *Penicillium* species produce lightweight conidia (spores) that are easily dispersed through the air. These spores contribute to indoor contamination and can spread quickly throughout a building, especially in environments with water damage.

- **Moisture Requirement**: *Penicillium* species thrive in environments with moisture, such as water-damaged or humid areas. They require some level of moisture for growth, although some species can survive in relatively dry conditions. *Penicillium* is commonly found in damp areas like bathrooms, basements, and poorly ventilated spaces.

- **Temperature Tolerance**: They can grow in a range of temperatures, from cold to warm environments. Some *Penicillium* species, responsible for food spoilage, can grow at refrigeration temperatures, making them common contaminants in food storage areas.

- **Organic Material Utilization**: *Penicillium* species use organic materials as a food source, growing on a wide range of substrates, including wood, drywall, carpet, insulation, and food products. They are also known for playing a significant role in the decomposition of organic matter, helping to break down cellulose-based materials.

- **Health Risks**: Many *Penicillium* species are known to produce allergens and mycotoxins, which can pose health risks, particularly to individuals with asthma, allergies, or compromised immune systems. Exposure to high levels of *Penicillium* spores or mycotoxins can lead to respiratory issues and other health complications.

- **Survive Diverse Conditions**: *Penicillium* molds are highly resilient and can survive adverse conditions, including low nutrients. They thrive in both indoor and outdoor settings, making them common in homes, especially in areas prone to moisture.

Penicillium brevicompactum

The HUD/EPA BASE Study found *Penicillium brevicompactum* in 52% of U.S. homes, typically at low levels of around five spore equivalents per milligram of dust, with a maximum recorded level of 6,200 spore equivalents per milligram. It colonizes indoor materials such as composite woods, paper-clad gypsum board, Kraft paper vapor barriers, and cellulose-based products like cardboard. Thriving in moderate moisture conditions with an A_w range of 0.81 to 0.88. (Pitt, 2009) (Flannigan, 2001) (Hung, 2005) (ACGIH, 1999) It can also grow in areas affected by saltwater flooding. In the outdoors, it is found in soil, decaying plant matter, and compost. Exposure can irritate the respiratory system, causing coughing, wheezing, and allergic reactions. Additionally, it produces mycotoxins such as patulin, citrinin, and mycophenolic acid, which may lead to more severe health effects with prolonged exposure. (Gravensen, 1994) (Abbott, 2002) (Bennett, 2003)

Penicillium chrysogenum

The HUD/EPA BASE Study found *Penicillium chrysogenum* in 66% of U.S. homes, typically at low levels of around five spore equivalents per milligram of dust. However, in some cases, levels can reach up to 38,000 spore equivalents per milligram, indicating severe contamination. *P. chrysogenum* can colonize indoor materials like wood, drywall, and cellulose-containing substrates, especially in areas with elevated moisture or water damage. It thrives in moderate moisture conditions, with a water activity range of 0.79 to 0.95, and exhibits rapid growth when conditions are favorable. (Pitt, 2009) (Flannigan, 2001) (Hung, 2005) (ACGIH, 1999) Outdoors, it is commonly found in soil, decaying organic matter, and on plant surfaces. Although *P. chrysogenum* is not typically considered a significant health concern, it may produce allergic reactions and volatile organic compounds (VOCs) contributing to musty odors. It is more widely known for its role in producing the antibiotic penicillin and other biotechnological applications rather than for causing adverse health effects.

Penicillium corylophilum

The HUD/EPA BASE Study found *Penicillium corylophilum* in 17% of U.S. homes, typically at low levels of around two spore equivalents per milligram of dust, with occasional higher concentrations reaching up to 2,600 spore equivalents per milligram, indicating significant contamination in some cases. This mold is less common indoors but can grow under favorable conditions, such as areas with elevated moisture and organic materials like wood, drywall, and cellulose-based products. *P. corylophilum* thrives in environments with moderate water activity, ranging from 0.90 to 0.95, and exhibits moderate growth rates under suitable conditions. (Pitt, 2009) (Flannigan, 2001) (Hung, 2005) (ACGIH, 1999) Outdoors it is found in soil, on plant surfaces, and in decaying organic matter. Although *P. corylophilum* is not typically considered a major health concern, it may produce volatile organic compounds (VOCs) that contribute to musty odors but are generally not considered highly toxic.

Penicillium crustosum

The HUD/EPA BASE Study found *Penicillium crustosum* in 8% of U.S. homes, with typically low levels of around one spore equivalent per milligram of dust. However, some homes showed much higher contamination, reaching up to 8,275 spore equivalents per milligram. While uncommon indoors, *P. crustosum* can colonize materials such as wood, drywall, and other cellulose-based substrates, particularly in moisture-damaged areas. It thrives in environments with moderate to high water activity, ranging from 0.85 to 0.95, and can grow relatively quickly under suitable conditions. (Pitt, 2009) (Flannigan, 2001) (Hung, 2005) (ACGIH, 1999) Outdoors, *P. crustosum* is found in soil, plant surfaces, and decaying organic matter. Although not typically associated with significant health concerns, *P. crustosum* may produce volatile organic compounds (VOCs) that contribute to musty odors, but it is not widely known for biotoxin production.

Penicillium spinulosum

The HUD/EPA BASE Study found *Penicillium spinulosum* in 20% of U.S. homes, typically at low levels of around one spore equivalent per milligram of dust, although higher levels reaching up to 1,901 spore equivalents per milligram indicate potential contamination in some cases. *P. spinulosum* is commonly found growing on home surfaces with high humidity, particularly on painted, varnished, or other organic materials where condensation can form. It thrives in environments with moderate to high water activity, ranging from 0.80 to 0.95, and grows at moderate rates, with visible colonies forming under suitable conditions. (Pitt, 2009) (Flannigan, 2001) (Hung, 2005) (ACGIH, 1999) Outdoors, *P. spinulosum* is found in soil, plant surfaces, and decaying organic matter. While it is not typically considered a major health concern, *P. spinulosum* is not well studied for its potential health effects and is not primarily known for producing biotoxins.

Talaromyces variabilis (formerly Penicillium variable)

The HUD/EPA BASE Study found *Talaromyces variabilis* in 50% of U.S. homes, typically at low levels of around three spore equivalents per milligram of dust. However, in some cases, levels reached up to 1,023 spore equivalents per milligram, indicating contamination. *Talaromyces variabilis* can colonize indoor materials like wood, drywall, and cellulose-based substrates, especially in areas with elevated moisture or water damage. It thrives in environments with moderate to high water activity, ranging from 0.85 to 0.95, and forms visible colonies relatively quickly under suitable conditions. (Pitt, 2009) (Flannigan, 2001) (Hung, 2005) (ACGIH, 1999) Outdoors it is commonly found in soil, on plant surfaces, and in decaying organic matter. While *Talaromyces variabilis* is not generally considered a major health concern, it may produce volatile organic compounds (VOCs), contributing to musty odors. However, it is not primarily known for biotoxin production.

SCOPULARIOPSIS AND *MICROASCUS*

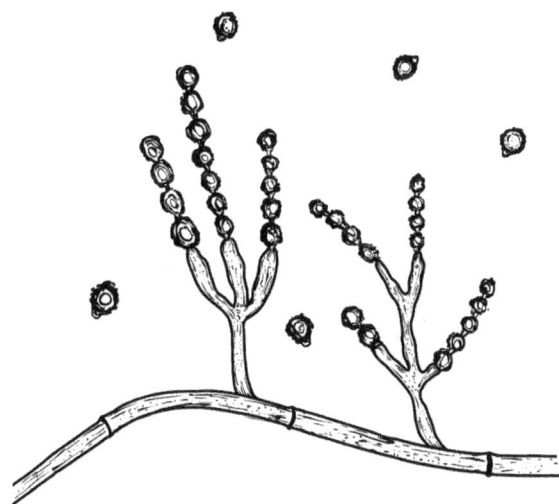

Figure 2-5: The genus Scopulariopsis consists of approximately 40 species. These molds are widely distributed in various environments, including soil, decaying organic matter, and indoor settings.

Scopulariopsis brevicaulis

The HUD/EPA BASE Study found *Scopulariopsis brevicaulis* in 53% of U.S. homes, typically at low levels of around two spore equivalents per milligram of dust, with some homes showing significantly higher contamination levels of up to 5,200 spore equivalents per milligram. This mold can colonize a variety of construction materials in homes, such as wood, drywall, wallpaper, and other cellulose-based substrates, especially in damp or high-humidity environments. It exhibits moderate growth rates when moisture conditions are favorable. (Pitt, 2009) (Flannigan, 2001) (Hung, 2005) (ACGIH, 1999) Outdoors, it is found in soil and plant debris but is more commonly associated with indoor environments. *S. brevicaulis* is believed to contribute to allergic reactions in sensitive individuals, and higher concentrations have been found in the homes of asthmatics. *Scopulariopsis brevicaulis* is an opportunistic pathogen that can cause infections in immunocompromised individuals. Infections can range from superficial conditions, such as nail infections, to more severe respiratory systemic infections in vulnerable individuals. These systemic infections can be challenging to treat due to the organism's resistance to standard antifungal treatments, making them potentially life-threatening in severe cases. This mold produces the biotoxin scopularide A, which may have antibiotic properties, though its biotoxin production has not been extensively studied. (Sandoval-Denis M, 2013)

Microascus chartarum (formerly Scopulariopsis chartarum)

The HUD/EPA BASE Study found *Microascus chartarum* in 38% of U.S. homes, typically at low levels of around two spore equivalents per milligram of dust, though some homes showed significantly higher contamination levels of up to 1,429 spore equivalents per milligram. This mold can colonize a range of indoor construction materials, such as wood, drywall, wallpaper, and cellulose-based substrates, particularly in damp or water-damaged environments. It thrives in areas with high water activity (A_w) and elevated humidity, exhibiting fast growth under favorable conditions. (Pitt, 2009) (Flannigan, 2001) (Hung, 2005) (ACGIH, 1999) While *M. chartarum* can also be found outdoors in soil and plant debris, it is more commonly associated with indoor environments. Exposure to *M. chartarum* may pose health risks, including respiratory problems and allergies, though more research is needed to fully understand its health effects. Additionally, this mold produces biotoxins like chaetoglobosins, which may have potential health implications. (Sandoval-Denis M, 2013)

||||||||||||||||||||||||||||||||||||||||||||||||||||||||||||||||||||||||||||||||||||||||||||||||||||||||||||||||||||||||||||||||||

Was Napoleon Poisoned?

The claim that Napoleon Bonaparte was killed by arsenic poisoning, potentially caused by *Scopulariopsis* mold, is a subject of historical debate and speculation. This theory arose from analyses conducted on samples of Napoleon's hair. Various studies have found elevated levels of arsenic in these hair samples, leading to theories that he was poisoned, either intentionally or accidentally.

The mold-related aspect of this theory involves wallpaper. During Napoleon's time, some wallpapers were colored with Scheele's Green, a pigment containing copper arsenate known to be highly toxic. It has been suggested that mold growing on such wallpaper under damp conditions could convert copper arsenite into a more volatile and toxic form of arsenic gas. In the confined space of Napoleon's residence during his exile on the island of Saint Helena, such gas could have been harmful. (Sandoval-Denis M, 2013)

However, it's important to note that this intriguing theory is not universally accepted. Some historians and scientists argue that the levels of arsenic found in Napoleon's hair samples were consistent with levels common in the general population at that time due to the widespread use of arsenic in products and medicines. Additionally, other factors, such as stomach cancer, have been suggested as more likely causes of his death. (Jones, 1982)

This topic remains an interesting intersection of history, forensic science, and speculation, but definitive conclusions about the exact cause of Napoleon's death are still elusive. The mold on wallpaper theory is just one of several surrounding this historical mystery.

||||||||||||||||||||||||||||||||||||||||||||||||||||||||||||||||||||||||||||||||||||||||||||||||||||||||||||||||||||||||||||||||||

SAROCLADIUM STRICTUM (FORMERLY *ACREMONIUM STRICTUM*)

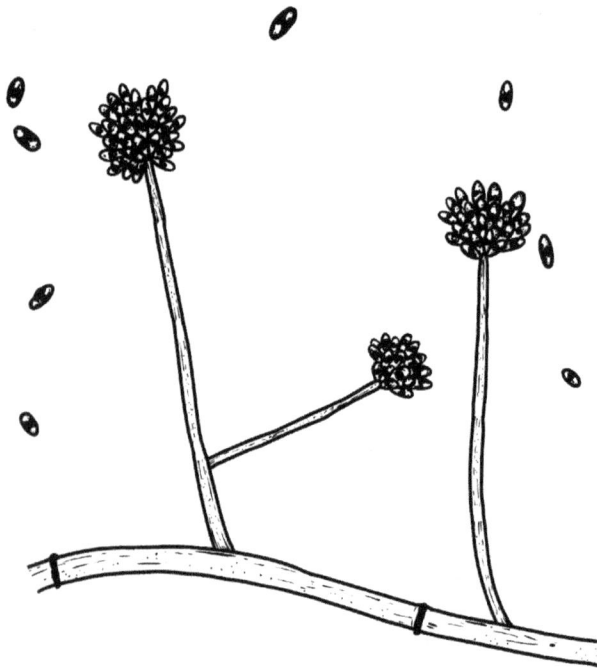

EPA/HUD BASE Study: *Sarocladium strictum* was identified in 57% of house dust sampled using MSQPCR. It is a common outdoor mold. While most homes have low indoor levels of this organism, a few sometimes experience severe contamination. This variability implies that *Sarocladium strictum* can grow indoors under favorable conditions, such as moisture and nutrient availability, but is also commonly introduced from outdoor sources such as soil and decaying plant material like leaves, wood, and other plant debris.

Moisture Conditions: Sarocladium is a group of molds that typically requires high moisture levels for growth. It is often found in environments with chronic moisture conditions, similar to *Stachybotrys*, which is also associated with wet, water-damaged materials. *Sarocladium* generally thrives in very wet conditions but can grow more slowly when moisture is not ideal.

Indoor Nutrient Sources: *Sarocladium* species can utilize a variety of substrates for nutrients, including painted gypsum board and plaster. They may also thrive on dirty surfaces in humidifiers where organic material can accumulate, providing a nutrient source. Reports indicate that *Sarocladium* has been found growing on artwork, likely due to organic material in the paints and accumulated substances in dust providing the necessary nutrients.

Temperature Requirements: *Sarocladium strictum* thrives at room temperature and above but cannot grow at body temperature (37°C, 98.6°F) and is therefore not considered a pathogen.

Presence of Growth in Outdoor Environments: Growth on common outdoor materials indicates that poorly maintained indoor plants or fireplace wood stored indoors may be a likely indoor source for this organism to be brought into the home.

Additional Species: The genus *Sarocladium* includes more than 80 species, with *S. strictum* being one of the more commonly identified and well-studied species found in homes.

Health: Exposure to *Sarocladium strictum* primarily exacerbates allergies and can cause irritation of the respiratory system, leading to symptoms like coughing and wheezing. Systemic effects from biotoxin illness are considered rare.

Biotoxin Production: *Sarocladium strictum* has not been found to produce significant levels or types of biotoxins. However, *Acremonium chrysogenum* is well-known for its role in producing cephalosporin, a class of β-lactam antibiotics used to kill a wide range of bacteria.

ALTERNARIA *ALTERNATA*

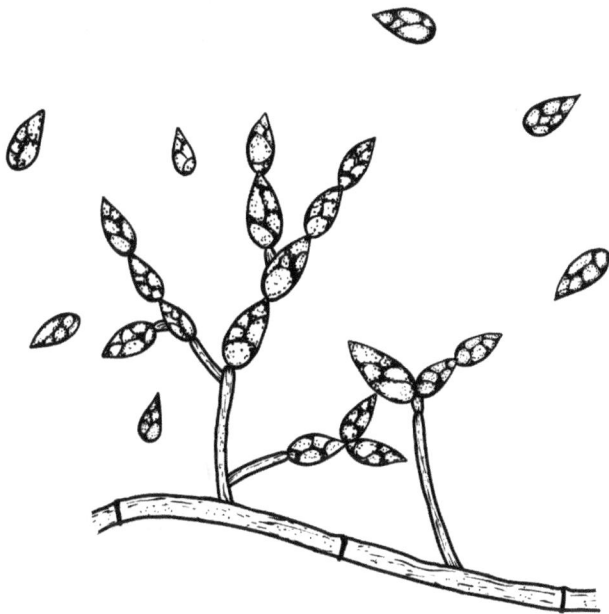

EPA/HUD BASE Study: *Alternaria alternata*, identified in 88% of sampled homes, is a common outdoor mold that sometimes grows indoors. While most homes have moderate levels, a few sometimes experience severe contamination. This variability implies that *Alternaria alternata* can occasionally grow indoors under favorable conditions when appropriate moisture levels and nutrients are available rather than only being introduced from outdoor sources. High concentrations in some homes point to occasional active indoor growth that could necessitate testing and targeted remediation if sources are not obvious.

Indoor Nutrient Sources: Appears as a black discoloration. Sources include indoor stored firewood. Some textiles, foodstuffs, wood, and gypsum board in areas affected by water leaks or flooding, carpet, especially in damp or humid conditions, and paper products such as cardboard or wallpaper in areas with moisture issues. Condensation growth on window framing (Pitt, 2009)

Moisture Conditions: optimum water activity (A$_w$) ranging from 0.90 to 0.99

A$_w$=0.85-0.88 (minimum for various species) (Flannigan, 2001)

Temperature Requirements: It thrives at a wide range of temperatures from 36 degrees to approximately 89 degrees F but grows best at (25°C, 77°F), which allows it to colonize in less than a week. (Flannigan, 2001) *Alternaria alternata* Does not grow at body temperature.

Presence of Outdoor Growth: Decaying wood, leaves, plant debris, decaying fruits and vegetables, cereals, grains, grasses, and animal droppings.

Additional Species: The genus *Alternaria* includes over 40 species, with *A. alternata* being one of the more commonly identified and well-studied species found in homes. (Flannigan, 2001) Based on genetic sequencing, the genus *Ulocladium* has now been reclassified as *Alternaria*.

Health: Exposure to *Alternaria alternata* is most significant for allergies. (Kurup V. P., 2000)

Biotoxin Production: Has not been well studied. (Pitt, 2009) Alternariol is an antifungal produced by *Alternaria* that may contribute to the suppression of culture organisms but would not influence the ability for detection by MSQPCR. Tenuazonic Acid: Another biotoxin produced by *Alternaria* species with potentially toxic effects. (Gravensen, 1994) (Abbott, 2002) (Bennett, 2003)

AUREOBASIDIUM PULLULANS

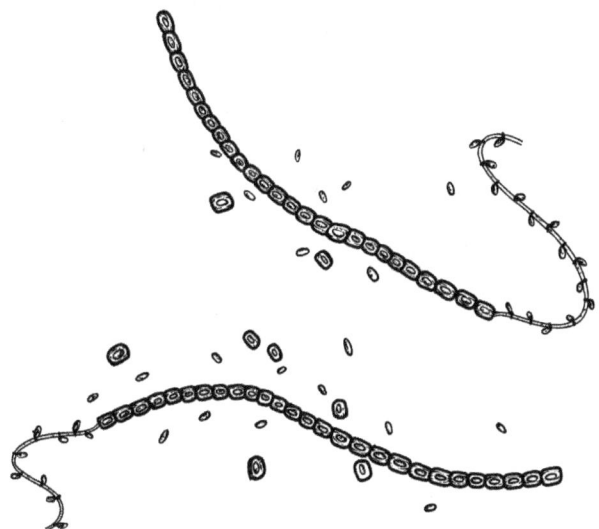

EPA/HUD BASE Study: The HUD/EPA BASE Study found *Aureobasidium pullulans* in 94% of U.S. homes, indicating it is almost always present indoors. With an average concentration of 1,719 spore equivalents per milligram of dust and a standard deviation of 178, most homes show moderate levels of this mold. However, some can experience significantly higher contamination, reaching up to 130,000 spore equivalents per milligram. *A. pullulans* typically grow indoors when conditions like moisture and nutrient availability are favorable. Still, it is likely introduced from outdoor sources, where it is commonly found on plant surfaces. The geometric mean of 263 spore equivalents per milligram suggests moderate levels in homes without water damage, underscoring the importance of thorough testing and targeted remediation when high concentrations are detected.

Indoor Nutrient Sources: *Aureobasidium pullulans* can grow using the nutrients found in house dust. It is commonly found in refrigerator condensate pans, air conditioning condensate pans, dehumidifiers, and humidifiers that are not kept clean. It can colonize a variety of construction materials commonly found in homes, including wood, painted surfaces, and damp areas such as bathrooms. *Aurobasidium* is sometimes called shower curtain mold and grows inside toilet tanks.

Moisture Conditions: *A. pullulans* is relatively adaptable to varying water activity (A_w) levels, but it typically thrives in environments with moderate humidity.

Temperature Requirements: *Auerobasidium pullulans* typically thrive in a wide temperature range. It can grow in temperatures as low as 5°C (41°F) and as high as 35°C (95°F), although its optimal growth temperature is around 20°C to 25°C (68°F to 77°F).

Presence of Outdoor Growth: *Auerobasidium pullulans* is commonly found outdoors in sources such as soil and decaying plant material like leaves, wood, and other plant debris.

Health: Exposure to *A. pullulans* is generally not considered a significant health concern. However, in individuals with mold sensitivities or compromised immune systems, it may lead to respiratory issues or allergic reactions.

Biotoxin Production: *A. pullulans* is not primarily known for producing biotoxins. However, it may produce some Microbial Volatile Organic Compounds (mVOCs) that contribute to musty odors and stimulate adverse vagal nerve system responses.

CHAETOMIUM GLOBOSUM

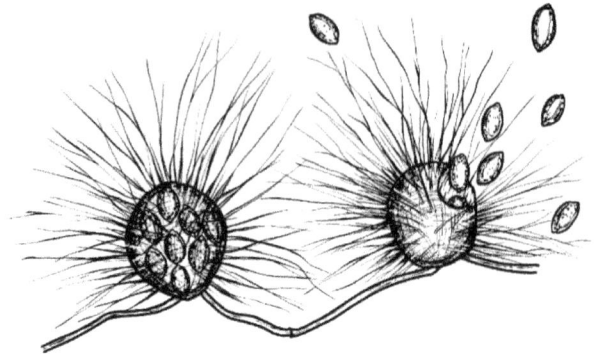

EPA/HUD BASE Study: *Chaetomium globosum* is a water damage indicator mold species found in 51% of sampled homes, making it a common indoor mold. The large standard deviation of 709 compared to the average of 45 spore equivalents per milligram of dust (sp eq/mg) indicates significant variability in mold levels across different homes, suggesting that while most homes had low levels, some experienced significantly higher concentrations. The highest concentration detected was 21,000 sp eq/mg, suggesting the potential for severe contamination representing actual growth in certain environments. This supports the idea that *Chaetomium globosum* can grow indoors under favorable conditions, such as adequate moisture and nutrient availability, and that it is less likely to be introduced from outdoor sources. The geometric mean of 2 sp eq/mg indicates that low levels are typical for homes in the United States that have not been water damaged. This highlights the importance of thorough testing and targeted remediation in cases where sources are not obvious or when high concentrations are detected.

Indoor Nutrient Sources: It can colonize a variety of construction materials commonly found in homes, especially in areas with chronically elevated moisture levels or water damage. Materials that support its growth include processed wood such as oriented strand board, paper-faced gypsum board, cardboard, and cellulose-containing substrates.

Moisture Conditions: *C. globosum* typically thrives in environments with a moderate to high water activity (A_w) of around 0.90 or higher, making it prone to growth in conditions with excess moisture.

Presence of Outdoor Growth: *C. globosum* is commonly found at low levels in various natural environments, including soil, decaying plant material, and plant debris.

Health: Allergic reactions, nail and skin infections.

Biotoxin Production: Chaetoglobosin A, C, from *Chaetomium globosum,* is common on damp building materials. (Gravensen, 1994) (Abbott, 2002) (Bennett, 2003)

EPICOCCUM NIGRUM

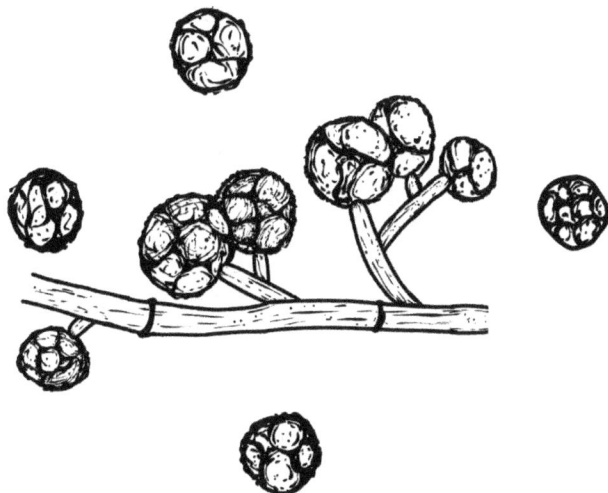

EPA/HUD BASE Study: *Epicoccum nigrum* is a common outdoor mold found inside 93% of sampled homes, making it almost always present indoors. The significant standard deviation of 12,291 compared to the average of 2,394 spore equivalents per milligram of dust (sp eq/mg) indicates significant variability in mold levels across different homes, suggesting that while most homes had moderate levels, some experienced significantly higher concentrations. The highest concentration detected was 250,000 sp eq/mg, suggesting the potential for severe contamination in certain environments. This supports the idea that *Epicoccum nigrum* can grow indoors under favorable conditions, such as adequate moisture and nutrient availability, even though it is likely to originate from outdoor sources. The geometric mean of 117 sp eq/mg indicates that moderate levels are typical for homes in the United States. This highlights the importance of thorough testing and targeted remediation in cases where sources are not obvious or when high concentrations are detected.

Indoor Nutrient Sources: While it is more commonly an outdoor mold, it can colonize organic materials found in homes with elevated moisture. Materials that may support its growth include wood, drywall, and cellulose-containing substrates.

Moisture Conditions: It typically thrives in environments with moderate water activity (A_w) ranging from 0.80 to 0.90, making it adaptable to various moderate-level moisture conditions. *Epicoccum nigrum* exhibits moderate growth rates, with visible colonies forming within days under suitable conditions.

Temperature Requirements: Ideal temperature requirements are between 70 to 86 degrees F, but can grow slowly at much cooler temperatures.

Presence of Outdoor Growth: It is commonly found in various natural environments, including soil, decaying plant material, and plant surfaces.

Health: Exposure to *Epicoccum nigrum* may lead to respiratory issues and allergies, especially in individuals with mold sensitivities. While it is generally considered less toxic than some other molds, addressing moisture issues in homes is essential to prevent its growth and maintain a healthy indoor environment.

Biotoxin Production: *Epicoccum nigrum* is not primarily known for biotoxin production. However, like many molds, it may produce some volatile organic compounds (VOCs) that contribute to musty odors.

FUSARIUM SOLANI

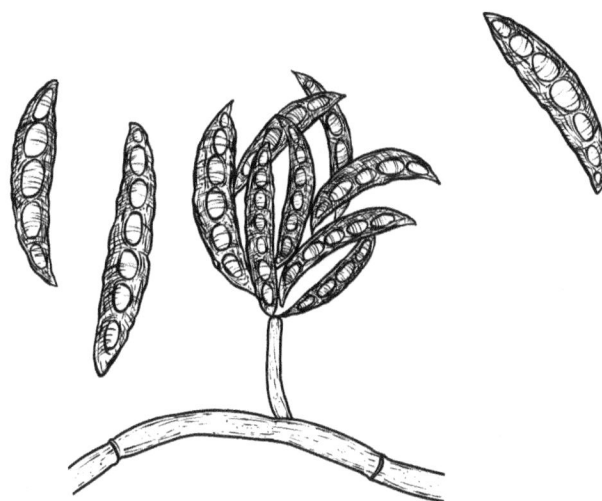

EPA/HUD BASE Study: *Fusarium solani* was not included in the 2007 study on mold prevalence in homes, so extensive statistical data and values are unavailable for this organism within that research context. Although it is not perceived as common, *Fusarium solani* can occur in indoor environments and is known for its potential health risks, particularly for individuals with weakened immune systems. This mold can cause infections in humans and plants, affecting various tissues and leading to conditions like fusariosis. While MSQPCR (Mold-Specific Quantitative Polymerase Chain Reaction) analysis for *Fusarium solani* is not typically part of standard testing, it may be available from specialized laboratories upon request. Monitoring indoor environments for the presence of *Fusarium solani* should be considered, especially in settings where vulnerable individuals reside. This highlights the importance of thorough testing and targeted remediation in cases where sources are not obvious or when high concentrations are detected.

Indoor Nutrient Sources: *Fusarium solani* can colonize a variety of construction materials commonly found in homes, especially in areas with elevated moisture levels or water damage. Materials that may support its growth include wood, gypsum board paper, and cellulose-containing substrates.

Moisture Conditions: It typically thrives in environments with a moderate water activity (A_w) ranging from 0.95 to 0.98, making it well-suited for conditions with ample moisture. It exhibits rapid growth rates, with visible colonies forming within days under suitable conditions.

Presence of Outdoor Growth: It is a significant agricultural pathogen, causing diseases in various crops and leading to substantial economic losses for farmers. It has outdoor sources, such as soil and decaying plant material like leaves, wood, and other plant debris.

Health: It is a major allergen (Gravensen, 1994)

Biotoxin Production: *Fusarium solani* is known to produce a variety of biotoxins in the trichothecene group. It also can make a compound that mimics estrogen called zearalenone. These can have various health effects when inhaled, ingested, or come in contact with skin. (Gravensen, 1994) (Abbott, 2002) (Bennett, 2003)

MUCOR AND RHIZOPUS

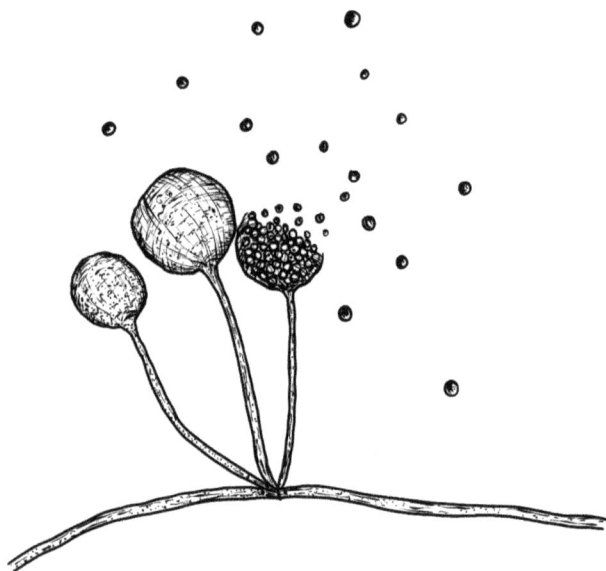

EPA/HUD BASE Study: *Mucor racemosus* is a very common outdoor mold found in 92% of homes. Most levels were moderate, but some reached 22,000 spore equivalents per milligram of dust, indicating severe contamination. The geometric mean of 15 sp eq/mg suggests low levels are typical in U.S. homes, though indoor growth can occur under favorable moisture conditions.

Indoor Nutrient Sources: While they are not typically associated with growth in homes, they can potentially colonize organic materials indoors, especially in areas with elevated moisture levels or water damage. Materials that may support their growth include wood, gypsum board paper, and cellulose-containing substrates.

Moisture Conditions: *Mucor* thrives in environments with a moderately high water activity (A_w) ranging from 0.90 to 0.99, making them well-suited for conditions with excess moisture. *Mucor* and *Rhizopus* species exhibit rapid growth rates, with visible colonies forming quickly under suitable conditions.

Presence of Outdoor Growth: *Mucor racemosus* is commonly found in soil and organic matter. *Mucor amphibiorum* is often found in soil and aquatic environments. *Mucor circinelloides* is commonly isolated from soil and plant debris and is used in the biotechnology industry for its potential in bioconversion processes. *Mucor hiemalis* is found in soil and decaying vegetation. *Mucor indicus* is utilized in the production of fermented foods and beverages. *Mucor mucedo* is found on decaying plant material and is known for its rapid growth.

MSQPCR Species-Level Identification Limitations: *Mucor racemosus*, along with *Mucor amphibiorum, Mucor circinelloides, Mucor hiemalis, Mucor indicus, Mucor mucedo, Mucor ramosissimus, Rhizopus azygosporus, Rhizopus homothallicus, Rhizopus microsporus, Rhizopus oligosporus*, and *Rhizopus oryzae*, are genetically similar and cannot be reliably identified to the species level using MSQPCR. Species identification would require a specialty laboratory capable of identifying by culture techniques.

Health: Exposure to *Mucor* and *Rhizopus* species may lead to allergic respiratory problems, skin irritation, and, in some cases, invasive fungal infections, particularly in individuals with compromised immune systems. *Mucor* can sometimes cause mucormycosis, a rare but severe fungal infection that can manifest in forms affecting the sinuses, lungs, skin, or multiple body systems. It's most common in immunocompromised individuals and those with uncontrolled diabetes. (Huang, 2023)

Biotoxin Production: Some species within these genera can produce biotoxins, such as *Rhizopus stolonifer*, which may produce rhizonins and rhizoxins. These biotoxins can pose health risks when ingested or in contact with the skin. (Gravensen, 1994) (Abbott, 2002) (Bennett, 2003)

Rhizopus stolonifer

EPA/HUD BASE Study: *Rhizopus stolonifer* was found in 29% of homes, with most levels low but some higher, reaching 530 spore equivalents per milligram of dust, indicating potential contamination. The geometric mean of 1 sp eq/mg suggests very low levels are typical in U.S. homes, emphasizing the need for thorough testing and remediation when high concentrations are detected.

Indoor Nutrient Sources: While it is not typically associated with indoor growth, it can potentially colonize organic materials in homes, particularly in areas with high humidity or water damage. Materials that may support its growth include food and cellulose-containing substrates.

Moisture Conditions: Rhizopus stolonifer thrives in environments with high water activity (A_w) and is commonly associated with damp or decaying organic matter. This fungus exhibits rapid growth and can quickly colonize substrates under favorable conditions.

Temperature Requirements: *Rhizopus stolonifer* grows well at temperatures from about 41 to 98 degrees F.

Presence of Outdoor Growth: *Rhizopus stolonifer* is commonly found in nature on decaying fruits, vegetables, and organic debris.

Health: Exposure to *Rhizopus stolonifer* is generally not considered a major health concern for humans. However, it can be a source of food spoilage and may contribute to allergic reactions in some individuals.

Biotoxin Production: *Rhizopus stolonifer* can produce biotoxins, such as rhizonin, which may have antimicrobial properties. However, its biotoxin production has not been extensively studied compared to that of other molds. (Gravensen, 1994) (Abbott, 2002) (Bennett, 2003)

PAECILOMYCES VARIOTII

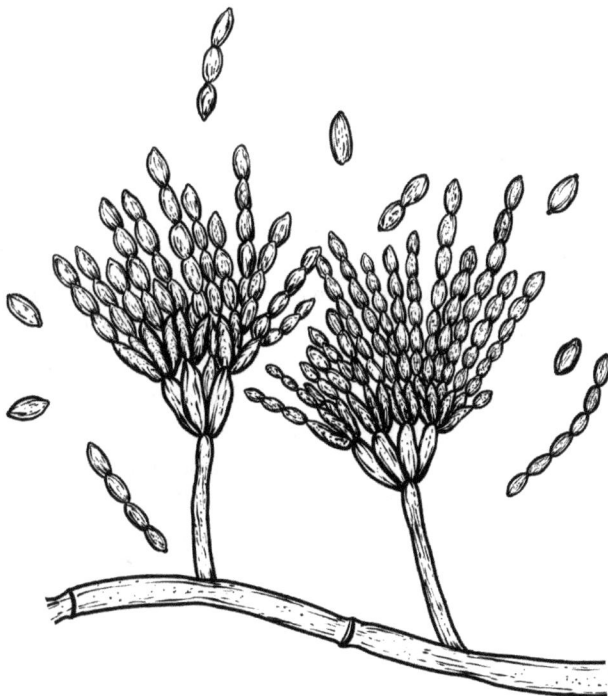

EPA/HUD BASE Study: *Paecilomyces variotii* was found in 46% of homes, with most levels moderate but some reaching 204,539 spore equivalents per milligram of dust, indicating growth and severe contamination. The geometric mean of 2 sp eq/mg suggests low levels are typical in U.S. homes, emphasizing the need for thorough testing and remediation when high concentrations are detected.

Indoor Nutrient Sources: While it is not typically associated with indoor growth, it can potentially colonize organic materials indoors, especially in areas with elevated moisture levels or water damage. Materials that may support its growth include wood, paper, and cellulose-containing substrates. Gypsum board wetted by salt water from storm surges in marine environments is often contaminated by the growth of this salt-tolerant xerophilic mold.

Moisture Conditions: Water Activity is 0.84 at 25°C. It typically thrives in environments with moderate to high water activity (A_w) ranging from 0.85 to 0.95, making it adaptable to conditions with moisture levels below saturation. *Paecilomyces variotii* exhibits rapid growth rates, with visible colonies forming within a few days under suitable conditions.

Presence of Outdoor Growth: It is commonly found in various natural environments, including soil, plant debris, and decaying organic matter.

Health: Exposure to *Paecilomyces variotii* is generally not considered a major health concern. It is generally considered less harmful than other molds.

Biotoxin Production: *Paecilomyces variotii* is not primarily known for biotoxin production. However, like many molds, it may produce some microbial volatile organic compounds (mVOCs), contributing to musty odors and possibly stimulating vagal nervous responses, but generally not considered highly toxic.

STACHYBOTRYS CHARTARUM

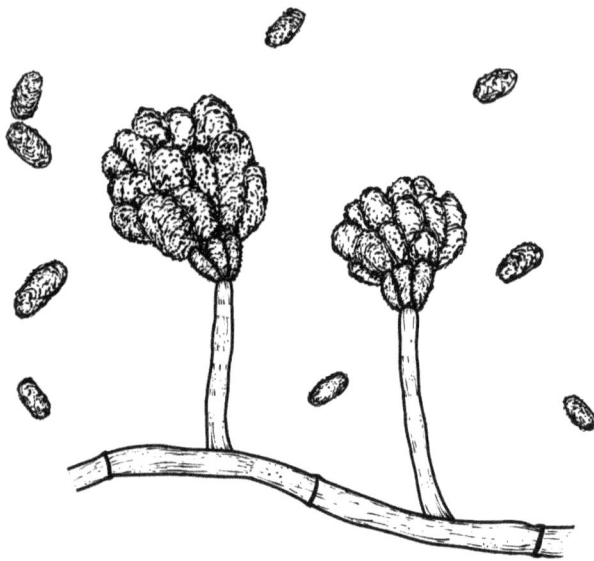

EPA/HUD BASE Study: *Stachybotrys chartarum* was found in 35% of homes, with most levels low but some reaching 2,000 spore equivalents per milligram of dust, indicating growth and severe contamination. The geometric mean of 2 sp eq/mg suggests low levels are typical in U.S. homes. Often referred to as "black mold," it is gray when immature and develops a dark greenish-black slimy texture as it matures. This highlights the need for thorough testing and remediation when high concentrations are detected.

Indoor Nutrient Sources: While it is not typically associated with indoor growth, it can colonize organic materials in homes, particularly in areas with high humidity or water damage. Materials that may support its growth include wood and cellulose-containing substrates. This mold is typically found growing on cellulose-rich materials such as paper, drywall, and fiberboard that have been subjected to chronic water damage. However, its nutrient requirements are such that it tends to grow poorly on wood, except in those locations where the wood is directly in contact with paper or cardboard, such as where gypsum wallboard meets wood framing.

Moisture Conditions: Water Activity is above 0.94. It is typically considered a slow-growing mold that requires chronic moisture, with surfaces needing to be continuously wet for 7–12 days for germination. It thrives at temperatures above room temperature, but its growth significantly slows or stops at colder temperatures.

Temperature Requirements: *Stachybotrys chartarum* grows best at 68–77°F but can grow very slowly at 59–98.6°F.

Presence of Outdoor Growth: It tends not to grow well on outdoor sources of materials unless they are very wet for an extended period of time. It has been observed growing inside hay bales, rice straw, and corn silage.

Species: The genus *Stachybotrys* includes multiple species, with over 50 recognized to date. Some of the most significant and well-studied species include:

- **Stachybotrys alternans**: Less common but similar to *S. chartarum* regarding habitat and health implications. It is also found in water-damaged buildings and can produce biotoxins.

- **Stachybotrys cylindrospora**: This species is known for its cylindrical spores. It can also be found in damp environments and has potential health risks associated with its spores and biotoxins.

- **Stachybotrys echinata:** Formerly *Memnoniella echinata,* this species has spiny spores produced in dry chains. It thrives on damp, cellulose-rich materials like drywall and wood. The second most common *Stachybotrys* (after *S. chartarum),* its mycotoxins and spores have similar toxicity risks, but it was not in the HUD BASE study.

- **Stachybotrys elegans**: Found in soil and decaying plant material. It is less common in indoor environments but is still significant due to its ability to produce biotoxins.

- **Stachybotrys kampalensis**: This species is found in soil and decaying vegetation. It is notable for its unique morphological features and ecological role in decomposing plant matter.

- **Stachybotrys microspora**: This species is characterized by smaller spores than other species. It also has potential health impacts.

Health: Exposure to *Stachybotrys chartarum* can cause respiratory issues, coughing, skin irritation, brain fog, and chronic fatigue. In severe cases, neurological symptoms may occur. Those particularly at risk include infants, the elderly, and people with pre-existing respiratory conditions.

Biotoxins: Much research on *Stachybotrys chartarum* has focused on its toxic compounds and their effects on human health, highlighting the mold's ability to produce over 200 different toxic compounds under various conditions. **These include the Trichothecenes**: Satratoxin H, Satratoxin G, **Roridins**, and **Verrucarins. Sporidesmins, Cyclosporins, Phenylspirodrimanes,** and **Isosatratoxins.** (Gravensen, 1994) (Abbott, 2002) (Bennett, 2003) (Jarvis, 2005) (Bennett, 2003)

TRICHODERMA VIRIDE

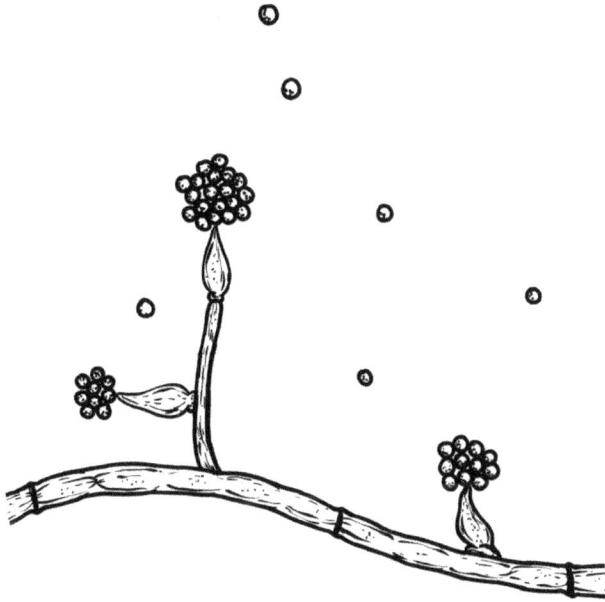

EPA/HUD BASE Study: *Trichoderma viride* was found in 27% of homes, with most levels low but some reaching 236 spore equivalents per milligram of dust, indicating likely growth and contamination. The geometric mean of 2 sp eq/mg suggests low levels are typical in U.S. homes, emphasizing the need for thorough testing and remediation when high concentrations are detected.

Indoor Nutrient Sources: *Trichoderma viride* can grow on a variety of construction materials that retain moisture, such as wood, wallpaper, carpet, and insulation materials. Any area that sustains water damage or elevated humidity levels can support its growth. It is especially common on water-damaged hardwoods and sometimes softwoods. It is frequently seen on the base of hardwood cabinets or hardwood veneer at the base of cabinets when they have sat in water.

Moisture Conditions: *Trichoderma viride* thrives on moderate to relatively high moisture levels. It typically needs a water activity level (a measure of water available for microbial growth) above 0.8. Damp environments, especially those with persistent moisture, are ideal for its growth. *Trichoderma viride* is a fast-growing mold species known for its aggressive colonization and ability to outcompete other microorganisms.

Temperature Requirements: *Trichoderma viride* has an **optimal temperature range of** 77–86°F but can grow between 50–95°F, though growth is slower at the extremes of this range.

Presence of Outdoor Growth: *Trichoderma viride* is commonly found in soil, decaying wood, and other organic matter. It plays a role in nutrient cycling and is adept at breaking down complex organic compounds.

Health: *Trichoderma viride* had significantly ($P < 0.05$) higher concentrations in asthmatics' homes compared with control homes. Exposure to this mold and its spores can cause allergic reactions and respiratory issues.

Biotoxin Production: *Trichoderma* species produce sesquiterpenes, gliotoxin, koninginin, and trichodermin. (Gravensen, 1994) (Abbott, 2002) (Bennett, 2003)

WALLEMIA SEBI

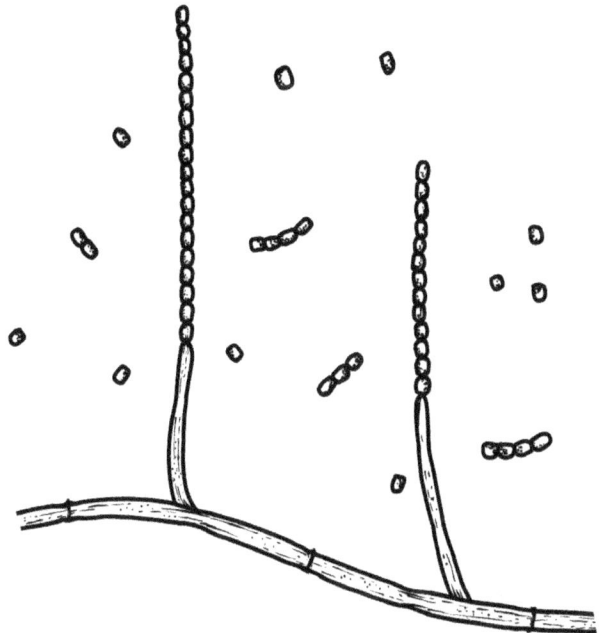

EPA/HUD BASE Study: *Wallemia sebi* was found in 75% of homes, with most levels moderate but some reaching 400,000 spore equivalents per milligram of dust, indicating severe contamination. The geometric mean of 18 sp eq/mg suggests low to moderate levels are typical in U.S. homes, highlighting the need for thorough testing and remediation when high concentrations are detected.

Indoor Nutrient Sources: This organism is frequently found growing in moldy mattresses. This may be because sleeping occupants' perspiration provides approximately 3.5 ounces of moisture per person each night. The salt in perspiration and skin cells as nutrients may make mattresses an ideal environment for growth. While less common indoors, it can still colonize a number of construction materials in homes.

Moisture Conditions: *Wallemia* sebi is a xerophilic (dry-loving) fungus known for its ability to thrive in low-moisture environments, making it well-suited for dry conditions. Water Activity is 0.70 at 25°C. It can grow at extremely low water activity (A_w) levels of 0.70 to 0.75, which sets it apart from many other molds and allows it to colonize dry and salty substrates. *Wallemia sebi* exhibits relatively slow growth compared to other molds, which may contribute to its preference for dry conditions.

Temperature Requirements: *Wallemia* sebi grows best at temperatures around 77° F and does not tolerate very hot or very cold conditions.

Presence of Outdoor Growth: It is commonly found in diverse environments, including arid and salt-laden environments.

Health: This organism had significantly higher concentrations in asthmatics' homes compared with control homes. While less studied than some other molds, exposure to *Wallemia sebi* may pose health risks to individuals, particularly those with sensitivities to mold.

Biotoxin Production: *Wallemia sebi* generates several metabolites, including walleminol, walleminone, azasteroid UCA1064-B, and the highly toxic compound wallimidione. (Gravensen, 1994) (Abbott, 2002) (Bennett, 2003) (Jančič S, 2015)

SERPULA LACRYMANS

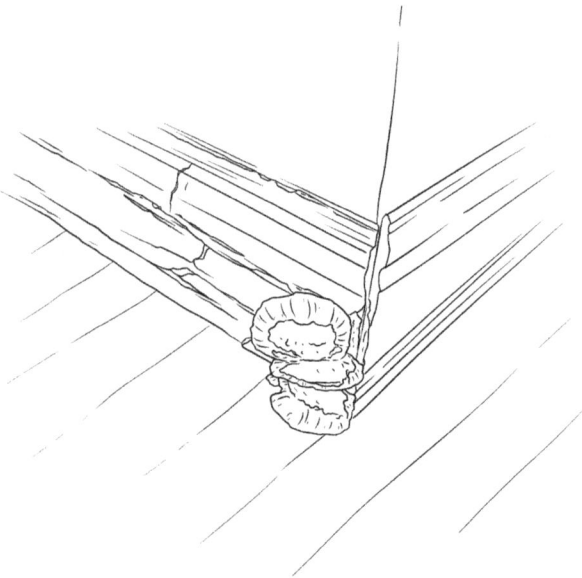

Figure 2-17: Serpula lacrymans is a form of dry rot that forms on wood; this is a costly fungus attacking construction wooden elements

Serpula lacrymans is a notorious fungus belonging to the Basidiomycetes class, known for causing dry rot in buildings. Its adaptability is alarming; it thrives even in dry conditions and has highly resilient mycelial cords. These cords can spread far from the central growth, even transporting water over long distances.

This fungus doesn't just mar surfaces; it jeopardizes the structural integrity of the wood it infects, sometimes leading to significant lumber structural failure. When you notice its musty odor or fruiting bodies, immediate and extensive restoration is often needed, which is neither easy nor cheap.

As for state regulations, wet and dry rot fall under the category of wood-destroying organisms. Many states require licensing for companies inspecting or treating wet rot or dry rot. The enforced control measures are administered through the state structural pest control regulations. While these fungi may not present health risks like harmful molds, wet rot, and dry rot, fungi can lead to structural collapse or instability. (Palfreyman, 1998)

LUMBER YARD MOLD

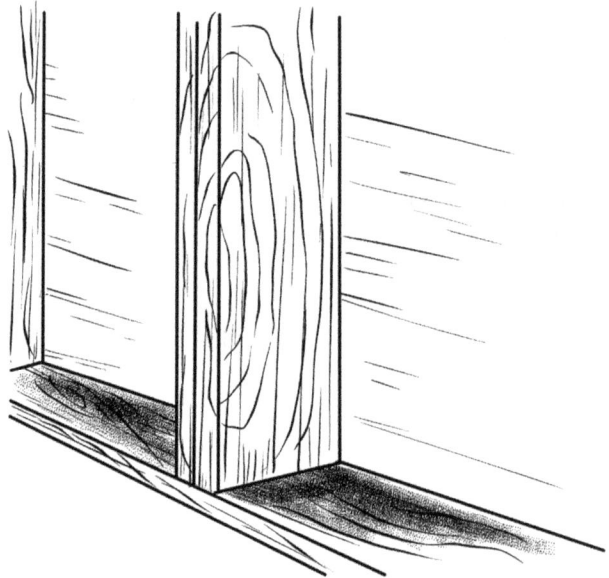

Figure 2-18: Lumber yard molds often grow on poorly managed green lumber while it is curing. This group of molds is generally considered a cosmetic issue but cannot be distinguished visually from more problematic surface molds.

The *Ceratocystis* and *Ophiostoma* group of fungi is commonly associated with lumber yards and wood-processing facilities. Although they are common in nature, they get much more attention when observed on lumber used to construct homes. These are saprophytic fungi, which means they feed on dead or decaying organic matter, primarily wood. They're generally not considered problems for human health but can contribute to wood decay and spoilage. In a lumber yard setting, they can be problematic because they can lead to staining or degrading the quality of the wood, affecting its market value. Proper lumber drying and storage are key measures to minimize the growth of these fungi. Once lumber has cured, these molds do not grow further. Even if the wood gets wet again, other mold types, such as *Penicillium* and *Aspergillus* species, may grow and co-exist on the same surface. This is problematic because visual inspection makes it impossible to tell when other molds have invaded the space.

MILDEW

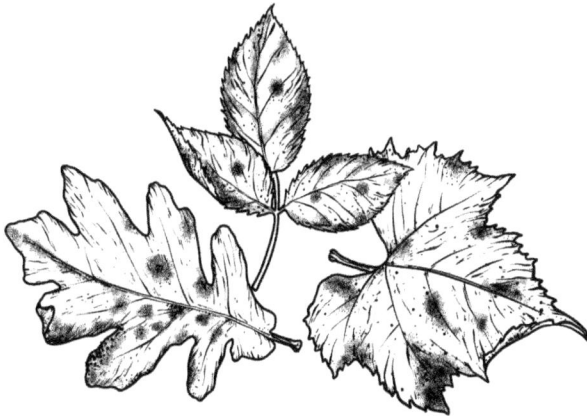

Figure 2-19: Mildew on rose (top), oak(left), and grape leaves (right)

Mildew is a common term for molds that grow on plant leaves while the plant is alive. It is commonly found on grapes, roses, and trees. The term "mildew" is sometimes used to downplay mold issues in buildings, but this is misleading. While all mildews are molds, not all molds are mildews. Whether you call it Mildew or Mold, if it is growing on any type of building materials or personal possessions, it needs to be properly addressed.

||||||||||||||||||||||||||||||||||||||||||||||||||||||||||||||||||||||||||||||||||||||||||||||||||||||||||||||||||||||||||||||||||||||||||||||||||||||||||||||||||||||||||||||||

MSQPCR Species-Level Identification Limitations

The following organisms are genetically similar and cannot be reliably distinguished from one another at a species level by using MSQPCR. Accurate identification requires the organisms to be viable (alive or dormant), and a specialized lab using culture methods is needed to distinguish the organisms from one another. This highlights the importance of thorough testing and targeted remediation in cases where sources are not obvious or when high concentrations are detected.

- *Aspergillus flavus* cannot be distinguished genetically from *A. oryzae,* which is used for food like soy sauce and sake.

- *Eurotium Amstelodami* is now known to be the sexual form of *Aspergillus amstelodami* and cannot be distinguished genetically from *A. chevalier, A. herbarium, A. rubrum, and A. repens.*

- *Aspergillus fumigatus* cannot be distinguished genetically from *Neosartorya fischeri. Neosartorya fischeri* is known for its heat-resistant ascospores and is studied in food spoilage and heat sterilization processes, as its spores can survive pasteurization and affect food safety.

- *Aspergillus niger* cannot be distinguished genetically from *Aspergillus foetidus* and *Aspergillus* phoenicis. *Aspergillus foetidus* is known for its pungent odor and is sometimes found in decaying organic matter. *Aspergillus phoenicis* is often isolated from soil and can be involved in the decomposition of plant material, but it is less commonly encountered in indoor environments compared to *Aspergillus niger.*

- *Aspergillus ochraceus* cannot be distinguished genetically from *Aspergillus ostianus. Aspergillus ostianus* is often isolated from soil and plant debris and has been noted for its ability to produce enzymes that are useful in the degradation of plant materials.

- *Aspergillus restrictus* cannot be distinguished genetically from *Aspergillus conicus. Aspergillus conicus* is found in soil and organic matter, contributing to the breakdown of plant materials.

- *Penicillium crustosum* cannot be genetically distinguished from *Penicillium camemberti, Penicillium commune, echinulatum,* and *Penicillium solitum. Penicillium camemberti* makes soft rind cheeses like camembert and brie. *Penicillium commune* is used in cheese production, contributing to ripening and flavor. *Penicillium echinulatum* is known for producing a variety of enzymes and is being studied for biofuel production. *Penicillium solitum* causes rot in apples and pears.

- *Penicillium spinulosum* cannot be genetically distinguished from *P. glabrum, P. lividum, P. purpurescens,* and *P. thomii. P. glabrum* causes rot in strawberries; *P. lividum* is commonly found in soil containing peat and can grow on brown algae. *P. purpurascens* has been isolated from soil in Canada, and *P. thomii* is found growing on brown algae.

- *Trichoderma viride, Trichoderma atroviride,* and *Trichoderma koningii* are genetically similar and cannot be genetically distinguished. *Trichoderma atroviride* is also used for biocontrol and is known for promoting plant growth and suppressing soil-borne diseases. *Trichoderma koningii* is frequently found in soil and decaying organic matter and is

used in agriculture for its beneficial effects on plant health and soil quality.

|||||||||||||||||||||||||||||||||||||||||||||||||||||||||||||||||||||||||||||||||||||||||||||||||||||||||||||||||||||||||||||||||||||||||||||||||||||||||||||||||||||||||||||

References

Vesper, S., McKinstry, C., Haugland, R., Wymer, L., Bradham, K., Ashley, P., Cox, D., Dewalt, G., & Friedman, W. (2007). Development of an Environmental Relative Moldiness Index for US homes. *Journal of Occupational and Environmental Medicine, 49*(8), 829–833.

Pitt, J. I., & Hocking, A. D. (2009). *Fungi and food spoilage.* Springer Science & Business Media.

Flannigan, B., Samson, R. A., & Miller, J. D. (Eds.). (2001). *Microorganisms in home and indoor work environments: Diversity, health impacts, investigation and control.* Taylor & Francis.

Hung, L.-L., Miller, J. D., & Dillon, H. K. (Eds.). (2005). *Field guide for determination of biological contaminants in environmental samples* (2nd ed.). American Industrial Hygiene Association.

American Industrial Hygiene Association. (1999). *Bioaerosols: Assessment and control.* American Industrial Hygiene Association.

Gravensen, S., Frisvad, J. C., & Samson, R. A. (1994). *Microfungi* (1st ed.). Munkgaard.

Kurup, V. P., Shen, H. D., & Banerjee, B. (2000). Respiratory fungal allergy. *Microbes and Infection, 2*(9), 1101–1110. https://doi.org/10.1016/S1286-4579(00)01249-7

Abbott, S. P. (2002). Mycotoxins and indoor molds. *Indoor Environment Connections, 3*(4), 14–24.

Stevenson, A., Hamill, P. G., O'Kane, C. J., Kminek, G., Rummel, J. D., Voytek, M. A., Dijksterhuis, J., & Hallsworth, J. E. (2017). Aspergillus penicillioides differentiation and cell division at 0.585 water activity. *Environmental Microbiology, 19*(2), 687–697.

SEAS Communications, The Harvard Gazette Science & Tech. (n.d.). *Tut, tut! Microbial growth in pharaoh's tomb suggests burial was a rush job.* Retrieved from https://news.harvard.edu/gazette

Shoemaker, R., & House, D. (2006). SBS and exposure to water-damaged buildings: Time series study, clinical trial, and mechanisms. *Neurotoxicology and Teratology, 28*, 573–588.

Ma, L.-Y., Zhang, H.-B., Kang, H.-H., Zhong, M.-J., Liu, D.-S., Ren, H., & Liu, W.-Z. (2019). New butenolides and cyclopentenones from saline soil-derived fungus *Aspergillus sclerotiorum. Molecules, 24*(14), 2642. https://doi.org/10.3390/molecules24142642

Sandoval-Denis, M., Sutton, D. A., Fothergill, A. W., Cano-Lira, J., Gené, J., Decock, C. A., de Hoog, G. S., & Guarro, J. (2013). *Scopulariopsis*, a poorly known opportunistic fungus: Spectrum of species in clinical samples and in vitro responses to antifungal drugs. *Journal of Clinical Microbiology, 51*(12), 3937–3943. https://doi.org/10.1128/JCM.01927-13

Jones, D. (1982, October 14). The singular case of Napoleon's wallpaper. *New Scientist, 101.*

Bennett, J. W., & Klich, M. (2003). Mycotoxins. *Clinical Microbiology Reviews, 16*(3), 497–516.

Jančič, S., Nguyen, H. D., Frisvad, J. C., Zalar, P., Schroers, H. J., Seifert, K. A., & Gunde-Cimerman, N. (2015). A taxonomic revision of the *Wallemia sebi* species complex. *PLOS ONE, 10*(5), e0125933. https://doi.org/10.1371/journal.pone.0125933

Jarvis, B. B., & Miller, J. D. (2005). Mycotoxins as harmful indoor air contaminants. *Applied Microbiology and Biotechnology, 66*(4), 367–372.

Institut national de santé publique du Québec. (n.d.). *Acremonium spp.* Retrieved from https://www.inspq.qc.ca/

Palfreyman, J. W. (1998). *The domestic dry rot fungus, Serpula lacrymans, its natural origins and biological control.* Dry Rot Research Group, University of Abertay Dundee.

Huang, S.-F., Wu, A. Y.-J., Lee, S. S.-J., Huang, Y.-S., Lee, C.-Y., Yang, T.-L., Wang, H.-W., Chen, H. J., Chen, Y. C., Ho, T.-S., Kuo, C.-F., & Lin, Y.-T. (2023). COVID-19 associated mold infections: Review of COVID-19 associated pulmonary aspergillosis and mucormycosis. *Journal of Microbiology, Immunology, and Infection, 56*(3), 442–454. https://doi.org/10.1016/j.jmii.2022.12.004

Part Two: Navigating the *Mold Controlled* Plan

Finding, fixing, and preventing mold and other water-damage organisms that degrade your home's environmental quality is a journey. If you're already dealing with water damage, mold, or related microorganisms, you may feel overwhelmed by the many perspectives on this issue. The mold remediation field is complex, filled with experts whose biases and areas of expertise may not always align with your desires or needs. This section provides a hands-on roadmap to help you anticipate and navigate the challenges.

My book focuses on a non-chemical approach, designed especially for those sensitive to organisms associated with water damage but practical for anyone interested in maintaining a mold-controlled home while avoiding chemicals stronger than soap or detergent.

Creating and maintaining a healthy home environment isn't just for those with mold sensitivities or specific health concerns—it benefits everyone. This approach aligns with the principles of ALARA (As Low as Reasonably Achievable) and the precautionary principle, advocating for the least invasive and safest methods. The methodologies promoted here aim to make homes life-enhancing spaces free from potentially harmful substances. By adopting non-toxic, preventative measures, we safeguard the health of sensitive individuals while promoting overall well-being, making it a wise choice for all households.

The guides that follow acknowledge the uniqueness of each person's situation and the variety of confusing options they may encounter. A mold-controlled environment benefits everyone, not just those with sensitivities. Living in spaces free from water damage enhances quality of life, brings economic advantages, and reduces stress. This approach empowers a wide range of people—from family members to professional caregivers—to contribute effectively to creating a wellness-supportive environment.

IT ALL BEGINS WITH EXCESS WATER

The next sections are divided into four parts:

Section One: Emergency Water Damage—How to prepare and respond when things go wrong.

Section Two: Finding a Home to Rent or Buy—Guidance on selecting a new place and recognizing conditions that could lead to mold issues in your current residence.

Section Three: My Five Stage, 25 Step Program—A structured approach to addressing mold and water damage issues that have already developed.

Section Four: Contents and Personal Possessions—Strategies for managing and protecting your belongings."

YOUR PROJECT DIARY

Effective planning and coordination are key to a successful outcome. Keeping a **Project Diary** will be instrumental in this process.

Look for the diary symbol, which prompts you to use your Project Diary. Here, you can log structured, factual details from your remediation plan to inform and document your progress. The Project Diary will help you prepare for, respond to, and track emergencies. It's a fundamental tool to guide you through each stage, keeping your path organized and well-documented.

USING A PROJECT DIARY TO DOCUMENT YOUR DECISIONS

As you work through each exercise of this section, keeping a project diary helps chart and document the many decisions you'll need to make. This diary will serve as your reference point, helping you stay organized and ensuring no important details are overlooked.

❏ For each boxed entry, you should make one of three types of decisions:

🚫 Doesn't Apply: If a section doesn't apply to your situation, you can move on.

☑ Relevant: If the facts of your situation indicate that a section is relevant, be sure to record it in your diary. Note any details that need to be considered, whether briefly or in more detail, depending on what's necessary to trigger your memory about the essential points.

◙ Uncertain: If you need clarification on whether a section applies to your situation, this is where your project diary becomes particularly valuable. Record the section in your diary with a circle around the box.

Using your diary in this way will help you keep track of the complexities of your project, from simple decisions to those requiring more in-depth consideration. This organized approach will help evaluate all aspects of your situation, making your decision-making process smoother and more effective.

CONSIDERATIONS FOR CALLING EMERGENCY 911

By preparing in advance, including identifying who to call in an emergency, you can minimize the impact of water intrusion and prevent the secondary damage caused by the growth of harmful microorganisms.

In the face of a water damage problem in the home, the absolute priority is the safety of all occupants. Taking immediate action is vital, not just for mitigating potential damage and limiting expenses but also for ensuring the well-being of everyone involved. Protecting individuals from immediate harm must always be the first step preceding any property damage assessment or restoration activities. By the time you begin to implement this 25 Step program. The rapid and uncontrolled deterioration of the building should have been arrested. The emergency phase discussed in this first section should have resulted in a dry building with measures to mitigate the risk of continuing water entering or causing rewetting.

A sewage or contaminated water damage emergency in your home not only damages property but also poses serious health risks due to the presence of harmful pathogens. Prepare by learning how to respond. This includes developing contact information for local sewage authorities, emergency services, and professional cleanup and remediation teams. You must immediately evacuate the household members from the affected area, avoiding direct contact with contaminated water, and shut off utilities if necessary. Knowing who to call will make a difference in managing the situation.

When to Dial 911

❏ **Life-Threatening Situations:** If someone is injured or any time you feel that your safety or the safety of others is at immediate risk, do not hesitate to evacuate and call 911.

❏ **Unsanitary Water Conditions:** If unsanitary water from floods, sewer lines, or other sources enters your home, posing serious health risks and property damage, evacuate and dial 911, especially if the situation is extensive and uncontrolled.

❏ **Electric Shock Hazards:** If you suspect water has come into contact with electrical outlets, appliances, or wiring, evacuate immediately and dial 911. Do not attempt to turn off power or use electrical devices.

❏ **Structural Instability:** If water damage has caused walls, ceilings, or floors to bulge, sag, or crack, or if you hear creaking or shifting, these could be signs of imminent collapse. Evacuate the area and dial 911.

❏ **Fire Hazards:** If you smell gas, see sparks, or notice smoke, evacuate immediately and dial 911. Water damage can exacerbate fire hazards by short-circuiting electrical systems or compromising gas lines.

❏ **Gas Leaks:** If you suspect a gas leak, such as smelling gas or hearing a hissing sound, evacuate immediately and dial 911. Do not turn on or off any electrical devices, as they can trigger an explosion.

❏ **Inaccessible Water Shut-offs:** If you cannot reach or turn off the main water shut-off valve due to flooding or debris, and the water continues to flow uncontrollably, evacuate and call 911 for assistance.

❏ **Uncontrolled Water Rise:** If water levels are rising rapidly and uncontrollably inside your home, threatening to trap you or cause significant damage, evacuate immediately and dial 911.

❏ **Chemical Spills:** If flooding causes chemical containers to spill, creating hazardous conditions, evacuate the area and dial 911 for professional assistance.

❏ **Frozen Burst Plumbing:** If a burst pipe has caused significant flooding and you cannot control the water flow, evacuate and call 911, especially if the flooding poses a risk to electrical systems or structural integrity.

Personal Protective Equipment and Respirators

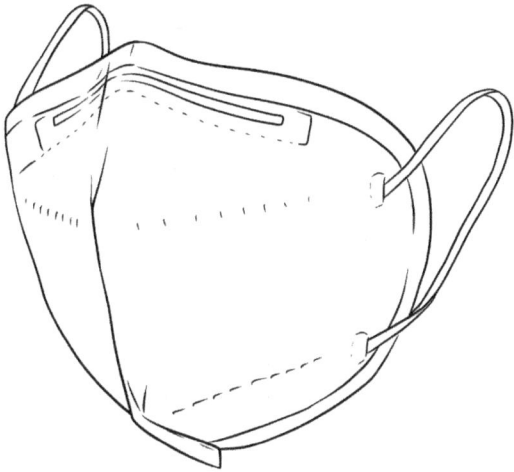

Figure 3-1: N-95 Face Piece Respirator

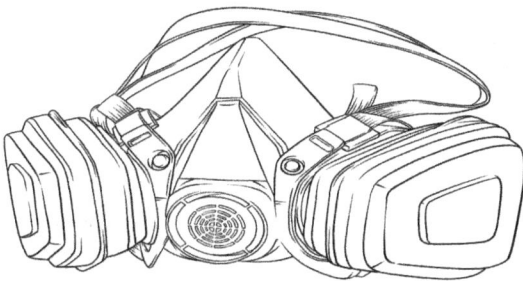

Figure 3-2: Half-Face Respirator

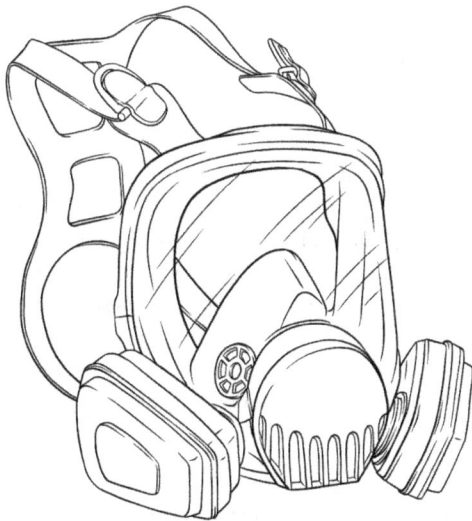

Figure 3-3: Full-Face Respirator

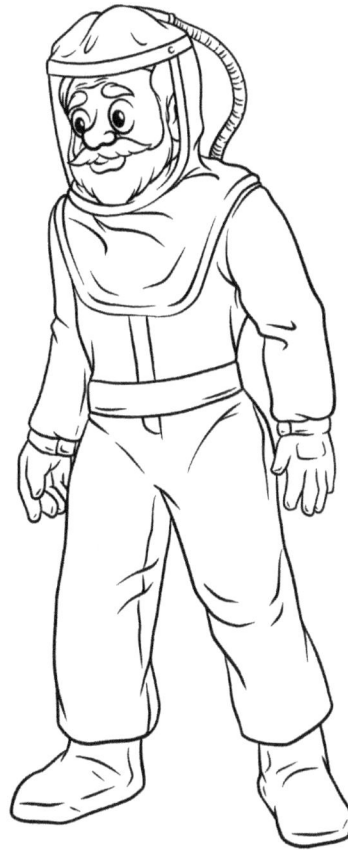

Figure 3-4: Hooded Powered Air Purifying Respirator with Full Personal Protective Equipment (disposable suit, gloves, and shoe covers)

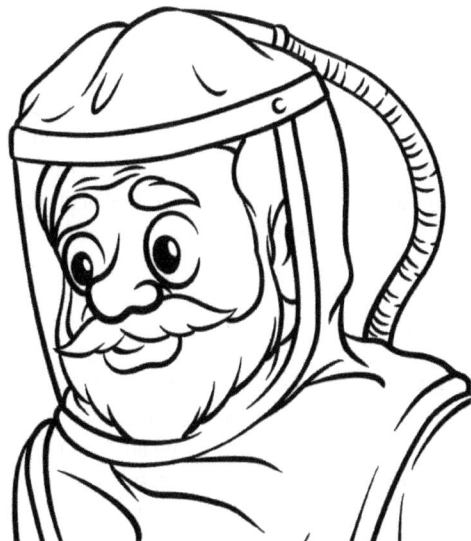

Figure 3-5: Powered Air Purifying Respirators or air-supplied respirators are the only types that can effectively be worn by someone with a beard.

Using Respiratory Protection When Entering a Water-Damaged Building

If you're sensitive to mold or water damage and experience adverse health effects when entering your building, the best choice is to avoid entering entirely. However, I understand that this may not always be practical. For those situations where entry is necessary, this guide provides options for respiratory protection to help reduce exposure to harmful particles and organisms. However, it's important to note that no respirator can offer complete protection.

Types of Respiratory Protection

This section covers several respirator types, each with different levels of protection. These include:

- **N-95 Respirators**: These are basic, disposable masks that filter out some particles but provide limited protection in highly contaminated areas.
- **Half-Face Respirators**: These reusable masks with replaceable filters offer better protection than N-95 masks but still allow exposure around the edges.
- **Full-Face Respirators**: With full coverage of the face and added eye protection, full-face respirators provide a stronger barrier, though they may still have some gaps.
- **Powered Air Purifying Respirators (PAPR)**: These battery-powered units deliver filtered air to a hood or facepiece, creating positive pressure that helps to prevent contaminants from entering. PAPR is the only practical option for individuals with facial hair since it does not rely on a tight seal against the face.

Each type has a specific **protection factor**, indicating its effectiveness in reducing exposure to airborne contaminants. However, no respirator completely blocks all particles, especially those smaller than the mask's filtration limit.

Respirator Considerations for Sensitive Individuals

Wearing a respirator can be challenging for individuals with sensitivities, significantly if lung capacity is reduced. Respirators, particularly those with higher filtration levels, require increased breathing effort, leading to discomfort or even dangerous breathing difficulties. For these reasons, children and babies should not be placed in situations requiring respiratory protection, as they lack the lung capacity to wear these devices safely.

Practical Precautions

If you must enter a contaminated building, ensure that you are properly fitted for your respirator, follow the manufacturer's guidelines for use, and limit your time in the affected area. Remember, while respiratory protection can help reduce exposure, it does not eliminate all risks. Use these tools as temporary aids and prioritize leaving the area as soon as possible to minimize exposure.

One day of beard growth can reduce the effectiveness of a negative pressure respirator—which relies on your lung power to pull air through the filter—by as much as 50%. In cases where facial hair interferes with the respirator's seal, only a Powered Air Purifying Respirator (PAPR) can provide adequate protection, as it does not rely on a tight facial seal. While neatly trimmed facial hair that does not affect the respirator's seal may be acceptable, it's essential to consult and strictly follow the manufacturer's instructions to ensure proper fit and protection.

The challenges of lung capacity and respirator use are serious enough that OSHA mandates comprehensive training and precautions for workers who need respirators. Employees must be trained annually, fit-tested to confirm a proper seal, instructed on proper wear and maintenance, and evaluated to ensure they are medically fit for respirator use. These and other protocols highlight the importance of understanding respirator limitations and following correct usage guidelines for effective protection.

Additional Personal Protective Equipment

When entering a water-damaged environment, additional protective equipment can be essential to minimize exposure to contaminants. **Tyvek™ suits** are a recommended option for protective clothing, as they provide a durable, non-porous barrier that effectively prevents particles, mold spores, and other microorganisms from contacting your clothing and skin. In contrast, cheap disposable coveralls may lack adequate protection, allowing contaminants to penetrate and potentially expose you to harmful particles.

Gloves are another component, as hands frequently come into contact with contaminated surfaces. Select gloves that are waterproof and resistant to tears for the best protection. Additionally, **heavy-duty shoe covers** and **head covers** should be worn to prevent contaminants from collecting on shoes and hair, reducing the risk of carrying spores and debris into clean environments. Using high-quality protective gear like Tyvek™ suits, sturdy gloves, and durable covers for your shoes and head adds a layer of safety, helping to contain contaminants and support a cleaner, healthier home environment.

For added protection in contaminated environments, consider **double-gloving** with an inner barrier glove and an outer heavy-duty glove. The **inner glove** should be made of a protective material like nitrile or polyurethane, which provides a strong barrier directly against the skin to shield it from contaminants. If you're performing heavy-duty work that could risk tearing or abrasion, use a sturdy outer glove over the inner one for added durability and protection.

Specialty **outer gloves** are also available for specific tasks; for example, **Kevlar®** gloves offer exceptional cut resistance and are ideal for work where sharp objects or rough surfaces could compromise regular gloves. This double-layer approach enhances safety by providing a secure inner layer and a tough outer layer, giving you the resilience to handle challenging tasks in water-damaged environments.

**Ensuring Safe and Effective Use of PPE
in Sensitive Environments**

In conclusion, properly using personal protective equipment (PPE) is essential for minimizing exposure to harmful contaminants in water-damaged environments. Using PPE effectively requires understanding how to properly wear, fit, and maintain each piece. While many resources are available on PPE use, it's important to note that these guidelines often assume the wearer is in good health and can tolerate its use. Consulting with a healthcare provider is strongly recommended for individuals with health sensitivities or concerns about their ability to wear PPE safely or enter a contaminated building. This professional guidance can help ensure that any protective measures are appropriate for their specific health needs and limitations, adding an essential layer of safety to the remediation process.

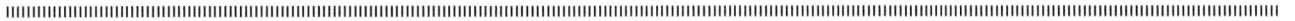

Being Prepared for Water Emergencies

Water damage can range from subtle to severe. This guide prepares you for the inevitable, helping you respond rapidly to prevent or limit damage. For situations where severe water damage occurs or goes unnoticed, you'll find guidance on following the 25 Steps to Recovery later in the book.

BEFORE DAMAGE

Water damage emergencies can affect anyone, regardless of location or the area's perceived flood risk. In fact, according to FEMA, a surprising 25% of flood-related water damage emergencies occur in regions with low flood risk. Consider the national averages: According to the Insurance Information Institute, In the United States, approximately 14,000 individuals experience a water damage emergency in their homes or workplaces every day. This statistic underscores the commonality of water damage incidents on a national scale.

The first objective is to equip you with the knowledge and strategies to protect your home and belongings from water or excess moisture. Early recognition of potential water damage and proactive planning are key to facilitating a rapid response. Water damage can strike at any time, and when it does, a swift and well-coordinated response helps prevent or limit damage.

When water damage results in mold growth in homes, the volume of mold spores and fungal fragments increases dramatically as they reproduce.

Secondly, this section will help you understand whether and how likely past or current water incidents relate to subvisible damage. Recognizing these signs early allows one to anticipate and address pending issues. Reviewing past incidents and how they were addressed and the need for follow-up with the 25 Steps Program that follows.

Thirdly, you'll develop a three-dimensional understanding of how water and moisture flow through a home. Water intrusion in one area can easily migrate to adjoining areas, creating conditions for additional hidden damage.

This awareness is vital for comprehensive water damage management.

The "standard of care" sufficient for healthy individuals can be devastating for those sensitive to mold and bacteria contamination. For medically hypersensitive individuals, an inadequate response can lead to severe health issues. Since an immediate professional response may often be unavailable, this section emphasizes the need to be prepared with an action plan tailored to the specific health needs of the occupants for when "things go wrong."

Finally, this section assists in determining whether you can manage water damage on your own or if professional assistance is necessary by knowing when and where to seek help, particularly in cases involving hypersensitive individuals, where professional expertise may be required to ensure a thorough and safe cleanup.

WHY IS WATER DAMAGE AN EMERGENCY?

Water damage is a swift destroyer of homes. While it may not be as immediate as fire, its effects can be as devastating. The deterioration of wet materials can commence within seconds and escalate rapidly. Understanding the visible flow of water and its unseen progression as it seeps into cracks and crevices and is drawn deeply into materials through capillary action helps understand the level of response that is needed. Wet areas often extend well beyond what is immediately apparent. Water will flow horizontally and downward. Within minutes, water saturates carpets, underlay, and subflooring. Furniture resting on these wet surfaces can leach discoloration and stain adjoining surfaces. Wood furniture absorbs water, causing it to swell, weakening joints and fasteners, and undermining the item's structural integrity. Other personal items, such as photos and documents, will bleed inks and emulsions almost immediately, and the paper they are printed on weakens.

After a few hours, the dormant bacteria that were once harmless emerge from their dry state and begin to multiply at an alarming rate. The number of bacteria cells at room temperature can double every 15 minutes. In eight hours, a single dormant bacterium in a water-saturated carpet will easily have multiplied to a million, but it doesn't stop there. The following chart shows a theoretical progression of bacteria:

Hours 1 through 3—Dormant or Lag Period	A single wetted bacteria remains dormant but begins to imbibe the surrounding moisture. Nutrients dissolve and are released from dirt and microscopic particles accumulated in the home.
Hour 4.0 – the first division	One bacterium divides and becomes two.
4 hour 15 minutes – 2nd division	2 doubles to become 4
4 hour 30 minutes – 3rd division	4 doubles to become 8
4 hour 45 minutes – 4th division	8 doubles to become 16
Fifth Hour – 5th division	32
Sixth division	64
Seventh division	128
Eighth division	250 (rounding begins here)
Sixth Hour – Ninth division	500
Tenth division	1,000
11th division	2,000
12th division	4,000
Seventh Hour – 13th division	8,000
14th division	16,000
15th division	32,000
16th division	64,000
Eighth Hour – 17th division	125,000
18th division	250,000
19th division	500,000
20th division	1,000,000
Hour Nine – 24th division	2,000,000
Hour Ten – 28th division	4,000,000
Hour Eleven – 32nd division	8,000,000
Hour Twelve – 36th division	16,000,000
24 hours	1,208,925,820,000,000,000,000,000 Or "One sextillion, two hundred eight quintillion, nine hundred twenty-five quadrillion, eight hundred twenty trillion."

Experimental Evidence

Of course, the above is a theoretical calculation of what could occur under a given circumstance. In real life, it is often far more complex. In 2011, several colleagues and everyone at RestCon Environmental embarked on a significant research endeavor, which led to the publication of a paper titled *Bacterial Amplification and In-Place Carpet Drying: Implications for Category 1 Water Intrusion Restoration*, published in the esteemed peer-reviewed "Journal of Environmental Health." Within scientific publications, an abstract serves as a succinct summary and a glimpse into the study's essence. Our abstract stated:

"The study described in this article investigated whether in-place carpet drying processes resulted in bacterial amplification following water intrusion from a clean water source (category 1) in a residential indoor environment. Bacterial amplification was examined after wetting a 10-year-old carpet and pad that had no history of water intrusion. Three test areas were extracted and dried using industry-recommended procedures for in-place drying and compared to a control area that was not extracted or dried. Results from carpet, pad, and subsurface dust demonstrated that bacterial amplification occurred in all test areas. CFUs of bacteria per gram of carpet surface dust and subsurface dust prior to water intrusion were lower than levels in subsurface dust after in-place drying. The authors' study contributes information regarding the restoration of water-based carpet damage by

professional water damage restoration companies, building maintenance personnel, and housekeeping managers. Results suggest that the appropriate response time for carpet pad salvage is considerably shorter than the current industry recommendation of 72 hours." (Holland, 2012)

Our effort to understand the timing and necessity of water damage restoration led us to design and conduct a practical experiment. We set up four carpeted areas that were intentionally flooded—one was left wet as a control, while the other three underwent standard drying practices. We monitored all four areas hourly, around the clock, collecting samples to determine how quickly mold and bacteria developed after water damage.

The industry consensus was that drying an area within 72 hours of clean water entering a building was sufficient to prevent significant mold and bacteria growth amplification. To test this, we created four areas in our warehouse that could be flooded. We lined the concrete slab with plastic, added a donated 10-year-old carpet and pad, and flooded the three test areas and one control area with an inch of water.

The experiment was carefully scheduled for a 72-hour duration, with hourly data collection. The first 24 hours proceeded smoothly as per our plan. The three test areas were flooded and allowed to sit for 12 hours, then extraction and drying were begun using air movers and dehumidification. However, by hour 30, an unexpected development occurred. The three extracted areas were drying nicely; however, the fourth still-saturated control area developed a terrible stench. Despite the negative air we had established using the warehouse ventilation system, a foul odor was filling the warehouse, emanating from the wet control test area. We surrounded the control area by constructing a containment chamber and added HEPA-filtered Air Filtration Device, which was exhausted in the adjacent parking lot. But the odor worsened, filling the parking lot and eventually reaching our office area on the other side of the building. Despite the physical separation, the impact on the office staff was swift and pronounced. In addition, complaints from neighboring businesses also arose as the odors around our building became intolerable. Within 36 hours, the situation had deteriorated to the point where several staff members were genuinely ill. The control part of our experiment was terminated, and office workers were told to leave work early. The technical staff donned respirators, collected a final set of samples for analysis, extracted the standing water from the contained control area, and disposed of it in the sewer system. The saturated carpet and pad were double-bagged and discarded along with the plastic-lined control chamber.

This real-world experience served as a stark reminder that the consequences of water damage extend far beyond mere numbers and data. It was a tangible lesson that the urgency of addressing water damage promptly and effectively could not be overstated. The impact of this experiment in our published study was profound. We concluded that the research strongly indicated that the 72-hour Standard of Care established for mold was insufficient and needed adjustment to reflect the reality of bacterial amplification in water-damaged environments. This revelation would significantly shape our understanding and recommendations to the water damage restoration industry, emphasizing the need for swift and effective responses to control bacteria and mold in the face of water damage challenges.

In retrospect, this incident provides further evidence that exposure to biotoxins, such as endotoxins from gram-negative bacteria and exotoxins from gram-positive bacteria such as Actinomycetes, would occur not just from sewage but also from any delays in a prompt response to water-damaged buildings. The ten-year-old carpet used in our study had no evidence of previous water damage and appeared well-maintained. The initial test results from our analysis agreed and showed it to have been from a normal building. It became apparent that the influence of biotoxins from bacteria in water-damaged environments could have far-reaching consequences, eventually for everyone, not just the hypersensitive. Whereas mold takes several days to germinate and grow, bacteria numbers increase exponentially, beginning a few hours after flooding. Those with genetic predispositions to mold and biotoxins provide early warnings of the impact of water damage for everyone. This real-world experience, ever-present in our conclusions, underscored the urgency of addressing water damage promptly and effectively. It strongly suggested that the 72-hour Standard of Care in place at the time needed adjustment to align with the reality of bacterial amplification in water-damaged environments. These insights profoundly shaped our understanding, emphasizing the need for swift and effective responses to water damage challenges.

WHEN TO ACT AND WHEN TO CALL FOR HELP

Rapid drying is undoubtedly the primary goal in any water damage situation. Fast and aggressive drying methods are necessary to prevent mold and bacteria amplification and the deterioration of the building's structure.

If effective drying is completed before mold and microbial problems set in, the likelihood of a complete building recovery increases significantly. However, immediate action limits further damage even if a preemptive response is no longer possible. Remember, deterioration will continue until the wet areas are thoroughly dry. However, many factors involved with understanding and intervening in water damage are counterintuitive.

- While rapid response is essential, attempting to dry a building too quickly can block the flow of moisture, impeding drying and resulting in a condition known as Case Hardening, which can trap moisture deep in the materials.

- Humidity levels depend as much on temperature as the amount of water present. This means that a cold item or surface may have reached dewpoint temperatures demonstrated by the formation of liquid water. This results in a higher relative humidity at the surface than in the surrounding air.

- Over-drying will damage wood, resulting in shrinkage, and under-drying will result in swelling.

- Just because a surface feels dry to the touch doesn't mean it is dry. Monitoring the moisture conditions with meters and understanding their readings is the key to establishing and maintaining a balanced drying system.

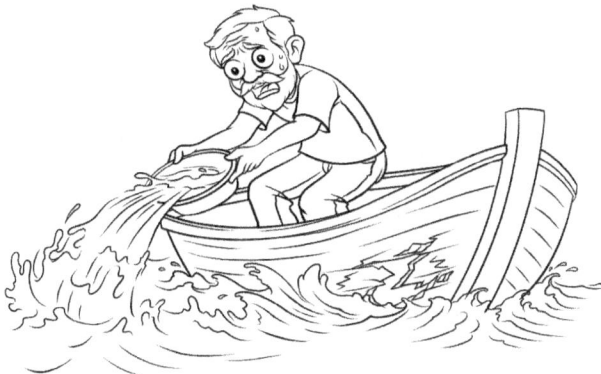

Over time, the levels of spores and fungal fragments that develop due to excess moisture will build up. Think of it this way: Your home is like a boat with a hole in its bottom. If the hole is small, the amount of bailing needed to keep the boat afloat is minimal. Similarly, regular cleaning can help remove spores and fragments when mold contamination is low, keeping the environment under control. But as the hole gets bigger—or as mold growth increases—it becomes necessary to bail faster, or in this case, clean more frequently and thoroughly.

At some point, just as the water may start coming in so fast that no amount of bailing can keep the boat afloat, and the boat sinks! This is analogous to when the level of mold contamination reaches a point where routine cleaning is no longer enough. This is when professional remediation becomes essential to restore the balance and health of your home.

One square inch of mold growth can contain over a million spores. It doesn't take much indoor mold growth to disrupt the balance of your home's environment.

Essay: Understanding the Nature of Structural Drying
by Ken Larsen, CR®, WLS®, FLS®, CLS®, ERS®, CMP®, CSDS

Water damage isn't just about the visible pooling of water; it involves moisture that penetrates deep into building materials. Proper structural drying helps prevent the growth of microorganisms such as mold and bacteria, which can compromise structural integrity and occupant health. It is essential to act swiftly, as microbial growth can begin within a few hours if conditions are right.

Unlike superficial drying, which often only addresses the water you can see, structural drying targets the unseen moisture within materials. Effective drying is about understanding

building assemblies and moisture behavior and controlling the drying environment to return materials to their normal, equilibrium moisture content, preventing future complications.

Preparation Before Water Damage Happens
Proactive preparation is key to mitigating the impact of water damage. Homeowners and renters can take several steps to make their property resilient and ensure that emergency response is fast and effective.

Know Your Property's Risk Areas: Understand where potential water ingress could occur. Basements, attics, roofs, and areas near plumbing lines are typically the most vulnerable. Keep a map or list of your flood risk. These risks are being increased due to extreme weather events becoming more common.

Equip Yourself with Basic Tools: Invest in tools like moisture sensors, water alarms, and a high-quality wet/dry vacuum. Moisture sensors can help you understand where water has penetrated, while water alarms provide an early alert to leaks. Thermal imaging cameras are becoming very inexpensive and can be useful in identifying wet materials by seeing temperature differences.

Establish Relationships with Professionals: Engage with a qualified structural drying contractor and vet them before disaster strikes. Ensure they are IICRC, ACAC, and/or RIA certified and employ best practices beyond merely "standard practice" to a "state of the art" understanding.

Approaches to restorative drying by competent restorative drying firms are much more than simply a *"Clean up on aisle three!"* service. It's a skilled trade, and there are many imposters out there. You can get help locating qualified people:

Institute of Inspection, Cleaning and Restoration Certification (IICRC)
Phone: 1-844-464-4272
Email: CertifiedFirms@iicrcnet.org, Standards@iicrcnet.org
Address: 4043 S. Eastern Ave., Las Vegas, NV 89119
Website: [IICRC.org]

The IICRC provides foundational education and certification for professionals in the cleaning and restoration industries, comparable to an entry-to-intermediate level of training suited for field technicians, helpers, and crew leaders. The organization also develops and maintains industry standards for cleaning and restoration practices.

American Council for Accredited Certification (ACAC)
Phone: 888-808-838
Email: info@acac.org
Address: PO Box 1000, Yarnell, AZ 85362
Website: [acac.org]

The ACAC offers third-party accredited certifications for professionals in cleaning and restoration, providing an advanced level of training comparable to college-level education. These certifications are designed for department managers and leadership roles, emphasizing credibility through rigorous training and testing. ACAC credentials are government-recognized, allowing certified professionals to display their designation after their names (e.g., "John Smith, CSDS").

Restoration Industry Association (RIA)
Contact Information:
Phone: 856-439-9222
Email: info@restorationindustry.org
Address: 1120 Route 73, Suite 200, Mount Laurel, NJ 08054
Website: [restorationindustry.org]

The RIA is the leading trade association in the restoration industry, offering the highest level of professional education available, akin to a university-level program. RIA's advanced certifications are suited for consultants, expert witnesses, and other top-tier roles. Prerequisites for RIA certification include significant field experience and foundational credentials from IICRC or ACAC. RIA-certified professionals are highly respected across the industry.

Registered Third Party Evaluator (RTPE)
Contact Information:
Phone: 817-542-1189
Email: Ken@drystandard.org
Address: 363 Loblolly Bay Drive, Santa Rosa Beach, FL 32459

The RTPE is a global registry of cleaning and restoration professionals recognized by their peers as experts who prioritize objective assessments in their evaluations, often guided by the principle of "speaking for the structure." RTPE registrants typically hold advanced RIA certifications and/or university degrees, underscoring their commitment to unbiased analysis, separate from the interests of property owners, contractors, or insurers.

Document Your Home's Condition: Take detailed photos of your home and keep good notes in your diary. This documentation can help contractors assess the changes caused by water damage and assist in insurance claims.

Read Your Insurance Policy: Don't assume you are covered for "everything." Property insurance policies have more exclusions or limits to coverage than ever—a "rider" to your policy coverage may be available for an additional charge. A good insurance broker can be very useful in helping you get the correct coverage.

Immediate Response to Water Damage
The swiftness of response to water intrusion in the first few hours following a water damage event will determine the extent of mold risk. However, bacteria and water-born microorganisms are likely to explode in the population far faster than mold will. Here's what to do:

- **Ensure Safety First**: Shut off the water source, if applicable, and electricity in affected areas. Water intrusions near electrical outlets or appliances can be dangerous, so safety should be your priority.

- **Document the Damage**: Take Lots of photos and videos of the affected areas. Digital photos are cheap—but so valuable for future use. Accurate documentation is necessary for insurance purposes and provides useful information for the restoration contractor to develop a drying plan. Record important information in your project diary.

- **Remove Standing Water**: Use wet/dry vacuums to remove as much standing water as safely possible—only if it is safe to do so and there is a place to safely / legally dispose of it. Remember that removing standing water is only the first step—materials must be dried thoroughly to prevent mold growth.

- **Isolate the HVAC system:** By sealing off ducts into and out of the affected areas, cross-contamination can often be limited to the water-damaged areas. When sealing off ducts, avoid trapping moisture in them is important. If water has entered the duct or system, it should be turned off and will need professional attention to prevent deterioration and biological growth.

Facilitating the Drying Process

Engaging a professional is always recommended for effective drying, but understanding the process can help you recognize whether the necessary steps are being taken. The following key practices help ensure successful drying:

- **Utilization of Proper Equipment and Techniques:**

  › **Extraction as the First Step**: Physically removing the liquid water from the structure is many times more efficient than trying to evaporate it. This means thorough extraction is the foundation of any competent drying project.

  › **Using Dehumidifiers and Air Movers:** Air movers help evaporate liquid moisture from surfaces, turning it into vapor, which industrial-grade dehumidifiers then collect. Effective coordination between airflow and dehumidification using air movers "transitions" moisture from the material surface into the air while dehumidifiers capture and remove it, ensuring the air-drying rate outpaces the rate of evaporation.

- **"Monitoring" and Adjustments:**

  › **Moisture Mapping:** Contractors should be using moisture meters and thermal imaging cameras to identify moisture in building materials and ensure drying progresses appropriately. Make sure professionals take initial moisture readings and conduct daily inspection, documentation, and modifications (sometimes called "Monitoring") until materials reach their "dry standard."

  › **Controlled Environment**: Drying should occur in a controlled environment to limit damage to building materials. This involves closing windows and doors and potentially sealing off affected areas to create a drying chamber. The goal is to prevent humid air from entering or leaving, thereby optimizing drying efficiency.

- **Evaluating Drying Success:**

  › **The Dry Standard**: *"Begin with the end in mind,"* says Franklin Covey. In restorative drying, a target dryness in materials is called a "dry standard," which means returning the moisture content of affected materials to what is normal for the given environment and material type. Make sure that your contractor is not simply estimating dryness by touch or feel; they should be using scientific methods to establish when materials are acceptably dry.

  › **Validation of Drying:** Request that contractors provide proof of successful drying through final moisture readings. Ask for detailed documentation, including moisture maps and photographs, showing that moisture levels are back to normal.

Preventing Mold and Long-Term Health Risks

For individuals with hypersensitivities, even small amounts of mold can have significant health implications. To protect indoor air quality and prevent mold, ensure the source of excessive moisture is controlled and that excessively wet materials are removed.

- **Use Non-Toxic Cleaning Methods**: Once drying is complete, any residual microbial risk should be managed using non-toxic, evidence-based remediation methods. Avoid harsh chemicals that could exacerbate sensitivity. Look for contractors who understand and utilize such approaches, ensuring that safety for occupants, especially those with health sensitivities, is prioritized. Be skeptical of "silver bullet" cures for biological risks. *(e.g., light bulbs, oxidizing gas-phase generators, oxidizing stain removers, fogging products, heating protocols, encapsulants/sealants)*

- **Replace Materials When Necessary**: Not all materials can be fully dried or remediated after water damage. Porous materials like drywall and insulation are often better replaced if significantly affected, as they can harbor moisture and microorganisms/mold spores even after the drying process. An experienced and educated contractor will help determine what must be replaced versus what can be restored.

- **Ventilation and Humidity Control**: After the structural restoration, maintaining appropriate humidity levels is key to preventing future mold growth. Use dehumidifiers, especially in naturally damp areas like basements, and ensure that bathrooms and kitchens are well-ventilated. Be aware of cold surfaces in your home, as they can sometimes condense the necessary water from the air to support the growth of mold.

Recognizing Competence in Water Damage Restoration Professionals

Choosing the right restoration contractor can make all the difference. A competent contractor will:

- **Demonstrate Advanced Knowledge**: They should discuss their plan with you in clear terms, highlighting not only their use of equipment but also their drying strategy based on scientific principles.

- **Document Everything**: Proper documentation, including photographs, moisture readings, and drying logs, should be a part of every project. This shows a commitment to accountability and transparency.

- **Practice Safety and Hygiene**: The contractor should wear appropriate personal protective equipment (PPE)—even when nobody is watching. If the contractor who does this for a living doesn't take the subject seriously, why would they expect you to?

Proper water damage restoration is essential to prevent mold growth and protect the health of those living in the home. By understanding the basics of structural drying, preparing in advance, and ensuring the correct procedures are followed during drying, homeowners and renters can significantly reduce the risk of mold and maintain a safe, healthy living environment.

Effective restoration is not about simply using the right tools but involves a thorough understanding of how moisture behaves and the best strategies to control it. Engaging knowledgeable professionals, equipping yourself with basic tools, and monitoring the drying process will go a long way in ensuring the integrity of your home and the health of its occupants.

The restoration industry has evolved significantly over the decades, with modern practices focusing on scientific and evidence-based drying methods. By taking the appropriate actions outlined in this guide, homeowners and renters can not only mitigate damage but also contribute to a restoration process that fosters long-term resilience and health in their living spaces.

THE CHALLENGE OF RAPID EMERGENCY DRYING

Professional restoration contractors play a pivotal role in the drying process. The longer you wait to address a water damage emergency, the more expensive and extensive the restoration process becomes. However, not all companies offering restoration or remediation services are created equal. Some may lack the qualifications, responsiveness, or knowledge to meet your needs, while others may engage in predatory pricing. Proactively researching and choosing a reliable service provider before a crisis can save you from these pitfalls.

Even with the best preparation, unknown pre-existing conditions can become problematic during the restoration process. Rapid air movement, essential for speeding up drying, can inadvertently spread pre-existing mold and bacteria spores throughout the home, causing cross-contamination. Balancing the need for quick drying to prevent further damage with the risk of spreading existing contaminants is a significant challenge. Using containment and airflow controls can help minimize dust spread to unaffected areas, which also helps with controlling the spread of organisms if they are present.

ACTION PLAN: IDENTIFYING A WATER DAMAGE RESTORATION COMPANY BEFORE NEEDED

Not all companies are equipped to handle emergencies, and some may not be sensitive to medical issues related to mold and water damage. It's essential to choose a company that can respond promptly and effectively.

Identify a reputable water damage restoration company and note their contact information. Ensure the company has a 24-hour emergency contact number so you can reach them anytime. Additionally, check if the company is an IICRC (Institute of Inspection, Cleaning and Restoration Certification) Certified Firm, which indicates they adhere to industry standards and practices. The search function at IICRC.org will help you locate certified firms and technicians in your area who are ready to help.

There comes a tipping point when controlling moisture and mold growth can no longer be easily handled as a DIY project, and professional assistance becomes necessary.

FINDING AN EMERGENCY WATER DAMAGE RESTORATION CONTRACTOR

1. Use the Institute of Inspection, Cleaning, and Restoration Certification website at IICRC.org

2. Use the site "IICRC Global Finder" finder to search by zip code for Firms within a reasonable distance of your home.

3. Under 'Locate a Certified Pro, ' indicate you are looking for a Certified Firm.

4. Search for Active Certifications. The ideal certification is the "**Master Water Restorer**". These people have proven by training and experience that they understand the wide range of water damage issues that may need to be addressed. If there are no Master Restorers available in your area, then the most important individual certifications would be the

   a. Water Damage Restoration Technician (WRT)

   b. Applied Structural Drying Technician (ASD)

5. These are likely to be the on-site technicians handling the day-to-day work at your home to help you adequately address your emergency water damage needs. Having this information readily available ensures

that in an emergency, you can quickly contact a qualified and reliable company to address the water damage, helping to mitigate further issues and ensuring a swift and effective response.

LIST EACH COMPANY YOU IDENTIFY WITHIN YOUR SERVICE AREA

Record the following information in your Project Diary

- Company Name
- Technician Names and Certifications
- 24-hour Emergency Contact Information and Number
- Website Address
- Confirmation of IICRC Firm Certification

The Institute of Inspection, Cleaning, and Restoration Certification (IICRC) is a globally recognized organization that establishes and maintains high standards within the water damage and mold remediation industries. With a network of over 50,000 certified technicians and 6,000 Certified Firms worldwide, the IICRC provides essential guidance and certifications to uphold industry practices and ensure a consistent standard of care. To become an IICRC Certified Firm, restoration contractors must meet specific requirements and follow rigorous procedures, demonstrating their commitment to quality and professionalism.

The ANSI/IICRC S500 and S520 standards are among the most important guidelines in water damage restoration and mold remediation, applicable across diverse settings from residential to commercial buildings. The ANSI/IICRC S500 outlines effective processes for water damage restoration, emphasizing the control of emergencies, prevention of further damage, and protection of occupant health and safety. The ANSI/IICRC S520, meanwhile, provides a structured approach to mold remediation, detailing the methods needed to remove mold contamination and restore affected areas.

While these standards offer extensive guidance for most water damage and mold remediation scenarios, they may not fully address the needs of homes occupied by individuals with medical sensitivities to water damage and the associated microorganisms. For these situations, the emergency drying steps in the S500 should be applied immediately to stabilize the environment and prevent further deterioration. However, if these initial emergency measures are insufficient to address health concerns fully, the next stages in the recovery process involve a more detailed, medically

sensitive approach. This is where the 25 Step Program becomes essential, guiding additional, thorough stages necessary to support recovery and protect the well-being of sensitive occupants.

PRE-QUALIFYING A PROFESSIONAL

I recommend using the 'Locate A Certified Pro' feature on the IICRC's website for assistance. Not every company is equipped to help with special medically essential needs, so do your best to vet companies before you need them—then keep them on speed dial!

The following will help you interview each firm you are considering:

Key requirements

For a restoration firm to be registered as a certified firm by the IICRC, they must agree to comply with the following:

- **Employee Certification:** Restoration firms must employ at least one technician with individual IICRC certifications in relevant areas of expertise. Technicians typically earn these certifications through training and passing exams in water damage restoration, mold remediation, fire and smoke restoration, carpet cleaning, and more.

- **Insurance:** Registered firms must carry the appropriate insurance coverage, including liability and workers' compensation insurance, as local regulations and IICRC standards require.

- **Code of Ethics:** Firms must agree to abide by the IICRC's Code of Ethics, which outlines the principles of honesty, integrity, and professionalism in the industry.

- **Written Contracts:** Firms are required to use written contracts that clearly define the scope of work, pricing, and other terms and conditions of the restoration services provided to clients.

- **Compliance with Standards:** Certified firms must adhere to the IICRC's industry standards and best practices for restoration and cleaning services. These standards provide guidelines for performing work to industry-accepted quality levels.

- **Continuing Education:** The IICRC requires technicians and firm owners to undergo ongoing education and training to stay current with industry advancements and best practices.

- **Inspection:** The IICRC may conduct inspections or audits to ensure that registered firms continue to comply with the organization's standards and requirements.

By meeting these requirements, restoration contractors can become registered as certified firms with the IICRC. This certification is a valuable credential that demonstrates the owners' and management's commitment to professionalism and industry standards in cleaning and restoration services. It seeks to assure clients that they are working with a reputable and qualified firm.

Basic Considerations Selecting a Water-Damage Restoration Firm

During water damage, time is of the essence! It is too late to expect you to be able to select a quality service after water damage has occurred. The more you can do in advance to identify and choose a reliable water damage restoration company, the better your chances of maintaining the habitability of your home—especially if you or a family member are genetically predisposed or have health conditions that make you more vulnerable to the organisms associated with water damage.

You can choose a qualified service provider who meets your needs by asking potential emergency drying companies comprehensive questions and considering various factors. With over 6,000 Certified Firms nationwide, a company is within a reasonable distance. Still, they may also need to be trained in medically important remediation to address pre-existing hidden mold contamination if it is present. Beginning your search early can provide the time necessary to help them better understand the specialized services you need and help them become educated so they can improve their services. If they show no interest, you can eliminate them from consideration and look elsewhere to find a suitable alternative before an emergency arises. This is particularly crucial for households with members who have environmental sensitivities. Here are essential questions and considerations to guide your decision:

1. Insurance and Licensing

Before hiring a restoration company, ensure they are licensed and insured to work in your area. Verify that the company is legally authorized to conduct restoration work, as this helps avoid potential liability issues. Reputable companies should be able to provide proof of insurance and licensing upon request, so ask for these credentials to confirm they meet necessary legal and professional requirements.

2. References and Reviews

When evaluating a restoration company, ask if they can provide references from past clients who have used their emergency services. Speaking with previous clients, especially ones with medical hypersensitivities, can offer valuable insight into the company's reliability and service quality. Additionally, check online reviews and ratings to gauge their reputation and customer satisfaction.

3. Equipment and Technology

Consider the equipment and technology the restoration company uses. Advanced tools can significantly enhance the efficiency and effectiveness of the restoration process. Check if they can access essential equipment such as drying and dehumidification machines, moisture meters, and thermal imaging cameras. These tools can aid in detecting moisture and ensuring a comprehensive restoration is performed.

4. Training and Certifications

Ensure the restoration company's technicians are regularly trained and certified in the latest water damage restoration techniques. Ongoing training keeps their knowledge and skills current, which is essential for high-quality service. Confirm that they stay up to date with industry advancements and best practices, as this commitment to industry standards reflects their dedication to excellence. Look for IICRC certifications in Water Damage Restoration Training (WRT) and Applied Structural Drying (ASD) as indicators of their expertise.

5. Response and Availability

Check if the restoration company is available 24/7 for emergency water damage, as round-the-clock availability is essential for effectively handling emergencies. Ask about their typical response time, especially after-hours, since a quick response can significantly minimize damage and costs. Additionally, find out if they offer same-day or next-day service for non-emergency situations, as prompt service is beneficial even for less urgent needs.

6. Pricing and Fees

Ask the restoration company if they can provide a detailed estimate or clear pricing structure for their services. Transparent pricing helps prevent unexpected costs. Inquire about any potential hidden fees or additional charges that might apply during emergencies to ensure full financial clarity. Additionally, confirm what payment methods they accept, as knowing your options can help you plan your finances accordingly.

7. Guarantees and Warranties

Find out if the restoration company offers any guarantees or warranties on its workmanship or the materials used. While assurances may provide greater peace of mind about the quality of its work, many firms may not be familiar with working with people suffering from sensitivities. Ask about its policy in the event you are unsatisfied with the restoration so you understand its process for addressing any issues or concerns.

8. Environmental Considerations

Ask if the company follows eco-friendly practices and uses environmentally safe products, especially if you have specific needs based on your medical conditions and desire specific medical preferences. Eco-friendly practices benefit both health and environmental impact but may need to go further for your particular situation. Confirm if they have experience handling medically important mold remediation and other potential hazards related to water damage, as specialized knowledge is essential for a safe and comprehensive restoration.

9. Communication

Inquire about how the company plans to keep you informed throughout restoration. Clear communication is essential for staying updated. Ask if there will be a designated point of contact for any questions or concerns, as having a single, reliable contact ensures consistent and effective communication.

10. Emergency Preparedness

Ask if the company has a plan for handling large-scale disasters or community emergencies. Preparedness for such events indicates that they can manage significant incidents effectively. Additionally, find out if they are part of any local or national emergency response networks, as this can enhance their ability to respond promptly and efficiently during widespread emergencies.

QUALIFYING A MEDICALLY IMPORTANT RESTORATION COMPANY

Finding an emergency drying company that performs high-quality, medically sound restoration or remediation would be ideal. However, the focus of these services can differ significantly. In an emergency drying situation, time is of the essence—your wet building can't wait for someone to fit you into their schedule. On the other hand, when selecting a company for medically necessary restoration or remediation, additional considerations often extend beyond the traditional standard of care.

The urgency shifts once the immediate emergency is over and the building is dry. Speed of response becomes less critical, allowing you to focus more on the quality of work, especially in relation to the health needs of the occupants. With the building stabilized and no longer in rapid deterioration, you can transition to the next phase, guided by the 25 Steps in this book. In this stage, you can plan thoughtfully, ask questions, and carefully consider the best options to address your unique situation, desires, and needs.

Certification

- Look for IICRC Certifications to become an Applied Microbial Remediation Technician (AMRT) or Mold Remediation Specialist (MRS) and that their training certifications are current. These are the premiere certifications for people performing remediation for households that do not have special medical needs.

- Have any company employees received specific training in Medically Important Remediation, including advanced training in water damage restoration and mold remediation, as offered by CIRSx.com?

- Ensure the company has other specialized training relevant to your needs. Confirm their qualifications.

- Have company employees received specialized training or certifications for working in environments with people with multiple chemical sensitivities or other medical conditions?

- If they have IICRC certifications but no specific medically important restoration or remediation training, are they willing to attend online continuing education training offered by CIRSx.com?

- Their willingness to further educate themselves demonstrates a commitment to your health needs.

Experience with Sensitive Clients

- Can they provide examples of projects where the company has successfully addressed the needs of individuals with mold or chemical sensitivities? Ask for specific case studies or examples to gauge their experience.

- Is the company willing to adapt restoration and remediation practices to accommodate sensitive clients? Flexibility in their approach is needed to meet the unique health requirements when medical issues are involved.

Expertise

When choosing a restoration company, consider their experience and expertise in water damage restoration. Companies with more years of experience often provide better service and a higher level of knowledge. Determine whether the company specializes in specific types of water damage to ensure they can handle your unique needs. Additionally, confirm that their technicians have experience managing various water damage scenarios, including floods, leaks, and sewage backups, as this breadth of experience enables them to address any situation that may arise effectively.

Health and Safety Measures

- What precautions are taken to ensure the safety and well-being of individuals with mold sensitivities during restoration and remediation?

- Do they advocate the physical removal of non-restorable materials, environmentally friendly soap or detergent methods, and avoid biocides and other chemicals, essential oils, and other killing agents? Eco-friendly methods can reduce health risks.

- Do they seek informed consent before using any chemicals on worksites? Transparency and consent are vital for trust and safety.

- Do they provide SDS and product information sheets upon request for every project? Advanced Access to Safety Data Sheets informs you about the chemicals used.

Communication and Customization

- How do they communicate with clients who have mold sensitivities to tailor the restoration plan to their specific needs? Clear communication ensures that your concerns are addressed.

- Are they open to client input and concerns regarding the choice of materials and products used? Their willingness to listen to your preferences is important for customized care.

Product Selection

- Do they use building materials and products that are safe for sensitive individuals? Ensure they choose low-VOC and non-toxic options.

- Are their cleaning agents and chemicals selected with sensitivity in mind? Opting for safe products can minimize health risks.

Ventilation and Air Quality

- How do they address indoor air quality concerns to ensure the environment is free of excess mold spores and contaminants? Effective air quality management is essential for a healthy environment.

Monitoring and Follow-Up

- Do they help facilitate independent third-party post-remediation testing and follow-up to ensure the environment remains safe for sensitive clients? Qualified independent verification adds an extra layer of assurance.

- What is their process for addressing any issues arising after the restoration work is complete? Understand their follow-up procedures to ensure continued safety.

References and Testimonials

- Do they provide references from clients with mold sensitivities who can speak to their experience? Client references can offer valuable insights into their service quality.

- Are there any testimonials or reviews from clients in similar situations? Testimonials can help validate their expertise and reliability.

Cost Transparency

- How do they structure their pricing for medically important remediation, and are cost breakdowns transparent? Transparent pricing helps you understand and plan expenses.

- Are any additional costs or fees associated with catering to sensitive clients? Clarify any extra charges to avoid surprises.

By asking these questions, individuals with mold sensitivities can find a qualified and empathetic restoration and mold remediation contractor who can provide specialized care and attention.

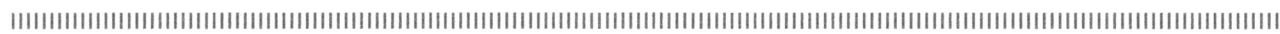

||||||||||||||||||||||||||||||||||||||||||||||||||||||||||||||||||||||||||||||||||||||||||||||||||||||||||||||||||||||||||||||||||||||||||||||

CIRSx.com Medically Important Remediation Training for Professionals

CIRSx was Founded by physicians working with patients with chronic inflammatory response syndrome and other medical conditions related to mold and other water damage-related organisms. I am a strategic partner with CIRSx and, along with other experts, have helped develop a two-day course for remediation technicians. This program integrates the ANSI/IICRC Standards with an additional focus on medically important aspects of water damage restoration. More information about their

Medically Important Remediation (MIR101) course is available on CIRSx's website, cirsx.com/cirsx-institute

Course Goal: The "Medically Important Remediation— Professional Version (MIR101)" course is designed to equip indoor environmental professionals, remediators, and restorers with advanced knowledge and skills essential for working in medically sensitive environments. The goal is to ensure that professionals can confidently bridge the gap between traditional remediation practices and the specialized needs of environments occupied by individuals with chronic health conditions, particularly those affected by mold-related illnesses.

Course Content Overview: This course offers 16 hours of in-depth, self-paced training developed by industry experts and reviewed by medical professionals. The curriculum is crafted to provide a comprehensive understanding of how to conduct remediation that meets industry standards and supports the health and recovery of individuals with sensitivities to water-damaged environments.

Participants will explore advanced remediation techniques with a strong emphasis on environments where health sensitivities are a concern. The course covers interdisciplinary collaboration with healthcare providers, ensuring that remediation practices are aligned with patient health needs. Medical considerations are integrated into the training, offering insights into how environmental factors influence health and how remediation efforts can be tailored to promote healing.

In addition to learning from seasoned experts in indoor environmental quality, participants will benefit from guest lectures delivered by medical professionals. These sessions will provide a medical perspective on remediation requirements and patient care, enhancing the learner's ability to manage sensitive cases effectively.

Upon completion, participants will earn a digital badge from CIRSx, recognizing their advanced expertise in medically necessary remediation. This credential acknowledges their specialized skills and counts toward 14 Continuing Education Credits (CEC) from the IICRC.

By completing MIR101, professionals will enhance their ability to collaborate effectively with healthcare providers and make a significant impact on the recovery journey of those affected by mold-related illnesses. This course empowers participants to extend their professional capabilities and provide the highest standard of care in the remediation industry.

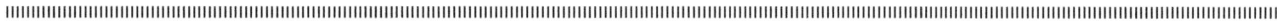

Emergency Water Damage: Immediate Actions Until Professional Help Arrives

SAFETY FIRST

You should only do the following if you know how and can do it safely!

• **Electrical and Water Safety:** Immediately turn off electricity to affected areas. Avoid contact with electrical outlets and devices near water.

• **Avoid Slip and Fall Hazards:** Be cautious of slippery, wet surfaces. Wear appropriate non-slip shoes and be careful.

• **Identify the Source:** Locate the origin of the water (e.g., burst pipe, leaky roof).

• **Protective Gear for Emergency Cleanup:** In cases where the water source is sanitary, such as a clean water pipe break, consider whether addressing the issue yourself with caution is appropriate. If you are going to perform any work yourself, wear protective gear, including gloves, masks, and waterproof boots, to minimize exposure to potential allergens and irritants. This precaution is particularly important for individuals with existing health issues or sensitivities, as even minimal exposure can exacerbate their conditions.

• **Dealing with Septic Water:** When the water intrusion is potentially septic, such as sewage backups or floodwater, it's a different scenario altogether. Septic water can carry a host of harmful microorganisms and toxins that pose serious health risks, especially to those with preexisting health concerns or hypersensitivities. In these situations, the safest action is to isolate the affected areas and seek professional assistance immediately. Professionals have the necessary equipment, protective gear, and expertise to handle such hazardous conditions effectively and safely. They should know how to contain and address this serious situation without using air movers for drying. They should ensure that the visible damage is addressed and the environment is thoroughly cleaned to prevent health risks. *(See "Essentials for Contaminated Water Emergency Response" on page 122)*

• **Stop the Source of Water (if possible) Shut Off Water:** Use the main water shut-off valve to stop water flow if the source is from within the home (like a burst pipe).

• **Contain the Spread (for sanitary water):** If you can do so safely—Use towels or mops to stop clean water from spreading to dry areas.

Know the Following Information Before You Need It

• **Municipal Waste:** If you are on a city or county sewer system and have had a backflow of water from the community sewer lines into your home or onto your property, Dial 911 to report the emergency immediately. This is considered a property damage emergency. The 911 operator should be able to contact the appropriate city or county department for emergency backflow services in your area. Universal safety precautions are essential in these situations since such waste may be carrying disease-causing organisms.

• **Septic Tank Backup:** If your home has a septic tank backing up into it or onto your property, it will likely be your responsibility. If you are renting, your landlord or management company needs to be notified immediately. The Emergency Water Damage Restoration company should be able to help if you don't know who to call.

• **Sewage Back-up in a Condominium or Apartment:** When sewage backs up from septic lines in multi-unit environments, Universal safety precautions are essential since the waste may be carrying disease-causing organisms from other occupants in the building. Notify the owner or manager as soon as possible.

Know Your Water Shutoff Locations— Limiting Damages

• **Familiarity:** Learn the locations of all water shutoff valves in and around your home. Every household member should know where these are and how to use them.

• **Know How to Stop the Flow:** Stopping the water is your first defense to limit water damage. Knowing how to use the individual fixture shut-offs, main house shut-offs, and the water main valve for your home can provide a triple level of understanding so you can act quickly and choose the best action. The main shut-off is typically found on the street or, in colder climates, under the home in the crawlspace cellar or in the basement. If the primary shut-off valve fails (due to corrosion or damage), have an alternative plan ready.

- **Tools:** Not all shut-offs can be controlled by hand. Keep the necessary tools for shutting off water in a dedicated and easily accessible spot and get training in how to use them. You may find the purchase of a universal shut-off tool helpful. These have been designed to shut off the gas and water for emergencies such as earthquakes, tornados, and hurricanes but can also be helpful for lesser emergencies.

Understanding Fire Suppression Systems

Fire suppression systems can save lives and limit fire damage to your home in case of a fire, but they can also create thousands of dollars of unnecessary damage if they malfunction and release water when there is no fire. The initial service visit or annual maintenance is an excellent time to ask lots of questions to ensure you understand how to keep your system in excellent condition and respond when something goes wrong.

- **Risk and Maintenance:** While homes with fire suppression systems are safer from fires, they face more significant risks of water damage. Regular professional inspections and servicing, at least annually, can help limit risks from malfunctions. If purchasing a home with such a system, ensure it's inspected during escrow.

- **Emergency Shutoff Devices:** Consider keeping emergency sprinkler head shutoff devices at home, especially if instructed in their safe and effective use. These can help limit the release of water in accidental activations.

EMERGENCY RESPONSE BY YOU AND YOUR FAMILY— BUT ONLY IF IT IS SAFE!

- **Multitask if you can:**
- **Call the Water Damage Restoration Company to get them on their way ASAP**
- **Mitigate Further Damage—if you can do so safely!**
- **Remove Water:** If safe, use buckets, mops, or wet/dry shop vacuums to remove standing water.
- **Move** Personal Belongings: To prevent further damage, relocate furniture, electronics, and other items above the water flow that have not gotten wet to a dry area. Items that have gotten wet should be left in the wet area. Moving items in areas with sewage backflow or damage will likely spread contamination.

- **Elevate Furniture:** If possible, lift furniture off wet flooring to prevent staining and swelling.
- **Document the Damage**—if you can do so safely! Keep track of the who, what, when, where, and why in your project diary. Diagram on a floor plan of your home how far the water traveled. Be aware that until the home is professionally extracted and drying begins, the water will continue to spread through capillary action, so add a date and time. Your version covers where you can tell it went based on seeing moisture. The professional water damage restoration company should prepare a moisture map based on meter measurements.
- **Take Photos and Videos:** Document the extent of water damage for insurance purposes. Take overview photos to provide perspective and close-ups to document damage. Include contaminated garments, stuffed goods, and foodstuffs.
- **List Damaged Items:** List all damaged personal property in your diary.

Ventilate and Start Drying

- **Open Windows and Doors**: If weather permits, ventilate the area to aid in drying.
- **Use Fans and Dehumidifiers:** If available, use fans and dehumidifiers to help prevent the spread of moisture to unaffected areas.

Prevent Mold Growth

- **Remove Wet Materials**: Take out items like wet rugs, carpets, and padding that can harbor mold.

Chemical Use in Sensitive Situations

- **Avoid Chemicals for Medical Sensitivities**: If occupants have medical sensitivities, avoid using chemicals or biocides. An approved detergent is usually sufficient for cleaning.
- **Misconceptions About Chemical Use:** Using toxic biocides, especially in septic or contaminated water, is not typically necessary and can worsen environmental sensitivities.

||||||||||||||||||||||||||||||||||||||||||||||||||||||||||||||||||||||||||||||||||||||||||||||||||||||||||||||||||||||||||||||

Myths, Misunderstandings, and Fallacies: The Chemical Treatment Fallacy

Fallacy: "Sewage and other contaminated water should be immediately treated with chemicals to kill microorganisms and make them safe."

The Reality: This widespread belief is a dangerous misconception. Sewage and similar contaminated water are loaded with organic matter. This organic content neutralizes the effectiveness of biocides and other antimicrobial chemicals. These chemicals are designed to work on surfaces that have been previously cleaned, not those heavily laden with organic matter. The label instructions on these chemical products are clear and should be adhered to strictly. They are intended for use on surfaces that have already been cleaned, ensuring the removal of organic matter that could otherwise impede their effectiveness.

Recommendation: When dealing with sewage backflow, **only properly trained and equipped restoration professionals** should come into contact with the contaminated areas. Handling sewage requires strict adherence to safety protocols to prevent health risks and cross-contamination.

Avoid Chemical Overuse:

Resist the instinct to rely on harsh chemical treatments. Instead, opt for a safer and more effective approach—using soap and water. This method thoroughly removes contaminants without introducing unnecessary chemical residues into the environment, supporting a healthier living space.

Discard Porous Materials:

Porous materials that have come into contact with sewage must be discarded. Restoration professionals should handle this step to ensure the proper removal and disposal of contaminated materials.

Thorough Cleaning of Organic Matter:

Restoration professionals should focus on **thoroughly cleaning and removing organic matter** using detergents. This step is critical to achieving a safe and effective restoration process while avoiding unnecessary chemical treatments that may not address the root problem effectively.

By following these guidelines, you can ensure the restoration process is both effective and health-conscious, prioritizing safety and the integrity of the living environment.

||||||||||||||||||||||||||||||||||||||||||||||||||||||||||||||||||||||||||||||||||||||||||||||||||||||||||||||||||||||||||||||

ADDITIONAL CONSIDERATIONS

Even after professionals have arrived to manage the emergency, your role is far from over. While the restoration team is focused on preserving your home and possessions, there are things that you can do to assist without getting in the way and slowing them down. Other times, your input is needed to help their work process and priorities. If you can think ahead and consider items requiring special handling, the time before the emergency team arrives is a good time to manage those situations.

Safeguarding Important Belongings

- Take a mental walk through your home and identify items essential to your daily well-being, such as prescription drugs, medical devices, or an EpiPen that might be needed immediately if a family member experiences a severe allergic reaction. If damaged or lost, these items could quickly escalate into an emergency.

- Additionally, consider other valuables that may need special attention, such as a tropical fish tank, a pet bird, or collections like stamps, comic books, coins, or baseball cards. Even if items are stored in a safe, that doesn't mean they're entirely protected. Humidity can still get in, potentially causing adhesive on stamp collections to stick them together, tarnishing coins, or promoting mold growth on comic books and cards.

Here are a few more things to consider:

- **Firearms and Ammunition:** Even if weapons are stored in a safe, they may still be at risk due to humidity. It's important to consider emergency storage options, such as taking them to a gun store, gunsmith, or firing range for safekeeping. Not every water damage technician will be versed in the safe handling of firearms. Accidental discovery could be awkward at best and potentially dangerous.

- **Valuables and Collectibles:** Items like jewelry, coins, and heirlooms may need to be moved to a bank safety deposit box, which can usually be set up quickly. Before storing them, ensure they're dried properly, and consider using silica gel desiccant packets to keep them dry.

- **Confidential or Sensitive Items:** If you have items of a confidential or sensitive nature, try to address them before the restoration crew arrives. Consider moving them to a secure location, a locked car trunk, or a specialty storage facility. If the item is directly damaged by water or cannot be safely retrieved beforehand, restoring it with professional help may still be possible.

Pet Safety During Water Damage Restoration

- **Birds:** Pet birds are highly sensitive to mold, water-damaged organisms, and fluctuations in temperature and humidity. Relocate birds to a safe, unaffected area or a trusted friend or relative's home. Ensure their environment remains within the average temperature and humidity range to prevent stress and health issues.

- **Cats:** Cats are often stressed by environmental changes and may attempt to hide in unsafe areas during restoration. Confine cats in a secure, quiet room with their essentials (litter box, food, water), or arrange temporary care at a friend's home or a boarding facility.

- **Dogs:** The noise and disruption caused by restoration activities can make dogs anxious or distressed. Keep dogs in a quiet, familiar space away from the work area, or consider temporarily boarding them at a trusted friend or relative's home to reduce stress and ensure their safety.

- **Fish Tanks:** Fish are highly sensitive to changes in water quality, temperature, and other factors during restoration. Consult with a local aquarium or fish supply store about vacation and emergency relocation services to ensure your fish are properly cared for during restoration.

- **Reptiles:** Reptiles require specific temperature and humidity levels, which can be drastically affected by commercial dehumidifiers used during restoration. Move reptiles to a controlled environment away from the restoration area, such as a separate room with a dedicated heat and humidity source, to prevent dehydration and potential fatality.

Communication is vital during all phases of restoration and remediation. However, this is especially true when someone in the household has environmental sensitivities. If you need to discuss a concern or confidential matter, speak directly with the lead technician to ask who in the company you should contact. If the employee doesn't have the authority to help or make decisions, they can likely connect you with someone who does. Taking these proactive steps can help you minimize unrestorable damage to your home and possessions, ensuring they are preserved while the professionals handle the emergency.

||||||||||||||||||||||||||||||||||||||||||||||||||||||||||||||||||||||||||||||||||||||||||||||||||||||||||||||||||||||||||||||||||

Essentials: Moisture Meters

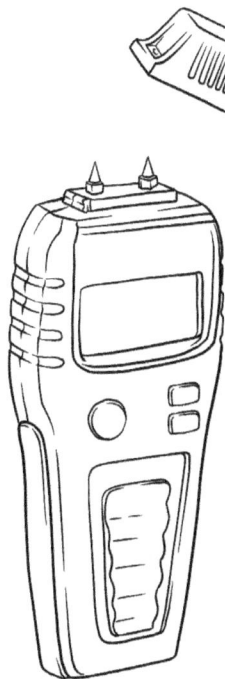

Figure 3-7: A Pin Probe Moisture Meter uses the electrical conductivity between the probes to approximate the moisture level. Pushing the probe into the material leaves small holes, which can cause unacceptable cosmetic damage to the surface of the measured material. Penetrating or Pin Probe moisture meters measure moisture based on the material's conductivity. Wet materials conduct more electricity than dry meters. The resistance or capacitance of the material is used to determine how much moisture it contains. The pins only measure the depth of the probe. Uninsulated probes measure the moisture at the wettest point. Insulated probes measure the moisture content at the depth of the uninsulated probe.

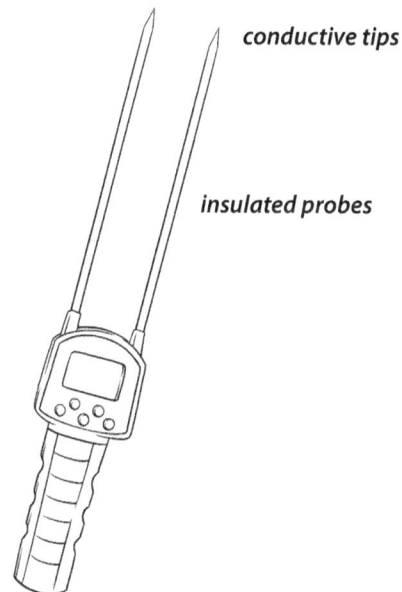

conductive tips

insulated probes

Figure 3-8: A Long Insulated Probe, Moisture Meter is used to measure the moisture content deep in materials. The length of the probes is insulated so that only the tips measure the moisture.

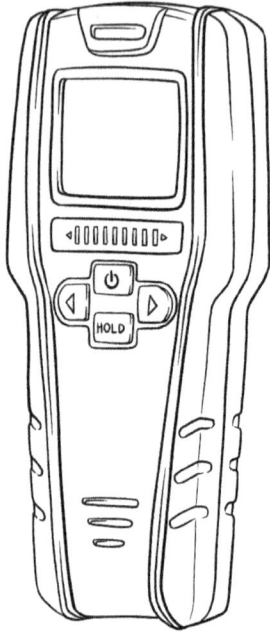

Figure 3-9: Non-Invasive Moisture Meter (front)

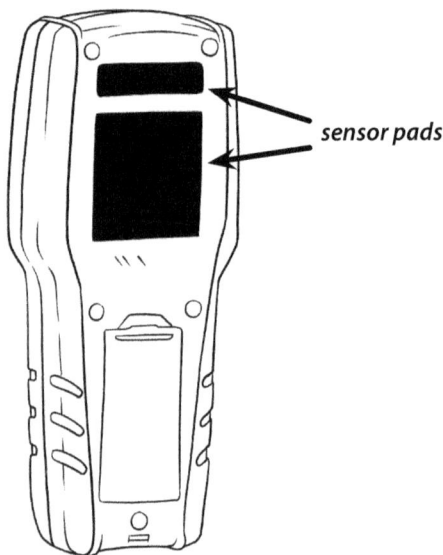

sensor pads

Figure 3-10: Non-Invasive Moisture Meter (Back). The meter does not cause damage because these meters measure moisture based on the conductivity of an electrical field or the impedance of a radio frequency wave.

Inexpensive moisture meters have become readily available. I have tested several of them and found that compared to expensive professional models, they are an adequate screening tool as long as precise calibrated measurements are not needed. The calibration issues are overcome by comparing known dry materials readings with the test materials to determine if the test surfaces are also dry.

Where inexpensive meters often fall short is in terms of longevity. My $800 moisture meter was durable. It lasted over

20 years, withstood dragging it into attics and crawlspaces and being dropped several times. Inexpensive (under $50) meters have tended to stop working in as little as a year. If you understand a few basic principles, you can use an inexpensive meter to monitor conditions over time. This helps provide information that can help you decide when it is time to bring in professionals. Owning a moisture meter can provide valuable information but is not a substitute for professional assistance when things go wrong.

- Moisture meters come in two basic types—Penetrating and Non-Penetrating. The Penetrating meters function by poking holes into the materials being tested. This means they damage surfaces by leaving pin holes in the surfaces. The meter only measures as deep as the pin probes penetrate. For most non-professional situations, I would suggest you get the non-penetrating type.

- Non-Penetrating Moisture Meters function based on either conductivity or radio frequency. Wet materials are more conductive of electricity. A Non-Penetrating Conductive Moisture Meter measures the conductivity of the material being measured. A radio frequency moisture meter uses radio waves. Either type of meter should provide sufficient information for an early warning or monitoring of a problem.

- Many people believe they can judge how wet a floor or wall is by touching it. While your hand can tell if something is very wet, it can't determine if it's dry. For instance, I've seen walls that felt dry to the touch, yet the wood moisture content was over 25%. Contractors are often taught that wood moisture should be below 19% to avoid structural damage, but this can be misleading. To prevent surface mold growth, which significantly impacts the health of a home, wood moisture needs to be much lower.

  › In most indoor environments, wood should ideally have a moisture content between 6% and 12%. This range is safe to prevent mold growth and structural damage like dry rot.
  › Wood moisture levels between 16% and 20% can support mold growth, and levels above 20% can lead to dry rot. Therefore, keeping wood moisture below these thresholds is necessary to maintain a healthy and structurally sound home. Begin acting well before moisture levels reach problematic levels.

- Moisture measurements can be complex and sometimes counterintuitive. For example, when measuring moisture in materials like wood attached to a gypsum board, you might find that while the wood is dry enough to prevent mold growth, the gypsum board paper may still be damp enough to support mold. To simplify moisture assessment, use the "dry standard" principle. Measure areas of the same material that you know to be dry, and use these readings as your baseline. This becomes your standard for determining if the same material in other areas is also dry. It's important not to compare moisture values between different types of materials, as each material has its moisture characteristics. For instance, compare Douglas fir framing to other areas of

Douglas fir and compare the gypsum board to other regions of the gypsum board. Go through your home now while it is dry and measure different areas during different seasons to become familiar with their normal readings.

- Most non-penetrating meters will measure a maximum depth of 0.5 to 0.75 inches. This means a wall cavity could be wet in the middle and not be able to be detected. Measuring at greater depths will require more expensive professional equipment and experience.

- Set the moisture meter to the appropriate material scale based on the underlying material you want to measure. For example, if you have a linoleum floor over wood, set the meter to the wood scale. If the linoleum floor is installed over a concrete slab, set the meter to the concrete or masonry scale.

- Hidden metal can give false readings on moisture meters, making it appear as though the material is wet. For example, metal flashing around windows or metal corner beads used to finish the edges of gypsum board installations may cause your meter to show inaccurately high moisture levels. Identifying these hidden metal elements beforehand can help avoid confusion when interpreting moisture readings.

- Pressure-treated lumber may have salts used to treat the wood, making it appear wet.

- Before using your meter, turn it on and touch it firmly with the palm of your hand. Because your hand is saturated with water, the meter should indicate it is wet. Practice with your meter now before you need it. This is a good double-check to see if your meter is functioning correctly.

- One of the most common reasons for inaccurate or erratic readings is low battery life. If things don't seem right, try changing the battery.

- Water Damage Restoration Technicians should have their WRT Certification from the Institute for Inspection, Cleaning and Restoration Certification (IICRC.org)

Essentials for Clean Water Emergency Response

*When a water damage restoration contractor responds to a clean water emergency in your home, they should **follow these steps:***

What to Expect from an Emergency Water Damage Restoration Contractor

❑ **Immediate Response:** Since time is a major factor in water damage, the restoration contractor should have a 24-hour emergency number and respond promptly. The cost of water damage increases rapidly with time—minutes matter. Don't be deterred by suggestions to wait until the next day to avoid an emergency fee; immediate action is essential.

❑ **Work Authorization:** Upon arrival, the restoration team will perform a comprehensive assessment, identifying the source of the water, the extent of the damage, and the contamination level (clean, significantly contaminated, or grossly contaminated water). Many companies now offer the option to review and sign work authorizations while the crew is en route, allowing them to begin work immediately upon arrival. Be sure to understand what you are signing.

❑ **Initial Health and Safety Assessment:** Before starting work, the contractor must ensure the work environment is safe and compliant with OSHA standards. The technician should wear appropriate protective gear and assess the water damage, categorizing it by source (clean, significantly contaminated, or grossly contaminated water), class (extent of absorption and evaporation needed), and mold condition (ranging from normal fungal ecology to actual mold growth as defined by IICRC S520 standards).

❑ **Control the Water Entry:** If water continues to enter the structure, the priority is to shut it off or control it to prevent further damage if you can do it safely.

❑ **Water Extraction and Initial Moisture Mapping:** Once the water source is controlled, technicians should begin extracting excess water using professional-grade equipment, which is more effective than DIY methods. I have known some situations where it is necessary to control the water source by beginning extraction even while the water is gushing into the property. As soon as it is reasonably possible, they should start moisture mapping to identify areas that need drying equipment. It's important to remember that water may spread further over time, so monitoring beyond initial boundaries is essential.

❑ **Establishing a Balanced Drying System:** Technicians will establish a balanced drying system by optimizing temperature, air movement, and dehumidification. This balance is needed to prevent over-drying or driving moisture deeper into materials. The HVAC system ductwork will likely need to be sealed to protect against additional system contamination.

❑ **Monitoring and Adjusting the Drying Process:** Minimum daily continuous monitoring is vital to ensure progress. The team will use moisture meters and other tools to assess humidity and moisture levels, adjusting equipment and strategies to achieve optimal drying results.

❑ **Inspection and Physical Removal of Wet Porous Materials:** The restoration team should inspect structural elements like walls, floors, and ceilings for signs of water infiltration. If necessary, wet porous materials such as gypsum board or cellulose insulation may need to be removed to access saturation pockets and prevent mold growth and structural deterioration. Emergency demolition might be required, especially in homes with occupants sensitive to organisms that thrive in wet conditions.

❑ **Atmospheric Stabilization:** A dry building should be maintained at 60°F to 80°F and 30% to 50% relative humidity. If this goal cannot be achieved, ongoing moisture control should be implemented to maintain the home in this condition.

❑ **End of Project Drying Check and Equilibrium Test:** At the end of the drying process, the equipment should be turned off while maintaining average room temperatures. The next day, moisture levels should be rechecked. If excess moisture is detected, select equipment may need to be reactivated. Since moisture migrates based on temperature (hot to cold), it is possible for a hot drying process to push moisture deeper into materials. Checking the next day after the temperatures have become more normal helps identify this condition early before the moisture migration does additional damage. This process is repeated until the building is confirmed to be thoroughly dry.

❑ **Avoiding Sanitizers and Antimicrobials:** Sanitizers and antimicrobials should be avoided whenever possible in homes with residents who have health concerns. This doesn't mean the house will be left with contamination that has not been addressed. Using soap detergent and surfactants helps physically remove contamination to facilitate the restoration. The decision does not need to be made immediately. Chemical treatments, fogs, sterilant, and other toxic chemicals are rarely necessary or useful if proper physical removal and cleaning have been performed.

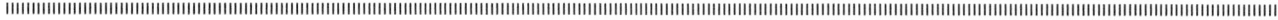

Professional restoration companies lift furniture off wet surfaces by inserting a rigid foam block under each foot to raise the item away from the damp floor and encourage air circulation around the surfaces of the item. Cardboard boxes on the wet or damp floor should immediately have the contents removed to a dry box with wet items separated for immediate, focused drying and the original box discarded. For other materials, such as linens and clothing, it may make sense not to wait for them to dry but to send them to a professional laundry or dry cleaners for immediate cleaning. Items labeled dry clean only may begin to shrink if they aren't blocked out to keep them in their original form. Specialty items like jewelry, coin collections, musical instruments, firearms, and artwork that gets wet may be immediately removed and transported to a specialist in the care and restoration of such items. The same is true for items like computers, where the stored information can be quickly backed up for preservation.

Specialists should know how to preserve the maximum value and appearance of the items to bring them back to the best possible condition. In addition, they will be able to store the specialty items in ways that will prevent them from being further compromised. An example would be a wine collection. Leaving bottles of wine in an environment undergoing rapid drying using dehumidification could "bruise" the wine by exposing it to elevated temperatures, and the process may dry out the cork, increasing the risk.

IMPLEMENTING MOISTURE CONTROL BARRIERS

When drying, moisture control barriers can be set up within the already affected area, preventing it from spreading to other parts of the building. This barrier is a physical partition, such as polyethylene sheeting, that isolates the affected areas from the rest of the home. Its primary intent is to reduce or prevent the spread of moisture and dust, containing the impact of water damage within a controlled environment. Think of these barriers as a "just in case" measure with significant advantages. They act as a defensive shield, containing moisture and serving as a containment strategy to limit the spread of potential contaminants, thereby preventing additional damage.

The barriers must be constructed far enough away from where the water to ensure that wet conditions remain contained within the controlled area. Sometimes, a simple barrier might involve keeping doors closed to isolate problem areas. More elaborate barriers can be combined with negative air controls to help isolate moisture. If mold growth has already occurred, these barriers offer the added advantage of containing contamination within the water-damaged area, preventing the spread of spores to unaffected spaces.

Professional drying companies should have access to HEPA-filtered equipment that can be deployed to further confine spores and other contaminants within the wet area, ensuring they don't contaminate the rest of the home. The rapid deployment of moisture control barriers, combined with HEPA-filtered air exhaust directed outdoors, can provide an extra layer of protection against cross-contamination.

Once the affected items and areas have been dried, they can be evaluated to determine whether they were addressed quickly enough to prevent mold growth or if preexisting mold has been contained. This careful approach helps maintain the integrity of the home's environment.

These barriers act as your first line of defense, containing the situation and providing you with the time needed to assess and address the full extent of the water damage. By following these measures, you'll be better prepared to handle the initial emergency phase and transition confidently to the more detailed remediation efforts that will follow.

A moisture control barrier and containment are similar and can provide dual benefits. However, the terminology used can significantly impact whether these measures are covered by insurance. Insurance adjusters may not understand the benefits of containment barriers and may refuse to pay for them if the policy doesn't explicitly cover such measures. However, they are more likely to approve moisture control barriers, which can save on emergency drying expenses. In this context, the intent behind the barrier and the specific language used to describe it can make all the difference.

PHYSICAL REMOVAL OF POROUS MATERIALS FOR WATER DAMAGE REMEDIATION

In water damage restoration, physically removing wet or previously wet porous materials is a faster way of removing water from buildings and speeding the ability of evaporation to address residual moisture. If emergency drying procedures are not implemented within a few hours of occurring or if water damage is significantly widespread, the physical removal of wet materials can help in several ways.

1. Moisture Management: Porous materials like drywall and insulation are highly susceptible to absorbing water. Once wet, these materials can retain moisture, leading to prolonged dampness within the structure. Removing them eliminates sources of moisture that could lead to mold growth or structural damage.

2. Inspection and Assessment: Removing these materials facilitates a thorough inspection of the building's interior structure. Exposing the studs, joists, and internal cavities allows professionals to assess the extent of water penetration and damage. This step is vital to identify and address all affected areas.

3. Ensuring Cleanliness and Dryness: Post-removal, cleaning and drying the exposed areas becomes possible. This step allows confirmation that the building's structural elements are free from moisture and contamination. Ensuring the cleanliness and dryness of these areas is essential before any reconstruction or restoration work can commence.

4. Preventing Mold Growth: Removing wet, porous materials significantly reduces the risk of mold growth. Mold thrives in moist environments, and eliminating wet materials disrupts its ability to establish and spread.

5. Restoration Readiness: Finally, removing damaged materials prepares the site for the restoration phase. It provides a clean, dry foundation for rebuilding affected areas with new, undamaged materials.

EFFECTIVE DRYING DECISIONS

Making effective drying decisions is crucial in the aftermath of water damage. While it may be tempting to tackle the drying process yourself, hidden moisture and structural complexities often make this better left to professionals. The following guidelines are designed to help you make informed decisions, choose qualified professionals, and recognize the difference between quality and substandard work.

1. Deciding How to Handle Hidden Moisture Under Appliances and Cabinets

- **Understanding Water Migration:** Water can migrate underneath floor-mounted cabinets and appliances, often reaching wall cavities and other hidden spaces. This knowledge should guide your decision to thoroughly inspect these areas or seek professional help.

- **Access and Inspection Requirements:** Effective drying decisions involve understanding if moving appliances like refrigerators and dishwashers is necessary to assess the full extent of moisture.

- **Choosing Professional Help:** Given the complexity of detecting hidden moisture, this may be the point at which you decide to involve a professional. Restoration experts have the tools to inspect these areas thoroughly and can help prevent issues from missed moisture.

- **Decision Point:** If moisture has traveled to difficult-to-access areas, consider hiring a restoration professional who will check under and behind appliances, as skipping these areas could lead to hidden mold growth.

2. Evaluating the Need to Access Built-Ins and Hard-to-Reach Areas

- **Determining the Extent of Moisture Damage:** In rooms with sloped or uneven floors, water can accumulate in unpredictable areas. Making an informed drying decision means evaluating whether moisture measurements should extend beyond immediately visible wet spots.

- **Deciding on Cabinet Removal:** Sometimes, it may be necessary to remove cabinetry to access wall cavities. When choosing a professional, ensure they are willing to take this step if required, as skipping it may leave hidden moisture.

- **Recognizing Water Flow Paths**: To make informed decisions, consider clues like water stains, which may indicate how far water has traveled. This awareness will help you communicate effectively with professionals and verify they are following a thorough process.

- ❏ **Decision Point:** Quality work often involves checking beyond the immediate wet area. Be cautious of professionals who ignore potential hidden moisture, as this could compromise the drying process.

3. Assessing the Impact of Water Intrusion from the Upper Floors

- **Understanding Downward Water Flow**: Water from upper levels can travel through stairways, wall cavities, or utility chases. Recognizing this path will help you decide on the extent of inspection and drying necessary to prevent damage on lower floors.

- **Deciding on Wall Material Removal**: In some cases, removing the wallboard along the water's path is necessary to access all affected areas. If you choose to hire a professional, they should be willing to take this step for a complete restoration.

- **Ensuring Proper Containment**: Containment provides a failsafe measure if microbial contamination is suspected. This decision affects whether professionals must set up barriers to prevent contamination from spreading during the drying process.

- ❏ **Decision Point:** If water has traveled from an upper level, consider whether professionals have accounted for potential hidden damage on lower floors. Look for indicators that they're addressing the full scope of the problem, including using containment when mold is suspected.

4. Weighing the Need for Flooring Removal to Access Hidden Moisture

- **Considering Flooring Materials**: Different types of flooring—like carpet, hardwood, and laminate—react differently to water. To make an effective drying decision, you'll need to consider whether these materials could trap moisture underneath.

- **Evaluating the Need for Flooring Lifting or Removal**: Professionals may recommend lifting or removing flooring to fully dry the area in cases of extensive water exposure. This decision is key to preventing mold growth, and you'll want to ensure professionals are thorough.

- **DIY Limitations**: Attempting to dry flooring yourself without lifting it may lead to missed moisture and future issues. When deciding between DIY and professional help, consider whether you can detect moisture beneath the flooring.

- ❏ **Decision Point:** Quality restoration professionals often lift or remove flooring when necessary. If a professional suggests leaving damp materials in place, consider a second opinion, as this decision could impact long-term health and structural integrity.

Essay: Understanding Case Hardening: The Risks of Drying Too Quickly
by Ken Larsen

When it comes to emergency drying, it might seem logical to think that faster drying is always better. After all, who wouldn't want to get things dry as quickly as possible to avoid further damage like mold, right? Some people even insist that everything can be dried in as little as 3 days and are only willing to pay for such a timeline. However, when it comes to hygroscopic materials—materials that readily absorb and retain moisture, like wood, drywall, and certain fabrics—attempts to dry too quickly can actually delay the drying time. The most common issue, known as **case hardening**, is a phenomenon that restorers need to manage carefully to ensure long-term success in restorative drying.

What is Case Hardening?
Case hardening occurs when the outer layers of a material dry much faster than the interior. Imagine a piece of wood that has been soaked with water. If we apply overly intense heat, too much wind velocity, or overly dry air to the surface, the outermost layer will quickly lose moisture and begin to shrink, creating a "skin" that traps the moisture inside. The moisture deep within the material (often called **bound moisture**) cannot migrate to the surface and evaporate as readily as a slightly moist surface would. As a result, the outer layer forms a hard, dry "shell," while the inner layers remain wet. This condition locks in the moisture, making it difficult for the remaining water to escape. Furthermore, the shrunken, dried skin on the surface will be dimensionally smaller than the swollen center core and can develop surface cracks called "surface checking," which is considered a permanently damaged condition.

In effect, case hardening creates a moisture barrier that can trap water within the material. Over time, this trapped moisture can lead to mold growth, structural weakness, and other long-term problems—precisely the outcomes you want to avoid.

The Science Behind Moisture Movement

To understand why case hardening happens, it helps to know a bit about how water moves through materials. Water inside hygroscopic materials exists in two forms: **free water** (liquid water that flows freely through the cavities in the material) and **bound water** (water that is chemically bonded to the material's cell structure). During the drying process, free water evaporates first, which is relatively easy to remove. Bound water, on the other hand, requires a more gradual approach to drying because it's tightly held to, and within, the material.

For efficient drying, it's essential to maintain a moderate moisture gradient—a gradual difference in moisture levels that allows water to migrate from the wetter, internal parts of the material to the slightly drier outer layers. When drying is too aggressive, this balance is disrupted. The outer surface dries so quickly that it forms a hard "shell," effectively trapping moisture inside and preventing further evaporation.

A similar process can be seen when working with clay. If sculptors allow the outer layer of a thick piece to dry too fast, it becomes rigid and cracks, while the inside remains damp. The same issue, known as case hardening, occurs in wood and other hygroscopic materials, where a dried shell forms, locking in moisture.

Toasting a marshmallow over a campfire offers another analogy. If it's held too close to the flames, the outside gets crispy while the inside stays firm—not gooey. However, if you patiently let it heat more slowly, the marshmallow warms and melts evenly throughout. Similarly, rushing the drying process in materials leads to a hardened exterior and moisture trapped within.

Why Is Gradual Drying Important?

Searing a steak on a hot barbecue is a perfect example of how intense heat can lock in moisture. When the steak hits the grill, the high temperature causes the proteins on the surface to rapidly cook and form a flavorful crust. This quick searing process creates a barrier that traps the juices inside, preventing them from escaping during the rest of the cooking.

In essence, the outer layer hardens and seals, keeping the interior tender and juicy. This is why a well-seared steak remains moist inside, even when cooked over high heat. However, if the heat is too extreme or the searing is rushed, the outside can char while the inside doesn't cook evenly, highlighting the need for the right balance of heat and time to achieve the perfect result.

The same principle applies to drying materials like wood or drywall. The goal is to gently coax moisture from the inside to the outside by creating a consistent, even gradient, allowing bound water to make its way to the surface and evaporate.

Rapid or aggressive drying—whether by blasting with heat, using excessively powerful air movers, or reducing the ambient humidity too quickly—will break this process. Without a proper gradient, bound moisture remains locked within, increasing the risk of mold, rot, or dimensional distortions later.

The Moisture Gradient: A Key to Success

Creating and maintaining a proper moisture gradient is essential to prevent case hardening. When there are no more puddles on the surfaces and *no liquid on the surfaces,* then a controlled and gentle drying strategy is preferred to expedite the drying process. Professionals achieve this by carefully managing the balance between airflow, temperature, and humidity during the drying process. Here are a few strategies:

When moisture is trapped within a material, and there is no visible water on its surface, effective drying requires careful control of several factors:

6. **Controlled Air Movement**: Instead of using high-speed air, gentle airflow is more effective at drawing moisture out from the interior to the surface. Air movement that mimics the breeze you might create by waving a magazine in front of your face is sufficient; anything stronger won't significantly speed up evaporation. Excessive airflow can actually cause the outer layer to dry too quickly, leading to case hardening.

7. **Temperature and Humidity Management**: Adjusting temperature and humidity levels is crucial to avoid excessively rapid drying. Maintaining moderate temperatures (around 75°F to 85°F) and gradually reducing humidity (starting at 40% relative humidity and slowly approaching 20% as the material dries) creates an environment that promotes gradual evaporation without causing case (surface) hardening.

8. **Precise Dehumidification**: Industrial dehumidifiers play a key role in managing moisture levels. Instead of trying to dry the environment too quickly, dehumidifiers should gradually reduce humidity according to a planned strategy. This "drying plan" should be established before the drying begins, with specific atmospheric targets. Gradual dehumidification encourages moisture to move naturally out of the material, minimizing the risk of case hardening.

References and Practical Application

The concepts discussed here are supported by scientific principles of drying, including the **psychrometry** (the study of air-vapor mixtures) used by professionals to create drying plans tailored to each scenario. The Institute of Inspection, Cleaning, and Restoration Certification (IICRC) outlines these strategies in standards like the **IICRC S500**, which provides guidelines for safe and effective water damage restoration. Properly trained professionals will use tools like **moisture meters** and **thermal hygrometers** to measure and monitor moisture levels, ensuring that drying follows a gradual, controlled process.

For instance, Dr. John F. Siau's work on wood drying physics emphasizes that moisture must migrate through the cellular structure. (Siau, 1995) If external drying happens too quickly, the wood can warp or split because the interior moisture has no way to escape. This principle applies broadly to other porous materials as well, which underscores the importance of proper drying techniques are so critical.

Conclusion: Finding the Right Balance

Effective drying isn't just about getting rid of water as fast as possible—it's about doing it right. Like most things in life, balance is key. A careful, gradual approach helps create a moisture gradient that allows water to migrate from the inside to the outside without causing the problems associated with case hardening. By using controlled airflow, managing humidity levels, and working with qualified professionals, homeowners and contractors can ensure that drying is effective, thorough, and safe.

So, while it may be tempting to crank up the heat and blast the fans, remember that patience is your best ally. Proper structural drying is as much an art as it is a science, and when done correctly, it protects both the integrity of the building and the health of those who live inside.

DRYING BEFORE GROWTH BECOMES ESTABLISHED

Effective drying requires balancing Air Movement, Dehumidification, and Temperature control. It is necessary to find the sweet spot between attempting to dry too fast and causing case hardening that locks in the moisture versus drying too slowly and allowing microbial growth to proliferate.

Effective drying should begin immediately as soon as the water issue is discovered. Whenever possible, start drying within the first 24 hours. If the problem isn't found and effective drying has not started within the first 24 hours, bacteria will already have begun to grow.

You may be able to clean up small water spills and dry them effectively—but only if you are prepared to discover and address them immediately!

- Professional water damage services are likely needed to dry large delayed-response water damages successfully. If water has been present for more than 48 hours, mold will likely begin to grow, and bacteria will be out of control.

- Air movement is used to lift moisture off the surface of the wet item. If the surface of a solid item has a low enough level of moisture present, microorganisms will not be able to grow.

  › Too much air movement will result in the area's relative humidity being dried, rising to a level where drying slows or stops. The excess moisture in the air prevents evaporation of the excess moisture and results in the material's surface being too wet, which can promote growth.
  › Too little air movement will leave excess dampness on the surface of the materials, promoting growth.
  › During the first 24 hours of drying, the area's relative humidity should ideally be reduced to about 40%. If the drying does not reduce the RH to approximately 40%, then a reduction in air movement or an increase in dehumidification may be needed.

- Dehumidification is used to remove excess moisture from the environment.

  › If the amount of dehumidification is too much, then the excessive drying may result in uneven drying, resulting in cracking or damage to materials. The excess moisture is unable to migrate to the surface of the material rapidly enough to facilitate rapid drying. Too dry of a surface can result in excess moisture being trapped in the center of the material and not being able to migrate to the surface.
  › If the amount of dehumidification is too little, then excess moisture remains on the surface of the materials. This excess moisture can result in mold growth.

- Temperature Control is used to facilitate drying in a controlled fashion.

  › Too high a temperature will increase evaporation so that the humidity level is too high to promote rapid drying.
  › Elevated temperatures increase the rate of microbial growth.
  › Too low a temperature will slow evaporation so that materials won't dry as fast.

When is the Emergency Phase Complete

The emergency phase concludes when the building is dry and further deterioration of construction materials is arrested. The potential consequences leave no room for guesswork because missed areas of dampness will continue to fester. A more exacting approach to post-emergency recovery from water damage is essential for medically important environments where individuals have been diagnosed with sensitivities. This specialized approach now transitions into the Five Stage, 25 Steps, and involves several key components to ensure a safe and healthy living environment.

Determining Which Stage Fits the Home's Condition

The building is dry, and further deterioration has been halted. Now, you need to determine whether it is clean and ready for reconstruction, or did problems with bacterial or mold growth develop?

❑ **Evaluation** involves assessing and testing to determine if mold, bacteria, or other contaminants have developed due to the water damage and to gauge the extent of contamination. Knowing which areas were affected during the emergency will help you better understand where the post-emergency focus should be. A thorough pre-remediation assessment is necessary to identify potential sources of mold, including hidden and less obvious areas that may have developed while the building was wet. Because most people are not hypersensitive to mold, bacteria, or the biotoxins they can produce, sensitivities are often overlooked in a standard remediation process.

❑ **Collaboration with Healthcare Professionals:** Working closely with healthcare providers can help tailor the remediation, post-verification, and assessment process to the occupants' specific health needs, ensuring that the approach is aligned with medical recommendations.

❑ **Remediation:** If needed, remediation addresses mold and bacteria growth areas and any resulting contamination. This process may also involve the removal of materials to access hidden or inaccessible damaged areas. Enhanced remediation protocols require stringent measures and attention to detail, including enhanced containment to prevent cross-contamination and HEPA filtration to minimize exposure to airborne particles.

❑ **Restoration** of damaged materials, such as swollen, delaminated, or warped materials, and structural damage, such as weakened beams or supports, ensure the integrity and function of the building is restored.

❑ **Repairs** to the cause of the water damage will prevent future incidents and ensure the building's long-term stability.

❑ **Cleaning**: should return the building to a condition free of contamination. The team should use safe and effective cleaning agents and techniques to ensure the property is dry, clean, and healthy. The use of chemicals can be particularly problematic for sensitive individuals and will be discussed in detail in the 25 Steps part of this book. Avoid using treatments, sprays, or fogging agents to kill mold. Instead, emphasize physical removal and cleaning, as chemical treatments may trigger adverse reactions in sensitive individuals and could stimulate additional toxin and inflammation production by the organisms.

❑ **Post-Remediation Verification and Independent Third-Party Assessment:** After restoration and remediation are complete, but before reconstruction begins, the remediation contractor needs to perform a thorough cleaning and verification of cleanliness. This is an ideal time for Pathways™ Cleanliness Testing. Any independent third-party assessments by qualified Indoor Environmental Professionals should follow this. The assessments should include testing with a focus on the individual's sensitivities to ensure the building has been returned to a habitable and healthy condition, with complete physical removal and cleaning of any mold or bacteria amplified due to the water damage.

❑ **Reconstruction** to return the home to a habitable condition.

❑ **Ongoing Moisture Control and Inspection:** Preventing mold recurrence is vital, which means ongoing moisture control and regular home inspections should become a part of the maintenance plan to sustain a mold-controlled environment and ensure the building memory of the water damage is addressed.

By adhering to these enhanced procedures, professionals can help ensure that homes with medically sensitive individuals are not only remediated but also maintained in a way that supports the health and well-being of their occupants. This tailored approach goes beyond the standard practices outlined in the IICRC guidelines. However, significant work remains, and this is where the 25 Step Process becomes essential.

Additional Considerations

||||||||||||||||||||||||||||||||||||||||||||||||||||||||||||||||||||||||||||||||||||||||||||||||||||||||||||||||||||||||||||||||||||||||||||||||||||||||||||||||||||||||||||||||||

Essentials for Contaminated Water Emergency Response

Sewage Water Damage Emergency Response

When a home is affected by a significantly contaminated (Category 2) or grossly contaminated water (Category 3) emergency, such as widespread sewage contamination, it is rarely a do-it-yourself situation. Specific professional-level procedures should be followed:

1. **Health and Safety Prioritization**: The contractor must prioritize health and safety, adhering to OSHA standards and using personal protective equipment (PPE) to ensure the safety of the restoration team and the home's occupants.

2. **Comprehensive Damage Assessment**: A thorough Indoor Environmental Professional assessment can help determine the water's category and class and assess the potential for mold growth. Category 2 water contains significant contamination, while Category 3 is grossly contaminated and may contain harmful pathogens.

3. **Containment and Extraction**: Separating affected versus unaffected areas of the building using containment is an important step in helping prevent cross-contamination. If the entire home is contaminated, containment barriers may not be necessary. However, the contractor should immediately proceed with water extraction, using professional-grade equipment to remove sewage and water.

4. **Handling Personal Possessions and Building Materials**: Personal possessions should be lifted out of the sewage and placed on blocks. Contaminated items should not be moved to uncontaminated areas to prevent cross-contamination. Porous materials like gypsum board walls, insulation, laminate or floating floors, and carpets should be removed and disposed of, as they cannot be restored. Personal possessions contacted by sewage should be documented; only those with significant value or sentimental worth should be considered for costly restoration.

5. **Addressing Overhead Contamination**: If the contamination has come from above, such as through a ceiling, personal possessions and affected building materials need to be evaluated, and decisions made about whether to be discarded, unless they undergo major decontamination.

6. **Cleaning Over Disinfection**: While disinfectants can be used, they are not always necessary and should be carefully considered and specifically approved before being allowed to be used in the homes of people with chemical sensitivities. Cleaning with soap, detergent, surfactant, and water is usually very effective. Post-cleaning testing can be used to evaluate the effectiveness of cleaning. This approach is particularly important in homes where residents might be sensitive to the harsh chemicals found in disinfectants.

||||||||||||||||||||||||||||||||||||||||||||||||||||||||||||||||||||||||||||||||||||||||||||||||||||||||||||||||||||||||||||||||||||||||||||||||||||||||||||||||||||||||||||||||||

DRYING CONTAMINATED BUILDINGS IN WATER EMERGENCIES

For drying buildings affected by significantly contaminated (Category 2) or grossly contaminated water (Category 3) emergencies, such as sewage water damage, the approach requires specialized strategies:

Containment and Airflow Control: The first step in drying is to establish containment, which might involve setting up physical barriers or simply closing off affected areas to prevent the spread of contaminants. Proper airflow control using air movers should be contained and controlled to ensure the airflow does not spread contaminants to unaffected areas. The air should be directed toward HEPA filtration units or exhaust systems to help remove contaminated air from the building. The aim is to create an environment that facilitates effective drying without spreading contaminants. This requires balancing airflow with dehumidification or outdoor air when weather and humidity conditions are appropriate to maintain an adequate drying environment airflow within the contained area.

Use of Industrial-Grade Drying Equipment: Industrial-grade dehumidifiers and air movers should be manufactured to facilitate effective decontamination between jobs and help ensure that cross-contamination does not occur. used strategically.

Regular Monitoring and Adjustment: The drying process must be closely monitored. Moisture levels in the air and in building materials should be regularly checked, and the setup of the drying equipment should be adjusted as necessary to ensure efficient and safe drying.

Safety Precautions for Technicians and Occupants: During the drying process, safety precautions for technicians and any occupants in the building are paramount. This includes using appropriate PPE and ensuring that occupants do not enter contaminated and drying areas.

Verification of Dryness and Contamination Control: Once the drying process is complete, a thorough inspection is necessary to confirm that all surfaces are dry and that contaminants have been effectively managed. This may include additional testing to ensure the environment is safe and minimize the risk of mold growth or other microbial activity.

SEPTIC SYSTEM SEWAGE DAMAGE

If the water source is sewage from the septic system, thoroughly removing porous affected materials such as gypsum board and insulation is essential. Cleaning using an approved detergent such as Branch Basics All Purpose Cleaner will remove soils and not interfere with commonly used post-remediation testing methods. Only approved products should be used. According to the ANSI/IICRC S500 Standard and Reference Guide for Professional Water Damage Restoration, SDS sheets and product information for all chemicals used on a project should be made available for approval by the owner. No product should be used without authorization. Any contractors using chemical products must also have reviewed them following their Health and Safety plan before use. If visible or suspected mold is discovered as a part of this water damage restoration work, the ANSI/IICRC S520 Standard and Reference Guide for Professional Mold Remediation is the minimum standard of care that should be followed in addition to the ANSI/IICRC S500. When people with hypersensitivities to mold or water-damage organisms occupy the home and problem organisms have potentially already developed, recommended practices should be specified as the standard of care and not just be considered advised or suggested but implemented unless there is a valid reason for rejecting them.

Air Movers and Fans should not be used on contaminated water damage until the building has been returned to a sanitary condition.

Generic Protocol for Cleaning Air Movers and Dehumidifiers

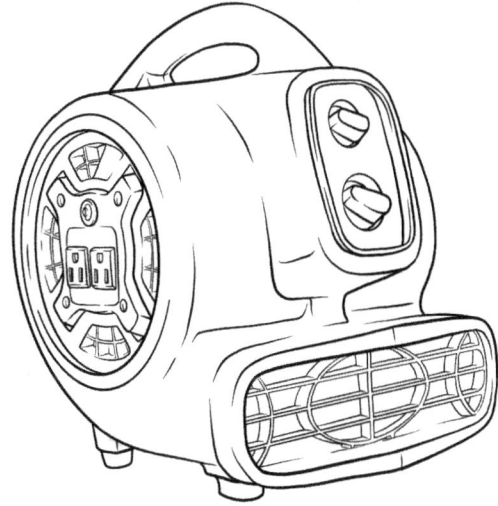

Figure 3-11: Air movers accelerate evaporation from materials' surfaces, "moving the moisture" into the air. This helps dry the surface but raises humidity levels.

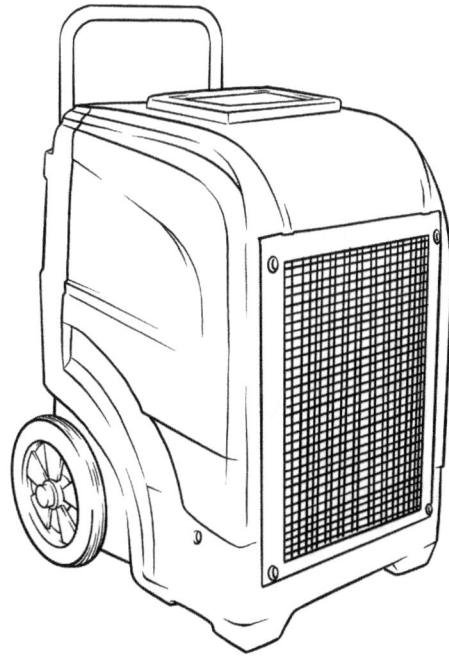

Figure 3-12: Refrigerant dehumidifiers remove the evaporated moisture by condensing it and draining it from the equipment. For dehumidifiers to work properly, the temperature needs to be correct. Too hot, and the moisture doesn't condense; too cold, and the moisture will freeze and cease to be removed. To function properly, the amount of evaporated moisture must be able to be removed by the drying equipment to provide a balanced drying system.

CLEANING PROTOCOLS FOR AIR MOVERS AND DEHUMIDIFIERS

Ensuring that only clean equipment enters a water-damaged home is crucial to safe and effective restoration. Contaminated tools can introduce bacteria, mold spores, and other pollutants, exacerbating damage and posing health risks. Many professional-grade air movers and dehumidifiers are designed with sealed components, allowing them to be cleaned thoroughly between jobs to prevent cross-contamination. However, these cleaning processes should be handled by trained professionals since using water on electrical equipment can result in severe shock or electrocution. In addition, dehumidifiers contain capacitors that can hold an electrical charge, increasing the risk of severe shock or electrocution if mishandled.

Here is a combined protocol for cleaning air movers and dehumidifiers that can safely be washed:

1. **Safety First**
   › **Read and follow the manufacturer's product instructions:** They are the ultimate authority on whether their equipment can be wet cleaned and how to perform the wet cleaning safely.
   › **Unplug the Equipment**: Ensure the device is disconnected from any power source to prevent electrical hazards.
   › **Wear Protective Gear**: Use gloves and a mask to guard against dust, debris, and potential contaminants.
   › **Dehumidifiers contain capacitors** that can hold an electrical charge; if you don't know how to discharge them, you need to learn from the manufacturer how to avoid severe shock or electrocution.

2. **Disassemble the Equipment:**
   › **Remove Detachable Parts**: Detach filters, grills, housing covers, water reservoirs, and other removable components for thorough cleaning.
   › **Discharge any capacitors that are present**.

3. **Prepare Cleaning Solution:**
   › **Soapy Water**: Use warm water with mild detergent, avoiding harsh chemicals that could damage the equipment. Do not submerge the equipment.

4. **Clean Each Component:**
   › **Filters and Reservoirs**: Wash filters and reservoirs in the soapy solution, using a soft brush if necessary. Rinse thoroughly and allow to dry completely.
   › **Grills, Fan Blades, and Housing**: Wipe down the fan blade, grills, and interior and exterior housing with a damp cloth or soft brush. Rinse to remove soap residue.

5. **Flush Sealed Components**:
   › For devices with sealed motors or other components, gently flush with soapy water. Avoid directing water forcefully to protect the seals. Rinse thoroughly to ensure no soap remains.

6. **Dry the Components:**
   › **Compressed Air**: Use compressed air to remove excess water from hard-to-reach areas.
   › **Air Dry**: Allow all parts to air dry completely before reassembly. A drying chamber with filtered, desiccated air can accelerate the process and prevent recontamination.

7. **Reassemble and Inspect:**
   › **Reattach Parts**: Once dry, reassemble by reinstalling all detached parts.
   › **Final Inspection**: Ensure cleanliness, secure parts, and test for functionality.

Following these steps helps maintain the longevity and effectiveness of air movers and dehumidifiers, ensuring they remain clean and safe for each restoration job. Always consult the manufacturer's guidelines in the manual or on their website for specific instructions.

Insurance: Review and Understand Your Insurance Policy

Review and Understand your coverage for water damage and the claims process before you need it. Your policy and company will typically have conditions and limitations. You should understand these before you need to call your carrier. Once you make the call—there may be ramifications for not knowing this information in advance.

The Importance of a Contingency Fund

Covering Shortcomings: Insurance may not cover all aspects needed for a healthy environment, especially for those with hypersensitivities. A contingency fund can help cover these gaps and ensure necessary measures are taken. For example, if you are hypersensitive or have other medical concerns, containment, and airflow controls should be used in water losses to minimize the spread of dust to unaffected areas. This helps control the spread of organisms as well as dust. But be aware that your adjuster may deny coverage for those expenses. Having and being willing to use your contingency fund can help avoid developing even more expensive issues. Most insurance policies have limitations, exclusions, or caps on the coverage they offer. Being in the middle of water damage is not the time to learn that you are underinsured or not insured. Coverage Caps and Exclusions may result in huge financial shortages between the cost of the loss and the reimbursement.

Essentials: Considerations for Water Damage, and Mold, Insurance:

Understanding home insurance in the context of water damage and mold is vital, particularly for mold-sensitive individuals. Whether you are a Homeowner or a Renter, you must know how insurance claims or inquiries can impact the property's insurability and premiums.

Key Considerations:

1. **Understand Mold Coverage Limits**: Most standard policies have mold exclusions, limitations, or caps that limit mold coverage. The caps are typically so low that it will be unusual for a person with environmental sensitivities to get the coverage needed to ensure they will achieve a healthy house post-water damage.

2. **Sudden and Accidental**: This clause in homeowners' insurance policies typically covers unexpected and abrupt incidents like burst pipes, excluding gradual damage like slow leaks. Understanding this clause is necessary, especially for mold-sensitive homeowners, as it determines what types of water damage will likely be covered by insurance.

3. **Understanding Pre-existing Conditions**: Homeowners' insurance policies typically do not cover pre-existing conditions. A pre-existing condition refers to any damage or defect present before the policy's coverage begins. This could include ongoing issues like slow leaks, gradual mold growth due to humidity, or any existing damage when the policy was purchased or went into effect after the condition developed.

4. **Understanding Pre-loss Conditions**: The term 'pre-loss condition' in homeowners' insurance policies typically focuses on restoring the property to its original structural and aesthetic state before damage occurs. This means repairs or replacements are intended to bring back the physical aspects of the property, such as walls, flooring, and fixtures, to their condition before the damage. However, this term often does not encompass the environmental healthfulness of the property, especially relevant in the context of mold damage. For individuals with mold sensitivities, restoring a property to its 'pre-loss condition' may not adequately address the potential health hazards of residual mold spores or unseen mold growth. The standard insurance restoration process might not include comprehensive mold remediation to the extent necessary for ensuring a healthy indoor environment free from mold. This can be a significant concern for mold-sensitive homeowners, as their health requirements might necessitate a more thorough remediation process than what the insurance policy covers under the scope of returning a property to its 'pre-loss condition.'

5. **Mitigate Further Damage Proactively**: After detecting water damage or mold, it's essential to immediately mitigate further damage. Quick steps like stopping the water

source, drying out wet areas, and removing affected materials can prevent the spread of mold and additional water damage. Insurance policies often require this to maintain coverage validity. Documenting these mitigation efforts is also important for supporting future insurance claims, showing that you've taken responsible actions to minimize the extent of the damage.

6. **Comprehensive Documentation**: Maintaining comprehensive documentation of all aspects of water damage and subsequent remediation efforts is vital. While detailed records might have limited influence on elements of the claim related to mold and health concerns, they can help clarify which parts of the claim are likely to be covered and paid for under the water damage part of the policy versus parts potentially excluded by the insurance. This documentation, including photographs, professional assessments, and repair receipts, can be instrumental in ensuring a fair and accurate claim process. For example, the cost of removing and replacing gypsum wallboard may be covered because it is water-damaged but excluded or capped if the reason for the removal is mold.

7. **Explore Additional Coverage Options**: Independent insurance advisors or brokers offer a wide range of options from multiple insurers due to their fiduciary responsibility to clients, not insurers. They provide personalized, expert guidance on various insurance needs, assist with claims, and foster long-term relationships for ongoing coverage assessment, all while upholding high professional standards as licensed, state-regulated professionals. They are particularly beneficial for individuals with specific insurance needs, such as those concerned about mold and water damage coverage. Their professional knowledge may also help make

important decisions regarding if and when to report a loss to the carrier.

8. **Comprehensive Approach to Insurance and Mold Management:** Regularly consult with mold remediation and legal experts to navigate insurance and health implications, review and update your insurance policy to align with current needs, and thoroughly understand all terms and conditions. Consider establishing a fund for potential mold remediation due to coverage limitations, proactively implementing preventive measures against mold, like controlling humidity and fixing leaks, and maintaining open communication with your insurance agent about how claims, inquiries, and the CLUE database can impact your policy.

9. **Considerations for Reporting Damage:** If you discover mold or water damage in your home, promptly assess the situation. Be aware that most insurance policies require timely filings and have specific time limits for submitting claims. Consider the severity of the damage and whether you can handle the remediation without an insurance claim. Even inquiries to your insurance company about potential claims can be noted and may affect your CLUE (Comprehensive Loss Underwriting Exchange) report. This information can influence future insurance renewals and premiums with your current carrier and other insurance companies that access the CLUE database. In cases of significant damage or uncertainty about the best course of action, consulting with a professional can provide guidance on whether involving your insurance company is advisable. This approach helps you make an informed decision without unintentionally impacting your insurance record or missing filing deadlines. (Consumer Reports, n.d.) (Insurance Information Institute, n.d.) (LexisNexis, n.d.)

Navigating the Influence of Insurance on Restoration Practices

The competition between restoration goals and unintended consequences is evident in the interplay between restoration practices and insurance policy coverage. Rapid air movement is essential for quick drying, but it can spread pre-existing mold spores, posing a risk to those with hypersensitivities. While containment methods to prevent cross-contamination during drying exist, they are often deemed unnecessary by insurance adjusters who prioritize cost savings. This undue influence can result in the rejection of extra measures necessary to protect sensitive individuals. While insurance policies typically require returning the building to a pre-loss condition for covered losses, they may not cover the health of the occupants. Owners should be prepared to cover costs that insurance refuses to cover, especially since most policies only provide coverage for sudden and accidental covered losses.

Therefore, maintaining a contingency fund to address these shortcomings in insurance coverage is prudent.

The Complexities of Insurance

Dealing with water damage is tough, but dealing with insurance companies can be even worse. This section addresses the harsh realities of insurance coverage for water damage and how it often falls short.

I remember meeting a woman in New Orleans after Hurricane Katrina. Her story hits hard. She woke up one morning to find her house flooded with water, which was beginning to soak her mattress. She climbed to her attic, hoping for the water to recede or someone to rescue her. Hours later, the water was up to the attic. She had to break through her roof with a discarded two-by-four she found to get out. Eventually, she was spotted on her roof and airlifted to safety by a helicopter.

You'd think her homeowner's insurance would help, right? She had paid for both homeowner's and flood insurance coverage for years. The homeowner's policy was supposed to cover wind damage from a hurricane, and the flood insurance was supposed to cover the water damage from the flooding. But here's the catch: the flood caused more than half of the damage to her home. Her homeowner's insurance policy had a clause that stated that if more than half of the damages were caused by a loss excluded from her policy (the flood), they wouldn't pay for the rest of the damage (wind from the hurricane). As for the damage she caused when she punched through the roof to save her own life, it was also not covered! Her adjuster

told her that if someone else, such as a guest, had punched the hole in her roof, they might have paid, but only if a police report had been filed that the guest had vandalized the property.

She was 78, widowed, and living on a fixed income. She and her husband had worked hard all their lives to buy the home, and now she couldn't afford to properly fix the home or pay the legal expenses to fight the insurance company. She was alive but left with an uninhabitable home that was continuing to deteriorate.

Essentials: Working with Insurance Adjusters

Navigating the claims process after water damage or mold infestation can be complex. Understanding the roles and responsibilities of insurance adjusters and your rights as a policyholder can help ensure a fair and efficient resolution.

Insurance Adjusters Have the Following Responsibilities:

- **Assess and Estimate:** Adjusters assess and estimate the extent of water damage or mold infestation.
- **Determine Coverage:** They determine insurance coverage and estimate repair and remediation costs.
- **Review and Approve Claims:** Adjusters review and approve claims in line with policy terms and conditions.
- **Coordinate with Contractors:** They coordinate with contractors for accurate repair estimates.
- **Guide Homeowners:** Adjusters guide homeowners on the claims process and expected timelines.
- **Collect Documentation:** They collect necessary documentation for claim processing.

Legal Responsibilities of Adjusters

- **Act in Good Faith:** Adjusters should act in good faith and ensure unbiased decision-making.
- **Comply with Laws:** They must comply with state and federal insurance claim laws.
- **Provide Accurate Information:** Adjusters must provide accurate information about policy coverage limits.

Regarding Contractor Recommendations

- **Recommendations, Not Demands:** Adjusters can recommend contractors but cannot demand that you use specific ones.
- **Policyholder's Choice:** As the policyholder, you have the right to choose your own contractor. This allows you to select a reputable, experienced professional who meets your needs.

Emergency Water Damage Drying Coverage

- **Mitigation of Damages Clause:** Under the "mitigation of damages" clause, insurers generally cover costs for emergency drying, but you are required to mitigate damages without any assurance that insurance will reimburse everything you pay.
- **Policy Terms:** The extent of coverage depends on policy terms, including deductibles and limits.
- **Document Damage:** Policyholders should document damage and necessary emergency measures.
- **Preferred Vendors:** Insurers may provide preferred vendors, but policyholders can choose their own.

Consultation for Policy Ambiguities

- **Consult Policy or Seek Advice:** In case of uncertainty, consult the insurance policy or seek independent advice.
- **Reservation of Rights Letter:** Insurers may issue a Reservation of Rights Letter when they believe there is uncertainty about policy coverage, reserving their right to potentially deny coverage after conducting further investigation. (Insurance Information Institute, n.d.) (IRMI, n.d.) (ABA, 2020)

PROHIBITED ACTIONS FOR ADJUSTERS

- **Avoid Legal Interpretations:** Adjusters should avoid providing legal interpretations or advice. (NAIC, n.d.(a))

- **Refrain from Discrimination:** They must not engage in discrimination or unprofessional behavior based on personal characteristics. (EEOC, n.d.)

- **Provide Accurate Information:** Adjusters must not misrepresent policy information or pressure for quick settlements. (IRMI, n.d.(b))

- **Maintain Professionalism:** They are forbidden from soliciting or accepting bribes or engaging in corrupt practices. (IRMI, n.d.(b))

- **Avoid Guarantees:** Adjusters must not make guarantees or promises about the outcomes of claims that cannot be substantiated. (IRMI, n.d.(b))

- **Respect Policyholder Rights:** They must not pressure policyholders to accept quick, potentially inadequate settlements. (NAIC, n.d.(b))

- **Adhere to Authority:** Adjusters must not overstep their authority by authorizing work not covered by the policy without agreement. (NAIC, n.d.(b))

- **Professional Conduct:** Harassment or unprofessional behavior toward any parties involved in the claims process is prohibited. (NAIC, n.d.(b))

- **Integrity in Documentation:** Adjusters must not alter, fabricate, or omit crucial evidence or documentation. (NAIC, n.d.(b))

References

Holland, J., Banta, J., Cole, G., & Passmore, B. (2012, May). Bacterial amplification and in-place carpet drying: Implications for Category 1 water intrusion restoration. *Journal of Environmental Health, 74*(9), 8–14.

Siau, J. F. (1995). *Wood: Influence of moisture on physical properties.* Virginia Polytechnic Institute and State University.

Consumer Reports. (n.d.). When to file a homeowners insurance claim. Retrieved June 28, 2024, from https://www.consumerreports.org/homeowners-insurance/when-to-file-a-homeowners-insurance-claim/

Insurance Information Institute. (n.d.). How to file a homeowners insurance claim. Retrieved June 28, 2024, from https://www.iii.org/article/how-to-file-a-homeowners-insurance-claim

LexisNexis. (n.d.). Understanding your CLUE report. Retrieved June 28, 2024, from https://risk.lexisnexis.com/insurance/claims/understanding-your-clue-report

Insurance Information Institute. (n.d.). What to do if your insurance claim is denied. Retrieved June 28, 2024, from https://www.iii.org/article/what-to-do-if-your-insurance-claim-is-denied

International Risk Management Institute (IRMIa). (n.d.). Reservation of rights. Retrieved June 28, 2024, from https://www.irmi.com/term/insurance-definitions/reservation-of-rights

American Bar Association (ABA). (2020). Why insurers issue reservation of rights letters. Retrieved June 28, 2024, from https://www.americanbar.org/groups/litigation/committees/insurance-coverage/practice/2020/why-insurers-issue-reservation-of-rights-letters/

National Association of Insurance Commissioners (NAICa). (n.d.). *Market conduct examiners handbook.* Retrieved June 28, 2024, from https://www.naic.org/prod_serv/MH-01.pdf

U.S. Equal Employment Opportunity Commission (EEOC). (n.d.). Prohibited employment policies/practices. Retrieved June 28, 2024, from https://www.eeoc.gov/prohibited-employment-policiespractices

International Risk Management Institute (IRMIB). (n.d.). Adjuster's code of conduct. Retrieved June 28, 2024, from https://www.irmi.com/term/insurance-definitions/adjuster-code-of-conduct

National Association of Insurance Commissioners (NAICb). (n.d.). Ethics for insurance professionals. Retrieved June 28, 2024, from https://www.naic.org/prod_serv/MH-01.pdf

Home Selection: Rent or Buy

A practical guide for readers to assess water damage and mold risk for potential homes, whether they rent or own.

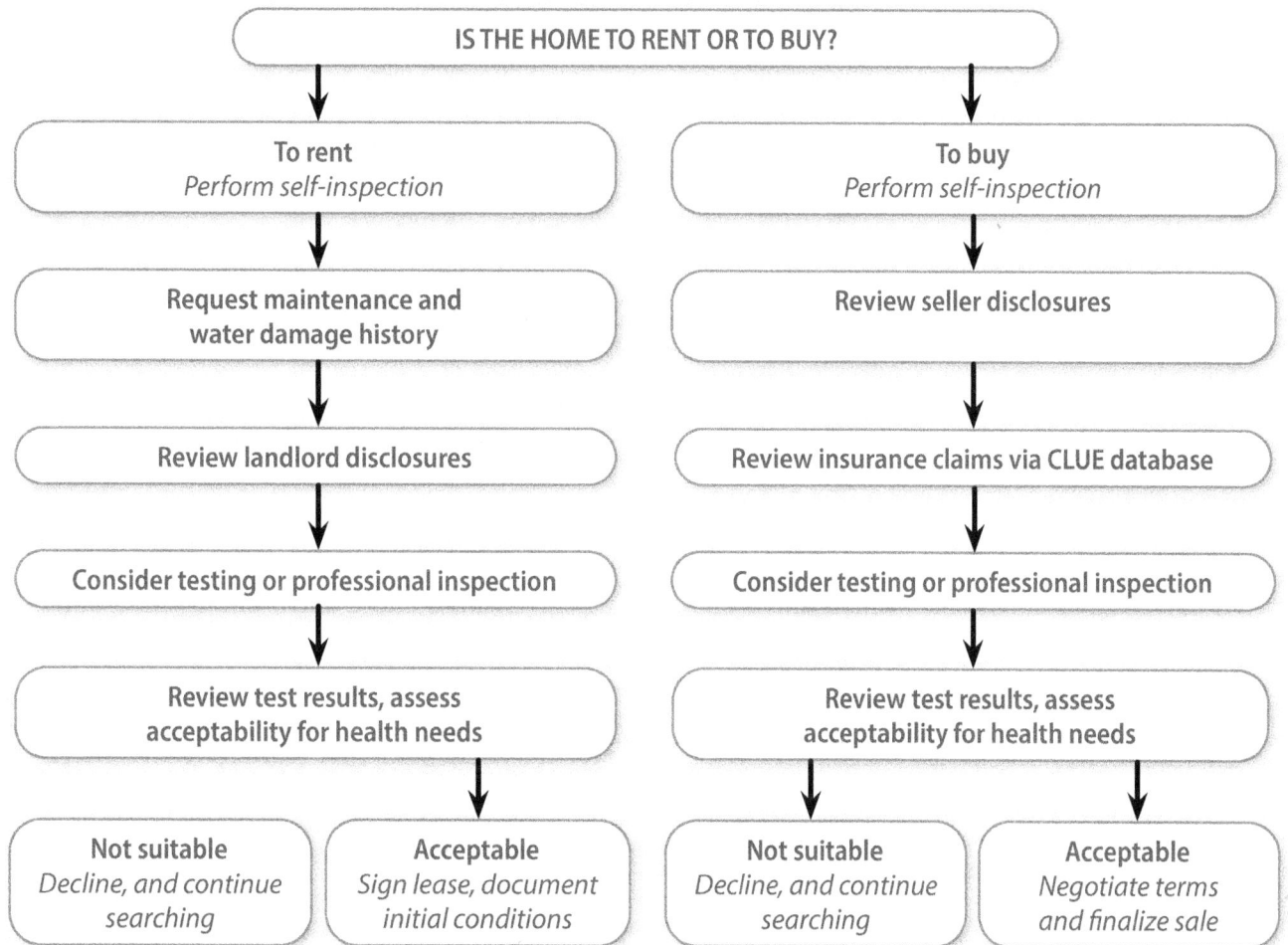

```
┌─────────────────────────────────────────────────────────────┐
│              IS THE HOME TO RENT OR TO BUY?                   │
└─────────────────────────────────────────────────────────────┘
              │                              │
              ▼                              ▼
┌──────────────────────────┐   ┌──────────────────────────┐
│         To rent          │   │          To buy          │
│  Perform self-inspection │   │  Perform self-inspection │
└──────────────────────────┘   └──────────────────────────┘
              │                              │
              ▼                              ▼
┌──────────────────────────┐   ┌──────────────────────────┐
│   Request maintenance    │   │  Review seller disclosures│
│ and water damage history │   │                          │
└──────────────────────────┘   └──────────────────────────┘
              │                              │
              ▼                              ▼
┌──────────────────────────┐   ┌──────────────────────────┐
│ Review landlord          │   │ Review insurance claims  │
│ disclosures              │   │ via CLUE database        │
└──────────────────────────┘   └──────────────────────────┘
              │                              │
              ▼                              ▼
┌──────────────────────────┐   ┌──────────────────────────┐
│ Consider testing or      │   │ Consider testing or      │
│ professional inspection  │   │ professional inspection  │
└──────────────────────────┘   └──────────────────────────┘
              │                              │
              ▼                              ▼
┌──────────────────────────┐   ┌──────────────────────────┐
│ Review test results,     │   │ Review test results,     │
│ assess acceptability     │   │ assess acceptability     │
│ for health needs         │   │ for health needs         │
└──────────────────────────┘   └──────────────────────────┘
        │            │              │            │
        ▼            ▼              ▼            ▼
```

Not suitable	Acceptable	Not suitable	Acceptable
Decline, and continue searching	*Sign lease, document initial conditions*	*Decline, and continue searching*	*Negotiate terms and finalize sale*

HOME SELECTION: FIRST STEPS

Consider this section the initial screening to help you decide whether a property is worth further consideration. Here, we focus on gathering non-invasive, non-destructive information about a property to help you decide whether to investigate further in your quest to buy or rent a home.

Since mold and water damage can pose significant health risks, particularly for those with heightened sensitivities or medical concerns, being vigilant and thorough in your home selection process and understanding the intricacies of building construction, maintenance, history, and climate impact is essential. Homes, much like living organisms, have life cycles and vulnerabilities:

Begin a new section of your project diary for each new property you consider. At a minimum, enter the site address, contact person, and abbreviated details. If you decide that the home is not for you, enter a brief explanation and place a single line through the entry with your initials and date. This will help you avoid looking at the sample place repeatedly. It also enables you to find It if you decide to reconsider. Place an entry in your diary for the Boxes to indicate if they are:

☑ Relevant

🚫 Doesn't Apply

◻ Uncertain

INITIAL CONSIDERATIONS

Begin by thinking about considerations that are off the table. The more you understand what is acceptable or unacceptable, the better you will be able to avoid wasting time, energy, and money evaluating places that are not worth considering:

- **Historic or Older Buildings:** Old Buildings might whisper tales of charm but could harbor threats like hidden water damage or hazardous materials such as lead-based paint and asbestos. Even those buildings that have undergone complete remodeling may not have considered all aspects of older construction.

- **New Construction:** While seemingly pristine, newer constructions are not without pitfalls. Often built with materials or methods that may not endure environmental pressures, minor construction or maintenance errors can compound into significant issues. Usually, brand-new buildings do not have a chance for issues to become apparent or sufficient dust to work its way into the living space for sampling to detect potential mold problems. Also, people with multiple chemical sensitivities may need a much longer period of time for materials to cure or off-gas and become acceptable.

- **Obvious Flawed Design or Construction:** The design and construction practices contributing to a home's architectural allure might also mask inherent flaws, predisposing it to moisture retention and microbial growth. Understanding these risks can differentiate between a haven and a health hazard.

- **Consider Local Climate Challenges**: Weather and our changing climate can play a crucial yet often underappreciated role in a building's health. The sultry humidity of the South, the freezing thaw cycles of the North, and the salt-laden air of coastal regions each present unique challenges that can affect a building's integrity and propensity for water damage. Awareness of these climate-specific risks can help you make educated decisions and recognize developing issues early on. Also, note any changes in the climate trend in the area.

- **Consideration of Professional Inspections and Specialized Assessments:** Investing in professional assessments can prevent future expenses and health issues by identifying and addressing potential problems before you commit to buying or renting the property.

- **Other Considerations:** Beyond the physical structure, the role of past owners in maintaining a healthy living environment is paramount. Regular maintenance, vigilance in observing changes, and proactive measures play a significant role in preventing the growth of organisms due to water damage. This means even the most diligent buyer or renter can be blindsided by hidden issues resulting from decades of owners' neglect, oversight, or even intentional concealment of problems. I am always amazed at what I have learned about a home and its history by talking to neighbors. Just be aware that whether or not they talk with you, there is a good chance they may talk about you, too!

CHOOSE AN AGENT

Engaging a buyer's agent who charges a fee for their service might offer more impartial advice, as their compensation is not solely commission-based. This can be particularly advantageous in prioritizing your interests throughout the property transaction process. A buyer's agent can provide a second opinion on inspection reports and may recommend additional inspections. They bring a wealth of knowledge and experience to the table, helping you navigate complex property evaluations and identifying potential issues that might be overlooked. Their expertise in interpreting inspection reports, understanding local disclosure laws, and recognizing subtle signs of mold or water damage can prove invaluable. Additionally, a buyer's agent can leverage their network to recommend reliable, independent inspectors, ensuring unbiased and thorough assessments. This relationship can also facilitate access to historical data, building permits, and past inspection reports, offering a comprehensive view of the property's condition. By having a dedicated professional, you can make informed decisions based on a blend of reported findings and broader contextual understanding.

Furthermore, consider the benefits of enlisting a buyer's agent, even if you want to rent. Unlike traditional real estate agents who often work on commission from the sale, you pay a buyer's agent directly, helping ensure their loyalty and motivation to secure the best outcome for you. This relationship can be particularly beneficial, potentially acquiring more transparent and detailed information about the property even if you are renting.

||||||||||||||||||||||||||||||||||||||||||||||||||||||||||||||||||||||||||||||||||||||||||||||||||||||||||||||||||||||||||||||||||||

Essay: Supporting Clients with Health-Related Sensitivities in the Home-Buying Process
by Jennifer Schrantz, Realtor

Health-related sensitivities, including reactions to water-damage organisms, fragrances, masking odors, and toxic chemicals, present unique challenges when searching for a home. A real estate professional's priority should be to guide clients through this process with empathy, expertise, and a commitment to finding an environment that supports their health. Below is guidance to ensure clients feel supported and secure throughout their home-buying journey.

Finding the right local Realtor® is the first step. This choice is crucial, as finding a suitable home for someone with sensitivities often requires patience and perseverance. It's not uncommon to view 30–50 homes before finding the right one. While this can be an exhaustive process for both the client and the agent, the satisfaction of securing a health-supporting home makes it worthwhile. An ideal Realtor® must be caring and compassionate, prioritizing the client's unique needs while maintaining the perseverance needed for this often-complex search. They should also have a deep understanding of the local market, enabling them to negotiate effectively on behalf of the client. Specific requests, such as extended inspection periods, can make a significant difference when evaluating homes for individuals with health limitations.

A thorough buyer consultation sets the foundation for the home-buying process. For clients with sensitivities, this conversation extends beyond typical topics like budget and location. Buyers should identify as many concerns as possible so the agent can incorporate these into the search and inspection process. Many clients already have some knowledge of testing and inspections, often guided by a clinician or Indoor Environmental Professional (IEP). During this consultation, the agent should aim to understand the client's comfort level regarding issues like visible water damage or potential remediation needs. Some clients may prefer to avoid homes with any signs of damage, while others might consider remediation or post-closing repairs as viable solutions. Together, the agent and buyer can strategize issues to address during the initial negotiation versus considerations to address once under contract. This nuanced understanding ensures that the agent's approach aligns with the client's preferences and limitations.

The search process begins with broad guidelines tailored to minimize risks associated with mold, chemical exposure, and other environmental triggers. For example, homes built within the last 2–10 years are often preferred for their lower likelihood of extensive water damage, though this is not guaranteed. Structural features, such as brick or block homes and pitched roofs, are often prioritized over wood frames or flat roofs due to their greater resilience to water intrusion. While these are helpful starting points, each property should be approached with an open mind, recognizing that even an older home with potential issues could work with proper mitigation.

New construction can be an excellent option for some clients, though chemical sensitivities may complicate this choice. Custom builds using low-VOC materials offer greater control over potential triggers. A framing or pre-drywall inspection for new builds can help identify issues like mold on lumber, while final inspections ensure that city or county inspections haven't overlooked significant concerns.

Virtual showings are an excellent option for clients who wish to minimize exposure to potential triggers like mold, chemical odors, or off-gassing. Using platforms like Zoom or FaceTime, agents can preview homes on behalf of the buyer, narrowing the list to a few top contenders for in-person visits. Some clients, however, may prefer to attend every showing to gauge how they feel in each space. There is no one-size-fits-all approach; the priority is an agent that can align with the client's comfort and preferences.

During showings, agents should pay close attention to signs of water damage or other potential health-related concerns. Subtle clues like mismatched wall textures, paint sheens, or unusual odors may indicate repairs, masking agents, or hidden problems requiring further investigation. While visible issues like mold or leaks might be deal breakers for some clients, others may consider remediation acceptable if the home meets other criteria.

Before making an offer, gathering as much information as possible about the property is essential. Seller disclosures, insurance claim histories, and other documentation can reveal past issues, though these records are not always comprehensive. In addition to a general inspection, specialized assessments such as termite evaluations, roof inspections, and HVAC reviews are often the most reliable way to assess a home's condition. For example, termite activity can indicate hidden water damage, while poorly maintained HVAC systems may harbor mold or allergens. When addressing roof conditions, obtaining multiple roofer opinions can provide a more accurate understanding of the property's condition. Additional tests for radon, lead-based paint, or microbial growth may also be appropriate, depending on the region.

Once inspections are complete, the second negotiation process begins. For repairs related to water damage or mold, clients are often advised to request a credit or price reduction rather than having the seller handle the work. This approach allows buyers to oversee the remediation, ensuring it meets their specific health and safety standards. Clear communication with the listing agent is key to reaching a solution that meets both parties.

Expecting a home to be entirely free of contaminants is unrealistic, but the goal is to find a property that supports the client's health and well-being. What works for one person may not work for another, making the process highly individualized. Clients can feel heard, understood, and confident in their decisions by prioritizing their needs, maintaining open communication, and leveraging the agent's expertise.

Serving clients with health-related limitations requires a compassionate, detail-oriented approach that goes beyond standard real estate practices. From identifying suitable properties to navigating inspections and negotiations, every step should prioritize their health and peace of mind. The ultimate goal is to help clients find not just a house but a home where they can heal and thrive.

August 2024 Nationwide Real Estate Industry Changes

In August 2024, significant changes were implemented in the real estate industry following a lawsuit involving the National Association of Realtors (NAR). These changes primarily affect how buyer-agent compensation is handled and require buyers to be more involved in negotiating fees with their agents.

Previously, compensation for buyer agents was often publicly disclosed and covered by sellers through the Multiple Listing Services (MLS). However, under the new rules, public offers of buyer broker compensation have been removed from the MLS. This means buyers must now negotiate directly with their agents regarding compensation and consider these costs when budgeting for a home purchase.

Buyers can ask the seller to pay their buyer agent's compensation as part of the negotiation process. However, this change makes it even more critical for buyers to carefully interview potential agents to ensure they find the right fit. With the possibility of being responsible for paying their agent's fees, buyers should weigh the services provided against the associated costs to ensure they receive value for their money.

In addition, agents who are members of the NAR and their local MLS boards must have a signed written agreement with buyers before showing them properties. This agreement formalizes the relationship between the buyer and the agent and outlines the terms of compensation and services provided.

Engaging with knowledgeable and experienced agents who understand the new rules will help buyers navigate this updated landscape smoothly and make informed decisions during the home-buying process.

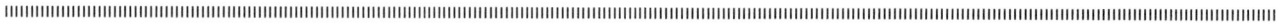

Keep notes about the agents you encounter, their contact information, and who they represent. If you are looking at open houses on your own and working with a buyer's agent, you should let the selling agent know who is representing you when you walk through the home.

YOUR PRELIMINARY LOW-COST SELECTION EVALUATION

The listing information provides an initial glimpse, but delving deeper into public records and other sources can reveal insights into the property's history and condition. By examining these resources, you can uncover potential water damage and mold issues that may not be immediately apparent.

Additionally, employing lateral thinking can be invaluable in this research process. For instance, a listing history might provide clues that a home was recently purchased as a fixer-upper to flip. Flipped homes often undergo cosmetic repairs to enhance their appearance, but underlying issues or deterioration may not be adequately addressed. Recognizing such patterns and thinking beyond the surface can help you identify hidden problems that could impact your decision. This section will explore listing details, public information, and lateral thinking to identify red flags and assess whether a property warrants further investigation or consideration.

Much of this section offers a user-friendly, self-guided preliminary evaluation at little to no cost. Home buyers and prospective renters can initially assess the potential mold and water damage risks in dwellings.

While this section provides a valuable starting point for recognizing apparent issues, it's important to remember that it cannot cover all potential risks associated with water damage and microbial conditions. Instead, it highlights visible issues and offers insights into subtler conditions that might exist or develop over time.

Disclosure Laws

You should understand local disclosure laws when pursuing a property, whether buying or renting, as they vary significantly across jurisdictions. States can be broadly categorized into "buyer or renter beware" regions and "full disclosure" states. In states with full disclosure, sellers and landlords must legally provide information about what they know regarding the property, including past inspection reports and any known issues. (NAR, 2021) (FindLaw., 2023) (Bagley, 2020) (Cornell, n.d.) (U.S.HUD, 2022)

However, even in states with less stringent disclosure requirements, asking specific questions regarding the property's history and condition is vital. While probing questions might make some sellers or landlords hesitant, you should persist tactfully. Withholding information in a "full-disclosure state" or providing false answers in a "buyer-beware state" can constitute fraud. Being aware of this can help protect you as a buyer or renter. Investigating the duration of the current owner's or property manager's involvement with the property can offer additional insights. Such information can hint at underlying issues not disclosed during initial discussions.

Determine the disclosure status of the property.

❏ Buyer Beware.

❏ Full Disclosure.

❏ Disclosure Exempt or sellers don't know.

||||||||||||||||||||||||||||||||||||||||||||||||||||||||||||||||||||||||||||||||||||||||||||||||||||||||||||||||||||||||||||||||||||||||

When the Past is Hidden: Disclosure Risks in Real Estate Transactions

- When a home is sold after the owner dies, there is usually no known history to disclose.

- Banks and lenders that foreclose and repossess homes usually don't know the history and will frequently not pass on what history they do know or even do what they can to avoid learning about the history.

- The housing crisis in the late 2000s resulted in foreclosures, and the number of homes flipped by do-it-yourselfers increased. Home flippers frequently don't adequately address mold for mold-sensitive people.

- Many state, county, and real estate guidance documents regarding mold only refer to "visible mold" regarding disclosure. This is often defined in different ways. Some assume it means only mold that you can see in the occupiable or accessible areas of a home, but visible mold may also be hidden and not become visible until materials are removed. Hidden or sub-visible mold may also be a health issue for hypersensitive people.

- In older homes, it is common for the water intrusion to have been fixed, but the mold that developed before the home dried has been left behind. Once dry, mold goes dormant. Over time, if no additional elevated moisture levels develop, the dormant mold dies off. As time passes, the mold begins to degrade into visually unrecognizable micro-fragments. Studies have shown that these tiny particles are often more problematic for sensitive individuals than intact mold spores. The fragments are so small that they elude the body's normal defenses. Allowing them to be inhaled deeply into the lungs, where they can be absorbed and cross directly into the bloodstream.

- Construction materials used in old homes may have reached the end of their useful life.

||||||||||||||||||||||||||||||||||||||||||||||||||||||||||||||||||||||||||||||||||||||||||||||||||||||||||||||||||||||||||||||||||||||||

Evaluating Existing Property Inspection Reports and Historical and Auxiliary Information

Embarking on the journey of buying or renting a home or evaluating the current state of a residence requires a thorough understanding of existing property inspection reports when available. These documents, often produced by real estate, pest control, or property inspectors, can provide a preliminary overview of a property's visible condition. Even if they are not offered, you can always ask if any are available, and if they are, for copies. However, a conscientious review of these reports should be made, and the circumstances of their availability and the transparency of their findings should be considered.

Past reports can be invaluable; they often focus on visible issues and typically include disclaimers about hidden hazards like mold. The true value in these reports often lies in reading between the lines. For example, a report noting poor drainage might indicate a greater risk that water damage has already impacted basements or crawlspaces. The drainage problem may have been corrected, but the damage it caused may have been cosmetically repaired or covered up, which hides the evidence. Such a repair may be adequate for most potential renters or buyers but be devastating for people actively suffering from sensitivities to organisms resulting from actions that eliminated the source of moisture and cosmetically repaired the damage but did not return the building to a clean and adequately mold-controlled condition.

Accessing Historical and Auxiliary Information—Strategies for gathering additional data about the property's past

Potential buyers should seek additional sources for more comprehensive property considerations.

❏ Explore the availability of existing reports or inspections that have already been performed. If you get a clean report that the seller has provided, you can ask about prior reports used to guide completed repairs.

❏ Historical reports, building permits, and records can sometimes be found in planning department files or through local historical archives.

❏ Digital resources such as Zillow, Realtor.com, and Redfin often list historical data and previous listings that can reveal property condition changes over time. Researching a rental as if you were planning to purchase it can provide valuable information about its suitability for your situation.

❏ Working with your insurance agent can help you explore flooding risks and past damage claim information. Buyers can obtain a Comprehensive Loss Underwriters Exchange (CLUE) database report for a property as part of their purchase agreement.

❏ Renters may face more difficulty obtaining this report, but you might be able to get a copy if you are getting renters insurance and your insurance agent is willing to help.

This information can help you and your agent understand if the property has had reported insurance claims that may affect the rates you would end up paying. Additionally, it can provide clues about damage losses that may not have been addressed adequately, which is crucial for individuals with mold sensitivities.

Local buyers' agents, familiar with neighborhood histories, can often provide insights not captured in official reports. Neighbors can also be valuable sources of information, offering anecdotal evidence or historical context that might not be documented elsewhere. These additional layers of information can prove crucial in identifying issues that previous inspections might have missed or that sellers might prefer not to disclose.

INTERPRETING OTHER INFORMATION

Interpreting other information often requires a discerning eye, as initial appearances can sometimes be deceptive. Visible signs hinting at more deeply hidden issues, combined with historical data and local knowledge, can be assembled to form a more complete picture of the property's condition.

❑ The age of a water heater may provide clues about its failure, leading to questions about what might have caused the failure. The nature of the failure may then offer insights into any water released. Thinking in three dimensions can help you understand which other areas of the home may have experienced water flow. Attic or upstairs water heaters that burst are more likely to affect multiple levels, whereas a ground-floor or garage-mounted water heater rupture may have caused damage to that level.

❑ Toilet tanks often have dates stamped inside. Learning the age of the toilet may merely indicate that it was replaced or updated during remodeling. Still, it may also indicate that it was damaged and had to be replaced because it released water.

❑ Room air fresheners can be telltale indicators that may hide indications of mold or water damage. Even freshly baked cookies may be a coverup for odor issues. If you are genuinely interested in a property, you will want to learn if odors are the issue by visiting it more than once when you have a fresh nose before committing to a purchase or rental.

❑ Evaluating pest control reports can be enlightening; conditions conducive to pest problems, like moisture issues, can also foster mold growth. Signs of past or current infestations might point to compromised structural integrity and potential moisture ingress points. Many states require pest companies to post termite inspection tags with company contact information, inspection dates, and treatment methods.

❑ Rot is caused by some wood-destroying fungal organisms that require elevated moisture. This may provide clues about additional problems with surface molds that could have developed due to the same water flow accumulation that caused the rot.

By paying attention to these subtle signs and seeking a deeper understanding, you can uncover hidden issues that might otherwise be overlooked.

PROFESSIONAL CONSULTATIONS, INDEPENDENT ASSESSMENTS, AND OTHER PAID ASSISTANCE

Given these complexities, if the free explorations you can perform based on available information are inadequate for your comfort level, you should seek professional advice for a more comprehensive evaluation. Though it involves some expense, consulting with an experienced building scientist, indoor environmental professional, or mold and water damage specialist can provide deeper insights.

It's also wise to consider the potential biases of inspectors, especially those who receive most of their work by being referred by real estate agents. Maybe they are really good, and your agent is looking out for your best interest. Still, there is always a risk that such an inspector might understate issues or identify them cryptically to maintain their referral relationships. Independent inspectors, who are not influenced by such relationships, are invaluable for their unbiased and thorough assessments. They can provide a more accurate picture of the property's condition.

A more detailed examination focusing on typically excluded areas may be necessary when significant concerns arise from a standard inspection. Professional specialized investigators can use advanced tools and techniques to detect issues that might not be visible to the untrained eye, such as thermal imaging to find hidden moisture and structural analysis to assess the integrity of the building. While air sampling is a common method used by mold inspectors, there are other ways to better inspect for mold and water damage, especially when someone is hypersensitive. The Five Stage, 25 Steps will discuss these investigation and sampling methods in greater detail.

Addressing Identified Issues

While inspection reports are foundational in evaluating a property's visible and superficial condition, a discerning review and reading between the lines can uncover more deep-seated, suspicious, or potentially hidden issues. Recognizing when to seek further professional advice and how to interpret and act upon the findings of these reports are key steps in making well-informed property investment, maintenance, and remediation decisions. By understanding the full scope of an inspection report and its limitations, you are better equipped to protect your investment and ensure a healthy living environment. (NAHI, 2020) (Kaplan, 2021) (Cornell, n.d.(b))

- Look for subtle hints in the report that might suggest more significant issues, such as minor water damage, which may indicate more significant hidden mold problems.

- Pay attention to the language used; vague or non-committal wording might be a red flag for underlying issues.

- Often, limiting statements will be made. They may conclude with a suggestion that a specialist inspection be performed, such as roofing, plumbing, and gutters, to provide additional information. This indicates potential issues without stating what they are. Pay attention to limiting language!

- If the report mentions any concerns, even minor ones, consider them as potential indicators of more significant problems. Always be aware that water spreads laterally outward and downward. It follows the path of least resistance. Capillary action may draw it deeper or higher into materials, and condensation can be expected on colder surfaces, sometimes without being obvious.

- Moisture-resistant or water-proof construction materials, while seemingly effective at preventing mold growth, can trap moisture, leading to significant mold growth and future issues in adjacent materials and hidden spaces.

- Follow up with specific questions or request a more detailed inspection by an expert in areas where concerns are noted. You must decide if you will be having these conversations in private! You may trust your agent, but the inspector may have reasons for disclosing more nuanced information to you if they have a sense of confidentiality.

- Consider what is present and observed and what may be concealed or developed over time.

Selecting Inspectors and Evaluating Credentials

Choosing the right inspectors is paramount for an unbiased and comprehensive property evaluation. Here are some key steps:

1. **Research and Recommendations:** Start by researching inspectors in your area. Look for professionals with a strong reputation and positive reviews from previous clients.

2. **Evaluate Credentials:** Ensure the inspector is certified by a reputable organization, such as the American Society of Home Inspectors (ASHI, n.d.) or the International Association of Certified Home Inspectors (InterNACHI, 2023). Verify their credentials, experience, and any specialized training they may have, particularly in areas like mold and water damage.

3. **Interview Inspectors:** Speak directly with potential inspectors to gauge their knowledge and approach.

Ask about their experience with similar properties and familiarity with common issues in your area. Clarify whether they are comfortable conducting a thorough evaluation that includes areas often overlooked, such as attics, basements, and crawl spaces.

Understanding the Benefits and Limitations of a Professional Home Inspection

A professional home inspection provides valuable insights into the property's condition but has certain limitations. To maximize its benefits, active participation and clear communication are essential.

1. **Directly Engage:** Addressing hypersensitivities means it's important that you vet, choose, and contact the inspector(s) directly to ensure they are working solely for you. Allowing the real estate agent to choose or suggest the inspector and set up the appointment can lead to potential conflicts of interest or give the impression that you are less invested in the process. Maintaining direct communication with the inspector demonstrates your commitment to a thorough and unbiased inspection, emphasizing that this is not a typical evaluation but a crucial step in ensuring the health and safety of your future home.

2. **Active Participation:** Accompany the inspector during the inspection and ask appropriate questions but avoid small talk that diverts their attention. Your presence can encourage a more thorough inspection. Set clear expectations about your goals for the home and request plenty of photos for documentation. Remember, you are the client, and the inspector works for you.

3. **Pre-Inspection Preparation:** Obtain a copy of the inspector's agreement beforehand to understand their service's scope, limitations, and terms. Review this agreement carefully to identify any aspects that require special attention or additional inspection.

4. **Private Communication:** Arrange to speak with the inspector privately, away from real estate agents, to express your specific concerns, especially about mold, water damage, or other health-related issues. This private conversation allows for candid insights and recommendations.

5. **Standard Practices and Fees:** Be aware that most inspectors have a standard rate and time limit for inspections. If you require more in-depth analysis, discuss this beforehand and be prepared to pay an additional consulting fee. This fee should be negotiated directly with the inspector.

6. **Direct Payment for Services:** Pay the inspector and any specialists directly for their services, including additional consulting fees, to ensure impartiality and commitment to your specific needs. Avoid including these payments in real estate transactions to maintain the independence of the inspection process.

7. **Post-Inspection Discussion:** If the inspector notes potential issues, ask for clarification on which findings are routine and which may indicate more serious concerns. Discuss any recommendations for additional inspections to understand whether these suggestions are standard procedure or prompted by specific observations.

Navigating Follow-Up Targeted Inspections

In some cases, initial inspections may reveal potential problems that warrant further investigation by specialists. Here's how to manage this process:

1. **Specialized Inspections:** Based on the initial inspection findings, consider hiring specialists for areas of concern, such as mold, structural integrity, roofs, siding, drainage, or plumbing. Discuss with the inspector the best approach for these additional inspections and seek recommendations from qualified professionals.

2. **Inspector Liability and Unseen Issues:** Understand that most property inspectors have liability limitations that restrict their responsibility for overlooked conditions, often capping liability at the cost of the inspection report itself. Recognizing these limitations highlights the importance of thorough and independent follow-up inspections.

THE IMPERFECT NATURE OF HOMES AND THE INSPECTIONS THEY RECEIVE

When considering the purchase of an existing home, recognize that no property is perfect. Understanding the common imperfections and how to address them can help you make a more informed decision.

Expecting Imperfections: Acknowledge that nearly all existing homes, regardless of their age, may have defects or signs of deterioration. Perfection is rare, and it's more realistic to anticipate some level of wear and tear. Recognizing these imperfections as a normal part of homeownership can help set realistic expectations.

Fixer-Upper vs. Hidden Issues: Consider the trade-off between purchasing a home with visible imperfections that you can address versus one with hidden or concealed problems. Sometimes, buying a less-than-perfect home and making necessary improvements can be a more transparent and cost-effective choice. Visible issues allow you to plan and budget for repairs, while hidden problems can lead to unexpected expenses and complications.

The Limitations of Mold Testing

When it comes to mold testing, it's essential to understand its limitations and how it fits into the broader inspection process.

Mold Testing Reliability: Avoid relying solely on mold testing to identify hidden issues. A thorough cleaning or surface treatment can temporarily mask mold problems, rendering tests inconclusive. Mold testing focuses on contaminants on surfaces or air during the test collection, so it will not be possible to identify mold growth confined to walls or under flooring. These hidden issues may require weeks or even months for the evidence to migrate from hidden locations to build up in areas where they can be non-destructively identified. Step 4 from the 25 Steps section provides additional information about mold testing and interpretation considerations.

Comprehensive Assessment: Mold testing should be just one part of a broader inspection process. Combine mold testing with a thorough visual inspection and any recommended specialized inspections to uncover potential problems. A comprehensive assessment that includes looking for signs of water damage, humidity issues, and ventilation problems is crucial for identifying and addressing mold risks. Step 4 provides additional guidance regarding these issues.

By understanding and accepting the limitations, you can better prepare for the realities of renting or owning. Recognizing which issues are easy preventative fixes versus those likely to result in hidden damage can help guide your decisions.

USING SAIIE TO ASSIST WITH HOME SELECTION (BUYING OR RENTING)

When selecting a home to buy or rent, the Sequential Activation of Innate Immune Effects (SAIIE) protocol can provide valuable insights into whether a property's environment supports health and is free from harmful exposures. This is particularly valuable for individuals with sensitivities to mold or other environmental contaminants, providing a systematic approach to screen for a home's suitability while supporting disability accessibility needs.

Overview of SAIIE for Home Selection

SAIIE involves a structured re-exposure process to monitor how a property impacts health markers such as symptoms, visual contrast sensitivity (VCS), and lab-based biomarkers. The protocol begins with establishing a baseline in a clean, controlled environment, followed by limited, monitored exposures to the prospective property over three days. This allows for the identification of potential environmental triggers that could affect long-term wellness.

Advantages and Disadvantages

One of the key advantages of SAIIE is its ability to objectively evaluate a home's suitability by measuring health impacts rather than relying solely on visual inspections or personal perception. This makes it particularly valuable for individuals with unique sensitivities, as it offers personalized insights into how the property might affect their health. Additionally, SAIIE may enable proactive prevention by identifying risks before committing to a property, potentially avoiding significant financial and emotional costs associated with moving into an unsuitable home.

However, the process has limitations. SAIIE is time-intensive, requiring several days for baseline and re-exposure testing, which may conflict with tight housing decision timelines. Recent property cleaning can also impact its effectiveness; if contaminants have not had sufficient time to accumulate, results may not fully reflect the property's typical environmental conditions. Implementing SAIIE requires informed consent and professional medical support to ensure safety, recognize when the exposure needs intervention to end the trial, select appropriate lab panels, ensure rapid turnaround of test results, and interpret the findings accurately—all of which may increase costs. Finally, landlords or sellers may resist allowing testing or extending timelines for decision-making, perceiving the process as burdensome or disruptive.

Overcoming Objections

❏ **Incorporate into Reasonable Accommodations**: Present SAIIE as part of a disability accessibility and reasonable accommodations strategy. Emphasize that providing time for SAIIE during the selection process is essential for determining whether the home is a suitable, health-supporting environment. This includes allowing sufficient time for contaminants to build up if the property has been recently cleaned.

❏ **Start with Preliminary Testing**: Use less invasive methods, such as MSQPCR and Pathways™ testing, to screen the property initially. This can help establish whether further testing with SAIIE is warranted.

❏ **Collaborative Communication**: Reassure landlords or sellers that the testing process is non-invasive and focused solely on health suitability, emphasizing that it benefits both parties by preventing future complications.

Further Guidance

For detailed instructions on implementing the SAIIE protocol, readers can refer to **Step 19** of the 25 Step guide. This section explains how to perform SAIIE effectively, including strategies for addressing the challenges of recently cleaned properties and ensuring accurate results. By integrating SAIIE into the home selection process and advocating for reasonable accommodations, prospective buyers or renters can make informed decisions, securing a property that supports their health and well-being.

Protecting Your Investment: Precautions When Placing an Offer

To safeguard interests, buyers might include contingencies in the purchase agreement. These contingencies generally allow inspection periods, providing an option to withdraw if the property fails to meet the desired standards. Yet, even comprehensive inspections come with limited or no guarantees. Simple cosmetic fixes like a fresh coat of paint or plaster can mask various issues, and inspection contracts often outline specific limitations. For instance, inspectors might not examine furniture-secure areas or engage in invasive evaluations that could damage the property.

A less-discussed yet significant challenge is inspectors' reluctance to speculate about potential hidden issues. An overly critical report might diminish future referrals from real estate agents and may influence their assessments. However, delving into such speculations can highlight the risks inherent in certain construction types. I'll also discuss environmental investigators' unique challenges, especially when assessing homes for individuals with sensitivities to mold and other water damage-related organisms. Various factors can obscure or complicate the detection of such issues.

The upcoming section delves into potential indicators and clues suggesting a higher likelihood of problems. Nonetheless, it's vital to understand that any home purchase carries the risk of undisclosed issues. Some of these problems might remain hidden or not be discovered until long after closing escrow, presenting unforeseen challenges to the new homeowners.

Looking For Red Flags in Property Transactions

When considering a property for purchase, especially one that has undergone significant renovations or flips, it's crucial to be vigilant for red flags that could indicate underlying issues that have been covered up or downplayed. This section discusses common warning signs and strategies for navigating potential problems, including seller misrepresentation and differing remediation standards. Also, look for past gaps in the record. Understanding the sales and ownership history can be helpful. Homes sold at a substantial loss from previous levels, foreclosed or distressed properties that were flipped are frequently indicators of poor maintenance or other disasters that may have affected them.

• When assessing a property, being vigilant about mold and water damage signs is crucial. A history of the home being flipped or extensively remodeled properties can be particularly concerning, as they might feature cosmetic updates that mask underlying issues. It is important to investigate the quality and extent of renovations thoroughly. Superficial improvements may hide inadequate mold or water damage remediation, so ensure that mold problems are properly addressed and not just painted over or superficially cleaned.

- Seller misrepresentation is another significant red flag. While sellers in some states are legally required to disclose known issues, they may avoid learning about certain problems to circumvent these requirements. Be alert for signs of concealment, such as vague or evasive responses to direct questions about water damage or mold history. Request detailed records of past water damage incidents and mold remediation efforts to verify the seller's claims.

- If the current owner has conducted repairs to prepare the home for sale, verifying the standards and quality of these repairs, particularly for mold and water damage, is essential. Were the repairs performed by a quality company with a good reputation? Was the work permitted? Requesting an independent re-inspection by a specialist after repairs to ensure all issues have been appropriately addressed and clarify whether the repairs meet current health code and safety standards, particularly those related to mold remediation. It is common for mold repairs to be performed at a level acceptable for most people but unacceptable for the hypersensitive population. Are you prepared to take on and address these issues?

- Unusual odors and stains are common indicators of hidden issues. Musty or damp smells can suggest hidden mold growth or water damage. Pay close attention to these odors as they often signal underlying problems. Look for stains on walls, ceilings, and floors, indicating past or ongoing water damage. Investigate the source of these stains to determine the extent of the problem.

- Attempts to mask musty odors with room air fresheners, deodorizers, heavy fragrances, or even freshly baked cookies can conceal significant underlying issues. A home should smell clean and fresh because it truly is clean and fresh, not because odors are being covered up.

- The lack of an odor doesn't necessarily mean everything is okay; the absence of active water can cause odors to disappear, but dormant or dead water-damage organisms may remain. Elevated levels of these harmful organisms can still pose significant problems for hypersensitive individuals.

- Inconsistent maintenance can also point to broader issues. Check for signs of deferred maintenance, such as water stains, rusted fixtures, or peeling paint. These signs can indicate broader water damage issues. Review maintenance records to assess how well the property has been cared for over time, as consistent maintenance reduces the risk of mold and water damage.

- Structural issues should not be overlooked. Be wary of cracks in the foundation, uneven floors, or doors and windows that stick, as these can signal significant structural problems related to water damage. Check for areas where water might intrude, such as basements, attics, windows, and doors. Ensure these areas are properly sealed and free from mold growth and elevated levels of spores and fragments that can migrate into the living space.

- Environmental factors, such as the local climate and geography, are also important. Properties in humid or flood-prone areas are at higher risk for mold and water damage. Investigate the area's and the property's flood history, as properties that have experienced flooding are more likely to have mold issues.

By being aware of these specific red flags for mold and water damage, you can better assess the condition of a property and make more informed decisions. Identifying these issues early can save you from future health risks and costly repairs.

Myth: Painting over mold will fix the problem.

Fact: Painting over mold with paint is not a solution. While some paints are marketed as mold-resistant, painting over mold without addressing the underlying moisture issue may temporarily cover It up but will not eliminate it.

LOOKING FOR A PLACE TO RENT

When looking for a rental property, specific considerations must be made to ensure a healthy living environment, especially if you have mold sensitivities.

Understanding the Real Estate Market for Renters

As a renter, it's essential to know that available rental homes are often properties with pre-existing problem conditions. Mold testing, while valuable, should be complemented with visual inspections to provide a comprehensive assessment of the property's condition. Accepting that nearly all existing homes have some defects can help set realistic expectations. It is often not about finding a good place but a place good enough to be worked with.

Buildings that allow water entry or have leaking plumbing are substandard regardless of visible mold, But navigating hidden conditions can be tricky. (Cornell, n.d.(c))

Legal Rights and Reasonable Accommodations

If you're living with mold sensitivities, understanding your rights under the Americans with Disabilities Act (ADA) is crucial. The ADA prohibits discrimination against individuals with disabilities, including those with severe mold allergies or sensitivities.

- **Reasonable Accommodations:** Landlords are required to provide reasonable accommodations. This might involve allowing you to make necessary modifications at your own expense, such as improving ventilation systems, installing air purifiers, or facilitating switching to an available unit in the same complex that satisfies the needs of the disabled renter. If the rental property has pre-existing mold issues that pose health risks for the general population, landlords must address these to ensure a habitable living environment. People whose medical need exceeds these conditions may need to pay for their own upgrades or modifications if the costs exceed reasonable accommodations to meet their needs.

- **Disclosure and Limitations:** Landlords are not required to address or disclose pre-existing conditions they are unaware of, and in "renter-beware" states, they may not need to disclose conditions they know about as long as these do not exceed levels of sanitation and habitability. However, telling a lie in response to direct questions can constitute fraud. While asking questions and expecting truthful answers can be helpful, landlords and management companies might decide that someone asking too many questions could be too much trouble and opt to rent to someone else. This is discrimination, but proving discrimination may be difficult, expensive, and time-consuming.

Regulations and Responsibilities for Rental Properties

Fair Housing regulations for rental units are overseen by the U.S. Department of Housing and Urban Development (HUD), which has specific guidelines and regulations regarding the health and safety of rental properties. These guidelines ensure that rental properties are safe, sanitary, and suitable for tenants. The Fair Housing Act and other components also play a role:

Fair Housing Act: This Act prohibits discrimination in the sale, rental, and financing of dwellings based on race, color, religion, sex, national origin, familial status, or disability. It ensures that all individuals have equal access to housing, including aspects of health and safety. (HUD, 2023)

Habitability Standards: HUD requires that rental properties meet basic habitability standards. These include structural safety, sanitation, water and heat availability, and freedom from hazardous materials like lead paint or asbestos.

Responsibility of Landlords: Landlords must maintain rental properties to meet these habitability standards. This includes prompt repairs, regular maintenance, and addressing health hazards such as mold, pest infestations, or structural issues.

Section 504 of the Rehabilitation Act: Administered by HUD, this section prohibits discrimination based on disability. It requires landlords to make reasonable accommodations for tenants with disabilities, which can include modifications to improve safety and accessibility.

HUD's Real Estate Assessment Center (REAC): REAC conducts inspections of properties that are owned, insured, or subsidized by HUD to ensure they meet federal standards of health, safety, and security.

Complaints and Enforcement: Tenants can file complaints with HUD if they believe their rights under the Fair Housing Act or other HUD regulations are being violated. HUD investigates these complaints and can take action, including fines and mandates for repairs or policy changes.

Steps to Help Ensure a Safe Rental Environment

Research and Initial Inspection: Thoroughly research potential properties before signing a lease. Inspect for signs of mold, musty odors, or dampness during property viewings. This helps identify properties that are less likely to trigger your sensitivities. However, understand that formal inspections are uncommon for rentals and might deter landlords from accepting you. This may be discrimination in the eyes of the law, but it can be difficult and expensive to prove.

Negotiating Accommodations: If you have mold sensitivities, it would be ideal to negotiate accommodations with your landlord before signing the lease. This would involve documenting all agreements in writing, discussing necessary modifications or accommodations, and agreeing on responsibilities. However, landlords may only address issues to a minimum level, which might not be sufficient for severe mold sensitivities.

Legal Rights Awareness: Familiarize yourself with fair housing laws. The United States Department of Housing and Urban Development administers the Fair Housing Act, which prohibits discrimination based on disability, ensuring your right to request reasonable accommodations without facing unfair or discriminatory treatment. You must have a doctor who will attest to your medical disability being adversely affected by the condition of the rental home. (Cornell, n.d.)

Open Communication: Maintain open and constructive dialogue with your landlord. Explain your situation and the necessity of the requested accommodation for your health. This can lead to a mutually agreeable solution, but be prepared for resistance.

Personal Preparations: Since landlords may not address mold issues adequately, consider personal measures such as:

- Use a dehumidifier to maintain optimal indoor humidity levels.

- Step 5: Pathways™ Testing may prove helpful in determining and maintaining cleanliness.

- Step 14: Using Approved Products for Effective Detailed Cleaning provides guidance for regularly cleaning with an acceptable soap or detergent product and keeping your living space dry.

- Step 22: Establish a Routine, Effective Cleaning Schedule. This step helps determine the cleaning frequency necessary to maintain control.

- Using portable air purifiers with HEPA filters can provide some limited assistance in reducing airborne levels, but it does not replace cleaning.

Addressing Mold Issues in Rentals

- **Pre-Move-In Testing:** Conduct mold tests before moving into the property. If mold is detected, negotiate when practical remediation with the landlord before signing the lease. Ensure that any mold issues are resolved satisfactorily.

- **Post-Move-In Testing:** If mold problems arise after moving in, document the issue and notify your landlord immediately. Request prompt, appropriate remediation and, if necessary, consider legal advice to help you understand your rights.

- **Breaking the Lease:** If the mold issue significantly impacts your health and the landlord fails to remediate it effectively, you may need to consider breaking the lease. This involves your doctor attesting to the mold exposure that exacerbates your condition. Consult a legal expert for guidance.

Understanding Reasonable Accommodations and Undue Hardship

A reasonable accommodation under the ADA refers to modifications that enable you to enjoy equal housing opportunities. Examples include:

- **Air Purifiers:** Allowing the use of air purifiers to improve indoor air quality.

- **Ventilation Systems:** Permitting the installation of additional ventilation or dehumidification systems.

- **Alternative Units:** Offering an alternative apartment unit if available and less prone to mold issues.

- **Allowing you to break your lease** without penalty. (HUD, 2023)

Accommodations become "undue hardships" for the landlord when they cause significant difficulty or expense. Factors include the cost relative to the landlord's resources, the impact on their operations, and whether it would fundamentally alter the nature of the housing provided. Navigating rental properties with mold sensitivities requires proactive measures, clear communication, and an understanding of your legal rights.

NEW CONSTRUCTION

Site, design, construction, and material choices all play a role in determining the overall health and safety of the living environment. From the location and layout to the quality of construction materials, every aspect can influence the potential for issues such as water damage and mold growth.

Our book, "*Prescriptions for a Healthy House: A Practical Guide for Architects, Builders, and Owners,*" co-authored with lead author and architect Paula Baker-Laporte, focuses on construction and remodeling to create healthy houses in general and contains significant information about siting, design, construction, and material choices related to mold and water damage considerations. It serves as essential reading, providing a comprehensive understanding of what should and shouldn't be included in your plans. Even if you're looking at existing homes, this knowledge will help you identify potential red flags and make informed decisions to ensure a healthy living environment. The rest of the information in this section is excerpted from *Prescriptions for a Healthy House:*

Site Considerations

The site of a home plays a crucial role in determining its long-term health and structural integrity, especially regarding moisture and location-related issues. Deficiencies in the site's conditions, such as poor drainage, expansive clay soils, or other geological factors, can significantly impact the building from the moment it is constructed. Even with remedial actions to improve or correct the site, mold or water-damage organisms that have developed are likely to remain, with dead mold posing health problems for sensitive individuals similar to those caused by living mold. While many sayings emphasize the importance of a good foundation, it is the site that dictates many of the factors necessary for establishing a solid and resilient foundation. Proper site drainage, understanding expansive clay soils, considering geological factors, and reviewing FEMA flood maps can help avoid expensive mistakes. These aspects, along with others, are covered in more detail in *Prescriptions for a Healthy House,* providing essential guidance for ensuring that the site is properly evaluated and managed to prevent water damage and mold issues, ultimately contributing to a healthier living environment. Regional Considerations include humidity and weather phenomena such as hurricanes and floods. These can greatly impact a home's susceptibility to water damage and mold.

Design Issues

Architectural designs significantly influence a property's health, and careful design consideration can help compensate for an imperfect site. Well-thought-out designs can incorporate long-lasting and low-maintenance features, reducing future problems and extending the building's lifespan. Conversely, when these elements are not integrated, the building may require major repairs sooner. If these repairs cut corners, issues may be covered up, making them even more challenging to repair and maintain. Effective design can mitigate site deficiencies, ensuring a healthier, more resilient living environment. Landscaping and vegetation are often not included as a part of the design and are instead frequently added or modified as afterthoughts. Installing patio slabs and concrete walkways too close to the bottom edge of siding materials or stucco frequently results in rising dampness entering the wall assemblies. The proximity of shrubs and trees often doesn't consider the mature height and damage they can cause to the building's ability to control moisture. Improper landscaping can affect drainage and moisture levels around the home.

Construction issues

The quality of construction plays a pivotal role in a property's long-term health and durability. Proper construction techniques and high-quality materials are essential to prevent issues such as water damage and mold growth. Certain architectural features and construction practices can increase the likelihood of mold problems, including below-grade spaces, flat roofs, inadequate roof overhangs, and complex roofing structures. If corners are cut during construction or if substandard materials are used, the building is more likely to suffer from structural weaknesses and moisture infiltration. These issues can lead to significant problems over time, often becoming hidden and more challenging to address.

KEY DESIGN AND CONSTRUCTION FEATURES TO CONSIDER

Basements and Below-Grade Spaces

❏ Basements, particularly those partially or fully below grade, are prone to moisture problems due to their proximity to the ground's dampness and the high pressures that can develop from hydrostatic pressure from water in the surrounding soils. The risk increases if the waterproofing and drainage around the foundation are not adequately implemented or have deteriorated over time. Even minor cracks can allow moisture seepage in such spaces, leading to mold growth. Look for homes without basements, crawlspaces, or cellars or well-designed waterproofing systems, proper drainage, and adequate ventilation in these areas.

Sump Pump and Backflow Valves

❏ Sump pumps and backflow prevention valves are often not installed until after the first time they are needed. Information on the presence and installation dates of sump pumps and backflow valves can help determine if they have been appropriately maintained or should be suspected of hidden damage. If the installation of these devices corresponds with a time during or shortly after heavy rainfall, it may indicate undisclosed water intrusion.

Roof Design: Flat and Low-Sloped Roofs

❏ Flat and low-sloped roofs can pose significant water drainage challenges. These designs often lead to water pooling, increasing the likelihood of leaks and subsequent mold growth within the home. These roof types can also experience additional stress in areas with heavy winds, exacerbating these issues. Choose homes with adequately sloped roofs that facilitate water runoff and ensure they are equipped with proper drainage systems.

Roof Overhangs and Eaves

❏ Adequate roof overhangs protect the home's walls from rain and snow. Insufficient overhangs can lead to water seeping into the walls and windows, creating a conducive environment for mold. Homes with generous roof overhangs that protect the building's walls and foundation are preferable.

Complex Roofing Structures

❏ Roofs with multiple valleys, pitches, and penetrations for ventilation, skylights, and other systems can present numerous challenges. The complexity of these designs often leads to a higher risk of leaks, especially at the junctions of different materials or roof angles. When considering a home with a complex roof, ensure it has been constructed with high-quality materials and waterproofing techniques.

Trees, Shrubs, and Climbing Vines

❏ Trees, shrubs, and climbing vines planted too close to the structure can cause extensive damage, resulting in water entry. Even if they appear properly pruned or controlled now, they may have already caused previous damage that was only cosmetically repaired.

Ventilation and Airflow

❏ Proper ventilation is essential in preventing moisture accumulation. Poorly ventilated spaces, especially attics and crawlspaces, can become hotspots for mold growth. Ensure the home has a well-designed ventilation system that promotes consistent airflow, particularly in damp areas.

Wall Construction and Siding

❏ The materials and construction methods used for walls and siding significantly affect a building's vulnerability to moisture. Certain materials, such as wood, are more susceptible to water damage and may require more maintenance.

- Look for homes with durable, water-resistant siding materials and construction methods that include effective moisture barriers that do not trap water vapor and that allow it to escape or dry.

- Smart membranes or moisture-resistant barriers that allow moisture to escape and prevent water from trapping within walls are now available and preferred.

- The sealing of all potential entry points for water, such as where cracks or openings for cables and pipes enter the home, must remain sealed and maintained.

Window and Door Installations

❏ Windows and doors are common points of water intrusion. Improperly installed or poorly sealed windows and doors can allow moisture to enter the home, leading to mold issues. Check for well-installed windows and doors with proper sealing and flashing to prevent water intrusion.

Plumbing and HVAC Systems

❏ Plumbing and HVAC systems are crucial to managing moisture within a home. Poorly installed or maintained systems can lead to leaks and excessive humidity, which are conducive to mold growth.

- Ensure the plumbing is in good condition and the HVAC system is correctly sized and well-maintained. It's also vital to check that the HVAC system is designed to handle the specific humidity challenges of the local climate.

- If inadequate HVAC systems have been present and supplemental seasonal portable dehumidification

has not been used, hidden dormant issues should be suspected and may not be recognized until the humid season returns.

- Window Units and PTAC Systems (packaged terminal air conditioner systems), common in hotels and apartments, are frequently poorly maintained and become a source of moisture and mold.

Insulation and Vapor Barriers

❏ Proper insulation and vapor barriers are essential to control moisture and prevent condensation within walls and ceilings. Inadequate or improperly installed insulation can create cold spots where condensation forms, leading to mold growth.

- Look for homes with comprehensive insulation and vapor barriers that are correctly installed and maintained, particularly in colder climates where condensation is a greater risk.

- Specifics regarding ventilation in different parts of the home, including attics and crawlspaces, properly vented, are crucial for preventing mold growth by reducing moisture accumulation.

- Cathedral Ceiling insulation methods are a special problem if improperly vented.

- Spray-in foam insulation presents multiple issues. It has often been touted as being superior at preventing condensation issues from forming. However, it is a major issue when the location of the condensation is shifted to an inaccessible space that cannot be inspected, such as the underside of the roof deck.

Foundation and Drainage

❏ A home's foundation must be designed to prevent moisture from entering the structure. This includes proper grading around the house to direct water away and the use of materials and methods that reject liquid water by allowing water vapor to evaporate and dry without becoming trapped.

- Check that the home has a solid foundation with no signs of water damage or cracks. The surrounding land should slope away from the house to facilitate proper drainage.

- Confirm proper grading, including a comprehensive property drainage plan, downspouts, gutters, drainage tiles, and surface grading to direct water away from the foundation.

Interior Materials and Finishes

❏ Choosing interior materials, especially in kitchens, bathrooms, and laundry rooms, can affect a home's vulnerability to mold. Materials like paper-faced drywall are more likely to harbor mold when exposed to moisture in these wet areas.

- Prefer homes with moisture-resistant materials in wet areas, such as cement boards or paperless gypsum boards.

- Flooring Materials: Various flooring materials, like hardwood and ceramic tile, are generally more resistant than laminate or luxury vinyl flooring. It is common for these to build up trapped moisture underneath when used over concrete slabs or damp areas. A meter can measure moisture from the finished floor to the slab below. It can tell you if it is wet but cannot determine if it was previously wet and then dried after hidden mold growth developed.

Other Considerations include

❏ Evidence of Termite damage or the post-construction installation of termite barriers or shields may indicate past infestations that may not have been properly addressed for moisture retention or concurrent growth.

❏ Evidence of wood rot or fungal damage identified in Termite and Wood Destroying Pests or Organisms Reports often indicates mold damage. The amount of moisture necessary to cause rot is more than enough to cause concurrent problems with hidden mold. Structural and pest repairs do not typically address mold contamination or growth. Surface mold is not a wood-destroying organism and is commonly omitted from wood-destroying pest and organism reports (Nor are most pest inspectors qualified to identify or offer opinions about mold).

❏ Buildings with a history of a fire event are often moldy due to the water damage from firefighting efforts and subsequent mold growth. The mold that results from a house fire is often not properly mitigated for someone with sensitivities.

❏ The inclusion of exterior utility closets when they are poorly protected from the elements is often a point of concern due to water intrusion and mold growth.

Conclusion: A Constructive Approach to Mold Prevention

In summary, when evaluating a potential home, it's essential to consider the construction practices and features. Understanding how these factors influence a home's susceptibility to mold can guide you in making an informed decision. Opting for a property that incorporates sound construction principles, appropriate materials for the climate, and quality workmanship is key to ensuring a healthier, mold-resistant living environment.

The overall quality of construction and attention to detail during the building process are as important as the design and materials used. Poor workmanship can negate the best design intentions, leading to gaps, cracks, and other deficiencies that allow moisture intrusion and mold growth.

Be cautious with homes that have undergone significant remodeling or renovations. While touted as improvements or features, these changes sometimes conceal previous water damage or improperly address mold issues. It's important to ensure that any past renovations were done properly, addressing the home's structural and environmental integrity.

MATERIALS LIFE EXPECTANCY

The life expectancy of materials used in home construction is deeply intertwined with moisture-related issues in buildings. Various materials respond differently to dampness, humidity, and water damage; some deteriorate rapidly, others show more excellent resistance, and a few may even thrive under wet conditions. Just because a home is built using materials that withstand organisms that thrive under moist conditions doesn't mean that so do materials that they cover or hide or that the occupants and their furnishings and personal possessions will thrive under the same wet conditions.

The resilience of a structure composed of these diverse materials often hinges on its most vulnerable elements. While sometimes deceptively resilient, exterior materials can inadvertently contribute to moisture entrapment, thereby accelerating the deterioration of hidden adjacent materials such as asphalt-impregnated building paper. Building life expectancy calculates beyond mere timelines; it offers a look into how the durability of different materials impacts longevity, but not necessarily the health of your home. Understanding the life spans of crucial construction materials should expand to adjacent materials. For example, the robustness of water-saturated concrete foundations is well recognized, but the vulnerability of the timber beams that sit on top of the wet concrete is often ignored. The material life expectancies are only as good as the entire system and how the materials interact. This is vital in illuminating their role in microbial growth and water damage susceptibilities. (NIST, 2020)

- **Lifetime Life Expectancy:** Sometimes, material things are expressed as having a "lifetime" life expectancy. This generally means the construction material will have an exceptionally long lifespan, often exceeding the typical duration of use for the building they're part of. It's important to clarify that "lifetime" doesn't imply that the material will last indefinitely but will likely outlast other structure components and not require replacement within a normal building's lifespan. Here's a more detailed explanation:

- **Duration Relative to Building's Life:** A material with a lifetime life expectancy is expected to last for the entire usable life of the building. This is commonly regarded as around 100 years or more for residential buildings.
- **Minimal Maintenance Requirement:** These materials typically require minimal maintenance to retain their integrity and functionality over decades.
- **Resistance to Environmental Factors:** They are usually highly resistant to environmental stresses like moisture, temperature fluctuations, and UV radiation.
- **Quality and Durability:** Such materials are often of superior quality and durability. They are designed to withstand wear and tear much better than standard materials.
- **Cost vs. Longevity Trade-off:** While these materials might be more expensive initially, their extended lifespan can make them cost-effective in the long term, considering the reduced need for replacements and repairs.

MATERIAL RESILIENCE AND LONGEVITY

Remodeling and maintenance decisions should consider both history and future projections. The Life Expectancy Chart offers insights into the anticipated lifespan of various building materials and components. However, it is crucial to recognize that these materials' actual performance and longevity are subject to multiple influencing factors, such as the quality of installation, environmental climate, exposure to ultraviolet (UV) light, and susceptibility to physical damage. Regular inspections and diligent maintenance are essential to ensure these materials achieve their full potential and function effectively throughout their intended lifespan.

Material Life Expectancy Considerations

Comparing a material's life expectancy with its current age can provide a starting point for evaluating its likely longevity and how soon you should anticipate needing to replace it. Some materials hold up well to moisture, while others begin to deteriorate immediately. If moisture can be trapped and accelerate deterioration, other materials may shorten the life expectancy of adjacent materials.

The following information integrates information, standards, and guidelines from organizations, including the American Society of Civil Engineers, (ASCE, 2021); Building Science Corporation, (Building Science Corporation, 2019); American Concrete Institute, (ACI, 2022); International Associations of Certified Home Inspectors, (InterNACHI, 2023); International Code Council, (ICC, 2023); and the author's experience.

Insulation
❑ Determine the type of insulation used and compare its life expectancy with the age of the building. Be aware that areas where new insulation is patched in with old may indicate previous damage underneath.

- Fiberglass Insulation: 80–100 years. Effectiveness may be reduced if damp or damaged. Kraft Paper facing can rapidly allow mold growth if it is on the insulation and gets wet. Asphalt emulsions impregnating the paper will slow the degradation but will still support the growth and deterioration resulting from *Stachybotrys chartarum* when these materials are chronically wet.
- Rock Wool Insulation 100+ years: It is also subject to similar considerations as fiberglass when faced with paper. Even asphalt-impregnated kraft paper facing on insulation will support mold growth if the insulation stays wet.
- Cellulose Insulation: 20–30 years. Vulnerable to moisture, requiring prompt replacement if wet.
- Spray Foam Insulation: It lasts over 80 years but needs protection from UV and physical damage. However, Spray foam can trap moisture behind it, resulting in rot or deterioration of the hidden material if it is moisture-sensitive, like building paper, wood, or paneling.
- Polystyrene (EPS and XPS) Insulation: 50–80 years. Environmental conditions impact lifespan. Polystyrene can trap moisture behind it, resulting in rot or deterioration of the hidden material if it is moisture-sensitive, like wood or paneling.

Foundation
❑ Determine the type of foundation that was originally used and its life expectancy. Be aware that areas where the new foundation is patched in with the old may indicate previous damage or a remodeling addition that may have incompletely repaired the damage.

- Poured Concrete: 80–100+ years.
- Concrete Block: 75–100 years.
- Structural Components
- Wooden Joists/Trusses: 80–100+ years.
- Steel Beams: 100+ years.

Exterior Materials
❑ Determine the type of siding or exterior materials used and compare its life expectancy with the age of the building. Be aware that areas, where new exterior materials are used as a patch, may indicate previous damage underneath.

- Brick Veneer: 75–100+ years.

- Wood Siding: 20–40 years.
- Fiber Cement Siding: 25–40 years.
- Vinyl Siding: 60+ years.

Caulk, Sealants, Adhesives, Paints

❑ Compare the age of the building with the condition of these materials. Unusual cracking deformation or deterioration may indicate hidden damage.

- Caulking: 5 to 10 years
- Construction Glues: 20+ years
- Paint (exterior): 7–10 years
- Sealants: 8 years

Roofing

❑ Compare the age of the building with the condition of the roofing materials. Unusual cracking deformation or deterioration may indicate hidden damage. Replacement should occur before failures have begun.

- Asphalt Shingles: 15–30 years.
- Wood Shingles and Shakes: 20–25 years.
- Metal Roofing: 40–80 years.
- Clay or Cement Tiles: 50+ years.

Windows and Doors

❑ Compare the age of the building with the condition of the windows or doors. Unusual cracking deformation or deterioration may indicate hidden damage. Replacement should occur before failures have begun. Mismatched windows and doors often indicate previous failures. The failed unit may have been replaced without remediating the hidden water damage.

- Wooden Windows: 15–30 years.
- Vinyl/Aluminum Windows: 15–20 years.
- Steel Doors: 20–30 years.
- Wooden Doors: 15–25 years.
- Fiberglass Doors: 20+ years.

Interior Finishes

❑ Compare the material's age and condition with the building's age and condition. Be suspicious of patches or repairs.

- Gypsum board: 40–70 years. Paper-faced gypsum board is especially prone to rapid mold growth if it gets wet.
- Interior Paint: 5–10 years, varies by quality and usage.

Flooring

❑ Compare the material's age and condition with the building's age and condition. Be suspicious of patches or repairs.

- Carpet: 8–10 years. Carpet frequently hides damage that can be discovered only with inspection during removal.
- Hardwood Floors: 100+ years with maintenance.
- Laminate Flooring: 15–25 years. Trapped moisture underneath causes hidden issues.
- Vinyl Flooring: 10–20 years. Trapped moisture causes patchy discoloration.
- Ceramic Tile or Stone Flooring: 75–100 years. May hide damage to subfloor.

HVAC, and Plumbing

❑ Monitor age and condition. Previous replacement may not have addressed water damage that led to the replacement

- Central Air Conditioning: 15–20 years.
- Furnace: 15–20 years.
- Heat Pumps: 10–15 years.
- Radiators: 15–25 years.
- Copper Pipes: 50+ years.
- PVC Pipes: Indefinitely.
- Water Heaters (Tank): 10–15 years.
- Water Heaters (Tankless): 20+ years.

Moisture Resistant Barriers

❑ Since these are often hidden under the exterior cladding, it is frequently challenging to know if they are present and have deteriorated due to past conditions.

- Asphalt-impregnated felt or Paper: 20–30 years, less if improperly installed or exposed to moisture.
- Tyvek (House Wrap): has a longevity of up to 50 years but must avoid prolonged sunlight exposure due to UV deterioration.
- Rubberized Asphalt Flashing: 20–40 years, affected by UV and temperature changes.
- Paper Covered Gypsum Board: Code has allowed this as an exterior base material for exterior cladding for fire resistance. Its use this way is short-sighted and particularly devastating when it gets wet and grows mold. This material should be avoided regardless of age.

Remember, these are general estimates. The actual lifespan can vary significantly based on the quality of materials, installation, environmental conditions, and how well the home is maintained. Regular maintenance and proper installation helps ensure these materials reach or exceed their expected lifetimes.

MAINTENANCE ISSUES LIST

The Homeowner plays a crucial role and is the first line of defense in maintaining a healthy home. Through homeowner awareness and vigilance, many problems can be avoided. Maintenance for renters can be more complicated. An astute landlord will recognize the value of a tenant concerned with property maintenance since a well-maintained property will have an extended life expectancy and fewer surprise repairs. Maintenance of a rental requires a balanced and cooperative effort from all parties. Frequent landlord inspections are often viewed as intrusive and violating privacy; however, they may help prevent significant problems.

Outside

❑ **Soil, mulch, or leaves piled against the house:** These materials allow insects and moisture to migrate into wall cavities and can clog weep screeds and screened ventilation pathways where exterior walls meet foundations. To prevent premature deterioration, soil, mulch, and leaves should be kept at least 6 inches below the bottom edge of the cladding. While clearing away accumulations can halt further deterioration, it does not address the hidden damage that may have already developed.

❑ **Irrigation faults:** Irrigation systems must be directed away from the building and constantly monitored to ensure they have not developed leaks or unintended spray patterns. It is crucial to avoid irrigation near the foundation or, if irrigation is in place, to consistently monitor it. Irrigation leaks, misdirected sprinkler heads, and breaks are common in garden irrigation systems. When these issues go undetected, water can accumulate at the foundation and on exterior walls instead of draining away, eventually seeping into garages and interior wall cavities. Sprinklers should be kept from the foundation and not allowed to spray on the house. A few weeks of overspray can cause rapid deterioration. Drip irrigation is preferable.

❑ **Keep planting away from the foundation.** Root growth can eventually threaten the integrity of damp proofing, and dense plant growth can create a visual and physical barrier that prevents the occupant from inspecting foundations. Landscape shrubs should be trimmed back so there are at least 12 inches between the plants and the structure. Very few modern buildings can withstand trellises or climbing vines like ivy growing up the walls. The areal roots will invade the substructure of the siding or stucco. They can enter wall cavities through cracks and small openings, increasing the likelihood of internal water entry, damage, and insect infestation. Raised planters should have sufficient space between them and the home to allow ventilation and

access to clean out accumulated debris. If they are too close to the home's walls, moisture accumulation will lead to mold growth in adjacent wall cavities.

❑ **Maintain drainage grading** so that water drains away from the home and doesn't enter the crawlspace, garage, or pond around the property. One of the more common changes to a yard that results in indoor mold growth is changes to the drainage slope or the direction of the water flow. Water should always be directed away from the foundations and not end up standing around or under a home.

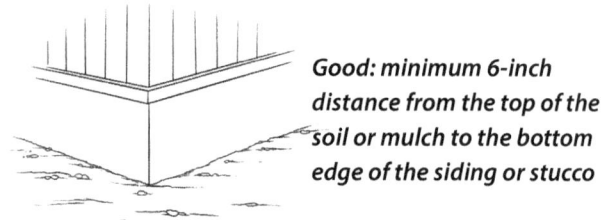

Good: minimum 6-inch distance from the top of the soil or mulch to the bottom edge of the siding or stucco

Bad: buildup of soil or debris promotes damage

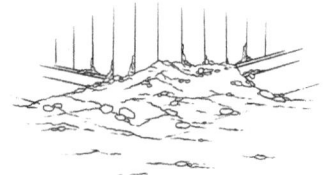

Figure 4-1: Maintain a minimum of 6" between the top of the soil and the bottom edge of the wall. Allowing soil, leaves, or other debris to accumulate against the foundation can direct moisture into the building, leading to rapid deterioration of the moisture-resistant barrier and mold growth within wall cavities. Removing this material can prevent further damage, but any existing deterioration and mold growth remains concealed.

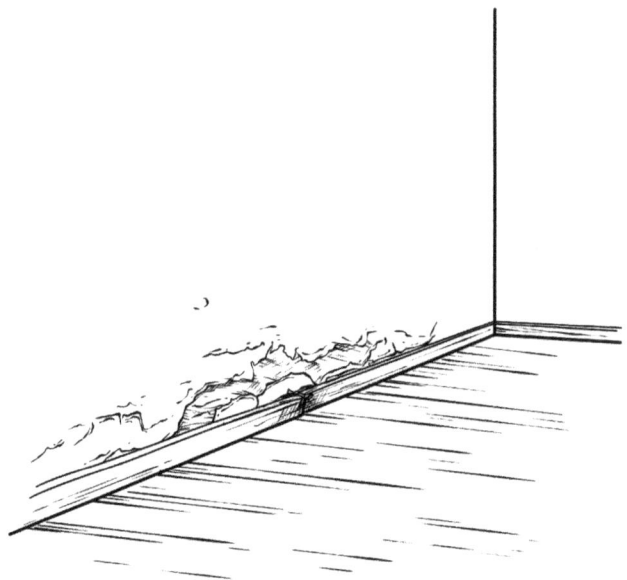

Figure 4-2: This illustration shows a severe amount of visible swelling or warping. Usually caused by the accumulation of moisture in the lowest part of exterior wall cavities, this is an extreme example. It is most commonly caused by dirt,

debris, or leaves piled above the level of the foundation and sill plate. Hidden damage is likely to be greater than the visible damage. Musty odors are often one of the first indicators that materials are wet and growing. These odors will disappear when the materials dry, but the damage remains, releasing contaminants into the living space.

Exterior Siding, Cladding, Stucco & Masonry Maintenance

❏ **Vigilance in maintaining good roof drainage and directing water away.** Gutters should be cleaned and repaired as a part of a regular maintenance schedule.

❏ **Remove standing snow:** Ensure that snow piling against the exterior siding, cladding, or stucco is removed from the perimeter before it melts and saturates the bottom edge of the structure.

❏ **Promote Drainage:** Observe and correct any changes in drainage over time through soil or debris build-up. One of the more common changes to a yard that results in indoor mold growth is changes to the drainage slope or the direction of the water flows. Water should be directed away from foundations and not saturate a slab, stand in the crawlspace under a home, or enter a basement.

❏ **Exterior siding or trim** should be frequently inspected and repaired to prevent water entry. Caulking must be replaced whenever openings that allow water entry develop but must never block intended drainage paths.

❏ **Damage to siding and trim:** Water entry can occur due to various factors such as pressure washing, acid cleaning, attaching decorative features, drilled holes, plant holders, and other fixtures. Ensuring these elements are properly sealed and maintained is crucial to prevent moisture infiltration.

❏ **Excess Mortar** inside brick, stone, or other masonry surfaces should not block drainage openings, vents, or weep holes.

❏ **Stucco:** should not block weep screeds or impede drainage.

❏ **Weep screed** is a metal flashing or trim placed at the bottom of the edge of the stucco to allow drainage. Soil, mulch, weeds, leaves, or debris should not come within 6 inches of the bottom edge of the siding or weep screed.

❏ **Window Weep holes** at the bottom of windows should be kept freely draining and free of dirt or other materials that would prevent water from draining freely. They allow condensation moisture and minor amounts of moisture to drain freely.

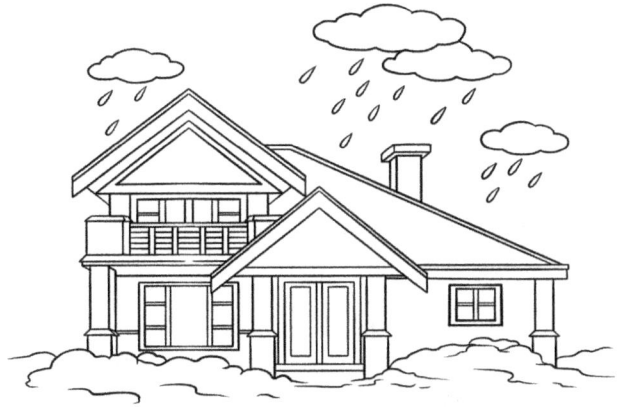

Figure 4-3: Naturally occurring outdoor water sources and weather events, like rain, snow, flooding, and wind-driven storms, can significantly impact a home's structure. Allowing snow to pile up against the foundation increases the risk of water seeping into the structure as it melts. Heavy rain, especially when driven by wind, can penetrate roof joints and walls, while flooding can overwhelm drainage systems and cause extensive water intrusion. Additionally, hail and strong winds can damage roofing materials, creating entry points for water. Regular maintenance, proper grading, and clear drainage paths help reduce these risks.

Crawlspace, Basement, Cellar Maintenance

❏ **Crawlspaces used for storage.** Crawl spaces should be kept clear of storage, especially wood, cardboard, or other digestible items sitting on the soil. Soil typically has enough dampness to cause mold growth in cellulose materials. Cellulose debris on soil also encourages termites and other insect infestations. Even non-cellulose items can trap moisture and provide a haven for rodents and other vermin.

❏ **Rodent damage.** For rodents to cause damage in hidden areas in a structure, they need an entry point. Owner vigilance in detecting and closing off potential entry points and dealing with an infestation as soon as there are any indications can save untold damage, including water leaks, electrical shorts, envelope damage, disease, and odor.

❏ **Failure to take action** or efforts to stop additional damage from worsening after a defect or problem develops will accelerate the repair cost. If you discover a water leak, you should immediately shut off the water and dry the area as best you can to arrest further damage. If you cannot dry the area completely yourself, you should have the area and materials professionally dried, remediated if necessary, and repaired. *(See section "Being Prepared for Water Emergencies" on page 98)*

❏ **Wear and tear** of building components and fixtures should be proactively evaluated and properly restored to proper functioning.

Roofs

❏ **Eave vents, attic vents, roof vents, weep holes, and other** openings must allow appropriate ventilation, but they must not permit rodents, insects, birds, or other pests to enter the building or associated areas. The damage they cause can lead to water entry.

❏ **Vigilance in maintaining good roof drainage** away from the building. Gutters should be cleaned and repaired as a component of a regular maintenance schedule.

❏ **Gutters** should be installed so they drain freely and do not direct water into wall cavities. Hidden gutters, concealed inside attics, or wall cavities may make leaks inaccessible for inspection and repair.

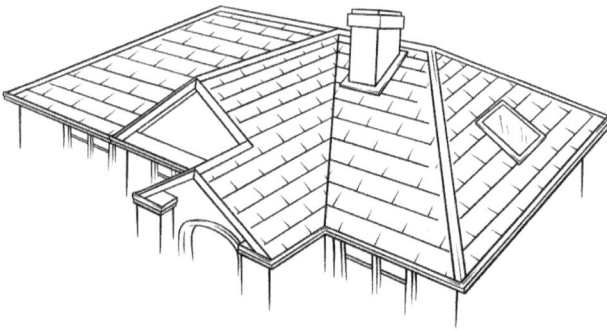

Figure 4-4: Complex roofs, with multiple slopes, valleys, and intersecting surfaces, are more prone to leaks due to the increased number of seams and joints where water can infiltrate. These intricate designs make it challenging to manage water runoff effectively, especially during heavy rain or snowmelt. Proper flashing, regular maintenance, and thorough inspections are essential to prevent leaks and ensure the long-term durability of complex roofing systems.

Interior

❏ **Plumbing traps** (U or P-traps) are present at every fixture to prevent sewer gases from flowing back into a home. The traps need to have water in them to prevent the gases. Normal use of fixtures will keep sufficient water in the trap. However, extended disuse, such as extended vacations or a failure to regularly use fixtures, will likely result in a foul odor entering the home. Adding water into the drain usually fixes the problem within a few minutes. Floor drains and others that do not have water flowing into them regularly should have water added.

❏ **Plumbing Vent Stack**: The vent stack is a vertical pipe that vents sewer gases out of the plumbing system, releasing them above the roofline to prevent odors from entering the home. Potential problems include blockages from debris or ice, which can lead to slow drainage, sewer gas backups, or gurgling noises in the plumbing.

❏ **Air Admittance Valve (AAV) / Cheater Vent**: If there are no Plumbing Vent Stacks, then there must be accessible AAV's at every drain. AAVs are under-sink valves that allow

air into the drain line, preventing a vacuum and ensuring proper drainage where traditional venting isn't possible. Potential issues include failure of the internal seal, which can lead to sewer gas odors and poor drainage. Cheaper AAVs often last less than five years; regular inspections and timely replacement can help prevent issues.

❏ **Condensation Drain Lines:** the air conditioning condensate pan should be kept clean and draining, and the overflow collection pan should be kept clean and free of debris.

❏ **Keep Ductwork Free of stored items**—they can collapse and restrict airflow or come loose and leak air.

❏ **Water should not infiltrate** the fireplace chimney. The junction between the fireplace and the house should be properly flashed and sealed to prevent water entry.

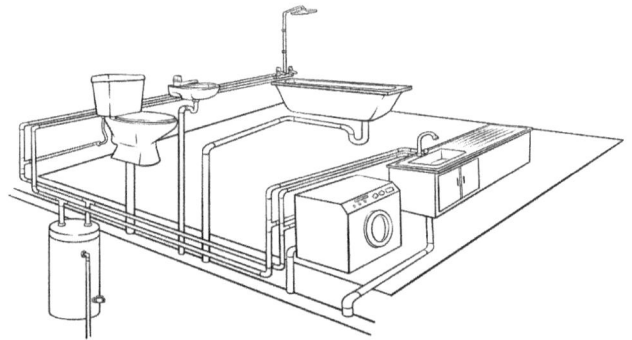

Figure 4-5: Plumbing systems are most prone to leaks or overflows at joints, fittings, and areas where pipes connect to fixtures or appliances. Common trouble spots include under sinks, around water heaters, at pipe elbows, and near valves. In bathrooms, leaks can occur around toilets, showers, and tubs, while kitchens are vulnerable around dishwashers and under-sink garbage disposals. Regular inspections of these high-risk areas can help identify early signs of wear or corrosion, preventing water damage and costly repairs.

Remodeling

❏ **Remodeling considerations:** When remodeling, follow the recommendations for walls, foundations, roofs, and other structural components as outlined in *Prescriptions for a Healthy House*. Special care should be taken at the junctions between old and new construction, as these areas are common trouble spots for water entry and may develop separations between the two structures.

❏ **Paper-covered gypsum board**, including treated paper, should never be used in frequently wet areas of the home, and if old walls have mold inside, they should be completely remediated.

❏ **Cardboard and Paper:** Remodeling and repairs frequently result in workers leaving debris in the crawlspace or attic. Cardboard or paper debris must never be allowed to remain, as it frequently becomes a food source for problem molds.

❏ **Damaged, settled, or missing insulation** should be repaired or replaced to help prevent hidden condensation moisture from developing.

❏ **Thermal** imaging may help identify cold spots hidden in wall cavities where insulation is inadequate or missing.

Seasonal

❏ **Anticipate problems** from frozen plumbing, ice damming, and roof overloading during heavy ice and snow conditions.

❏ **Maintain adequate indoor temperature** to prevent frozen plumbing or material stress crack separations due to expansion and contraction for fluctuating temperatures.

❏ **Vacant Homes** should be inspected, and any deficiencies should be repaired before the vacancy begins. Plumbing pipes should be winterized.

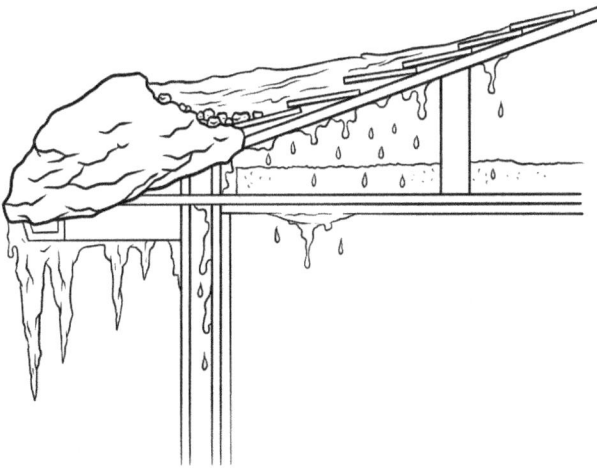

Figure 4-6: Ice damming occurs when snow on a roof melts due to heat escaping from the home, then freezes at the colder eaves, creating a "dam." This dam prevents proper drainage, causing water to back up under shingles and potentially seep into the home. Over time, ice damming can lead to water damage, mold growth, and structural deterioration in walls and ceilings. Proper insulation and ventilation can help prevent ice dams from forming.

Appliances

More information is included in the Contents and Personal Property section. The following are considerations when renting or purchasing a home.

❏ **Condensation pans** in refrigerators, HVAC systems, dehumidifiers, and other equipment should be cleaned and properly drained to prevent mold growth.

❏ **Humidifiers** built into HVAC systems should be avoided.

❏ **Dehumidifiers** are difficult to maintain and keep mold from growing when built into HVAC systems.

❏ **Refrigerator maintenance.** Refrigerator condensate pans require cleaning to remain mold-free, but homeowners often neglect this chore because the pans are inconveniently arranged, requiring that the refrigerator be pulled out. Many refrigerators have condensate pans that are bolted in place and can't be removed for cleaning, making maintenance even more difficult.

PREVIOUS REMEDIATION SHORTCOMINGS

In addition to removing the mold, it is crucial to address the source of moisture that caused the problem. When looking to buy or rent, the more you can do to screen for mold issues and eliminate homes with severe problems from your prospective list, the better. After over three decades of inspecting buildings for mold problems, I am still amazed by the unexpected issues that can arise. Because many construction materials have a limited life expectancy, hidden mold problems, and deteriorated materials are often buried within walls, ceilings, or floors, making them difficult to discover and repair. Some contractors ignore mold problems during repair work to stay on schedule and maintain their profit margins. Sellers and landlords can deliberately hide issues without properly fixing them or providing disclosure. For medically sensitive individuals, these hidden problems can have devastating effects. Identifying deliberate attempts to cover up issues can be challenging.

However, it is not hopeless. The deck may seem stacked against mold-sensitive buyers or renters, especially if they are not allowed to have the home inspected and sampled by a qualified professional. Many people are now performing their own stealth inspections and sample collections. This chapter aims to help level the playing field and provide an understanding of the situations that may be encountered.

Knowing about areas that have had prior remediation can help you check the effectiveness of the remediation. Verifying previous work before accepting that all is well is always a good idea. By being informed and vigilant, you can better protect yourself and ensure a healthier living environment.

PREPARING FOR A SHIFTING CLIMATE

Preparing for microbial problems and water damage requires adaptive strategies for home health due to changing climatic conditions. In a world where the climate is constantly changing, understanding and adapting to these shifts is not just reacting to changes; it's about anticipating and preparing for future trends. Consider each home you have decided to evaluate and how you can help it become more resilient to an evolving climate. You can regularly update yourself on local climate trends and predictions. This knowledge is crucial for anticipating new risks in your area that might not have existed previously. There are clues all around us that things are changing. If you have lived in a particular area for a while and you think back, you may be able to recognize many of these changes yourself. Still, if you don't have a history of an area, there are still available clues to follow up on what is changing in the local area.

- Flood Ratings: FEMA and other organizations have been upgrading flood maps, allowing you to explore what is changing.
- Planting zones are shifting
- Weather swings are becoming more pronounced.

We don't often consider increased drought or the risk of wildfires as factors that can heighten the risk of water damage, but they can have indirect consequences. These environmental conditions can lead to increased erosion and subsequent flooding, heat effects on construction materials, and shifting of buildings due to the rapid drying of expansive clay soils or earth movement. The expansion and contraction of the building can result in cracks or openings that allow water entry. All of these factors can elevate the risk of plumbing ruptures. When freshwater lines are damaged, they can cause immediate and extensive water damage. Septic lines can also be compromised, releasing unsanitary water, leading to further contamination and damage. Awareness of these potential risks is essential for maintaining the integrity of your home.

- **Building Resilience:** Consider what improvements or modifications will enhance the home's resilience to extreme weather. This can include improvements such as:
- **Upgrading roof resistance** to higher winds and water intrusion, plan to pay extra for a more resilient shingle or membrane and the best-flashing ice shields to reduce the potential for ice damming.
- **Thermal imaging** is used to determine where shortcomings exist in insulation, waterproofing, and ventilation systems.
- **Shifts in the External Environment:** Include how the immediate external environment, such as the type of vegetation, proximity to water bodies, and landscaping, can influence mold risks. Cyanobacteria and their associated toxins in freshwater bodies and other considerations
- **Seasonal Variations and Adaptations:** Discuss how changes in seasons within the same region can affect mold growth and water damage, requiring different strategies at different times of the year.
- **Emergency Preparedness:** Develop a comprehensive plan for emergency situations like floods or severe storms. This includes having a rapid response strategy for water intrusion to prevent or arrest bacterial and mold growth.

- **Regular Maintenance and Inspections:** Consistently inspect your home to identify and address vulnerabilities. Pay special attention to areas prone to moisture accumulation.
- **Community Resources:** Utilize community resources and guidelines for climate resilience in housing. Engage with local initiatives that focus on sustainable living and disaster preparedness.
- **Professional Advice:** Consult with building science, climate resilience, and mold prevention experts to get tailored advice for your specific situation. But also become an informed skeptic.
- **Climate Based Considerations**
- "The air of coastal locations is typically characterized by high salt content, resulting in metal corrosion. Corroded galvanized metal flashing and fasteners fail faster and can lead to a failure to divert water away from the building. Flashings are intended to direct water away from areas of the home where it may collect and cannot dry rapidly, leading to water intrusion into the building envelope.
- Areas that experience alternating freeze/ thaw conditions are susceptible to ice damming problems. Buildings will also be much more challenged by deterioration caused by water seeping into cracks and then expanding as it turns to ice.
- Wood products exposed to the elements in southwestern deserts will suffer from accelerated drying due to extreme UV exposure and low humidity.
- Moisture and mold problems associated with condensation caused by air conditioning are common in high-humidity climates such as those found east of the Rockies.
- Regionally atypical events such as floods, cold snaps, heat waves, high winds, hurricanes, tornados, and earthquakes are also subject to damage that may result in water damage or moisture entering and accumulating in the home, causing mold to develop.

Myth: Only Certain Climates Have Mold Problems.
Fact: Mold can grow in any climate. While it's more prevalent in humid climates, homes in dry climates can also have mold issues, especially if there are internal sources of moisture, like plumbing leaks.

Outdoor weather conditions have far less impact on whether homes will develop mold than faulty or non-adaptive construction practices. I have frequently talked with people who think moving to a desert community will solve their mold issues. Some of the moldiest homes I have ever inspected have been in desert communities such as Palm Springs, Las Vegas, Phoenix, and Albuquerque. Desert communities frequently experience a summer monsoon season with short-lasting torrential rains. These areas are just as prone to water damage resulting in mold when the construction and maintenance are not up to par.

In conclusion, a climate-conscious approach to home selection is vital for long-term comfort and health, especially for those with mold sensitivities. Each climate zone brings its unique set of challenges. By upgrading systems to be able to withstand greater fluctuations in weather and understanding these specific environmental impacts, you can make more informed decisions, choosing homes that are better suited to withstand the particular challenges of their local climates.

The following organizations and agencies have information available to assist in understanding and addressing the additional stresses on our homes.

- *Climate impacts on buildings and infrastructure.* U.S. Environmental Protection Agency (USEPA, 2022)

- *Climate resilience toolkit: Protecting homes from climate impacts.* National Oceanic and Atmospheric Administration. (NOAA, 2021)

- *Impacts, Adaptation, and Vulnerability: Effects of climate change on the built environment.* (IPCC, 2023)

- *Building codes and climate resilience: How to protect homes from climate change impacts.* International Code Council. (ICC, 2020)

- *Climate change and housing: Strategies for resilience.* National Institute of Building Sciences. (NIBS, 2021)

References

National Association of Realtors. (2021). *Real estate seller disclosure laws by state.* National Association of Realtors. Retrieved from https://www.nar.realtor

U.S. Department of Housing and Urban Development (HUD). (2022). *Disclosures upon sale of residential property: A guide for homeowners and homebuyers.* U.S. Department of Housing and Urban Development. Retrieved from https://www.hud.gov

Legal Information Institute. (n.d.). *Real estate disclosure requirements.* Cornell Law School. Retrieved from https://www.law.cornell.edu

Bagley, K., & Long, R. (2020). Real estate disclosure laws: A state-by-state comparison. *Journal of Real Estate Law, 57*(2), 102–121.

FindLaw. (2023). *Home sellers' disclosures: What you must reveal in every state.* FindLaw. Retrieved from https://www.findlaw.com

American Society of Home Inspectors (ASHI). (n.d.). *Standards of practice and code of ethics.* American Society of Home Inspectors. Retrieved from https://www.homeinspector.org

National Association of Home Inspectors (NAHI). (2020). *Ethics and professional standards for home inspectors.* National Association of Home Inspectors. Retrieved from https://www.nahi.org

International Association of Certified Home Inspectors (InterNACHI). (2023). *Code of ethics for home inspectors.* International Association of Certified Home Inspectors. Retrieved from https://www.nachi.org

Kaplan, D., & Wilson, L. (2021). Ethics and legal regulations for home inspectors: A state-by-state guide. *Journal of Home Inspection Standards, 46*(1), 15–29.

Legal Information Institute. (n.d.). *Home inspector licensing and regulatory laws.* Cornell Law School. Retrieved from https://www.law.cornell.edu

U.S. Department of Housing and Urban Development (HUD). (2023). *Tenant rights, laws, and protections by state.* U.S. Department of Housing and Urban Development. Retrieved from https://www.hud.gov

Legal Information Institute. (n.d.). *Landlord-tenant law.* Cornell Law School. Retrieved from https://www.law.cornell.edu

National Multifamily Housing Council. (2022). *Understanding rental housing regulations: A guide for property owners and tenants.* National Multifamily Housing Council. Retrieved from https://www.nmhc.org

American Bar Association. (2021). *Landlord and tenant rights and obligations.* American Bar Association. Retrieved from https://www.americanbar.org

National Low Income Housing Coalition. (2023). *Tenant protections and rental assistance programs.* National Low Income Housing Coalition. Retrieved from https://nlihc.org

National Institute of Standards and Technology (NIST). (2020). *Guidelines for resilient construction materials and their life expectancy.* National Institute of Standards and Technology. Retrieved from https://www.nist.gov

American Society of Civil Engineers (ASCE). (2021). Sustainable and resilient infrastructure: Life-cycle considerations for construction materials. *Journal of Infrastructure Systems, 27*(4), 100–115. https://doi.org/10.1061/(ASCE)IS.1943-555X.0000642

Building Science Corporation. (2019). *Durability and resilience of construction materials: Best practices for material selection.* Building Science Corporation. Retrieved from https://www.buildingscience.com

American Concrete Institute (ACI). (2022). Life expectancy and durability of concrete in resilient construction. *ACI Structural Journal, 119*(2), 75–88. https://doi.org/10.14359/51734523

International Code Council (ICC). (2023). *Evaluating material resilience and longevity in building codes and standards.* International Code Council. Retrieved from https://www.iccsafe.org

U.S. Environmental Protection Agency (EPA). (2022). *Climate impacts on buildings and infrastructure.* U.S. Environmental Protection Agency. Retrieved from https://www.epa.gov

National Oceanic and Atmospheric Administration (NOAA). (2021). *Climate resilience toolkit: Protecting homes from climate impacts.* National Oceanic and Atmospheric Administration. Retrieved from https://toolkit.climate.gov

Intergovernmental Panel on Climate Change (IPCC). (2023). *Impacts, adaptation, and vulnerability: Effects of climate change on the built environment.* IPCC Sixth Assessment Report. Retrieved from https://www.ipcc.ch/report/ar6/wg2/

International Code Council (ICC). (2020). *Building codes and climate resilience: How to protect homes from climate change impacts.* International Code Council. Retrieved from https://www.iccsafe.org

National Institute of Building Sciences (NIBS). (2021). *Climate change and housing: Strategies for resilience.* National Institute of Building Sciences. Retrieved from https://www.nibs.org

25 Essentials for Finding a Healthy Home to Rent or Buy

1. **Historical Buildings**: Older buildings are at an increased risk of hidden water damage or hazardous materials like lead paint and asbestos. Even completely remodeled structures often have hidden issues that were missed or covered up. Inspect thoroughly.

2. **Newer Constructions**: Ensure that newer homes are built with durable materials and proper construction methods to avoid issues from environmental pressures.

3. **Understand Local Climate**: Each region has unique climate challenges that can affect a building's integrity. For instance:
   › **Southern regions**: High humidity can lead to mold.
   › **Northern regions**: Freeze-thaw cycles can cause structural damage.
   › **Coastal areas**: Salt air can corrode materials.

4. **Architectural Design**: Evaluate designs for potential moisture retention and microbial growth risks.

5. **Construction Quality**: Inspect the quality of construction and materials used, focusing on durability and resistance to environmental factors.

6. **Past Owners' Maintenance**: Investigate how well past owners maintained the property. Regular maintenance reduces the risk of hidden issues.

7. **Thorough Inspection**: Look for subtle hints in inspection reports that might suggest larger issues. Pay attention to limiting language and recommendations for specialist inspections.

8. **Follow-up**: Always follow up on any concerns noted in reports and consider additional expert inspections if necessary.

9. **Seller Misrepresentation**: Be alert for vague responses and incomplete disclosures. Request detailed records of past water damage and mold remediation.

10. **Quality of Repairs**: Verify the standards and quality of any repairs made, especially for mold and water damage.

11. **Unusual Odors**: Musty smells or heavy use of air fresheners can indicate hidden mold. Investigate thoroughly.

12. **Visible Stains**: Look for water stains on walls, ceilings, and floors and determine their sources.

13. **Check for Cracks**: Foundation cracks, uneven floors, and sticking doors/windows can signal significant structural problems.

14. **Proper Sealing**: Ensure windows and doors are properly sealed and flashed to prevent water intrusion.

15. **Site Conditions**: Evaluate drainage, soil conditions, and potential flood risks. Ensure proper grading to direct water away from the home.

16. **Geological Factors**: Be aware of expansive clay soils and other geological factors that can impact a building's stability and cause plumbing to rupture.

17. **Roof Design**: Opt for homes with well-sloped roofs and adequate overhangs to facilitate water runoff and protect walls.

18. **Ventilation**: Ensure proper ventilation in attics, crawlspaces, and other areas prone to dampness.

19. **Moisture-Resistant Materials**: Use moisture-resistant materials that won't trap moisture. These are especially useful in wet areas (e.g., kitchens and bathrooms). Avoid paper-faced drywall and other materials that provide the nutrients for microorganisms to grow.

20. **Durable Siding**: Look for homes with breathable or well-drained water-resistant siding and construction methods that prevent moisture trapping.

21. **System Integrity**: Ensure plumbing and HVAC systems are in good condition and properly maintained to manage moisture.

22. **Proper Insulation**: Verify that insulation and vapor barriers are correctly installed and maintained to prevent condensation and mold growth. Avoid cellulose or other insulations that provide nutrients that support growth.

23. **Regular Inspections**: Consistently inspect and maintain the property, addressing any issues promptly to prevent mold growth.

24. **Proactive Repairs**: Quickly repair any damage to prevent further deterioration and potential mold issues.

25. **Prepare for Weather Extremes**: Upgrade systems and materials to withstand extreme weather conditions and anticipate increased cracking and separation of materials due to increased expansion and contraction and other new risks due to climate change.

Guided Notations

The following symbols will be used throughout the 25 Steps as a visual cue, indicating how your insights or information gathered from the exercises should be recorded.

The pencil symbol directs you to make a journal entry in the Project Diary, where you log the factual or objective details from your remediation process and plan to document your path forward.

The caduceus is the icon that signals the use of your health diary, a place to journal health-related notes, observations, and action items. It's where you record any physical symptoms, medical appointments, findings, and healthcare steps you plan to take.

The floor plan symbol guides you in recording information on your home's diagram or floor plan. This information will include specific sites of water damage, visible mold presence, areas of suspicion, containment strategies, and other information best represented on a diagram.

The heart on this icon indicates that this diary is more personal. It's a space for your speculations, musings, daydreams, and other thoughts that are important to you but may not yet be fully developed. Writing here can help you process and clarify your ideas, which may later form the basis for facts and decisions recorded in your project diary, floor plans, or medical journal.

Symbols for Tracking Navigation and Decision-Making

Marking boxes ❑ can help you chart where you are in the process, what steps come next, what can be ignored or omitted, and if you need to return to take care of something missed.

- A box that is left blank means you have not decided if an action is needed (If necessary, you can always change your mind).
- If you have already begun taking action with your home, place an arrow in front of the box that indicates what part of the process you have already reached. →❑
- Draw a circle around the box if you have read the exercise and need to consider it further. ❍
- Placing a checkmark in the box indicates you have completed the Stage or Step. ✓
- Crossing the box out means you have determined the Step does not apply. ✗

Five Stage, 25 Step Instructions

Tips for Achieving Your Desired Results

Establishing Your Vision: Reflect on what a healthy, mold-controlled environment means and consider the importance of indoor environmental quality, comfort, and overall well-being. Are you looking to address known mold issues, discover hidden conditions, prevent future problems, or, ideally, all the above?

- **Be Realistic:** Set achievable goals based on your current situation and resources.
- **Consider Health Impacts:** Prioritize by focusing on outcomes that create a healthy living environment.
- **Be Flexible:** Remember, your objectives might evolve as you progress through the steps. Stay adaptable.
- **Regular Check-ins:** Regularly revisit your goals as you move through the steps. Are they still relevant? Do they need adjustments based on new or changing conditions or information?
- **Document Changes:** Keep a log of any changes requiring adjustments. New information may result in changes to your plans.

INTRODUCTION TO STAGE AND STEP EXERCISES

This book section is designed to guide you using Stage and Step Exercises. Stage Exercises are the broader, strategic components that help you outline your overall strategy for achieving a mold-controlled home. They set the direction for understanding the big picture. On the other hand, Step Exercises are more tactical and detailed. They involve specific actions and decisions that contribute to fulfilling the objectives laid out in the Stage Exercises. Together, these exercises form a more comprehensive approach to mold control in your home.

UNDERSTANDING THE BALANCE OF COST, SPEED, AND PRECISION

In the journey to create a mold-controlled environment, every decision pivots around three factors: cost, speed, and precision. Your budget and timeframe will often guide the

depth and thoroughness you can afford at each step. Here's how these elements interact:

- Cost vs. Precision: Greater precision typically demands higher costs and more time. For instance, thorough moisture mapping might increase expenses but significantly reduce the risk of recurrent mold issues.
- Cost vs. Speed: Aiming for cost-effectiveness may require longer timelines and potentially less precision, leading to possible overlooked problem areas.
- Speed vs. Precision: Faster execution increases the risk of missing critical details, potentially resulting in repeated efforts and higher costs.

Achieving the perfect balance between cost, speed, and precision in addressing mold and water damage is more than a mere logistical challenge; it's a decision-making process with far-reaching implications. Opting for speed over precision might appear efficient in the short term, but it risks overlooking crucial moisture areas, potentially leading to recurrent mold problems. Such oversight increases long-term costs and can compromise the building's structural and environmental health. On the other hand, an initial investment in a thorough and precise approach mitigates these risks and contributes to the overall well-being of the building and its occupants. As you navigate through these decisions, it's essential to assess each situation carefully, considering the immediate and long-term health impacts, the environmental quality of the indoor space, and the level of sensitivity of the individual occupants. This book provides a comprehensive framework to guide you in making informed, balanced decisions prioritizing your home's integrity and its inhabitants' health.

NAVIGATING THE FOG: A JOURNEY TO CLARITY AND CONTROL

Whether you're establishing a 'forever home' or making do with temporary housing to navigate a health crisis exacerbated by water-damaged conditions, I aim to demystify a process that can often be confusing and overwhelming. I intend to provide the tools necessary for evaluation and decision-making, empowering you to make choices that align with your goals. Along this journey, you'll likely need to seek assistance. Recognizing potential helpers' inherent biases is necessary to clarify your health-related and environmental issues. By understanding your unique challenges and needs, you'll be better equipped to navigate the complexities of remediation and create a plan that truly addresses your and your family's well-being.

The Intertwined Emotional and Physical Journey

Physicians specializing in mold sensitivities agree that the first step toward healing is to either remove the patient from the exposure (temporary or permanent relocation) or the exposure from the patient (fixing the building). The path to the home's recovery is often paralleled by the experiences of the people traumatized by illness. Often, the stages of grief—denial, anger, bargaining, and depression—are each amplified by the physical symptoms of exposure, such as memory loss, brain fog, and chronic fatigue. These emotional and physical challenges are entwined, complicating the pursuit of clear, decisive action for remediation and relocation. Successfully navigating the 'stages of grief' results in acceptance. This does not mean stagnation or that you are stuck accepting your situation as unchanging. Confronting this internal resistance is crucial, as understanding and overcoming your personal and health-related hurdles are just as vital as the practical steps required for mold remediation. This emotional journey is intertwined with the physical healing process, and together, they form a comprehensive path toward recovery.

The Impact of External Influences

Support from friends and family can be a pillar of strength, providing emotional and practical assistance. However, it's not uncommon for someone within your inner circle to inadvertently challenge your efforts, perhaps minimizing the seriousness of your circumstances or suggesting oversimplified solutions. It's vital to assemble a knowledgeable team, including your physician, environmental consultant, and mold remediator. Yet, fostering a support network that genuinely comprehends and supports your cause is just as helpful. Seek individuals who not only acknowledge the complexities of your situation but also share your commitment to achieving a safe and healthy living environment. A knowledgeable health coach or group led by an experienced professional can help build a support network that aligns with your goals and will prove invaluable as you navigate the challenges of remediation and recovery.

BECOMING YOUR OWN BEST EXPERT

Empowerment on your journey to a healthier home begins with self-education. The information landscape regarding mold and water damage can be vast and sometimes overwhelming or misleading. However, by arming yourself with knowledge, you become the foremost expert on your situation and home. This book is designed to help guide you through the steps but cannot make decisions for you. Your willingness to become your own best expert will help facilitate your transformative process.

1. Understanding Your Home's Environment: Each home has distinct challenges. Learn about your home's construction, ventilation, moisture levels, and repair history. This foundational knowledge is key to understanding potential water damage, mold growth, and other water-damage organisms.

2. Learning Mold Basics: Understanding how water-damage organisms affect your home and health may seem complex. However, understanding growth conditions, common types of contamination found in homes, and health implications helps ensure the accuracy of your assessment.

3. Navigating Remediation Options: Mold remediation varies by situation. Learn about different strategies to make informed choices for your home. Working with knowledgeable professionals can help facilitate the process, but understanding DIY options can help you be prepared to provide or oversee quality control that will prevent missing important measures from being implemented.

4. Developing a Critical Eye: As your understanding grows, you will grow in your ability to evaluate the advice you encounter. Learn to identify credible sources and trust your judgment. Being your best expert can help you recognize and step in when someone is unwilling or unable to work in your best interests.

5. Preventative Strategies and Maintenance: Knowledge equips you to implement preventative strategies and regular maintenance, significantly lowering mold and water damage risks and expenses.

6. Creating a Personal Action Plan: Use your newfound understanding to develop a tailored action plan for your home's maintenance and mold management.

By becoming your own best expert, you will not only gain control over your home's health but also develop a sense of confidence and assurance in managing its well-being.

HOW TO BEGIN WHEN YOU HAVE ALREADY BEGUN

If you have already embarked on the journey of remediating mold and water damage in your home, the question arises, "Where do you go from here if you've already begun?" It's a common concern, and it's important to understand that it's never too late to reassess your path. The key is to step back and see the bigger picture, ensuring that the steps you've already taken align with the comprehensive strategy laid out in this book.

Reassessing Your Journey: Adjustments Along the Way

If the remediation process has started without this guide, review your actions against the Five Stages and 25 Steps outlined below. You may be relieved to learn that the original approach is proceeding well and needs little or no adjustment. Should this reflection reveal any overlooked areas or highlight where your plan might require fine-tuning, understanding the entire process provides context to the steps you've already taken and guides you in effectively integrating any missed elements into your existing plan.

Re-Evaluating Your Current Plan— Correcting the Course When Necessary

Begin by conducting a thorough assessment of your current situation. Ask yourself: Have I set clear goals as recommended in Stage One? Have I collected all the necessary health information to tailor my remediation plans? Ideally, these foundational steps should be completed before moving on to actual remediation. If you discover any gaps, it's crucial to address them to ensure the effectiveness of your overall plan.

When you identify areas that need improvement or steps that were omitted, you will be able to correct the course. This may involve revisiting earlier stages or incorporating new measures, such as additional inspection or testing, to determine if problem areas have been missed. You may bring in or consult with different professionals to help with a more nuanced approach to remediation.

- Remember, most mistakes or oversights can be corrected or controlled, although they may require additional time or expense.
- Be aware, however, that certain errors can significantly set back the project or substantially increase costs, and a few may ruin the home or significantly delay occupancy by people with medical hypersensitivity. Some of the most problematic include:
- Using inappropriate chemicals for remediation, especially in health-sensitive cases, is a mistake. This includes antimicrobials, biocides, or chemicals that claim to eliminate or control microorganisms. These often adversely affect remediation efforts, especially when health-related hypersensitivities are a concern. It is always best to avoid allowing these situations to develop, but a reasoned approach can often help once they have occurred. Trying things at random doesn't help, which can often compound the issues or even make them worse.

- In cases where encapsulants or sealants have already been applied that can inadvertently trap moisture, they may need to be carefully sanded back off to restore the ability of water vapor to escape and prevent further issues. When moisture becomes trapped, and additional organisms have already begun to grow, adopting a well-reasoned approach to remediation is essential. Attempting random interventions can often exacerbate the problems or even worsen the situation. Instead, it is advisable to carefully assess the situation and follow a systematic plan for addressing the moisture issue caused by encapsulants or sealants. This thoughtful approach, which may include the careful removal of the encapsulant or sealant, is more likely to yield positive results and contribute to the successful resolution of the problem.
- Neglecting to identify and rectify the source of the moisture that caused the original problem can lead to ongoing deterioration.
- Reconstructing the affected area without being sure issues have been adequately addressed can result in needing to remove and replace brand-new materials. However, more frequent maintenance cleaning may be able to address the increased building memory.

PRELIMINARY EXERCISE, AN OVERVIEW OF THE FIVE STAGES AND 25 STEPS

This preliminary exercise is for everyone and will help determine where your home's situation fits within the *Mold Controlled* 25 Steps. There are likely multiple motivations for addressing water damage or mold issues in your indoor environment, and your circumstances will guide your approach. This pre-exercise aims to help you see the big picture while organizing your thoughts and concerns into a prioritized action plan. I want to help you manage your process so that what you want to accomplish harmonizes with what you need to do. The most effective way to do this is by understanding the overall process, which is what this pre-exercise is about.

If you are already in the midst of a remediation project, this is also the place to assess where you are in the process. You may have skipped steps along the way, which can lead to confusion or leave gaps in essential information. By clearly identifying your current stage and reviewing the steps you may have missed, you can gain clarity on what needs to be done to get back on track. Remember, with many skipped steps, it's never too late to make new determinations or change your mind. While some missed steps may mean lost guidance or information, recovery is still possible. You may encounter minor inefficiencies, additional costs, or missed opportunities. Still, most of the time, you can find ways to continue successfully or at least know where increased vigilance is required moving forward.

Stage One: Is There a Problem?

This stage is all about assessment and planning. It is about determining if there is a problem for you or someone in your household. The home could have an issue that is severe enough for everyone or possibly only for people with sensitivities.

❑ **Use this pre-exercise to evaluate your progress and decide which part of the process you have already reached, marking it with an arrow to track your path.**
Also, Indicate all that apply:

❑ **Step 1: Establish Your Goals:** Set your goals to effectively address what you need to do to care for yourself, your family, and your home. Step 1 is designed to help you establish the journey that lies ahead. You may need to manage a crisis, assess damage, find temporary housing, or locate a durable, healthy home to rent or purchase. This Step aims to help you plot your path from wherever you are in your current situation to recognize or create a durable, healthy, and manageable home.

❑ **Step 2: Gather Medical Information to Tailor Remediation Plans:** The focus is to develop a plan to protect the most vulnerable household members and guide informed decisions on occupancy. Most family members will never experience medical issues based on the presence of hidden mold at elevated levels in their household. However, when mold illness is an issue, the help of an experienced and knowledgeable physician working with you on your specific challenges is an important ally. This Step may require a separate entry for each sensitive household member.

❑ **Step 3: Home History and Initial Assessment:** This step involves assembling and combining your knowledge with any new information you can uncover to inform your decisions regarding mold and water damage. It's essential to continuously evaluate this information to determine if additional details are needed for your decision-making process, planning your path forward, or establishing your plan. Step 3 of this process is designed to be relatively inexpensive or free, providing cost-effective ways to gather crucial insights. The information you compile in this step may be sufficient to decide if you want to proceed. Consequently, if this early step leads you to an early decision, it does so without significant economic impact.

❑ **Step 4: Investigation, Testing, and Next Steps:** You'll learn to select and collaborate effectively with an Indoor Environmental Professional and other inspection experts in this step. You'll gain insights into various testing methods and how to customize them to address specific issues within your home. Reflecting on the information gathered in Steps 1 to 3 will guide your decisions regarding the depth of investigation required and the budget you're willing to allocate to assess the suitability of the house for your needs. This includes a discussion of the advantages and disadvantages of performing certain types of sample collection on your own versus hiring a professional indoor environmental consultant. Depending on your circumstances, you may combine this Step with the more comprehensive 'Stage Two, Step 5' evaluations to help identify hidden issues. After completing this Step, you should also have sufficient information to determine a strategy for your possessions and contents.

Stage Two: Develop Strategy, Team Assembly, and Locating Hidden Problems

Here is where you select your team and collect the additional information needed for a plan. Before moving into Stage Two, you should review all the information you assembled in Stage One and clearly understand if your indoor environment does have a problem that needs to be addressed! By the time you have completed the four steps in Stage Two, you should have gone from a generalized understanding that there is a problem to a more focused understanding of which general areas have well-defined problems needing remediation and which areas can be controlled by other less invasive means.

❑ **Step 5: Screening for Hidden Sources of Contamination:** This step introduces various screening methods, weighing the pros and cons of destructive investigation, wall-cavity sampling, mold dogs, and non-invasive Pathways™ Testing. Establishing baseline and follow-up levels of hidden organisms associated with water damage can help differentiate areas of mold growth from areas with an accumulation of spores and fragments from elsewhere. In addition to mold, Pathways™ Testing also screens for any protein-based contaminant, such as peptide bonds and proteins from rodent feces and urine, cockroach and insect frass, dust mites, and other potential protein-based contaminants that you don't want or need in your home. Understanding these distinctions is another clue for assisting with targeted remediation and ensuring the health of your home.

❑ **Step 6: Integrate Known and Suspected Issues into a Plan.** This Step is where you will combine all the information gathered so far to determine how to continue. Additional rounds of Pathways™ Testing can determine the extent to which effective cleaning might be used to create sanctuary areas to keep exposures under control and the degree of remediation needed. Often, a hybrid approach can be practical. This is where the information is gathered, and the previous steps will be assembled into a draft plan.

❑ **Step 7: Team Assembly:** Not every remediation firm is qualified or trained to address homes where water damage results in medical issues. This step guides assembling a mold remediation team attuned to health concerns to ensure expert and health-conscious remediation.

❑ **Step 8: Hidden or Unidentified Issues: Attics, Crawlspaces, and Basements:** This step adopts a detective-like approach to reveal and incorporate hidden or unforeseen issues into your remediation plan and develop contingency strategies.

Stage Three: Remediation Planning and Execution

Stage Three transforms the plan into action, focusing on mold and water damage remediation to enhance overall living conditions.

❑ **Step 9: Implementing the Remediation Plan:** This Step emphasizes executing the remediation plan, focusing on non-toxic methods and team hierarchy for effective project management and a healthy living environment.

❑ **Step 10: Containment, Negative-Air, and Local Exhaust Ventilation:** Establishing precise containment zones and ventilation systems is essential in remediation to control mold spore spread, monitor particle levels, and maintain barrier integrity.

❑ **Step 11: Physical Removal of Contaminates:** This step emphasizes non-chemical mold remediation by physically removing damaged materials or using HEPA-filtered abrasive cleaning methods to eliminate embedded mold growth structures.

❑ **Step 12: Special Attention to HVAC and Air Conveyance Systems:** In medically necessary remediation, this step prioritizes inspecting and cleaning HVAC systems and ductwork to ensure indoor environmental quality, especially for sensitive individuals, by thoroughly addressing mold and contaminants in components like the systems cooling coils, ductwork, and other parts of the system.

❑ **Step 13: Special Attention to Enclosed Spaces:** This step underscores the importance of addressing mold in enclosed spaces, such as unfinished basements, cellars, crawlspaces, and attics.

❑ **Step 14: Using Appropriate Products and Methods for Detailed Cleaning:** This step focuses on selecting non-toxic cleaning products to ensure a healthy, chemical-irritant-free environment, particularly for those with sensitivities.

❑ **Step 15: Avoidance of Trapped Moisture Problems Caused by Sealants and Encapsulants:** Here, I emphasize avoiding sealants and encapsulants that can trap moisture. I will introduce methods for use in Stage Five for airtight yet moisture-managing installations and focus on long-term building health and mold prevention through effective moisture control.

Stage Four: Quality Control and Monitoring

Quality control methods like visual inspection and testing are reviewed to confirm successful mold growth removal and cleaning. A thorough evaluation is prioritized to avoid premature reconstruction that could trap mold, emphasizing remediation effectiveness, safety, and healthfulness.

❑ **Step 16: Visual Surface Evaluation for Cleaning Effectiveness:** Step 16 involves using visual inspections during and after cleaning to monitor surface cleanliness and identify potential hidden conditions needing further attention.

❑ **Step 17: Progress Monitoring Using Theatrical Fog, Surface, and Pathways™ Testing:** This step emphasizes conducting thorough surface evaluations post-cleaning, using Pathways™ and theatrical fog testing methods to objectively verify that surfaces meet or exceed health and safety standards, ensuring successful mold remediation and identifying potential hidden issues.

❑ **Step 18: Third-Party Verification:** This step focuses on balancing the unique needs of medically important remediation with legal, real estate, and insurance requirements, ensuring safety for sensitive individuals while adhering to external standards.

Stage Five: Post-Remediation Reconstruction and Maintenance

Stage Five transitions to post-remediation reconstruction and maintenance, focusing on sustaining long-term environmental health by maintaining remediation gains and establishing preventive practices against future mold and water damage.

❑ **Step 19: Confirmation of Remediation Success before Reconstruction:** This step uses Pathways™ Testing to confirm reduced mold levels and establishes a maintenance testing schedule for early detection of new issues.

❑ **Step 20: Water Source Identification and Management:** This step focuses on identifying and managing moisture sources, such as finding and repairing leaks and balancing ventilation with moisture control, before reconstruction to prevent future water damage and mold, ensuring comprehensive repair and minimizing recurrence risks.

❑ **Step 21: Reconstruction:** This step emphasizes using mold-resistant materials and water management strategies during reconstruction, drawing insights from *Prescriptions for a Healthy House* for health-conscious, sustainable, and mold-preventive building and remodeling.

❑ **Step 22: Establish a Routine Effective Cleaning Schedule:** This Step shows how to use Pathways™ Testing to establish a cleaning schedule for long-term mold control of building memory and to maintain a safe, healthy building environment.

❑ **Step 23: Establishing a Maintenance Plan and Periodic Monitoring Schedule:** In this step, you are guided to create a maintenance plan and periodic monitoring schedule to proactively detect and address new issues. The plan focuses on regular inspections of moisture-prone areas to maintain the integrity of the remediation work and prevent future costs.

❑ **Step 24: Revise Your Maintenance Plan as Needed:** Step 24 focuses on regularly updating the maintenance plan to accommodate climate change and environmental shifts, ensuring long-term responsiveness and effectiveness for the health and safety of your living space.

❑ **Step 25: Develop a Budget and Contingency Fund:** This step emphasizes developing a comprehensive budget and contingency fund for routine maintenance and unexpected mold-related expenses. These are crucial for long-term property health and stability.

LIMITATIONS, COMPLICATIONS, COMPLEXITIES, AND CONFLICTS

The ANSI/IICRC S520 Standard and its companion document, the ANSI/IICRC S500 Standard, establish the industry benchmarks for professional mold remediation and water damage restoration, respectively. Referred to as "Standards of Care," these guidelines are instrumental in defining the procedures to swiftly mitigate water damage and revert properties to their pre-loss condition, as outlined by the S500. The S520 focuses on returning a home's environment to normal by effectively addressing mold and related organisms.

These standards guide safe and effective practices in mold remediation and water damage restoration. They accommodate the need for flexibility in special cases, like Medically Important Remediation, by incorporating sections on Limitations, Complications, Complexities, and Conflicts. This ensures that remediation efforts can be customized to suit the specific requirements of each scenario, providing a framework for informed decision-making and appropriate adjustments where standard procedures may fall short.

However, for situations labeled as "Medically Important Remediation," the conventional approach outlined in these Standards of Care might not always be adequate. Drawing on over two decades of leadership in developing these standards, particularly in areas addressing project challenges, it's clear that while the S500 and S520 provide a foundation, they must sometimes be supplemented with additional considerations to fully meet the needs of those with significant health concerns related to mold and water damage.

The American National Standards Institute (ANSI) plays a critical role in the standardization process across various industries in the United States. While ANSI itself does not develop standards, it accredits standards developed by other organizations, such as the IICRC, ensuring they meet specific criteria for openness, balance, consensus, and due process. Here are the basic principles that an ANSI-approved standard adheres to:

1. **Consensus:** Standards must be developed through a consensus process involving parties interested in the standard. This means that all views and objections must be considered, and an effort must be made to resolve any objections.

2. **Due Process:** The standard development process must be open to all parties affected by it, providing equal opportunity to participate and express views. Clear, documented procedures for submitting comments and mechanisms for resolving differing opinions should exist.

3. **Openness:** Participation in the standard development process is open to all persons directly and materially affected by the activity in question. Any single interest category, individual, or organization should not dominate the process.

4. **Balance:** The standards development process should have a balance of interests without any single interest group dominating the process. This ensures that the standard reflects a broad range of interests and is not biased towards any particular party.

5. **Public Comment and Right to Appeal:** Draft standards must be made available for public review and comment so that a broad audience can provide input. Additionally, there must be a process for addressing and resolving appeals regarding the standard or the standards development process.

6. **Evidence of Compliance:** There must be a clear and accessible process to demonstrate that the principles of due process, consensus, and other requirements are being followed in developing the standard.

7. **Harmonization:** Efforts should be made to avoid duplicating other standards. Where possible, developing new standards should be harmonized with existing international and national standards to contribute to global standardization.

8. **Clarity and Objectivity:** Standards should be written in clear, concise language with objective criteria for compliance to facilitate understanding and application.

By adhering to these principles, ANSI ensures that the standards it approves are developed in a manner that is equitable, accessible, and responsive to the requirements of various stakeholders, thereby enhancing their credibility and acceptance both nationally and internationally.

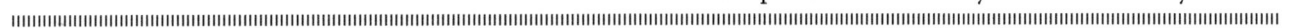

Here's a closer look at what the S520 says about Limitations, Complications, Complexities and Complaints:

Limitations

A "limitation" is a restriction placed by others upon a remediator that limits the scope of work, the remediation activities, or the expected outcomes. Before beginning non-emergency work, known or anticipated limitations and their consequences should be understood, discussed, and approved in writing by remediators and the owner or owner's agent. —IICRC, 2024

Examples:

- **Health-related Limitations:** If the property owner or occupants have health issues, especially chemical sensitivities, mold remediation chemicals and methods may not be suitable. Instead, remediators might need to use soaps or detergent cleaning agents instead of more aggressive, unnecessary strategies that are often problematic for people with environmental sensitivities or medically important issues.

- **Structural Limitations:** Some buildings, particularly historic ones, may have structural limitations that prevent standard remediation activities. For instance, removing mold-infested plaster without damaging historical features may be impossible, requiring less invasive mold stabilization or cleaning methods.

- **Financial Limitations:** Budget constraints might limit the extent of remediation or restoration efforts that can be undertaken. As a result, a remediator may need to target some areas for more frequent cleaning if mold removal and repair are delayed.

- **Equipment Limitations:** Access to state-of-the-art remediation equipment may be limited due to availability or cost. This can restrict the remediation process to more manual methods, potentially reducing efficiency and effectiveness.

- **Space Limitations:** Tight spaces like crawlspaces or attics may not be easily accessible for standard remediation equipment and crews. This could necessitate using smaller, portable equipment and may limit the thoroughness of remediation work.

- **Time Limitations:** Time constraints may limit the scope of remediation. For instance, if a property needs to be habitable quickly after water damage, drying methods might need to be accelerated, possibly affecting the long-term efficacy of the remediation.

- **Regulatory Limitations:** Local regulations or building codes may restrict the methods or disposal of materials used in mold remediation and restoration, potentially limiting the choices for a remediator.

- **Availability of Professionals:** The availability of qualified mold remediation professionals may be limited in each area, affecting the timing and possibly the quality of the remediation work.

Each limitation requires a customized approach to address mold or water damage as effectively as possible within the constraints presented. Each limitation may result in conditions that could render mold remediation ineffective for people with hypersensitivities to mold.

It's crucial to recognize that the Standard stipulates a clear understanding of the dynamics of project limitations. The property owner exclusively has the authority to consent to any limitations. All constraints on the remediation's scope, practices, or expected outcomes should be transparently communicated to the owner for explicit agreement. While this protects both the remediator and the owner, it can occasionally result in remediation being temporarily on hold during negotiations of these specifics.

When a third party with a material interest but does not represent the owner attempts to impose limitations, remediation professionals are obligated by the Standard of Care to decline such directions. Instead, they should immediately consult with the property owner or their representative to relay the proposed limitations. An insurance adjuster, for instance, is not authorized to prescribe how remediation work should be executed. Their role is to assess the claim according to the policy's terms, determining a payout that reflects the insurance company's obligations based on the policy details. It is then incumbent upon the owner to understand that if the insurance does not cover work essential for the health and safety of the occupants, they reserve the right to finance those aspects of the work independently.

This procedure guarantees alignment among all involved parties, with limitations that are carefully evaluated, formally approved, and duly documented. Such a measure is instrumental in maintaining the integrity of the remediation process and ensuring the property owner's rights are respected.

Complexities

A "complexity" is a condition that causes a project to be more difficult or detailed but does not prevent remediators from performing work adequately. Before beginning non-emergency work, known complexities and their consequences should be understood, discussed, and approved in writing by remediators and the owner or owner's agent. —IICRC, 2024

Examples:

- **Historical Properties:** Remediation in historical buildings can present complexities due to the need to preserve original architecture and materials while effectively addressing mold.

- **Multiple Stakeholders:** Projects involving multiple stakeholders, such as tenants, property management companies, and condominium Homeowners' Associations, can complicate decision-making and communication.

- **Advanced Mold Infestation:** Mold infestation penetrating structural elements may require sophisticated remediation techniques, engineering input to prevent building shifting or collapse, and additional protective measures for workers and occupants.

- **Environmental Regulations:** Navigating environmental regulations regarding the use and disposal of chemicals and materials can add complexity to a project, particularly in areas with strict environmental protection laws.

- **High-Risk Occupants:** Properties housing individuals with compromised immune systems or hypersensitivity to exposure that could result in anaphylaxis or other emergency conditions require additional controls and precautions, complicating standard remediation practices.

- **Concurrent Construction:** Performing mold remediation in an environment where construction or renovation is also happening can be complex due to dust, debris, and the coordination of different work crews.

- **Difficult Access:** Locations with difficult access, such as high-rise buildings or remote areas, can introduce complexities in transporting equipment and crew, affecting the remediation timeline and methods.

- **HVAC Systems:** Remediation involving HVAC systems can be complex because of the potential for cross-contamination and the challenge of accessing ductwork throughout the property.

- **Materials with High Porosity:** Addressing mold in highly porous materials like carpet or insulation, which are difficult or impossible to clean, often requires complete removal, adding complexity in logistics and ensuring thorough remediation.

- **Insurance Coverage Disputes:** When insurance coverage is involved, complexities arise in aligning the remediation work with what is covered under the policy. This requires careful negotiation and documentation of disputes and what each party agrees to pay for.

These complexities necessitate a well-thought-out approach that considers the implications and incorporates appropriate adjustments to standard remediation and documentation procedures to ensure effective and efficient project completion.

Complications

A "complication" is a condition that arises after the start of work and causes or necessitates a change in the scope of activities because the project becomes more complex, intricate, or perplexing. The owner or owner's agent should be notified in writing as soon as practical regarding complications that develop. The presence of project complications can necessitate a written change order. —IICRC, 2024

Examples:

- **Unexpected Structural Damage:** Discovering hidden structural damage, such as weakened floors or walls, can significantly complicate remediation efforts, requiring additional repairs and potentially altering the project scope.

- **Secondary Mold Infestations:** Uncovering additional mold infestations in areas not initially identified can complicate the remediation process, expanding the scope and duration of the project.

- **Water Source Identification Difficulties:** Identifying the precise source of water intrusion can be complicated, as effective remediation depends on addressing the root cause of moisture.

- **Hazardous Material Discovery:** Finding asbestos, lead paint, or other hazardous materials during remediation can complicate the project, necessitating specialized removal procedures and potentially halting work until proper safety measures are implemented.

- **Technological Failures:** Equipment malfunctions or failures, such as dehumidifiers or air filtration devices breaking down or power failures, can complicate the drying and cleaning process, delaying project timelines and potentially resulting in a release of contamination to otherwise unaffected portions of the building.

- **Adverse Environmental Conditions:** Extreme weather conditions, such as high humidity or temperatures, can complicate drying efforts and mold control, requiring adjustments to the standard remediation strategies.

- **Occupant Health Issues:** If occupants experience health issues during or after the commencement of remediation work, this may necessitate reassessing the remediation strategy and additional safety measures.

- **Legal or Regulatory Hurdles:** Encountering unforeseen legal or regulatory requirements can complicate the project, particularly if additional permits or inspections are required that were not initially anticipated.

- **Cross-Contamination Risks:** The risk of cross-contaminating other areas of the property during remediation efforts can introduce complications, necessitating the implementation of containment measures and possibly expanding the project scope.

- **Communication Breakdowns:** Miscommunications between the remediation team, property owner, and other stakeholders can lead to complications, especially if there are misunderstandings regarding the scope, expectations, or progress of the project.

Addressing these complications often requires prompt communication, flexibility in project management, and sometimes a change order to account for scope, timeline, or budget adjustments.

Conflicts

"Conflicts" are defined as limitations, complexities, or complications that result in a disagreement between the parties involved about how the remediation project is to be performed. Mutual agreements to resolve conflicts should be documented in writing, and releases, waivers, and disclaimers should be reviewed by a qualified attorney. —IICRC, 2024

Examples:

- **Scope of Work Disagreements:** Conflicts can emerge when the property owner and the remediation team differ in opinion regarding the extent of the work required. For instance, the owner may need more extensive remediation than initially agreed upon or push for less to save costs, contrary to the remediator's professional assessment.

- **Methodology Differences:** There might be conflicts over the remediation methods employed. For example, the remediation team might recommend a method the owner believes is too disruptive or expensive, or the owner might request a specific technique that the remediator deems ineffective or unsafe.

- **Financial Constraints:** Conflicts often occur when the remediation cost exceeds the owner's budget or the amount covered by insurance. This can lead to disagreements over which aspects of remediation are essential and which can be postponed or eliminated.

- **Scheduling Issues:** Timing conflicts may arise if the property owner needs the remediation completed by a certain date, but the remediators find that a thorough job requires more time, possibly due to unforeseen issues like hidden mold or structural challenges.

- **Insurance Company Disputes:** There can be conflicts with insurance adjusters concerning coverage limits and what constitutes necessary remediation. Adjusters may deny certain claims the remediation team and owner feel are crucial for a comprehensive resolution.

- **Health and Safety Standards:** Disagreements may arise over the need for certain health and safety measures, such as the level of containment or personal protective equipment required.

- **Third-Party Recommendations:** Conflicts can surface when a third-party consultant or expert recommends a different course of action than the one proposed by the remediator, leading to confusion and potential disagreements on how to proceed.

- **Quality of Work:** The property owner may be unsatisfied with the work's quality, perceiving it as substandard or incomplete, which conflicts with the remediator's belief that the work meets industry standards.

- **Communication Breakdowns:** Misunderstandings or lack of clear communication can lead to conflicts about project expectations, updates, and outcomes.

- **Post-Remediation Concerns:** Even after the remediation is completed, conflicts may arise if new mold issues appear, leading to disputes about the efficacy of the remediation and who is responsible for additional work.

Although the ANSI/IICRC S500 and S520 standards do not specifically address Medically Important Remediation, the Limitations, Complications, Complexities, and Conflicts Section provides a framework for navigating the intricacies when people are being made ill by their home. This provides an important way to ensure that all parties are informed, consent is obtained, and any necessary deviations from standard practices are carefully considered and applied, prioritizing the health and safety of individuals with specific needs.

PERSONALIZING THE PROCESS: WHEN THE 25 STEPS AREN'T A PERFECT FIT

We've already explored strategies for rehabilitating properties affected by mold for those planning to retain ownership. Yet, your intentions for the property might vary. As you begin working with this book to resolve issues particular to your situation, it helps to reassess the 25 Steps, recognizing that your distinct objectives may require customized adjustments. The applicability and enactment of each step can differ greatly, highlighting the need for an individualized plan. The pertinence and execution of each step can vary widely, underscoring the need for a personalized plan. Following are scenarios that may necessitate a distinctive approach to implementing the steps:

If You are Mold Sensitive and Already Own the Property, But Plan on Never Returning

Fixing and Selling Your Moldy Property: The focus here shifts to addressing mold issues concerning any potential buyer. While personal health sensitivities are less of a direct consideration, ensuring the property is remediated to a legally compliant and marketable standard is important. Getting full market value likely means investing in remediation that significantly reduces mold levels and repairs any water damage that could deter buyers, but not necessarily to the level that a mold-sensitive individual would require for their own habitation. Selling a home with mold intertwines legal obligations with ethical responsibility. Some states' "buyer beware" policies may not mandate disclosure, but honesty and transparency remain paramount. When asked, directly lying about mold issues or water damage may constitute fraud with severe legal and ethical implications. This ethical complexity deepens in a competitive market where homes often sell "as is," potentially disadvantaging buyers with mold sensitivities.

Moreover, the Federal Fair Housing Act's requirements for reasonable accommodations when selling to individuals with disabilities, including mold sensitivities, emphasize the need for sellers to avoid discriminatory practices. Sellers are encouraged to disclose known issues and permit buyer due diligence, aligning with both ethical standards and legal requirements. This fosters a transparent, equitable housing market that respects the rights and needs of all parties, especially those with disabilities.

Other Scenarios That You May Consider Include:

- Fixing and Renting Out Your Moldy Property
- Selling Your Moldy Property 'As-Is'
- Considerations for Purchasing an Existing Home
- Considerations for Buying a Condominium
- Scouting for a Mold-Controlled Rental Home
- Considerations for Renting a Condominium
- Scouting for a Mold-Controlled Apartment
- Temporary Measures for Motels, Hotels and Air B&Bs:
- Motor Homes, Vehicles, Tiny Homes, Cabins.
- Buying and Flipping a Moldy Property
- Restoring an Apartment Affected by Mold
- Scenario Twelve—Short-term Emergency Mold-Controlled Housing
- Building a Mold-Controlled Home

Each scenario requires a nuanced understanding of the 25 Steps, with adaptations made to suit the unique challenges and goals of the situation. This flexibility ensures that your mold control approach is practical and situationally appropriate whether you're selling, renting, flipping, or building.

Stage One: Is There a Problem? Assessment and Planning

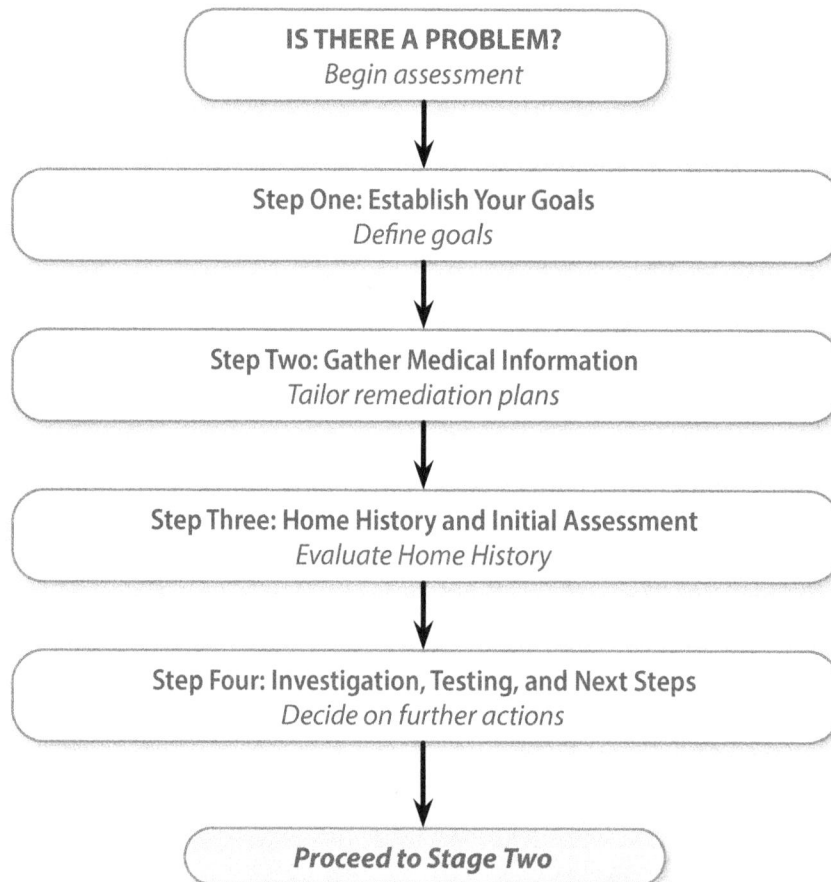

```
┌─────────────────────────────────┐
│      IS THERE A PROBLEM?        │
│        Begin assessment         │
└─────────────────────────────────┘
                │
                ▼
┌─────────────────────────────────┐
│   Step One: Establish Your Goals │
│          Define goals           │
└─────────────────────────────────┘
                │
                ▼
┌─────────────────────────────────┐
│ Step Two: Gather Medical Information │
│      Tailor remediation plans    │
└─────────────────────────────────┘
                │
                ▼
┌─────────────────────────────────┐
│ Step Three: Home History and Initial Assessment │
│       Evaluate Home History      │
└─────────────────────────────────┘
                │
                ▼
┌─────────────────────────────────┐
│ Step Four: Investigation, Testing, and Next Steps │
│       Decide on further actions  │
└─────────────────────────────────┘
                │
                ▼
┌─────────────────────────────────┐
│       Proceed to Stage Two       │
└─────────────────────────────────┘
```

Empowered Decisions: Your Home, Your Health, Your Plan

In this foundational stage, whether you're a homeowner, renter, or looking for a different living arrangement, you'll evaluate the living space for signs of mold or water damage. It's about collecting and organizing essential information regarding the history and current condition of the property. This stage equips you with the tools to document and interpret these findings, empowering you to make informed decisions about your living environment. The focus is on your needs and goals for you and your family, guiding you to formulate a clear action plan. While you might seek assistance from family, friends, neighbors, or professionals, the emphasis is on fulfilling your objectives for a healthy and safe space. This stage also introduces the concept of an 'exit plan'—a crucial consideration if the severity of issues suggests that moving might be a more viable option than attempting remediation. By the end of this stage, you'll have a solid foundation for either embarking on a remediation journey or making a well-informed decision to find a healthier environment that better suits your needs.

STAGE ONE GOALS: BIG PICTURE STUFF – WHAT MOTIVATES YOU TO MOVE FORWARD?

Once you have completed the four Steps in Stage One, you should be prepared to answer these questions:

- Is there a problem with water damage, mold, or other water damage-related problems in your home?

- Is the information collected sufficient to help a physician, well versed in mold and water damage exposure, determine if the condition of your home is likely to be impacting the health of one or more occupants?

- Do you need to proceed to Stage Two to determine the sources and locations of any hidden issues in the home and see what will likely be involved in resolving them?

- Do you want or need to begin the search for another place that presents better temporary or permanent options for health and well-being for you and your family?

Step 1: Establish Your Goals

Shaping Your Mold Control Strategy

This marks your initial step in navigating the 25 Step process tailored for effective mold control in your home. Use this Step to help you determine what you want to achieve and how to tailor this process to meet your specific needs and achieve your mold control goals. This process can also help you set your levels of expectation for yourself and your situation to effectively address mold and water damage, guiding your journey from urgent crisis management to a lasting, healthy home.

Exercise 1.1: Begin a Project Diary

Objective: Starting a project diary to document your experiences and findings while performing the exercises is an invaluable step toward mastering your indoor environment. By keeping a detailed record, you create a personalized reference tool that tracks your progress and helps identify patterns, triggers, and practical solutions specific to your situation. This project diary should be kept separate from a medical diary, which you will begin in Step 2. There are compelling reasons for maintaining these diaries independently: to delineate indoor environmental quality observations regarding your home from health symptoms and help facilitate a clear, effective, more targeted analysis and intervention strategy for each. Keeping the entries in the project diary factually objective and goal-oriented is essential. If you need to vent or express personal frustration, anger, or other emotions, consider keeping those reflections in a separate personal diary. This approach ensures the project diary remains a focused and professional tool for analysis and communication, providing clear and organized information to share with selected professionals while maintaining your ability to decide when medical confidentiality should be maintained.

Begin by recording the Property Identification information such as address, rent, own, and other special considerations or arrangements.

Exercise 1.2: What is Your Role?

Define your role in the 25 Step remediation process and record your responsibilities in your project diary accordingly.

❑ **Homeowner:** As a homeowner, you are responsible for making decisions regarding the property and will likely bear the ultimate financial burden of remediation. You or members of your household are directly affected by the outcome of the remediation process. You are also responsible for maintaining communication with all parties involved.

❑ **Tenant:** If you are a tenant, you experience the issue firsthand but may not have the authority to make remediation decisions. Your responsibilities include communicating problems to the landlord or property manager and coordinating with them for access to facilitate remediation efforts. In cases where the landlord or property management company is unwilling or unable to help, you might need to negotiate or consider an exit strategy.

❑ **Family Member/Significant Person:** As a family member or significant person involved with someone affected, you might be directly or indirectly responsible for remediation decisions and could be a primary caregiver or support person for the affected individual. Your role includes advocating for the health and safety of the affected family member and possibly coordinating remediation efforts.

❑ **Health Coach/Assistant/Friend:** For those in the role of a health coach, assistant, clergy, or friend, it is unlikely that you will bear the financial burden of remediation or be responsible for property-related decisions. However, you may still significantly impact the outcome of the remediation process. Your responsibilities might include supporting the affected individual, advocating for their health and safety, and helping coordinate efforts as needed.

By clearly identifying and understanding your role, you can better navigate the remediation process and ensure that all necessary steps are taken to address mold issues effectively.

Exercise 1.3—What Is Your Current Situation?

This exercise encourages you to concisely articulate the concerns, challenges, and problems you're facing in your current living situation due to water damage or mold. The aim is not to find immediate solutions but to clearly define and acknowledge the issues. This understanding will serve as the foundation for the subsequent steps, guiding you toward effective strategies to address these challenges.

❑ **Health Concerns:** Begin by briefly describing any health issues you, your family, or household members are experiencing that might be related to current or past mold or water damage conditions. Provide a general overview of the information someone not immediately and directly involved with your health care would need to know to assist you. This is not the place for noting specific symptoms or medical diagnostics, but general information, such as listing the affected individuals in the household and a general synopsis of their condition (CIRS, Asthma, Allergies, Multiple Chemical Sensitivities, and other general relevant information).

❑ **Home Environmental Issues:** Outline the conditions in your home that are causing concern or the purpose for the evaluation. List immediate triggers such as musty odors, visible mold, dampness, and humidity issues. Note any observations that make you believe mold or water damage is present. This should be a general overview, as more in-depth analysis will follow in Step 3.

❑ **Interactions with Others:** It is important to document your interactions with others, such as contractors, landlords, property maintenance workers, property managers, or others regarding home environmental issues.

Use the **Project Diary** to record facts, observations, and professional-level considerations. Keep it objective and free from emotional or unprofessional comments, as contractors, insurers, or legal professionals may review it. Reserve the **Personal Diary** for venting, anger, and personal musings to ensure the project diary remains credible and useful while giving yourself a space to process emotions privately.

❑ **Current Impact on Your Life:** Reflect on the Non-Health impacts of these issues on the daily life of each person living in the affected home. Determine if this is factual information that should go in the project diary or thoughts that are more appropriate for your personal diary:

• **Family Dynamics:** Examine how tensions or changes in responsibilities have altered the interactions and harmony within the household.

• **Stress:** Note the increased stress levels stemming from the need to address and manage water damage, mold, cleanup, and mitigation efforts.

• **Anxiety:** Acknowledge worry or unease about the health implications, financial costs, and the overall remediation process.

• **Financial Strains:** Detail the economic burden caused by remediation costs, potential loss in property value, and unexpected expenses.

• **Legal & Insurance:** Document challenges include navigating insurance claims, understanding coverage limitations, and resolving legal disputes arising from the damage.

• **Living Conditions:** Reflect on disruptions or inconveniences in your living environment, including temporary relocations, loss of personal belongings, or living in a construction zone.

• **Work:** Consider how these issues have affected your professional life, whether through lost work, decreased productivity, or the need to take time off.

• **School:** Discuss the impact on children's learning environments, including distractions, absences, or the need to move to temporary accommodations.

• **Social Life:** Note changes in your ability to host or participate in social activities or feelings of isolation due to the situation.

• **Time:** Evaluate the significant time commitment required for insurance, contractors, and the restoration process.

• **Peace of Mind:** Consider how ongoing concerns have disrupted your sense of security and comfort in your home.

• **Overall Well-being:** Reflect on the cumulative effect of these issues on your mental, emotional, and social well-being.

• **Long-term Plans:** Consider how your plans, such as selling your home, undertaking renovations, or considering a change in living situations, have been influenced.

• **Personal Relationships:** Document the strain or support experienced in relationships with family, friends, and neighbors, highlighting any notable changes or challenges.

• **Other Impacts:** Identify any additional areas of your life affected by the water damage and mold issues that have not previously been covered.

Exercise 1.4: When Did You Begin this Journey?

Reflect on when you first became aware of the possibility of mold or water damage health issues. Understanding the timeline helps assess the problem's progression and the urgency of the required actions. Provide a general overview; a more in-depth analysis of the origins and path you have followed to address health issues will follow in Step 2 Exercises.

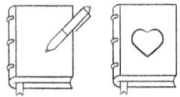

*(Use the **Project Diary** to record facts, observations, and professional-level considerations, keeping it objective and free from emotional or unprofessional comments, as it may be reviewed by contractors, insurers, or legal professionals. Reserve the **Personal Diary** for venting, anger, and personal musings to ensure the project diary remains credible and useful while giving yourself a space to process emotions privately.)*

❑ **Consider What You Suspect and What You Know:** The following will help summarize the history of the situation that has brought you to today. Try to begin each sentence with one of the following to indicate your degree of certainty:

I know that (objective comment):

I suspect that (subjective comment):

I wonder if (a question that remains to be answered):

› **First Suspicions Noted:** Identify the earliest signs or symptoms of potential mold or water damage. Consider the certainty of these signs or symptoms: What do you know, suspect, or wonder?

› **Initial Discovery:** Note the moment or event when mold or water damage was discovered. Evaluate the certainty of this discovery and whether it was conclusively identified as mold or water damage.

› **Seeking Information:** Reflect on when you began researching mold and water damage. Determine the certainty of the information found and its sources. Grade the value of this information in understanding your situation.

› **Professional Consultation:** Document your first consultation with a professional, if any. Consider the certainty of their assessment and the clarity of the next steps they provided. Evaluate the helpfulness of this engagement in advancing your action plan.

› **Taking Action:** Mark if actions to address the mold or water damage were initiated. Assess the certainty of these actions being the correct ones and their potential impact. Rate how valuable these steps were in mitigating the issue.

› **Awareness of Severity:** Determine when the severity of the issue and its potential impacts became clear. Evaluate the certainty of this realization and its implications. Assess how this awareness influences your decisions and actions.

› **Documentation and Evidence Gathering**: Note when systematic documentation began. Consider the certainty and completeness of this evidence and its usefulness in supporting your concerns. Rate the helpfulness of this documentation.

› **Broadening Understanding:** Reflect on moments of significant learning. Consider the certainty and reliability of this new knowledge. Grade its value in enriching your understanding and shaping your response.

› **Community Engagement:** If you joined support groups or forums, mark this engagement. Reflect on the certainty of the support and information received. Assess how valuable or supportive these communities have been in your journey.

SETTING YOUR GOALS

You have so far been reflecting on your situation. It is now time to look to the future and set some goals.

Exercise 1.5: Where Do You Want or Need to Live?

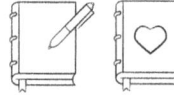

Start by considering your ideal living situation, both in the short and long term. Do you plan to stay in your current home post-remediation, or are you looking for temporary or permanent relocation?

❑ Begin by identifying your immediate needs for safety and comfort, such as finding a temporary place to stay or setting up a safe space or sanctuary within your home. Then, think about your longer-term goals: where you want to be in a month, a year, and even ten years. Use these reflections to guide your actions and decisions throughout the remediation process.

Exercise 1.6: Why Do You Want a Mold-Controlled Home?

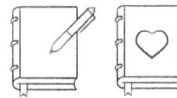

Understanding your core motivations will help you focus on creating a mold-controlled environment.

❑ Consider whether health concerns, the need for better air quality, protecting property value, or ensuring your family's well-being drive you. Identifying your primary motivations will allow you to prioritize the most important aspects of mold control and align your actions with your goals.

Exercise 1.7: How Motivated Are You to Achieve Your Goal?

Evaluate your commitment to creating a mold-controlled home.

❑ Consider how much time, effort, and financial resources you're willing to invest, as well as your willingness to learn and adapt. Reflect on your emotional resilience and the support you have from family and friends. Understanding your motivation level will help you set realistic goals and tailor your remediation plan to match your dedication.

Exercise 1.8: What Resources Do You Have?

Take stock of the resources available to you for your mold remediation efforts.

❑ Consider your financial resources, support networks, access to professionals, and the time you can realistically dedicate to the process. Document these resources in your diary, as this will help you plan effectively and identify any additional support or resources you may need.

REVIEW OF ESTABLISHING GOALS

By reaching this stage, you have diligently gathered and documented a wealth of information in your project diary. The journey is dynamic, requiring periodic reassessment of your goals and strategies based on new insights and evolving circumstances. It's essential to recognize that the goal-setting section is not static; it is expected to undergo revisions as you progress and your understanding deepens. Such revisions reflect your growing awareness and adaptability in managing your indoor environment.

This section has served as a foundational tool, enabling you to capture a snapshot of your current housing situation and set the stage for targeted action. Maintaining an accurate and up-to-date record cannot be overstated as you move forward. It will act as a roadmap, guiding your efforts and allowing you to measure progress over time.

Exercise 1.9: Clarifying Your Goals and Focus

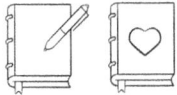

As you progress through this 25 Step process to achieve a *Mold Controlled* home, it's essential to clarify your primary goals and understand how they align with your circumstances. Each household's needs differ based on health considerations, genetic predispositions, and long-term aspirations for home stewardship; by identifying where you and your household fit among the following categories, you can better tailor this process to meet your unique needs.

Use the descriptions below to reflect on your priorities and establish a clear focus for your *Mold Controlled* journey:

❏ Normal, Resilient, or Unaffected Occupants

Individuals without known sensitivities to mold or water-damage organisms within their household. Concerns typically center on how water damage or mold affects the home's aesthetics and functionality. The primary goals are maintaining a resilient, dry, and functional home to prevent costly repairs and maintain a healthy living space for healthy people, focusing on prevention and general upkeep.

❏ Medically At-Risk Occupants

Individuals genetically predisposed to mold sensitivity or other health conditions who are not currently exhibiting symptoms but could be affected by external stressors in the future. The primary goal is to maintain a home free of environmental stressors that might activate latent sensitivities, with a focus on prevention and creating a safe, low-risk living environment.

❏ Medically Compromised Occupants

Individuals actively experiencing health conditions worsened by mold or water-damage organisms, often without full awareness of the environmental connection. The primary goal is to establish a safe and controlled living environment to prevent further health impacts and support recovery, focusing on rigorous remediation, ongoing monitoring, and tailored adjustments to the home.

❏ Home Stewards

Individuals who may belong to any of the previous categories but view home health as part of a broader commitment to life enhancement. You prioritize creating an optimal living environment while considering the future well-being of others who may occupy the home. Your goal is to achieve the highest level of environmental quality, emphasizing resilience, health, and sustainability, with a focus on excellence in stewardship for long-term benefits.

This book is written for individuals committed to creating healthy homes, whether for personal well-being, family health, or stewardship. While some property owners or managers may be disinterested in addressing these issues, neglecting mold and water damage not only compromises the health of occupants but also leads to long-term financial and legal liabilities. For those managing rental properties, it's worth noting that maintaining a mold-controlled environment benefits both tenant retention and property value.

Step 2: Gather Medical Information to Tailor Remediation Plans

Bridging Health & Habitat

This step is focused on collecting health information relevant to exposure to mold and organisms typically found in water-damaged environments. Documenting this information in a diary is highly recommended, as it aids in customizing your remediation plan to the needs of the most vulnerable individual in your household. This process will guide you in making informed decisions about your living arrangements before and during the remediation. Prioritizing health and safety is crucial, as well as ensuring that the remediation strategy aligns with the specific health requirements of each family member.

A team approach to medically important investigations and remediation often proves most effective in addressing mold and water damage-related health concerns. All parties involved must handle these situations with appropriate care. When a third party, such as an Indoor Environmental Professional or a remediation specialist, needs to discuss your health issues related to mold with your physician, strict adherence to privacy protocols is essential. These measures protect your medical information and ensure respectful, confidential communication in compliance with healthcare privacy laws.

Furthermore, as someone dealing with mold-related health issues for you or your family, your informed consent is paramount when third parties communicate with your physician. All parties, including environmental consultants, remediators, technicians, and physicians, need your permission to discuss sensitive health topics. The aim of these discussions is clear: to relate mold and water damage aspects of your health to your remediation requirements. Effective collaboration with your physician is achieved through a team approach, where each member, including you, plays a vital role in your health recovery and in ensuring your post-remediation home is healthful. Documenting all interactions ensures consensus and respects the primary patient-physician relationship. Legal compliance with healthcare privacy laws, such as HIPAA in the United States, is critical to safeguard your private information. By being informed and involved, you can ensure that communication with your physician maintains ethical standards and prioritizes your well-being in mold and water damage-related health issues. This collaborative and patient-centered approach is key to successfully resolving mold-related health concerns, benefiting the patient, physician, and all professionals involved.

Disclaimers and Limitations

Some exercises provided in this book are designed to assist readers in identifying aspects related to exposure-related symptoms of mold and water-damage organisms, such as conditions like Chronic Inflammatory Response Syndrome (CIRS), as well as in compiling information about other health conditions that may be caused by or exacerbated by such organisms.

It is important to emphasize that the exercises are not a substitute for professional medical advice, diagnosis, or treatment. They are intended for educational and informational purposes only and are focused primarily on your home. If you have concerns about your health, medical conditions, or potential exposure to mold and water-damage organisms, it is imperative to consult with a qualified healthcare provider or medical professional.

Individual health circumstances vary widely, and the exercises offer guidance and promote understanding. However, they should not be used as a basis for medical decisions. The author and publisher do not assume responsibility or liability for actions or decisions based on the book or its exercises. Always prioritize your health and well-being by seeking guidance from qualified healthcare experts when addressing medical concerns or conditions.

Exercise 2.1 Starting a Personal Health Diary

This is the symbol that will alert you to record entries in your health diary. Almost all of the information you develop during this step should be recorded in your health diary. Each affected person should have a separate Health Diary to help avoid confusing entries and records.

Objective: The aim of this exercise is to begin a detailed health diary that tracks your or your family member's health conditions concerning mold and water damage exposure. This is a different diary than the one you started in Exercise 1, which relates to the project with your home. This diary will be a valuable tool for observing changes over time, identifying what is working, and recognizing what isn't regarding health and environmental conditions.

❏ **Step-by-Step Guidance:** Select a diary format that suits your daily routine and ensures consistent use. Whether it's a traditional physical notebook, a digital document, or a specialized health-tracking app, choose the medium that you find most convenient and accessible. The chosen format should be adaptable enough to integrate the information from these 25 Steps Exercises. This integration is key for effectively correlating your personal health observations and actions with the changes and interventions made in your home environment. The goal is to create a comprehensive record that reflects your health journey and the evolution of your living space.

❏ **Daily Health Logging:** Each day, make a detailed record of any symptoms or health changes experienced by vulnerable individuals in your household. Be sure to note the time of day when symptoms occur, their duration, and the severity of each symptom. Upcoming Exercises 2.2 and 2.3 will provide further guidance on tracking and interpreting this health-related information effectively. This consistent daily logging is crucial for identifying patterns and triggers related to health changes and will be instrumental in tailoring your approach to creating a healthier home environment.

❏ **Environmental Observations:** Note any changes or events in your home environment that might correlate with health changes. This includes dampness, new water damage, or any remediation efforts undertaken.

❏ **Medication and Treatment Tracking:** Keep a detailed log of all medications, treatments, herbal remedies, and nutritional supplements used. Document the effectiveness of each and note any side effects experienced. This record will help understand the impact of these treatments on health conditions and provide valuable data to healthcare providers for optimizing treatment plans.

❏ **Physician Interactions:** Document key points from medical appointments, including advice given, changes in treatment, and any specific recommendations related to your living environment.

❏ **Regular Review and Reflection:** Set a regular schedule, perhaps weekly or monthly, to review the diary entries. Look for patterns or correlations between environmental changes and health symptoms.

❏ **Share and Collaborate:** Relevant sections of this diary may be shared with environmental consultants, remediation specialists, and healthcare providers to help guide the assistance they can provide. This collaborative approach allows for a more tailored remediation plan and better-informed decisions regarding your living environment. The insights gleaned from your diary entries can be invaluable in adapting strategies to suit your specific health needs and environmental conditions, ensuring a more effective response to mold and water damage issues.

❏ **Privacy Considerations:** Upholding privacy and complying with healthcare laws is imperative when handling personal health information. Such information should only be shared with authorized individuals, always with informed consent and clear communication that this information is confidential and not for dissemination. It should only be shared on a 'need to know' basis. While your physician is privy to detailed health information, Indoor Environmental Professionals (IEPs), Remediation Specialists, Restorers, and Contractors typically require only the information directly relevant to their role in improving your home environment. For example, disclosing instances of Multiple Chemical Sensitivities (MCS) in your household is essential for those working in your home. This knowledge allows them to take appropriate precautions, such as avoiding strong fragrances in personal care products or helping you select materials your family will tolerate, to ensure a safe and health-conscious environment.

Exercise 2.2 Working with Your Physician

The goal of Exercise 2.2 is to provide you with the tools and knowledge necessary to find and work with a physician who understands medically important exposure to water damage and the associated organisms.

Record the following in your medical diary

❏ If you already have a physician who specializes in exposure to mold and other water-damage organisms, start by recording their information: the physician's name, medical specialty, and contact information (phone/physical address/email). This ensures you have all the necessary details for future reference and communication.

❏ Discuss the importance of collaborating with specialists focused on mold and water damage exposures with your primary care physician. Ensure that your primary care physician is willing to work with functional medicine, integrative medicine, or other health professionals to provide comprehensive care tailored to your needs. This collaborative approach can help address your health concerns more effectively.

Local health departments may be an information resource, although the assistance they offer may vary. They typically recognize that visible mold and wet buildings must be properly addressed and consider these issues in rental housing as a sanitation concern, especially for normal, resilient, or unaffected Occupants. However, they may not offer adequate advice for Medically At-Risk Occupants or Medically Compromised Occupants.

If you are looking for a specialized physician, the following resources can assist you in finding professionals who are experienced in dealing with mold-related health issues. CIRSx.com
SurvivingMold.com
iseai.org/find-a-professional

Exercise 2.3 Summarize Medical Information

This is not a detailed medical record. Its purpose is to help compile information that may be important for selecting the appropriate 'Standard of Practice' level that can be used to target appropriate actions for the person occupying the home.

*Record the following in your medical diary
for each person with related health Issues*

This exercise will help you summarize medical information for each household member potentially affected by exposure to mold or other water-damage-associated organisms. The goal is not to create a detailed medical record but to compile essential information to guide the decisions that lead to an appropriate 'Standard of Practice' for addressing health concerns in your home.

❑ Begin by recording each individual's name and date of birth in the Health Diary. For each household member, document any relevant medical conditions. Indicate whether a healthcare provider has formally diagnosed these conditions or if they are suspected. This initial summary should serve as a general overview; a more detailed analysis will follow in subsequent steps.

Common conditions to consider: If a household member has allergies indicate whether this has been formally diagnosed or is merely suspected, and include the date of the diagnosis or when symptoms were first noticed. Repeat this for each listed condition. If you need help compiling this information, consult with your physician to ensure accuracy.

❑ allergies

❑ asthma

❑ aspergillosis

❑ hyperactive immune system

❑ compromised immune system

❑ hypersensitivity pneumonitis

❑ skin disorders

❑ toxicosis

❑ Chronic Inflammatory Response Syndrome (CIRS)

❑ Any other relevant conditions that may impact the individual's health due to mold or water damage.

By clearly summarizing this medical information, you can better target remediation actions to address the health needs of everyone in the household.

Exercise 2.4 Track Common Symptoms

This exercise will help you summarize medical information for each household member potentially affected by exposure to mold or other water-damage-associated organisms.

Date_____ / Year _____

Check Box if Applies on this Day		Sun	Mon	Tue	Wed	Thu	Fri	Sat
✓	Symptom:	Rate the level of severity from 0 (no symptoms) to 10						
❏	Chronic Fatigue							
❏	Sleep Disorders							
❏	Brain Fog							
❏	Aches, Pain							
❏	Joint Pain							
❏	Facial Pain							
❏	Migraines							
❏	Weakness							
❏	Muscle Cramps							
❏	Morning Stiffness							
❏	Headaches							
❏	Light Sensitivity							
❏	Red Eyes							
❏	Blurred Vision							
❏	Tearing							
❏	Sinus Congestion							
❏	Coughing							
❏	Shortness of Breath							
❏	Word Finding Difficult							
❏	Knowledge Retention Difficulties							
❏	Confusion							
❏	Disorientation							
❏	Rash, Eczema, Hives							
❏	Skin Sensitivity							
❏	Night Sweats							
❏	Mood Swings							
❏	Excessive Thirst							
❏	Static Shocks							
❏	Numbness/Tingling							
❏	Dizziness/Vertigo							
❏	Metallic Tastes							
❏	Abdominal Pain							
❏	Diarrhea							
❏	Tremors							
❏	Appetite Swings							
❏	GI Tract Issues							
❏	Night Urination							
❏	Depression							
❏	Anxiety							
❏	Infertility							
❏	Chemical Sensitivities							
❏	Exercise Intolerance							

Exercise 2.5 Assessment

Look at the subjective information you collected in this Step and share it with your physician. This may lead to additional recommendations for medical evaluation and testing. Have your physician help you integrate and understand the Subjective and Objective data together and use this information to assess the medical information that has been collected.

❑ **Update Your Diary:** As your situation evolves or as you gain new insights, make it a priority to update your diary. This ensures that your documentation remains relevant and reflects the current state of your journey. Consider this a living document, one that evolves alongside your understanding and experiences.

❑ **Advise Your Inner Circle:** The people who form your support network—your inner circle—play a crucial role in your journey. It is crucial to keep them informed of updates to your goals and strategies. Their support, understanding, and assistance can be invaluable, and ensuring they are up-to-date with your plans enhances their ability to provide meaningful help.

❑ **Your physician** can help you track and understand the health information and diagnosis and can help guide you regarding the multiple steps that may be needed. Not every medical condition is about water damage and mold. Coinfections and other medical conditions may have an impact not caused by water damage, but some of these conditions may be exacerbated. (Storey, 2004)

Step 3: Home History and Initial Assessment

Past to Present: Charting Your Home's Water Damage Evolution

This step involves compiling subjective observations and historical data regarding your home. You will begin by noting any visible signs of water damage, such as water stains, wet conditions, visible or suspected mold, musty odors, and documenting known remodeling or additions to the property. You will be guided in utilizing online and other resources to uncover any additional information that might not be immediately apparent. The more comprehensive your assessment, the more targeted and effective subsequent investigative steps will be, helping save time and money. Emphasizing the importance of thorough documentation, this step also highlights the necessity of regularly updating your records to reflect any new findings or changes in the condition of your home.

Exercise 3.1 Answer some basic questions about the home in question
Home Information Questionnaire

This is your first step in gathering details about your current or prospective home. If you're tracking one property, use your diary. For multiple properties, set aside space to track each one separately. A loose-leaf notebook with dividers can help you organize, allowing you to add or remove pages as you make decisions. When recording property information, start with the

❑ **Property Identification,** including the full street address, city, state, and zip code.

❑ **Type of Property**, specifying whether it is a single-family home, apartment, condominium, or a different kind of dwelling. These details are essential for clearly identifying and categorizing the property under consideration.

❑ **Property Facts:** Many facts are available online at real estate listing services such as Zillow, realator.com, or Redfin.

› **Estimate the Square footage of the home or unit:** While smaller buildings are not immune to mold issues, they generally have simpler systems, a smaller area to monitor, and fewer things to go wrong, potentially reducing the risk and cost of mold problems that develop.

› **Estimate the year of completion for the original construction of the building:** Over the years, buildings inevitably age, with different components reaching their useful life expectancy. Wear and tear can accelerate the deterioration, resulting in potential moisture problems like roof leaks or cracked foundations. Building codes and standards have also evolved, meaning older buildings may not meet current requirements for moisture control. Furthermore, the likelihood of past water damage incidents, which can lead to hidden mold growth, is higher in older buildings. Finally, older buildings may contain asbestos or lead-based paint, resulting in additional abatement costs when mold remediation that disturbs these materials is performed.

Past Issues and Repairs

- History of Water Damage or Mold Issues.
- Repairs or Remediation Efforts Undertaken (include dates).
- Maintenance and Inspection History.
- Frequency of Routine Maintenance (e.g., annual, bi-annual).
- Date of Last Professional Inspection (if applicable).

Why: Maintenance is the key to a home's longevity, regardless of age. A building's maintenance history strongly indicates its current condition and potential for future issues. Regular and thorough upkeep of areas such as roofing, plumbing, HVAC systems, and the building envelope is essential to prevent moisture intrusion and mold growth. For potential homeowners or renters, reviewing the maintenance history of a property is crucial. Red flags like frequent repairs in certain areas may point to ongoing issues. When possible, obtaining records of past repairs and maintenance can provide valuable insights into the condition of the building and the care taken by previous owners or tenants. Whether considering the charm and challenges of older homes or the modern appeal and potential rapid deterioration of newer constructions, a vigilant assessment of maintenance history and the property's current condition is vital. This understanding is foundational to choosing to align with your health needs.

Describe the area where the building is located

- Major City (over 100,000 population)
- Minor City (over 10,000 population)

- Town (under 10,000 population)
- Rural
- Other Details (Commercial Center, Industrial, Agricultural, Lake Home, and Mountain Homes)

Why: Understanding the location of your home is crucial in assessing mold and water damage risks. While mold problems can arise in any environment, specific regional characteristics significantly influence these issues. Each region requires a tailored approach to mold prevention and remediation, considering its unique environmental factors and challenges. Understanding these regional differences is key to effectively managing and preventing mold in homes. Some factors to consider:

- Local Building Practices and Materials: These can vary significantly and influence how homes respond to environmental conditions.

- Availability of Remediation Services: Urban areas might have more resources for mold remediation, while rural areas could face challenges in accessing specialized services.

- Community Awareness and Regulations: Local regulations and general awareness about mold can impact how communities manage mold issues.

Exercise 3.2: Consider Building Specific Dynamics and a Changing Climate

Each home faces unique water damage and mold-related challenges influenced by local environmental factors, design, construction practices, and conditions that can increase vulnerability. This section explores how these elements shape mold management issues and aims to equip homeowners and renters with the knowledge to navigate these risks. Climate plays a crucial role in the health and longevity of a building, with regional conditions posing distinct challenges for mold growth and water damage—challenges that are becoming more pronounced as climate change alters traditional weather patterns. Understanding how design, construction, and regional climate affect your home, you can implement targeted strategies to identify a healthier, more resilient living environment. Recognizing these differences is key, not just geographically but also in understanding the environmental dynamics that can make a home more or less vulnerable to mold. This knowledge is essential for selecting or maintaining a home suited to withstand local climate challenges.

Indicate all that apply:

❑ **Older buildings** may have materials that have outlived their useful life expectancy.

Older homes, often admired for their craftsmanship and character, come with unique considerations, particularly regarding hidden histories of water damage. Over time, these structures may have undergone repairs or renovations that failed to address underlying issues, such as water intrusion or mold growth. Homes built before the 1980s may also contain hazardous materials like lead-based paint and asbestos, which pose health risks and complicate mold remediation efforts.

When assessing a potential home, it's crucial to consider the building's age and maintenance history. Older homes are more likely to have experienced deferred maintenance or neglect, increasing the chances of water damage or mold. Additionally, outdated construction materials and methods can make these homes more susceptible to mold and water issues. In some cases, making necessary repairs may be complicated by historical preservation requirements that restrict modifications to the property's visual or architectural features.

❑ **Newer Homes: Modern Materials, Newer Risks**

Newer homes, while free from the historical issues of older constructions, are not immune to mold-related problems. Though advanced, modern building materials and practices often prioritize cost-efficiency and aesthetics over durability and longevity. This can lead to quicker deterioration and increased susceptibility to moisture issues, particularly if the construction does not emphasize proper ventilation or moisture barriers. Though newer homes are less likely to have suffered from neglect, the materials used may be of lower quality, leading to faster development of problems like mold, often hidden behind a seemingly flawless exterior. While these homes may have had less time for poor maintenance to cause issues, their reliance on less durable materials can result in quicker degradation, making them vulnerable to moisture-related concerns.

❑ **Coastal Regions** pose unique challenges for homes due to high humidity and salt-laden air, which accelerate the deterioration and corrosion of building materials, particularly metal components like galvanized flashings and fasteners. As these materials corrode, their ability to prevent water intrusion weakens, increasing the risk of moisture entering the building and promoting mold growth. Wind-driven rains, tropical storms, and hurricanes further exacerbate the problem, making homes in these areas more vulnerable to water damage and structural issues. Regular maintenance and inspections are essential, as homes in coastal regions also face elevated risks from storm surges, flooding, and other extreme weather events that can compromise building integrity and increase the likelihood of mold development.

❑ **Mountainous and forested areas** shaded by trees can limit sunlight exposure, resulting in prolonged dampness that fosters mold growth. Additionally, the cooler temperatures characteristic of such areas can extend drying times, further exacerbating mold problems.

❏ **Regions with ice, snow, and freezing conditions:** homes face unique risks from water seepage caused by snow melt and ice damming. Ice dams form when snow melts on warmer roof sections and refreezes at the colder eaves, creating barriers that prevent proper drainage. This water backup can seep under shingles, leading to water damage and mold growth. Additionally, the freeze/thaw cycle causes building materials to expand and contract, widening cracks and allowing more moisture to penetrate. This process weakens the structure and increases the potential for mold and other water-damaged organisms to take hold. The risk of frozen and burst pipes is also significant, potentially causing severe water damage inside the home.

❏ **Desert Climates and Dry, Arid Regions,** while typically perceived as inhospitable to mold, present unique risks. Substantial temperature fluctuations between day and night cause building materials to repeatedly expand and contract, leading to the early formation of cracks and crevices—potential entry points for moisture. Despite the dry conditions, infrequent but intense rainfall, such as monsoon rains, can overwhelm homes unprepared for water-related issues. The rapid accumulation of rainwater can lead to moisture penetration, providing ideal conditions for mold growth. Intense sunlight, UV exposure, and low humidity also degrade materials, compromising a building's ability to resist moisture.

❏ **Areas Prone to Extreme Weather and Other Anomalies** or events pose significant building risks. Floods, hurricanes, tornadoes, and even earthquakes can rapidly inflict severe water damage on a home. Other conditions, such as drought and high winds, take longer but often lead to compromised building envelopes and internal water intrusion, providing fertile grounds for mold growth if not promptly and adequately addressed. Understanding the local risk factors for such events and preparing for them through building resilience and rapid response plans is crucial. This might include reinforcing structural elements, ensuring proper drainage, and planning for rapid remediation during water intrusion.

❏ **Flood Plains, River Valleys, or Areas with High Flooding Risk** are at risk for bacteria and mold. Floodwater can introduce a variety of contaminants into homes, and lingering moisture provides a breeding ground. Regular inspections and emergency plans for flooding are essential.

❏ **High water tables or groundwater issues** may require specialized drainage, foundation, and basement waterproofing to prevent mold in homes. If adequate drainage wasn't installed when the home was first built, it was frequently installed after problems developed. Although the water intrusion was addressed, the mold that developed was frequently covered up cosmetically.

❏ **In densely populated cities** and urban environments, the heat island effect can lead to higher temperature fluctuations and a more rapid daily expansion and contraction of materials, causing cracks and allowing water entry.

❏ **Humid regions** are particularly prone to condensation and moisture, creating ideal conditions for mold growth. Even small amounts of liquid moisture from leaks or spills can accelerate mold development, challenging rapid drying. In these climates, moisture-resistant barriers must be carefully installed to avoid trapping moisture, which can lead to hidden deterioration. East of the Rockies, humidity levels remain consistently high in the summer, making moisture control a constant battle. Air conditioning is essential but can introduce condensation risks. HVAC systems are particularly vulnerable when not adequately maintained or designed to handle the area's high moisture load. Regular HVAC maintenance and vigilant moisture control are crucial to preventing these issues in humid climates. Adding supplemental dehumidification to HVAC systems frequently results in more significant problems with mold growth within the systems since built-in systems are difficult to access and complex to maintain. Portable dehumidifiers that can be used when necessary provide an option that is less expensive, can be easily moved around to address issues, and are easier to maintain and clean.

❏ **Homes near lakes or ponds** are at risk of toxic algae blooms. Changes in weather conditions, warmer temperatures, and altered rainfall patterns create ideal conditions for harmful algae to thrive, release toxins, and potentially cause health issues for residents in nearby homes.

❏ **Ranches, agricultural communities, and areas near livestock are at** risk of endotoxins from gram-negative bacteria, also exacerbated by moisture problems.

❏ **Shared Walls in Multi-Unit Buildings** may allow one unit's water damage and mold problems to spread to others, complicating remediation efforts. If you can smell cooking or other odors from an adjacent unit, a mold problem in that unit is more likely to permeate your unit. Limited or shared ventilation between units can create a less responsive, more humid indoor environment conducive to mold growth and the migration of contaminants between dwelling units.

Exercise 3.3 Higher Risk Design Issues
Indicate all that apply:

❏ **Below-grade finished spaces.** Basements and portions of a home installed below grade are prone to hidden moisture damage. Inattention to detail in the planning, design, and construction can result in long-term moisture seeping into unseen areas. Even well-thought-out and implemented moisture control measures have a life expectancy, after which they are likely to fail. Since the most effective measures are applied to the exterior of the foundation walls, repairs may involve extensive excavation. Avoiding designs that include living spaces that are partially buried is the best insurance.

❏ **Flat or low-sloped roofs.** Flat and low-sloped roofs are prone to roof leaks that lead to mold and other deterioration. A flat or low-sloped roof can also act like airplane wings in heavy winds and literally apply enough upward force to exert intense upward forces, which, in extreme cases, can lift a home off of its foundation. Even in lesser wind situations, repeated pressure changes can result in less extreme movement that can result in shifts and cracks.

❏ **No (or inadequate) roof overhangs.** Roof overhangs are an effective way of preventing water entry or accumulation on exterior walls. Rain, sleet, snow, and ice can beat directly against walls, windows, and doors without adequate overhangs.

❏ **Overcomplicated roofs**. Roofs with multiple valleys, pitches, and flashed connections to the house present many opportunities for failure. The most significant risk of roof leaks is at elevation changes or the joining of differing materials. These junctions must be properly installed with adequate flashing to prevent damage and mold from water intrusion. Penetrations for skylights, vents, fireplace chimneys, and roof lines meeting a vertical wall are places with a greater risk for water entry.

❏ **Zero or low clearance between homes**—In some communities, houses are built so close together that there is very little space between them on one or more sides. This makes maintenance on the exterior walls very difficult and requires the cooperation of the neighbors. These narrow, airless spaces between buildings are more vulnerable to debris build-up and receive little sunlight, often creating damp conditions ripe for mold growth.

❏ **Apartments or condo units.** Shared walls can provide pathways for neighbors to impact the air quality of adjoining dwellings. Chemicals, smoke, cooking odors, EMR frequencies, and mold contamination are just a few problems that may migrate directly from a neighbor's unit. Odors noted when the neighbor in a multi-family dwelling is cooking, smoking, or engaging in other smelly activities are an indicator that airflow pathways are present between units. The odors may be more than just unpleasant—they often indicate that the fire protection between units is also insufficient. Unfortunately, the conditions that lead to these issues are out of the direct control of the occupants. When repairs are required, they may involve the cooperation of the neighbors, landlords, or a condominium board. These other parties may not have the same level of health concern.

❏ **Internal gutters.** Gutters hidden inside the attic or walls can be problematic. If not installed correctly or if a problem develops over time, it is difficult to detect and, once discovered, difficult and costly to repair.

❏ **HVAC systems and components that are difficult to access.** Mechanical systems need to be routinely maintained, and if access is restricted or difficult, routine system maintenance will likely be ignored or shortcuts taken.

❏ **Multiple HVAC systems.** More than one HVAC system in a building can cause airflow imbalances that force unhealthy air from attics, basements, crawlspaces, and wall cavities into occupied spaces

❏ **Humidification.** Adding moisture via the HVAC system can cause the growth of mold and harmful bacteria unless the ducts are kept scrupulously clean with frequent inspection and maintenance

❏ **Duct plenums in floors**. Registers located on floors are more problematic because debris will fall into them. When duct registers are on the floor, they should have an adequate catch box in the plenum. If not, dirt and debris will fall directly into the ductwork and be carried by gravity into the depths of the ductwork, which is unable to be easily and routinely cleaned. Simple, inexpensive specification requirements can be the difference between expensive duct cleaning maintenance and simple routine do-it-yourself cleaning.

❏ **Attached garages**. Fumes from auto exhaust and stored chemicals frequently migrate into the living space if special precautions are not taken to ensure adequate sealing between the home and garage. The attached garage is often the weakest point in a catastrophic weather event. In a tornado, hurricane, or flood, the garage will frequently collapse first, bringing down the rest of the home.

❏ **Cantilevered porches.** Support beams under cantilevered porches provide a direct pathway for air and moisture infiltration where they pass through the building envelope.

❏ **Porches that are located over an occupied space or garage.** If not properly designed and built, the floors of framed porches, like flat roofs, are prone to leaks. When built over living spaces, they are usually more difficult and costly to repair and maintain.

❏ **Spaces that are inaccessible or difficult to access**: When moisture is present in out-of-sight areas such as enclosed soffits, under and behind built-in cabinets, and underneath enclosed stairwells, the damage can grow undetected and become a serious hidden health issue.

❏ **Paper-faced wallboard in wet rooms**. Walls in kitchens, baths, and laundry rooms are more likely to get wet, and paper-faced drywall in these areas is a common source of mold growth. Any gypsum board product with a paper facing, including "Green board" and other paper-faced products treated with antimicrobials, will develop mold if they stay damp for a sufficient period. The biocides wash out over time, and the developed organisms will tend to produce higher biotoxin levels. More durable, non-nutritive materials should be used for any area with the potential for repeated wetting. Paperless wallboard materials and non-nutritive interior wall framing products are better—but when searching for a home, they are often not able to be determined without cutting inspection holes.

- **Built-in wine rooms.** Wine rooms are prone to moisture damage because the cooler temperatures ideal for storing wine frequently result in condensation. Free-standing controlled wine cooler appliances are preferable, but they should have a condensate collection pan easily accessed for routine cleaning to prevent mold from developing.

- **Indoor pools, hot tubs, wet saunas, and steam rooms.** Typical HVAC systems are not designed to control the moisture generated in these areas. Special care in the design and construction and specialized mechanical equipment that can handle the extra moisture is necessary to avoid developing mold problems.

- **Unconditioned attics, basements, and crawlspaces.** When attics, crawlspaces, or basements are outside the insulated building space, they are called "unconditioned." Proper ventilation to the outside and moisture exclusion measures are required to prevent moisture accumulation, damage, and mold growth in these unoccupied areas. They should be isolated from the home's conditioned space with meticulous air sealing. They should not contain storage or mechanical equipment.

- **Metal framing.** Metal framing readily conducts heat. Unless properly isolated, this construction is prone to cold bridging, which results in condensation. Damage is especially common in areas with cold winters.

- **Fire suppression systems.** Homes with fire suppression systems have more plumbing, which increases the likelihood of water damage. These systems are currently mandated in many jurisdictions around the country. They are designed to save lives if a building is on fire, but they will quickly damage the building, creating major flood damage if the clean-up is not immediate, thorough, and professionally dried.

- **Drainage toward building.** This commonly occurs when the site selection and preparation are not followed or adequately considered.

- **Gutters that dead-end into walls (i.e., buried in stucco) or in contact with siding.** I have seen numerous instances where gutters were installed before the stucco, or siding was installed. This has resulted in the gutter extending into the cavity and dumping water directly into the wall when it rains. Gutters should be installed so the end cap has a gap between the gutter and the home. The gap allows the wall to dry. Also, if the end cap of the gutter develops a leak, it will drain outdoors, where it can be observed instead of being directed into the wall cavity.

- **Gypcrete or other lightweight concrete materials poured using gypsum wallboard or other mold-sensitive materials as the forms.** Ideally, concrete pours should occur before paper-covered gypsum wallboard is in place and never into stay-in-place paper-based formwork. If concrete is poured against a paper product, the moisture that remains after the pour will result in a severe mold problem. Shielding the paper product by applying a polyethylene or other plastic barrier is rarely successful. Minor pinhole-sized leaks or gaps result in capillary action, pulling excess moisture into the sensitive material.

- **Cover-up Remodeling:** Poorly executed remodeling may cover up deep-seated water damage. Some homes that appear to have been meticulously remodeled contain portions of older water-damaged materials left in place. The mold-containing dust often remains hidden behind the new construction. Over time, the contaminants work their way back out into the occupied parts of the building.

- **Dryer vent problems:** If the ductwork for a clothes dryer is too long or has a circuitous route to the outside, it will clog with lint and become a fire hazard. It is common but unacceptable for dryer ducts to be installed with duct tape joining the ducts at the seams. The heat running through the duct can cause the adhesive on the tape to fail after a few years. If the ductwork comes loose, it will leak moist lint-filled air, creating friendly conditions for mold growth.

- **Improperly installed or missing flashing:** Flashing at joints between different materials that expand and contract at different rates must be properly installed to adjust the movement. When movement widens the space between materials, the gap allows moisture to enter, resulting in mold growth. Since many of these flashing materials are hidden, this issue often won't be discovered until the deterioration is extensive. The use of galvanized metal flashing in marine

- **Poorly compacted soils:** If soil is insufficiently compacted under the structure, it can settle and crack. If a building settles, plumbing and gas pipes are stressed and may rupture.

- **Differential expansion and contraction.** Materials expand and contract at different rates. Solid wood expands more across the grain and less along the grain. Over time, these differential movements can create gaps in the building envelope, allowing moisture to enter.

- **Failure at sealed joints.** Even the best caulk or sealant has a shorter life span than properly flashed buildings. Junctures that rely on caulk or sealant must be frequently inspected and maintained.

- **Leaky ductwork** in HVAC systems will not only waste energy, it can also suck contaminants into the system and drive them into the living space. <2% leakage is considered to be acceptable for an energy-efficient home. This may not sound like much, but if an HVAC unit is moving 1000 cfm, it will leak up to 20 cubic feet of air each minute!

- **Damaged or missing insulation.** Damage and gaps can occur in insulation due to improper installation, settling, careless maintenance workers, or rodents, causing cold patches that lead to condensation inside the structure. When roof or attic insulation is missing, the heat from the house can melt the snow over the uninsulated area, resulting in water damage from ice dams.

Exercise 3.4 Visible Mold Growth Patterns

Understanding mold growth patterns is the first step in addressing the underlying causes of water damage. Each pattern tells a story—it's not just about the mold you see but what it signifies about your indoor environment. Each pattern provides clues, from condensation-induced growth to the hidden molds lurking behind walls.

Remember that not all mold is immediately visible. Some growths require microscopic examination, especially in their early stages. Invisible surface molds can often be eliminated by HEPA vacuuming, followed by cleaning with a dampened disposable microfiber cloth to clean exposed surface area. Minor visible growth, swelling, staining, or cracking may indicate deeper, hidden issues, but these are usually not identified until after significant damage has accumulated. Musty odors are a telltale sign of hidden active mold growth, implying that some nutritive material has elevated moisture. The absence of musty odors does not mean the mold growth has disappeared or been adequately addressed. Often, the disappearance of musty odors signifies that the mold has dried out and entered a dormant state where it no longer emits odors indicative of active growth.

Safety First: Protecting Health in Mold-Contaminated Areas

Engaging in activities that may disturb mold growth or by entering contaminated areas increases health risks, particularly for sensitive individuals. It is strongly recommended that sensitive people avoid exposing themselves to contaminated environments as much as possible. Mold-contaminated areas should best be approached by trained professionals with appropriate personal protective equipment (PPE), including a properly fitted N95 or higher-rated respirator, gloves, and protective clothing. For anyone entering such areas, time spent inside should be minimized, and the area should be under negative pressure with HEPA-filtered air filtration devices exhausting to the outside. More information on safety and personal protective equipment can be found in this book in the Emergency Water Damage Section, page 98–124.

Touching or rubbing mold should be avoided. A single square inch of visible mold can contain 1 to 10 million colony-forming units (CFUs), and physical contact disturbs the mold, significantly increasing the risk of inhalation. Some mold biotoxins, if present, can also absorb through the skin, adding to the exposure risk. Additionally, rubbing mold off a surface can compromise the integrity of testing, as removing spores or residues before collecting samples may skew the results downward. Avoid these practices to ensure accurate assessments and minimize health risks.

GENERAL OVERVIEW OF CONDENSATION-RELATED MOLD GROWTH

Condensation occurs when water vapor in the air cools and transforms into liquid, a common occurrence in environments with high humidity or where there's a significant temperature difference between surfaces and the ambient air. This phenomenon is particularly noticeable during colder months when warm indoor air rapidly cools upon contact with cold windows or poorly insulated walls, leading to condensation. Similarly, hot water steam in bathrooms or kitchens can condense on colder surfaces, such as mirrors, tiles, or walls. Inadequate ventilation in areas also contributes to surface moisture accumulation, creating conditions conducive to mold growth. If surfaces remain continuously wet for a couple of days without sufficient drying, mold germination occurs, and if dampness continues, growth becomes inevitable. Types of mold typically associated with condensation include *Cladosporium* and *Aureobasidium pullulans*. *Cladosporium* is often found on painted surfaces and window frames. At the same time, *Aureobasidium pullulans* commonly colonize painted wooden surfaces, wallpaper, and other continuously damp areas like toilet tanks, shower curtains, and condensate pans for refrigerators and air conditioners. These molds are known for their ability to grow at lower temperatures, with some species of *Cladosporium* even thriving at temperatures near freezing. The color of these molds varies, feeding on different nutrients, usually appearing as spots or streaks.

While molds from rapidly discovered and addressed condensation films usually present minimal health risks, they can cause allergic reactions, especially in sensitive individuals. The cold temperatures where such mold grows tend to slow its development, providing early detection and cleaning opportunities. Factors contributing to condensation-related mold growth include high indoor humidity levels from daily activities like cooking or showering, temperature differences causing warm air to lose moisture upon cooling, and inadequate ventilation that traps moist air. Recognizing these factors is key to managing moisture, preventing mold growth and water damage, and ensuring a healthier living environment.

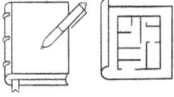

(Record the following in your diary and Floor Plan Diagram)
Indicate all that apply:

Condensation on Windows

❏ **Minor Mold Growth from Window Condensation**

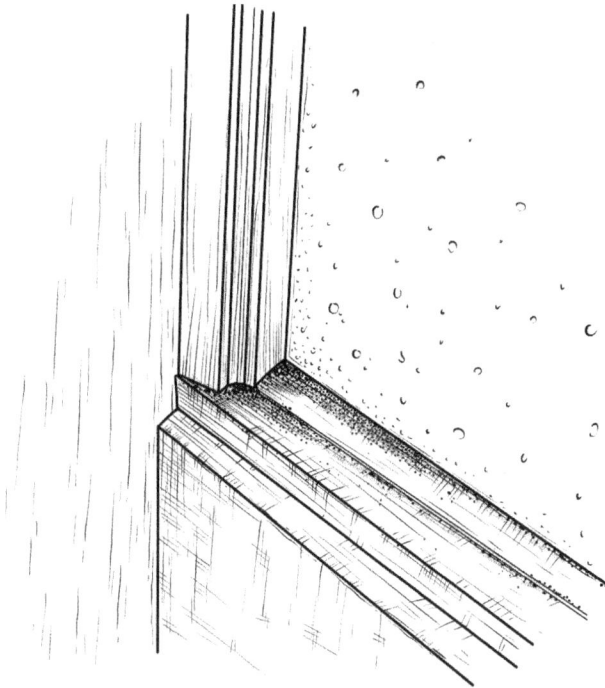

Figure 5-1: Minor Mold Growth from Condensation on the Windowsill: This illustration shows minor, streaky, and spotty mold growth on a painted windowsill surface, a typical result of condensation. This is surface growth and has not penetrated the paint layer (yet), making it possible to remove it through effective cleaning. Should any staining persist after thorough cleaning, using a peroxide-based stain remover or repainting may be necessary. The underlying causes of the condensation should be addressed to prevent the recurrence of such mold growth. This could involve identifying and correcting or managing moisture sources. Regularly drying the affected area, especially after identifying these conditions early, is a key preventive measure to ensure mold doesn't develop again.

❏ **Moderate Mold Growth from Window Condensation**

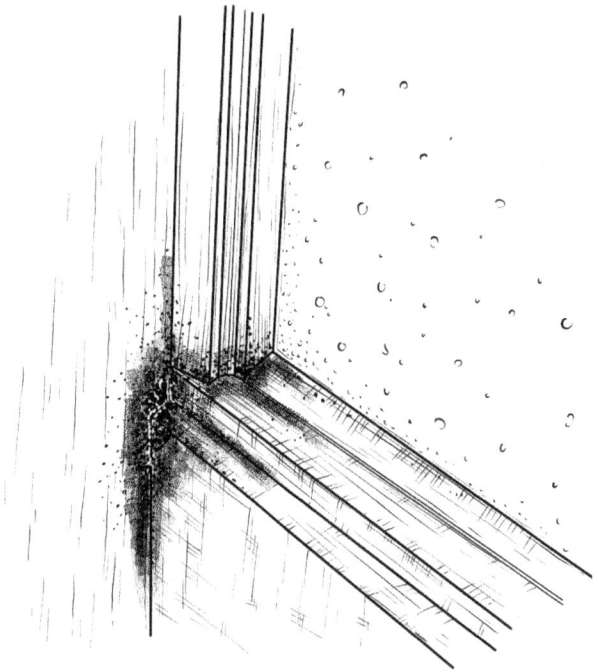

Figure 5-2: Moderate Mold Growth from Window Condensation: This illustration shows moderate mold growth on a painted window surface caused by condensation from elevated humidity. The mold has slightly damaged the paint but has not deeply penetrated. Remediation includes HEPA vacuuming, cleaning, sanding while HEPA vacuuming, and repainting with stain-blocking paint to prevent discoloration; avoid using biocides, antimicrobials, and encapsulant paints that trap moisture. Prevent recurrence by improving insulation, sealing gaps, managing indoor humidity, and regularly drying affected areas. Identifying this issue in one window suggests similar risks in others, so proactive inspection and humidity control can minimize future problems.

❏ **Major Mold Growth from Window Condensation**

❏ **Mold Growth on Draperies from Window Condensation**

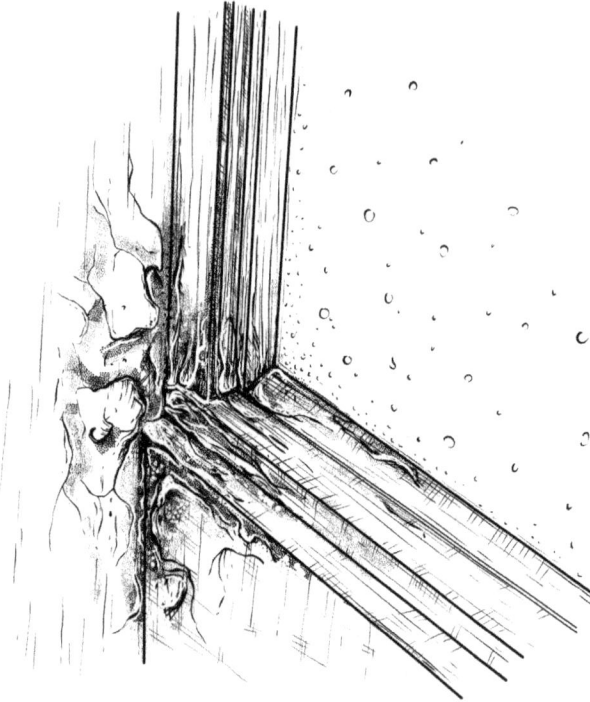

Figure 5-3: Major Mold Damage from Window Condensation This illustration shows significant mold growth at the top of a window, where it meets the gypsum wall, highlighting extensive damage due to condensation. The presence of cracks or openings has not only allowed cold air drafts to bring in moisture from outside but may also have enabled condensation water to seep deeply into the wall cavity.

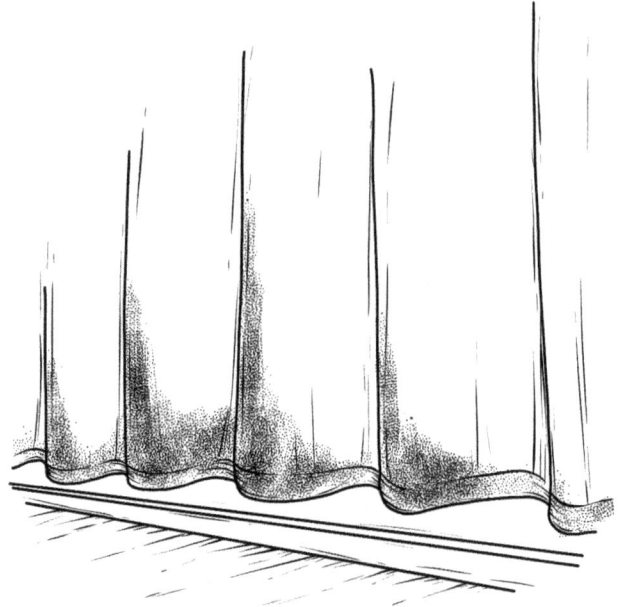

Figure 5-4: Moderate to Major Mold Damage on Window Draperies from Condensation This illustration highlights significant mold growth on window draperies due to condensation caused by cold air descending from poorly insulated windows. The heavier cold air accumulates moisture at the bottom of the draperies, creating an ideal environment for mold. This extensive growth has likely caused irreversible damage to the drapery material, indicating the need for replacement. Failure to address the source of moisture will result in a reoccurrence.

The visible mold is just the tip of the iceberg, suggesting considerable hidden damage. Remediation in such severe cases requires full-scale containment and airflow control to prevent mold spores from spreading during removal. The affected materials, having undergone swelling and cracking, will likely need replacement. It's crucial to address the underlying causes, such as cold surface conditions, high humidity, and potential exterior leaks, which might have contributed to this situation. The damage might extend to the building's exterior, allowing rainwater entry. Early measures like frequent inspections and sealing cracks could have mitigated this extensive damage. However, more extensive intervention is required to halt ongoing deterioration at this stage. The window may need new flashing or replacing the window itself to prevent further water entry.

The mold issue stems from factors like inadequate window insulation, the use of single-pane windows, and insufficient ventilation, all contributing to condensation. This moisture, trapped close to the window and wall by the draperies, exacerbates the mold problem. Specific strategies around windows are needed to address and prevent such mold growth. These include insulating drapery materials, improving insulation around windows to prevent cold-bridging to reduce condensation, enhancing air circulation by shortening draperies away from the floor, and keeping them open, particularly during the day, to facilitate air movement. Ensuring that the draperies are completely dried at least once every 24 hours prevents mold. Similar conditions can also develop with roll-up Venetian or vertical blinds, where restricted air circulation and moisture accumulation can lead to mold growth.

Examples of Other Mold Growth from Cold Surface Condensation

❑ **Mold growth due to steam from a tea kettle.**

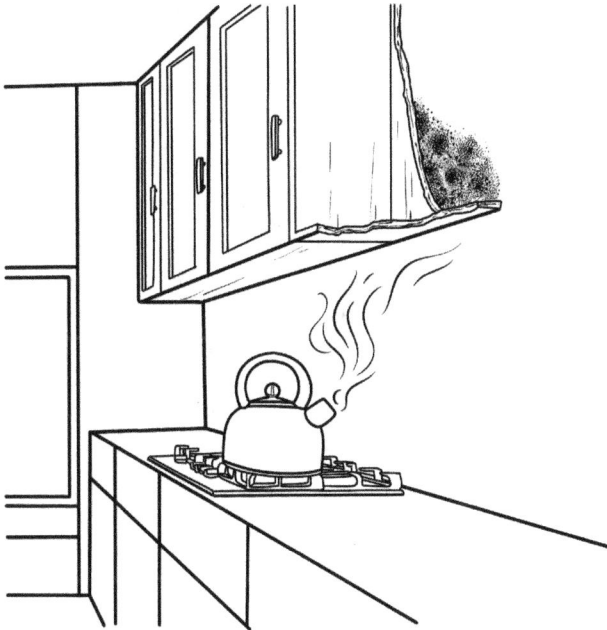

Figure 5-5: Mold has grown on the wall behind a cabinet due to condensation occurring on the colder wall behind the cabinet. This cutaway illustration reveals mold growth hidden behind an upper kitchen cabinet caused by steam from an uncontrolled boiling tea kettle. Steam, finding its way behind the cabinet through an unsealed bottom edge, condensed in the colder space, leading to hidden mold development. This situation highlights the potential for mold growth in obscured areas, which are not visible until the cabinet is removed. Preventive measures such as using a vent hood, keeping the kettle lid on, and sealing the cabinet's back edge to the wall with caulk could have prevented this issue, underscoring the importance of moisture control in mold prevention.

❑ **Minor mold in a tub or shower**

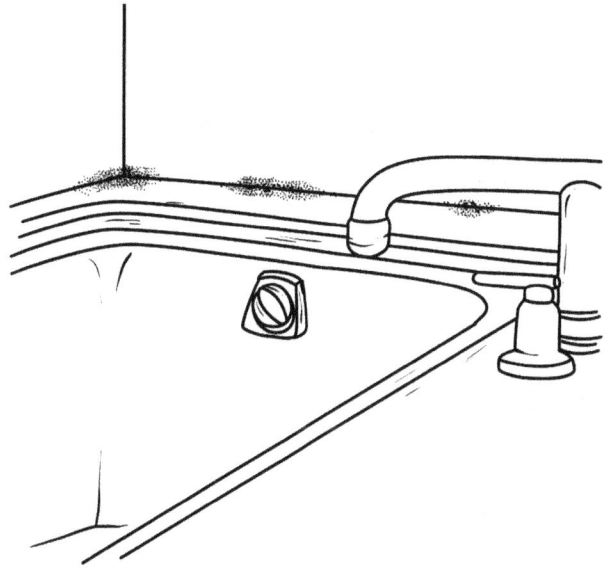

Figure 5-6: This illustration depicts minor mold growth on the caulk and grout in a bathtub or shower area. The mold appears as small, dark patches, primarily in the seams and joints where splashed water accumulates. Such growth is often due to persistent dampness in these areas and limited ventilation and lighting. The mold is on the surface, making it possible to clean effectively with Regular cleaning using a mild detergent or soap solution, ensuring thorough drying after each use, and improving air circulation can prevent recurrence. If the mold has begun to degrade the integrity of the caulk or grout, repairs to the grout or caulk may be necessary. If the water has already penetrated, the backing materials it can be identified by using a moisture meter. Cement-based backer is very resistant to mold, whereas a paper-covered gypsum wallboard is not. Although green and blue boards are advertised as moisture resistant, they also develop mold growth on the paper when exposed to water that gets behind the tile.

❑ **Moderate mold in a bathroom ceiling caused by condensation from missing insulation.**

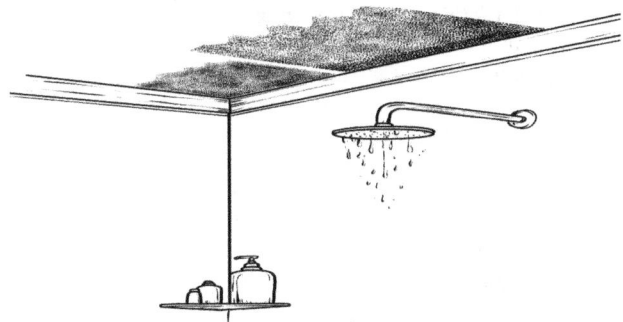

Figure 5.7: This illustration showcases moderate condensation-related mold growth on a bathroom ceiling due to missing insulation in the attic space above. The steam from hot showers rises and condenses on the colder, uninsulated ceiling area, especially in winter, creating a perfect environment for mold.

This condition, while surface-level, indicates the need for immediate attention. Effective cleaning might address the mold if the ceiling materials are intact and the moisture source is solely from condensation. It can be cleaned and repainted with stain-blocking paint. This measure can only be effective if no mold has developed behind the trim or in the attic. If these conditions are present, it would indicate long-term severe damage that should be remediated by physically removing the ceiling under containment and verifying that the condition did not extend into the wall cavity behind the shower.

❑ **Moderate mold growth in a closet from condensation**

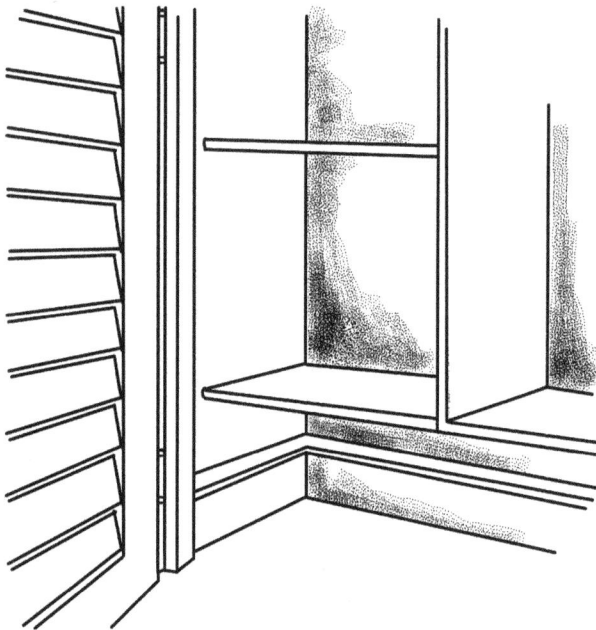

Figure 5-8: Moderate mold growth in a closet from condensation forming on the exterior uninsulated walls. This illustration depicts moderate mold growth inside a closet, typically caused by condensation on an improperly insulated wall. Mold often develops in closets or behind furniture pushed against exterior walls, usually hidden behind clothes or stored items. These items block air circulation, worsening the issue as the colder exterior wall collects condensation, creating a perfect environment for mold. Clothing in contact with moldy walls may become stained or have weakened fibers, making restoration difficult and often ineffective. Closets are especially prone to mold due to poor ventilation and storing damp or wet items, such as rain-soaked jackets. To prevent mold growth, ensure proper air circulation, avoid storing items until fully dry, and improve ventilation to better regulate humidity in the closet. In this case, the additional ventilation provided by the louvered doors was insufficient to prevent condensation from forming, but it might have been sufficient in a less severe situation.

❑ **Mold growth around an electrical outlet where cold air leakage has resulted in condensation resulting in mold growth.**

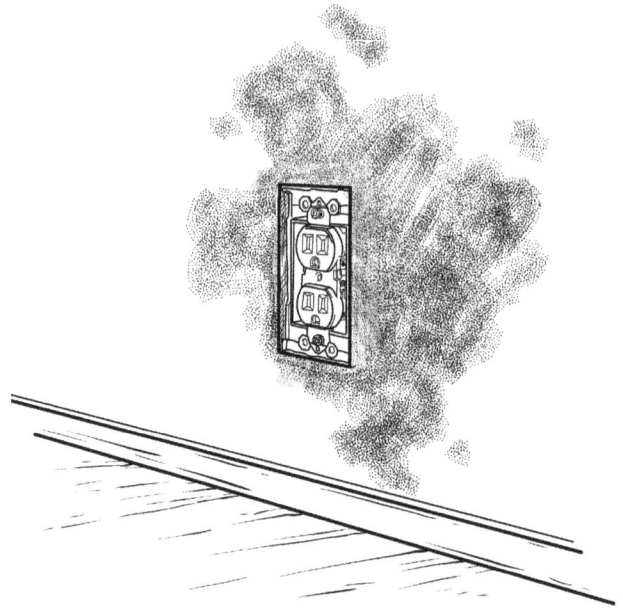

Figure 5-9: Mold growth around an electrical outlet where missing insulation has resulted in condensation moisture on the gypsum wallboard paper surrounding the outlet, resulting in visible mold growth. Patterns like this are often seen if the electrical outlet was installed as a retrofit on an exterior wall and the integrity of the insulation was damaged during installation. A growth pattern like this on the back side of the gypsum wallboard paper may not be observed from the room. It would likely develop from cold air leakage, causing moisture condensation inside the wall cavity and resulting in hidden mold growth. A strong musty odor will often be noted emanating from the electrical box.

❑ **Mold growth pattern from condensation moisture forming from cold-bridging**

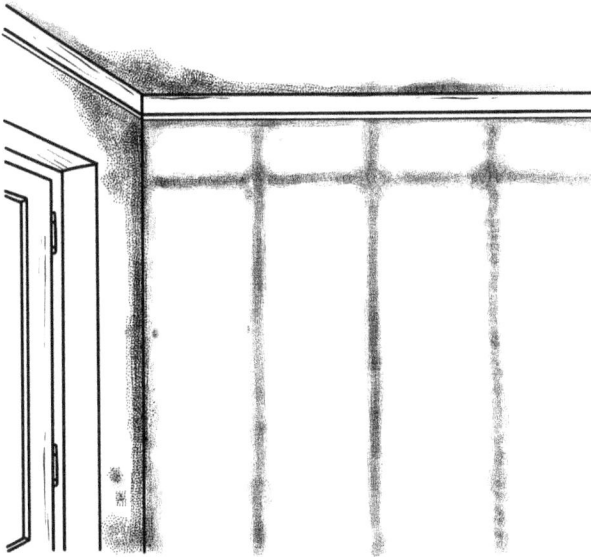

Figure 5-10: This pattern of condensation-induced mold growth illustrates the result of cold-bridging, a condition where the building's framing allows cold temperatures from outside to transfer indoors, causing moisture to condense on interior walls in areas with elevated humidity. Cold-bridging is more common in metal-framed buildings, as metal conducts temperature differences more effectively than wood. In this case, the wall cavities were insulated, but some areas of insulation were missing or damaged. A thermal imaging camera could have identified these cold spots before the damage appeared. Allowing for mitigation methods like dehumidification to reduce indoor humidity might have prevented the mold from developing.

❑ **Uninsulated cold water plumbing pipe or gas line with condensation moisture forming and dripping to the surface below.**

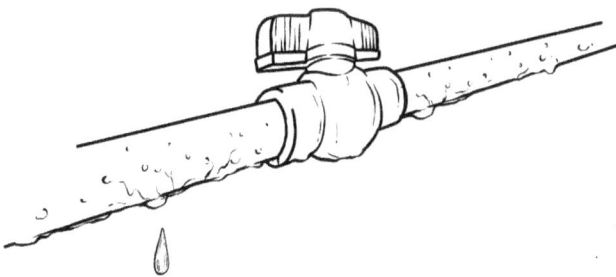

Figure 5-11: Dripping Condensation on Cold Water Pipes: This illustration depicts an uninsulated cold-water pipe with condensation forming and dripping, a common issue when moisture-resistant barriers are missing, allowing humid air to enter a wall cavity. The cold metal surface of the pipe causes moisture to condense, especially in areas where airflow from humid environments, like bathrooms, reaches the uninsulated cavity. The condensation drips onto adjacent surfaces, such as sill plates or gypsum wallboard, and spreads through capillary action. This hidden moisture

can persist for years, potentially leading to intermittent musty odors from mold growth within the wall cavity, even if mold isn't visible in the room. Insulating the pipes is essential to reduce temperature differences and minimize condensation. Additionally, managing ambient humidity through dehumidifiers or improved ventilation is crucial. Regular inspections of hidden areas are key to early detection and remediation of moisture accumulation, helping mitigate mold growth risk from condensation on cold water pipes.

COMMON STRATEGIES AND CONSIDERATIONS FOR ADDRESSING CONDENSATION-RELATED MOLD

Preventing condensation-related mold growth involves several key strategies. Insulating plumbing and gas lines helps minimize temperature differences, thereby reducing condensation. In addition, controlling ambient humidity through improved ventilation, regular inspections of hidden areas for early signs of moisture or mold, and using mechanical dehumidifiers when necessary are crucial for maintaining a healthy environment. These preventive steps should be part of a comprehensive maintenance routine to significantly lower the risk of mold growth caused by condensation.

Addressing the root causes of elevated dampness, humidity, and water damage is essential for long-term mold management. Key measures include improving insulation, enhancing ventilation, and ensuring proper sealing of building materials to prevent moisture ingress. However, caution is necessary when implementing upgrades, such as elastomeric encapsulation or other impermeable sealing techniques, as these can trap moisture and cause further damage. Also, double—or triple-glazed windows may reduce surface condensation on the window, but they can inadvertently shift moisture problems to other cold surfaces.

Historically, homes built before the 1970s energy crisis were often drafty and poorly insulated. Post-crisis energy efficiency upgrades, if not holistically planned, have sometimes led to increased condensation, moisture, and mold growth issues, highlighting the need for balanced solutions. Proper ventilation, humidity control, and managing indoor moisture sources like plants, aquariums, or kitchen activities—such as covering boiling pots—will help lower indoor humidity levels.

Incorporating comprehensive, non-toxic strategies into your mold management plan addresses existing mold issues and targets the underlying causes of condensation-related growth, promoting a healthier living environment. While this book focuses primarily on water damage and mold, I recommend my first book, *Prescriptions for a Healthy House: A Practical Guide for Architects, Builders,* and *Homeowners,* co-authored with architect Paula Baker-Laporte and Dr. Erica Elliott. It provides valuable insights into balancing healthy building practices with energy conservation goals.

Cleaning Instructions for Minor, Moderate, and Major Condensation-Related Mold

Addressing Condensation-related mold in its early stages, especially when it first appears as a minor patch, helps maintain a healthy living environment. Quick action prevents its spread and minimizes spore dispersal throughout the home. Early detection and prompt remediation are essential to prevent the need for more extensive measures.

The following cleaning suggestions are for mold growth resulting from a condensation film of moisture that does not damage the surface. They are not sufficient for use when addressing hidden or severe issues. In these cases, the rest of the Five Stage, 25 Step program is needed.

Minor Mold Growth

Sensitive individuals should avoid performing cleanup if there's a risk of triggering sensitivity reactions.

- **Preparation:** Wear protective gear, such as gloves, an N-95 mask, and eye protection, and ensure good ventilation. HEPA vacuum to remove loose mold and surface debris.

- **Cleaning:** Use a disposable microfiber cloth with a mild, fragrance-free detergent such as Branch Basics All-Purpose Cleaner to wipe the area.

- **Rinsing and Drying**: Rinse with water and dry thoroughly.

- **Stain Removal:** If stains persist, apply a paste of Branch Basics Oxygen Boost, let it sit, then rinse.

Moderate Mold Growth

Sensitive individuals should not handle moderate mold growth; consider professional or non-sensitive assistance using non-toxic methods.

- **Preparation:** Wear appropriate protective gear and ensure good ventilation.

- **Containment:** Consider setting up a mini-containment area and using a HEPA vacuum cleaner to create negative air pressure and prevent spore spreading.

- **HEPA Vacuuming:** Vacuum the moldy area before applying any liquid to capture loose spores.

- **Cleaning:** Scrub the area using a non-metallic abrasive pad with diluted Branch Basics All Purpose or other mild, unscented cleaner. Follow up with the same rinsing and drying steps as for minor mold.

- **Stain Removal:** Repainting may be necessary if stains are too deep.

Major Mold Growth

- **Preparation:** Professional remediation is strongly recommended. Sensitive individuals should not be involved.

- **Containment: Full**-scale containment and negative air pressure are usually required.

- **Remediation:** Even if the mold is on accessible surfaces, wallboard removal may be necessary, as significant damage often indicates hidden mold in wall cavities.

General Tips for All Levels

- Use disposable microfiber cloths for cleaning, as they effectively capture mold particles and other contaminants.

- Address the underlying moisture issue to prevent recurrence.

- Regular inspections and moisture control are basic for maintaining a healthy environment.

By categorizing mold cleanup into these levels, individuals can better assess the appropriate actions for their situation. Prioritizing health and safety—especially for sensitive individuals—is essential, and professional assistance should be considered for more severe mold issues.

CHRONIC LEAKS, DRIPS, WATER INTRUSIONS, AND FLOODS RESULTING IN MICROORGANISM GROWTH

Often found near plumbing fixtures, roofs, or windows, this pattern results from consistent, slow water intrusion.

Indicate all that apply:

❏ **Plumbing leaks under sink:**

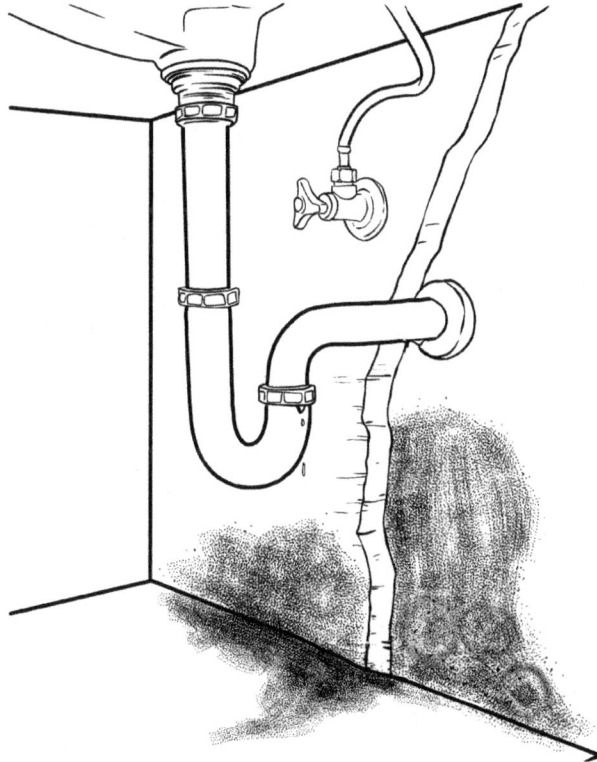

Figure 5-12: Major Mold Damage from a Drip or Slow Leak: Significant mold growth along the bottom edge of a wall shows extensive damage from a pipe leak. Hidden conditions will usually be worse than what can be observed. There is no way to remediate or treat a condition like this without removing the cabinet. A severe condition like this will often develop mold growth at floor level where water has flowed by capillary action so that the damage extends into the subfloor and into the areas behind adjacent cabinets. It is rare for the cabinetry to be able to be saved. Destructive investigation may result in a spread of spores—containment and airflow controls are highly recommended for inspections.

Here's the chart showing the amount of water that can flow in one day from different types of pipe leaks in both metric and English standard units:

Pipe Leak Amounts in English and Standard Units			
Type of Leak	**Rate of Leak**	**ml per Day**	**Gal per day**
One drop per minute	1 drop/minute	72 ml	0.02 gallons
One drop per second	60 drops/minute	4,320 ml	1.2 gallons
Pinhole spray leak	3,600 drops/minute	259,200 ml	68.5 gallons

These calculations are based on an average volume of 0.05 milliliters per drop. The actual volume can vary slightly depending on the viscosity and temperature of the water, as well as the size of the leak.

❏ **Window leaks: where water seeps through or around window frames.**

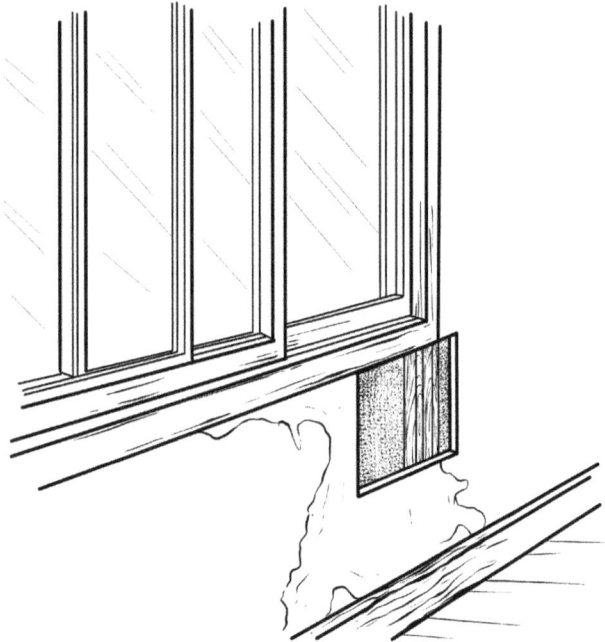

Figure 5-13: A window leak flowing directly into the wall cavity under the window may result in little or no visible water staining within the living space. With more water for a longer period, water stains may provide clues regarding the leakage. Eventually, visible mold will develop. Inspection holes would need containment and airflow controls to facilitate the inspection. Hidden conditions will usually be worse than what can be observed.

❏ **Severe water damage and mold caused by water leaking from above.**

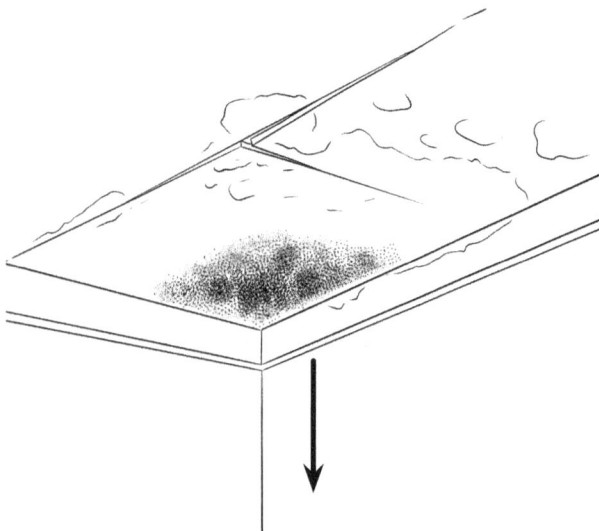

Figure 5-15: This illustration shows severe damage seen when water comes from above. In this case, the presence of a water stain with this pattern is close enough to the wall that it is likely that water also traveled down inside the wall cavity

and, with sufficient volume, reached the sill plate below. The weight of the water-saturated gypsum board has been enough to cause the ceiling to begin to sag and risk collapse. The underlying moisture cause must be identified and repaired to prevent ongoing mold growth and structural damage.

❏ **Roof Leaks: into attic spaces migrating to ceiling. shows the pattern of water coming from above**

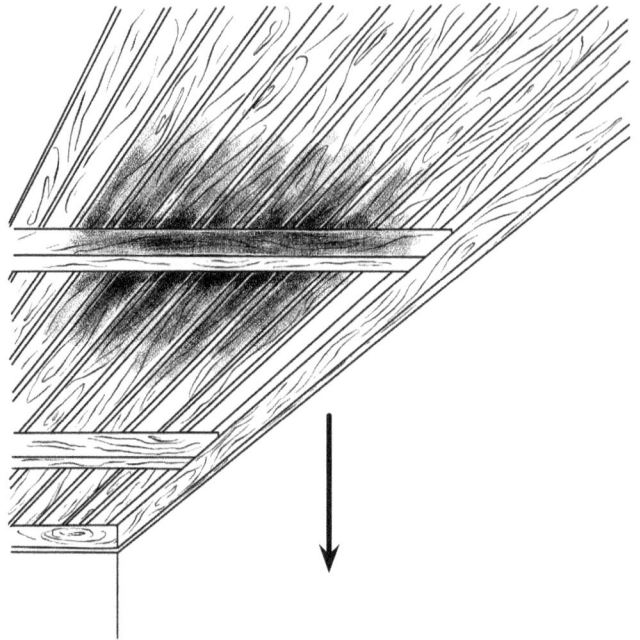

Figure 5-14: In this case, ceiling moisture from a roof leak may be close enough to the wall for mold to have developed in the upper and possibly lower wall cavity. Water should be investigated to see if it traveled downward from the ceiling space, migrated into the adjacent wall cavity, and then spread out when it reached the sill plate. Water that travels this way can also be drawn upward by capillary action in the gypsum board. Hidden conditions will usually be worse than what can be observed.

❏ **Flooding related growth**

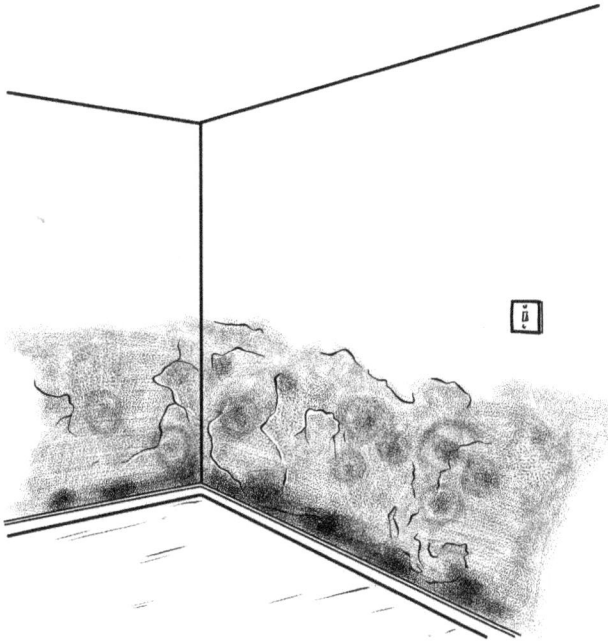

❏ **Water flow coming from above in a basement corner**

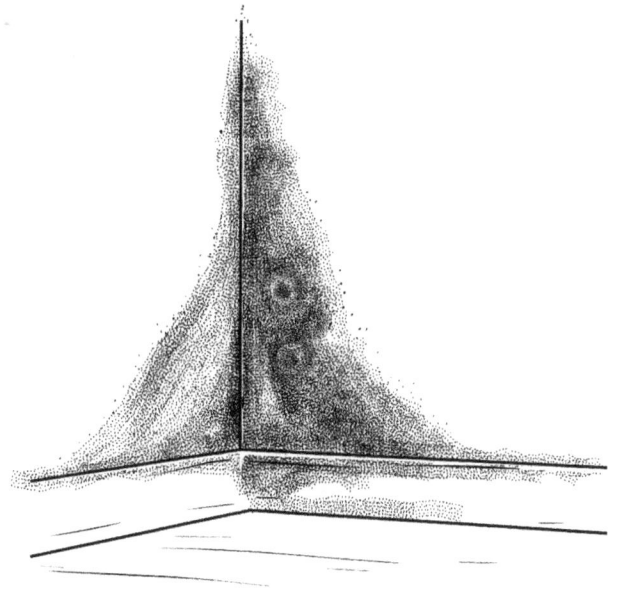

Figure 5-16: Flooding-Related Growth: Following significant water ingress events like floods, this pattern can be widespread across lower wall sections, floors, and basements. Lower Walls show the most significant amount of damage. This is often addressed by making a flood cut, typically up to 16 to 24 inches above the level of capillary rise. Hidden conditions will usually be worse than observed and may extend much higher. Elevated humidity within the wall cavity may cause subvisible mold to reach into upper sections of walls. Significant damage like this will often require the removal of wallboards from floor to ceiling and involve finish floors and potentially subfloors.

Figure 5-17: Moisture seeping through the foundation or basement walls can create ideal mold conditions. Exterior water from over-irrigation of landscaping flowing down an interior finished basement wall corner. The pattern shows the water flowing down from above; there is enough water to spread out, so the pattern widens as it travels to floor level. Once the water has reached the sill plate, it is drawn by capillary action along the area under it and behind the baseboard. Any excess water in contact with the bottom edge of the gypsum wallboard can then be pulled upward higher in the gypsum wallboard through capillary action. The mold condition that develops will be more significant in the hidden wall cavity than is visible in the room. Subvisible mold levels may be present on surfaces inside the wall cavity adjacent to the visible growth.

GROWTH IN HVAC SYSTEMS

❏ **HVAC system duct growth**

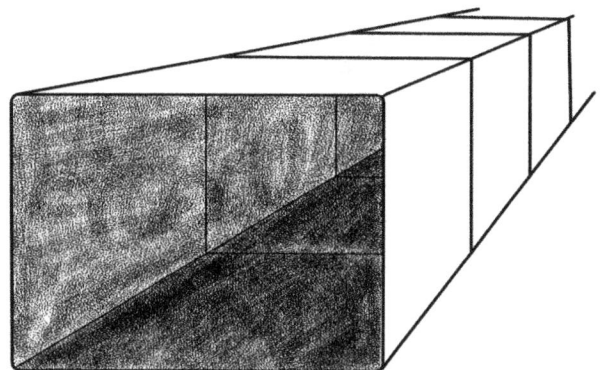

Figure 5-18: HVAC System Duct Growth: A relatively uniform layer of mold growth can occur in ductwork when Air Conditioning Systems are "Short-Cycling." This means cold air from the cooling coils passes into the ductwork too quickly

to remove excess moisture from the air stream. This excess moisture condenses on the interior of lined ducts, resulting in mold growth. Short Cycling can result from an oversized HVAC system, having blocked or partially blocked cold air returns vents, or inadequately sized cold air return ductwork. This is especially common in Hot, Humid parts of the country.

❏ **Filtration soiling of HVAC ductwork insulation:**

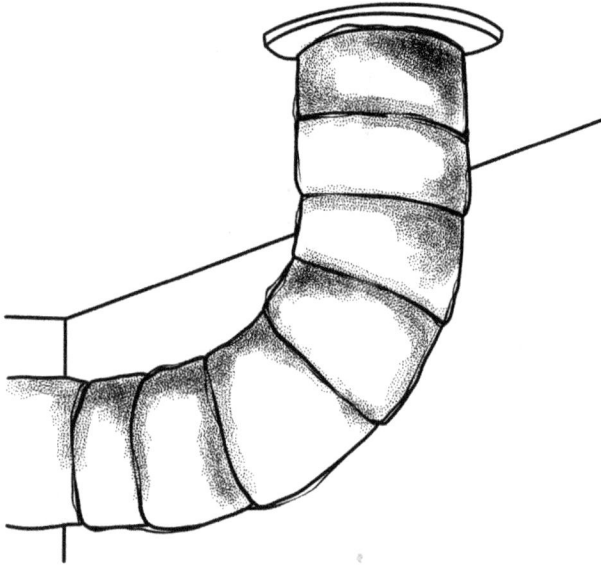

Figure 5-19: Dust Leakage Filtration Soiling: Dust leakage or filtration soiling on return or supply ducts indicates that dirty air is being filtered by insulation as it leaks into or out of the ductwork. This soiling may result from dust or mold. Its presence signals the need for further investigation to determine whether it consists of dirt and settled spores, which may be addressed through duct cleaning and sealing leaks, or if it points to a larger issue, such as mold growth within the system or ductwork.

❏ **Condensation on registers:**

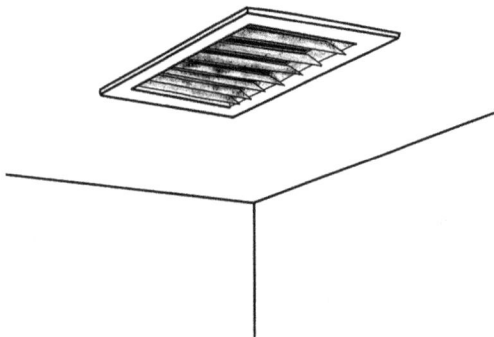

Figure 5-22: Moisture accumulation on registers results from elevated humidity in the room or the AC system operating at a too-cold temperature. It is most common when the system is oversized, turned down, or shut off when the home is unoccupied, then turned high to get the interior conditions under control when occupants return.

❏ **Unsealed duct plenum box:**

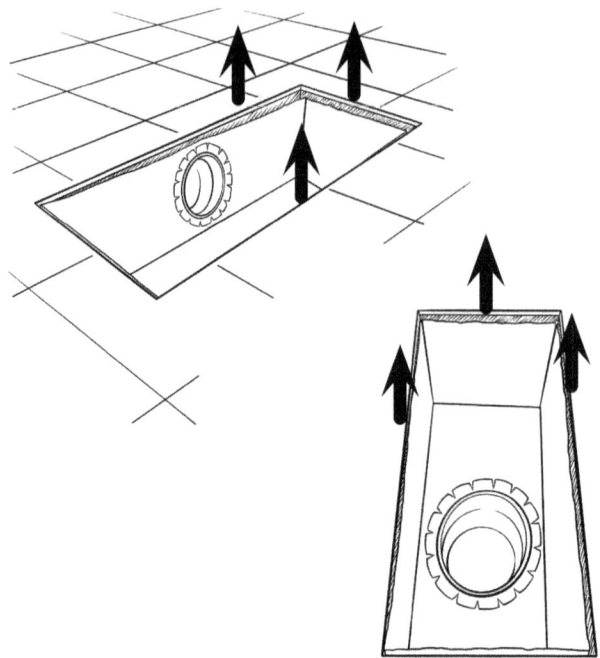

Figure 5-20: Plenum Leakage results in unintended dirty airflow from the crawlspace being pulled into the room through cracks or openings around the metal duct plenum.

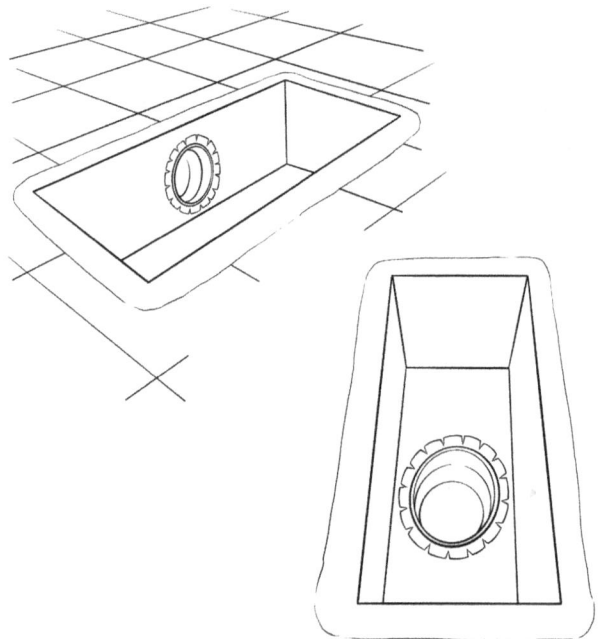

Figure 5-21: Sealing the metal plenum box to the subfloor with foil tape or mastic prevents cross-contamination from below.

SUBSTRATE-SPECIFIC GROWTH

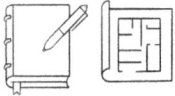

Certain materials like wood, drywall, or carpet can show distinct mold patterns due to their absorbency and texture. Wallpaper will show a characteristic blotchy look when mold is growing underneath.

❏ **Mold growth or water damage hidden behind wallpaper**

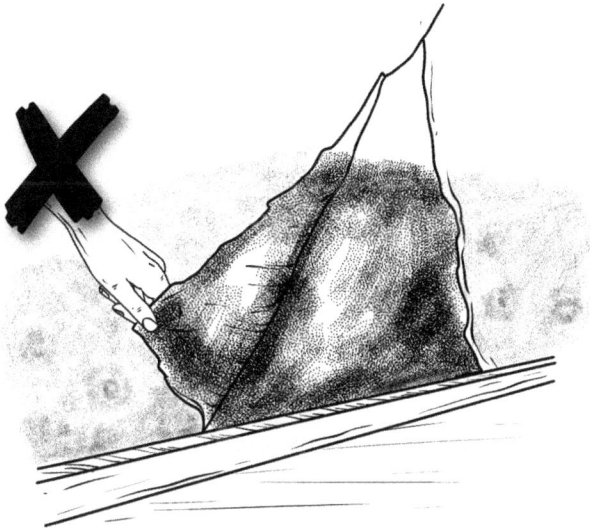

Figure 5-26: Mold Growth Behind Wallpaper Due to Trapped Water Vapor. Faint blotches and musty odors are common signs of mold growth when moisture accumulates behind wallpaper. Avoid peeling the wallpaper, as this can cause a massive release of spores and fragments into the home, significantly increasing remediation costs. Removing the gypsum wallboard with wallpaper intact functions like a barrier preventing the release of spores under the wallpaper. There is a risk that mold growth will also be present in the hidden wall cavities so all appropriate room containment and air flow controls should also be used.

❏ **Hidden mold growth or water damage on the floor and tack strip under the carpet**

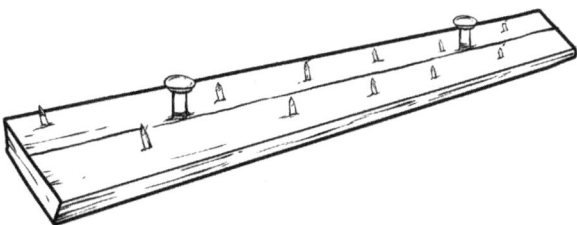

Figure 5-27: Normal carpet tack strip does not show signs of water damage or rusting of the nails. There will be no staining or discoloration that has transferred to the carpet backing or surrounding materials.

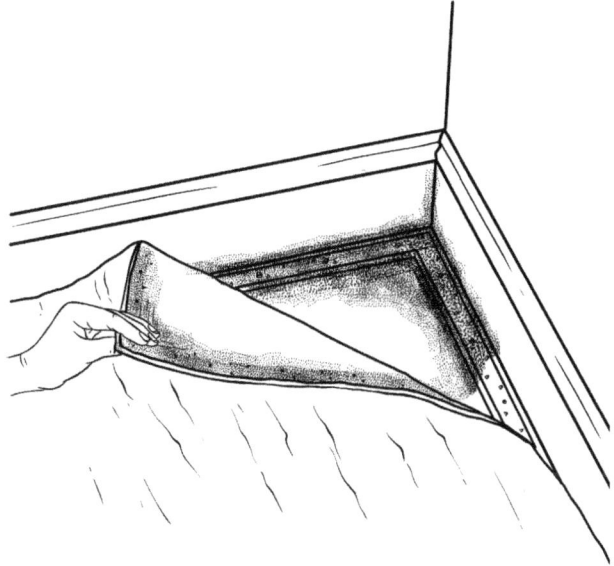

Figure 5-28: Carpet Staining and Growth are often not visible until the carpet is detached. Carpet installation technicians frequently ignore or don't recognize mold or water damage and can hide problem conditions by installing new materials over the top. Discovering and announcing a problem with mold or water damage problem can delay the job and cut their bottom line. The carpet should be removed by someone focused on preserving the evidence of what caused the damage and the source of the moisture. The pattern indicates that the water came from the wall cavity.

||||||||||||||||||||||||||||||||||||||||||||||||||||||||||||||||||||||||||||||||||||||||||||||||||||||||||||||||||||||||||||||||||||||||||||||||||||||||

Sealing an Unsealed Ceiling Can Light

Purpose: Blocks the passage of contaminated air through the penetrations present in can lighting fixtures. In winter, a reverse stack effect is common when heavier cold air can flow downward through ceiling openings or penetrations such as can lights. Sealing fixtures will help reduce the flow of contaminants into the living space, but if the source of moisture isn't addressed, then deterioration of the attic area will continue.

First Step: Unscrew and remove the old lightbulb.

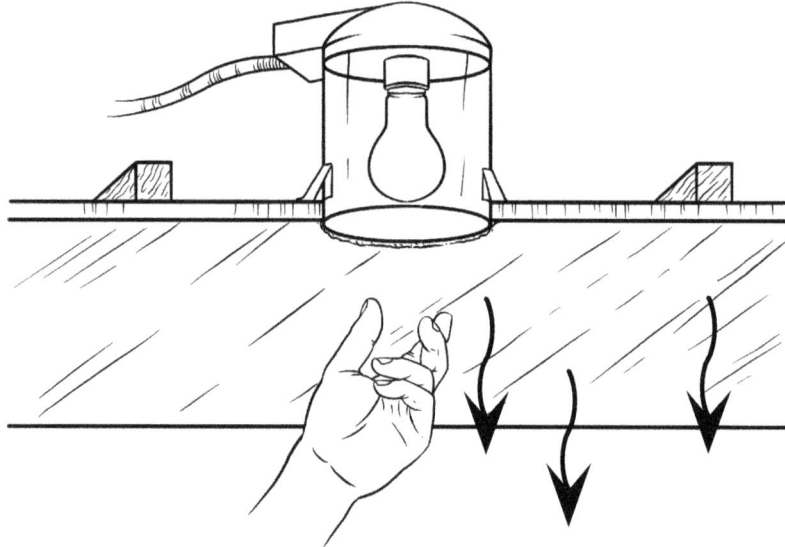

Figure 5-23: Unsealed can lights allow airflow from the attic or ceiling cavity to enter the room, bringing contaminants from those hidden spaces. Installing an LED retrofit light can help block this airflow, preventing contaminants from entering the living area. While this reduces exposure, it doesn't address the underlying cause of water damage and mold.

Second Step: Install a light-emitting diode (LED) retrofit unit according to the kit's directions.

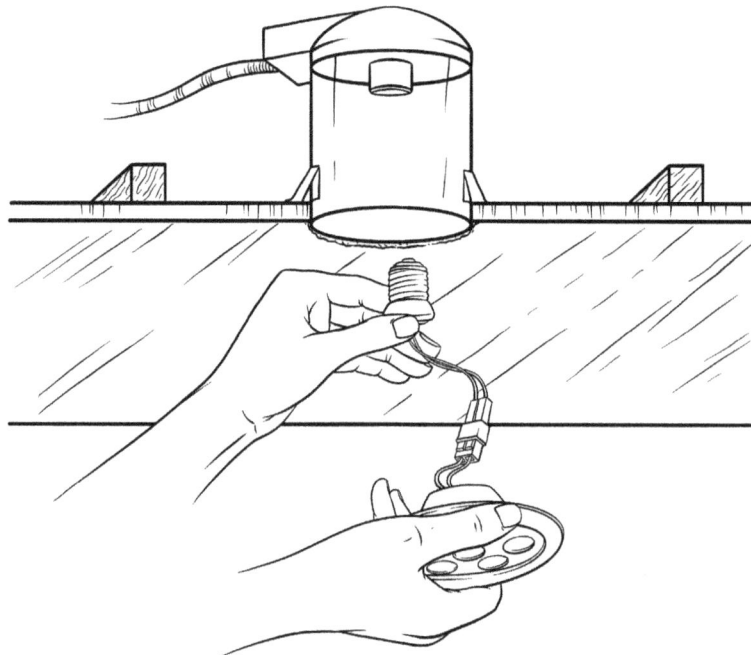

Figure 5-24: The old light bulb is removed, and the LED retrofit light is installed by screwing or wiring it into the existing can light fixture. It is then fitted securely into the receptacle according to the kit's instructions.

Third Step: Seal the LED retrofit around the edge where the decorative ring meets the ceiling using a thin bead of caulk. This prevents unintended air leakage and blocks cross-contamination.

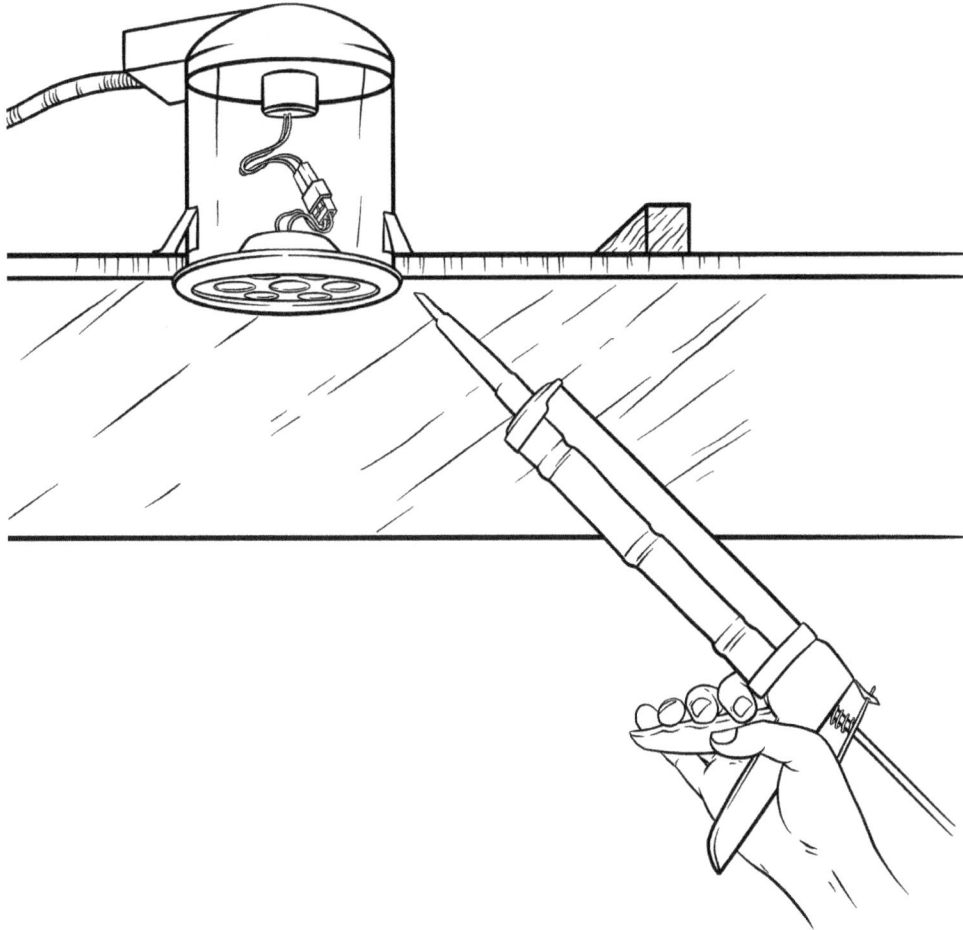

Figure 5-25: A thin bead of caulk is installed to seal the can light to the ceiling, blocking the unintended airflow.

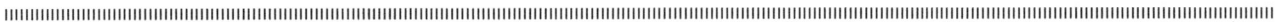

SEASONAL GROWTH

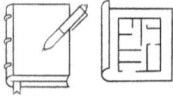

Patterns that emerge or intensify with seasonal changes are often linked to varying indoor humidity levels and temperature fluctuations.

- Summer Growth: In areas that form cracks or openings due to the expansion that occurs due to hot and humid conditions. The newly formed cracks or openings allow water entry.

- Winter Growth: Resulting in frozen plumbing breaks and ice dams.

- Transitional Growth: During fall and spring, repeated expansion and contraction occur due to temperatures and humidity levels fluctuating.

❏ **Major mold growth from burst frozen plumbing**

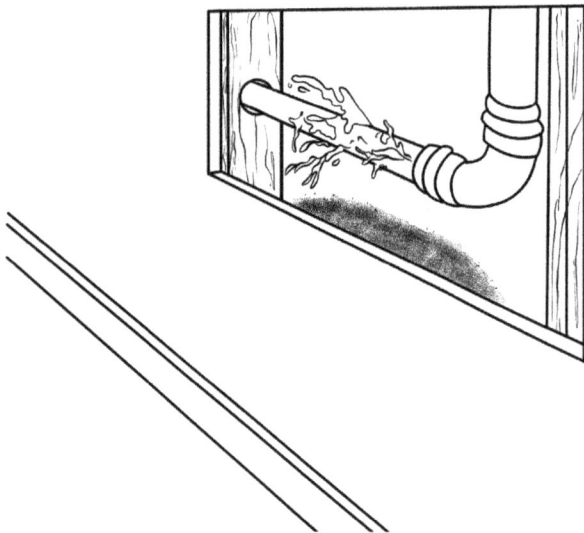

Figure 5-29: Frozen Plumbing: Significant mold growth can occur when frozen pipes lead to major water damage.

❏ **Ice damming**

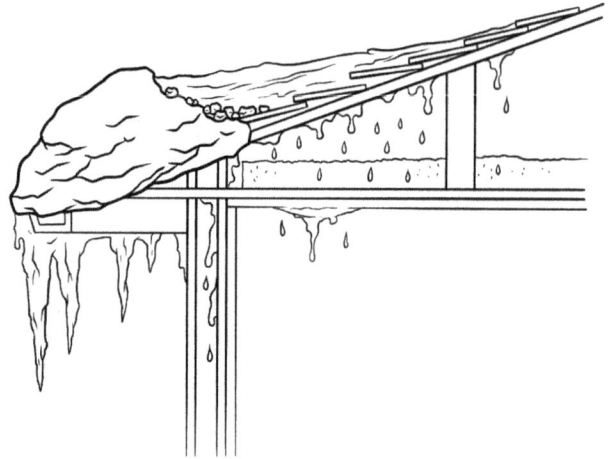

Figure 5-30: Ice Damming Forms when freeze-thaw conditions result in frozen ice preventing liquid water from draining freely off the room. The trapped or dammed water then seeps into the roof assembly. Significant mold growth can develop inside and at the base of walls, attic, and all along the path of water flow.

❏ **Subvisible or hidden growth**

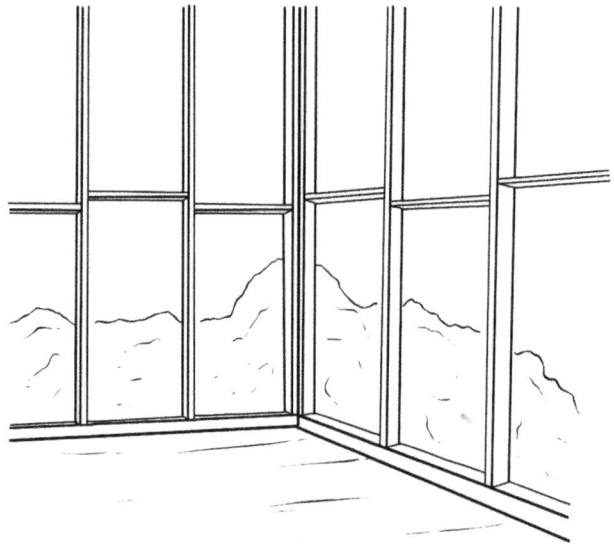

Figure 5-31: Water staining or mold growth is often found inside previously damp wall cavities, which cannot be visually observed until one side of the wall is removed. Even then, the amount of growth is often not dense enough to be visible. Mold growth can contain hundreds of thousands of spores and fragments per square inch and often cannot be observed without the aid of a microscope or sampling.

CONSTRUCTION RELATED GROWTH

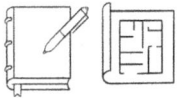

New Building Materials: Mold growth on improperly stored or freshly installed materials due to uncontrolled moisture during construction.

❑ **Mold growth on wood or framing lumber left out in the rain**

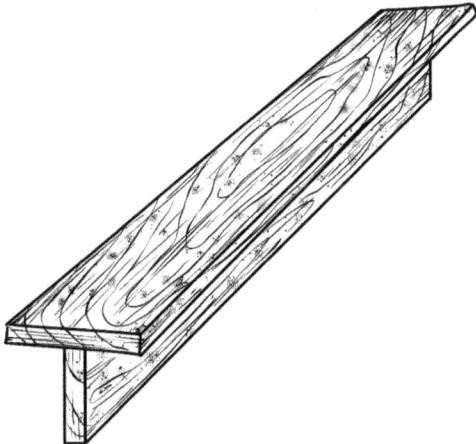

Figure 5-32: New Building Materials show visible mold growth beginning on newly installed wood due to a failure to control moisture before the building is weather-tight and controlled for condensation. The source of the moisture can be wetting from rain, high humidity, or being trapped, such as by enclosing the building without supplemental moisture ventilation or dehumidification when a newly installed concrete slab is releasing moisture due to inadequate curing.

❑ **Lumber-yard mold**

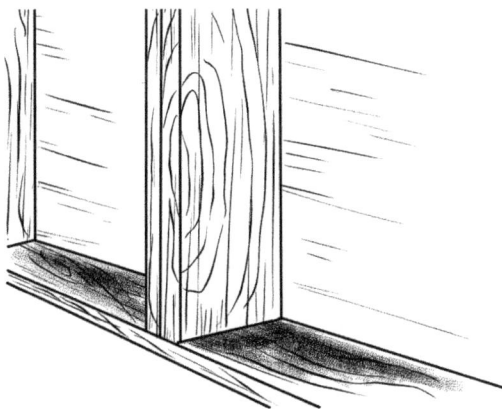

Figure 5-33: Lumbar-Yard: Mold from the Groups Ceratocystis and Ophiostoma commonly grows on green lumber, taking advantage of the natural moisture in freshly cut wood. However, these fungi stop growing once the wood is cured and dried, making it essential to distinguish between pre-existing growth and potentially ongoing mold issues. Notice how the mold on installed lumber does not spread or bridge to adjacent materials, indicating a condition usually associated with "Lumber Yard Mold."

Lumber Yard Mold

Lumber Yard Mold is not known to cause health issues on its own. However, when it is rewetted, such as when an unfinished, unprotected building is exposed to damp or rainy conditions, it can act as a source of predigested nutrients. This can support the growth of more problematic mold types, potentially leading to health concerns and structural damage. Rejecting lumber with significant amounts of *Ceratocystis* and *Ophiostoma* early can help prevent conditions that foster the growth of more harmful molds during construction.

Blue-Stain Mold: Blue-stain on lumber is caused by certain species of fungi from the *Ophiostoma* genus, commonly known as "blue-stain fungi" or "sapstain fungi." This discoloration often manifests as a blue or grayish tint, sometimes making the lumber more attractive and valuable. The stain is not caused by mold but by a fungal infection that targets the sapwood of lumber. These fungi grow in the water-conducting cells of the wood, causing a cosmetic change without affecting the wood's structural integrity. While they don't weaken the wood by rotting, they can impact its aesthetic value, especially in pine and other softwoods where the discoloration is unattractive. Such staining is more prevalent when wood is not adequately dried or is stored in moist conditions, making it susceptible to fungal growth.

❑ **Storage-induced mold**

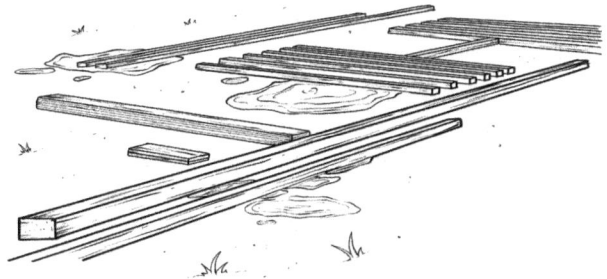

Figure: 5-34: Storage-induced mold occurs when lumber is stored in damp or wet conditions, leading to surface mold growth. Lumber used in construction often becomes moldy when it gets repeatedly wet without the opportunity to dry properly. This situation typically occurs during the building process when the lumber is exposed to elements, such as rain or high humidity.

Mold growth on lumber during construction can be a significant concern, as it can lead to several issues:

- **Health Risks:** Mold growth on lumber can pose health risks, especially for future mold-sensitive building occupants. Mold exposure can cause allergic reactions, CIRS, and respiratory issues, particularly in sensitive individuals.

- **Material Integrity:** While mold on lumber does not necessarily weaken its structural integrity, it can affect surface quality. Over time, persistent mold growth may lead to cosmetic damage and make the wood look unsightly.

- **Spreading to Other Materials:** Mold on wet construction lumber can spread to other building materials, such as drywall, insulation, or carpeting, potentially leading to broader mold issues in the completed structure.

- **Moisture Content and Durability:** Mold growth indicates excessive moisture content in the lumber, which can affect the durability and performance of the wood. High moisture content in wood can lead to warping. Long-term moisture can lead to the development of rot and other wood-destroying pests.

Covering wood with polyethylene plastic is a common practice in construction to protect it from rain and moisture. However, this method, if not managed correctly, can lead to several issues:

1. **Trapping Moisture:** Polyethylene plastic is impermeable, meaning it doesn't allow moisture to pass through. While this is beneficial for shielding materials during active rain, leaving the plastic in place when it's not raining can trap moisture against the wood. This trapped moisture can come from the wood itself (as it releases absorbed water) or from condensation, especially if there are temperature fluctuations.

2. **Promoting Mold Growth:** The trapped moisture creates an ideal environment for molds to thrive. Unlike breathable covers that allow moisture to evaporate, polyethylene keeps the moisture contained, increasing the risk of mold development on the wood.

3. **Staying Wetter Longer:** The impermeability of polyethylene means it doesn't allow the wood to dry out naturally between rain events. This can prolong the wood's exposure to moisture, which leads to mold. This can be especially problematic in construction environments where drying out is necessary before further building stages.

4. **Wood Degradation:** Over time, prolonged exposure to moisture can compromise the quality of the wood. It can lead to issues such as warping, rotting, or deterioration in the strength and integrity of the wood, which can affect the overall stability and durability of the construction.

To mitigate these issues, it's important to manage the use of polyethylene covers effectively. This means removing or ventilating the covers when it's not raining to allow the wood to dry out and, alternatively, using breathable, water-resistant materials such as Tyvek® or "smart membranes" designed especially for this purpose, as covers can protect from rain while allowing moisture to evaporate from the wood. Regularly monitoring covered wood is also crucial to ensure it remains dry and free from mold growth.

❏ **Improperly installed Gypcrete**

Gypcrete, a lightweight concrete used primarily in flooring applications, combines gypsum plaster and fibrous materials to create a versatile and fire-resistant material. It is frequently used to raise and level a floor and to cover the water distribution tubes for a radiant hot water heating system. The installation of gypcrete introduces large quantities of water into the building. While gypcrete itself does not typically provide the nutrients necessary for mold growth, its interaction with surrounding materials can lead to mold problems in adjacent moisture-sensitive materials. Moisture control measures are necessary for up to a month after installation and during the curing of the slab to prevent damage from condensation as the excess moisture evaporates and condenses on sensitive materials. Wicking or capillary action can also become an issue when the water travels from the newly poured slab into nutritive materials such as paper-based gypsum wallboard, resulting in mold growth on the wetted paper.

Step 4: Investigation, Testing, and Next Steps

*IEPs, DIY, and Getting Help: Who Do
You Want in Your Inner Circle?*

Introduction to Sampling

Understanding how an Indoor Environmental Professional (IEP) can assist in identifying environmental problems within your home is essential in evaluating if a consultant can help you address mold and other issues effectively. Many types of testing are available, but before deciding on any specific company, individual, or type of assistance, it is important to clarify the questions you want to answer about your home environment, potential exposures, and their effects. Each testing method has specific advantages, disadvantages, and limitations, often requiring expertise to navigate effectively. Not all consultants are well-versed in adapting testing strategies to meet the unique needs of their clients, particularly those with medical sensitivities.

Some consultants may primarily serve specific industries, such as insurance companies, real estate transactions, or public health concerns, without fully considering the implications of their methodologies for people with sensitivities. This underscores the importance of aligning your consultant's experience, philosophy, and strategy with your unique needs.

Collaborative Approaches to Sampling

When considering sampling, you have several options:

- **Do-It-Yourself Testing**: This approach may work for some initial screening sample collection, but the person collecting the sample will need to easily access both low and high areas. Sampling can unintentionally stir up dust, posing additional risks of exacerbating exposure for sensitive individuals during collection. Individuals may also face physical challenges, such as difficulty safely using a ladder or collecting floor-level samples.

- The reliability of reported results and their interpretation depends on the laboratory's quality and the expertise applied to analyze them rather than the sampling process itself. The expertise needed to understand building-related issues and the types of problems they develop often lies with experienced consultants, not laboratories. Choosing a professional who can make

laboratory recommendations and interpret results with a deep understanding of building dynamics and your unique needs is essential. The act of collecting samples may be challenging for people with mold illness.

- **Long-Distance Consulting**: Engaging a professional to provide guidance remotely can be a cost-effective way to receive expert advice tailored to your situation and help extend the capabilities of the locally available resources.

- **Local Professional Assistance**: Hiring a local IEP for on-site inspections and testing may provide the most comprehensive assessment, provided they have the necessary expertise and align with your specific goals and needs.

- **Cooperative Approaches**: Combining methods can be effective, for example, conducting initial sampling with assistance from a non-sensitive friend or family member while consulting remotely with an expert or supplementing local professional evaluations with online follow-ups has proven very helpful in many cases.

Each option can work depending on your circumstances, resources, and the complexity of the environmental issues you're addressing.

Avoiding Predatory Companies

Unfortunately, not all service providers, online or in person, operate with integrity or possess the necessary expertise. Be wary of companies that promise immediate solutions without a clear strategy, rely heavily on fear-based marketing, have predatory pricing practices, or employ testing methods designed more to sell services or products than to provide actionable insights. Look for companies that pay attention to your needs and help develop a personalized approach to your project. Avoid companies that have a one-approach-fits-all type of practice. Avoiding these pitfalls requires careful vetting. Ask potential consultants about their experience, strategy, and philosophy to ensure they align with your goals and sensitivities. Confirm that the information they provide will be actionable and worth the investment.

Incorporating Insights from Stage One

As you worked through Stage One: *Is There a Problem*, the insights gathered in Steps 1 through 3 should help guide your decisions about the level of investigation needed and the budget you're prepared to allocate. These steps help determine whether your home meets your needs and evaluate the benefits and limitations of conducting certain types of sample collection versus hiring a professional IEP.

Depending on your circumstances, you may choose to combine the on-site inspections or testing outlined in Stage One, Step 4, with the more detailed evaluations described in Stage Two, Step 5, which focuses on uncovering hidden issues. Completing both these Steps should equip you with the information necessary to make thoughtful decisions about addressing environmental concerns in your home and managing your possessions and contents effectively.

Moving Forward with Professional Collaboration

The exercises in this Step are designed to help guide you in selecting and collaborating with an IEP and other inspection experts or gathering your information to help you gain meaningful insights into addressing your home's environmental challenges. While this book offers guidance, it cannot fully provide all the necessary information to navigate mold issues in homes. Proper selection and collaboration with professionals will give a clearer picture of your home's condition and the steps required to restore and maintain a healthful living environment.

Exercise 4.1: Finding an Indoor Environmental Professional: Do Your Goals Align?

Indoor Environmental Professional or Consultant: Finding a suitable indoor environmental professional or consultant helps address mold and building-related issues, especially when health concerns are involved. A qualified professional should provide expert advice and guidance tailored to your specific needs and goals, ensuring their experience aligns with the unique challenges of your situation. In cases of medically important remediation, they may need to present evidence to counter advice from less experienced peers while remaining within their professional boundaries. It's essential to understand that while they can advise on how building conditions may impact health, they should never prescribe, diagnose, or make medical decisions for you. Ultimately, decisions about your goals, actions, and expenditures are yours to make, ideally with the consultant as a knowledgeable guide to help you make informed choices.

❑ **List Your Mold Investigation Goals**: Describe in detail what you aim to achieve with the process (e.g., health improvements, property value preservation).

❑ **Identify the Type of Professional Needed**: Based on your goals, determine whether you need a mold sampling technician, a building scientist, a Medically Important

Remediation-experienced and competent Indoor Environmental Professional, a construction-savvy contractor, or other specialists.

❑ **Screening Potential Consultants**: When screening potential consultants, it's helpful to consider questions that will help determine if their expertise aligns with your goals. Ask about their experience with cases like yours, their approach to testing and assessments, and whether they have the necessary tools and equipment to conduct the evaluation themselves. If they lack specific experience in medically important investigations, consider whether they show a willingness to learn and adapt to your unique needs. Resources such as this book and training through the CIRSx Academy (see "Medically Important Remediation (MIR101) – Advanced Training" on page 33) can help bridge knowledge gaps and bring an experienced consultant up to speed. If the scope of work requires specialized skills or equipment beyond their capabilities, inquire about their ability to collaborate with other professionals long-distance to help ensure a comprehensive assessment. This process enables you to identify a consultant who can effectively meet your needs, whether independently or as part of a cooperative effort.

Engaging the right IEP is about building a partnership to restore and maintain a healthy environment. Thoughtful preparation and collaboration set the stage for a thorough investigation and effective remediation strategy.

Exercise 4.2: DIY, Online Consultant Assistance, or Onsite Environmental Professionals

Assessing Capabilities and Limits: You and the consultant you are considering should evaluate the feasibility of creating an effective plan to address mold and water damage issues. Begin by listing the tasks you can realistically handle, considering whether the information in your project diary provides a solid foundation for further action. Evaluate your comfort level in performing or coordinating additional inspections, such as lifting carpets to check for clues or collecting primary samples, and identify where professional expertise is essential, such as conducting detailed assessments or interpreting test results.

❑ **Weighing DIY vs. Professional Guidance**: Consider the advantages and disadvantages of DIY versus professional guidance, weighing factors like your ability, cost, and time to decide the best approach. Plan your involvement based on your health, availability, and resources—deciding whether to oversee the process, provide input, or handle specific tasks.

❑ **Planning for Limited Involvement**: If your health prevents active involvement, determine whether a trusted friend or family member can assist onsite or explore what level of professional assistance you can afford to hire to ensure the job is done effectively.

Exercise 4.3: Finding Qualified Indoor Environmental Professionals

The Exercises in the Emergency Water Damage section of the book may have already helped you select a consultant to work with. If not, review that section and:

❑ **Research Potential IEPs**: Compile a list of IEPs with experience in mold investigation and remediation and other necessary attributes.

❑ **Check Credentials and References**: Verify the professionals' qualifications, certifications, and references to ensure they meet your standards and have relevant expertise.

❑ **Interview Prospective IEPs and Evaluate Their Proposals**: Assess the proposals from different IEPs based on how well they align with your goals and budget. Ask specific questions to determine their understanding of medically important remediation and whether their approach fits your needs.

❑ **Leverage CIRSx Resources**: CIRSx comprises healthcare providers, environmental consultants, and mold remediators. They are working diligently to identify, train, and establish a nationwide network of professionals skilled in Medically Important Mold Investigations and Remediation. Visit CIRSx.com and search for the CIRS Academy for resources to help you find qualified professionals.

Exercise 4.4: Types of Testing

In the intricate process of mold assessment, various types of testing are employed, each with unique advantages and limitations. This exercise focuses on helping DIY individuals understand what they can do independently and when professional assistance is necessary, such as for complicated projects, specialized medical, exposure assessments, or legal cases.

❑ **Tape Lift Sampling**

Purpose: Tape lifts focus on visible mold growth, providing direct evidence of surface contamination. They are especially useful for assessing visibly evident colonies but are less effective for detecting sub-visible mold levels. Some laboratories claim they can identify mold at densities as low as one spore per square inch. Still, practical experience shows a more realistic lower detection limit of around 1000–1500 spores per square inch.

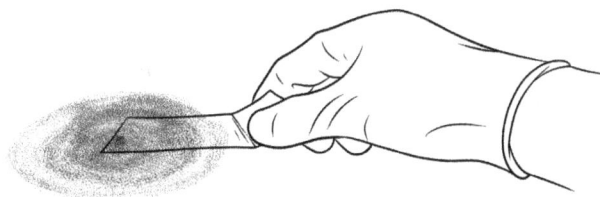

Figure 5-35: Tape lifts are used to collect a sample of visible mold growth to provide genus-level identification. They are ineffective for determining the types or quantities of individual Penicillium and Aspergillus spores. They cannot identify particles or fragments of mold or hyphae to determine the type of mold.

Instructions for Tape Lifts

1. **Use Appropriate Tape**: Use Scotch Brand Transparent Tape (red package).

2. **Prepare the Tape**: Tear a 2–3" strip of tape, avoiding contact with the sticky side.

3. **Proper Collection Technique**: Press the tape straight down onto the surface of the visible mold, ensuring it bridges the outermost inch of the colony to capture both new and mature growth. Press the tape gently into the area of visible mold being sampled. Avoid grinding the tape into the surface or smearing it across the sampling area, as this can destroy the mold structures, making identification more difficult.

4. **Peel and Secure**: Lift the tape straight up from the surface to preserve the sample's integrity. Attach the tape to the transparent, unlabeled portion of a resealable bag, sticky side down.

5. **Label and Double-Bag**: Label the bag with location details, then place it into a second resealable bag to prevent contamination during transport.

6. **Submit for Analysis**: Send the double-bagged sample to a lab with a completed Chain of Custody form.

Properly collected samples allow skilled analysts to visualize mold structures like *Penicillium* or *Aspergillus* and identify them at the genus level without the growth being smashed or torn apart.

❑ **Culture Sampling**

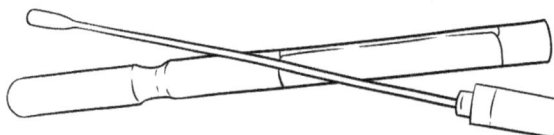

Figure 5-36: Culture, PCR, and direct exam can be used to analyze collected swabs. The type of analysis desired will determine if the swab is collected wet or dry, where it is sent, and how rapidly it must arrive. Swabs used to collect live or dormant mold deteriorate rapidly after collection, so next-day shipping with ice packs and advanced notice to the laboratory are often needed. Swabs only tell you what is

on the surface from which the swab is collected. Depending on your request, the identification can be done using direct examination at a non-specific level, especially for Penicillium and Aspergillus molds, a genus or a species level using culture (Not all laboratories can speciate a culture sample), or PCR for identification to a species level for hundreds of organisms regardless of viability. Swab samples are typically an advanced technique that requires special handling. Consider working with a qualified IEP if you need this type of sampling.

❏ **Surface Dust Sampling with Swiffer Wipes**

Swiffer wipes effectively collect dust from hard, horizontal surfaces like shelves, door frames, and baseboards. This method captures settled spores and fragments, offering a historical perspective of contamination. High and low sampling locations ensure a broader understanding of the environment. For example, some laboratories will instruct people not to collect anything below 3 feet or knee level. They are telling you this so you can collect an exposure assessment sample, assuming that is what you want. If you are trying to figure out information about contamination, then non-floor low surfaces are necessary to consider because heavy spores like *Stachybotrys* may not make it high enough into the air to identify.

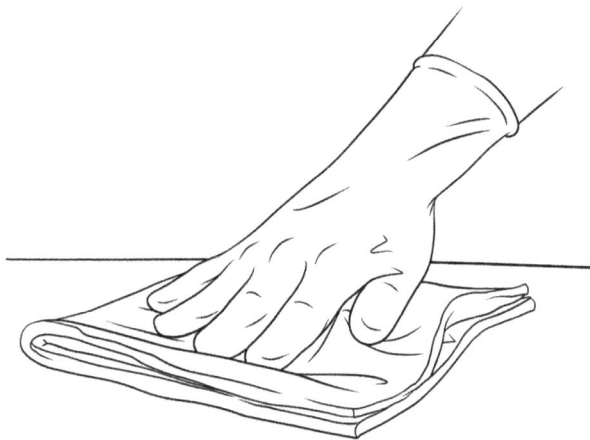

Figure 5-37: Dust collection using a Swiffer® wipe is used for either MSQPCR or culture analysis from hard or non-porous surfaces. The wipe is collected so that one side is completely dirty with dust. An inadequate amount of dust will result in skewed results.

Instructions for Swiffer® Wipes

1. **Use the Right Wipes**: Use new, unscented, electrostatic Swiffer dry wipes from a fresh box to ensure they are uncontaminated. You can usually purchase a sampling kit from the laboratory, but this means you have to wait for the supplies, and the shipping will cost a lot more than going to your local supermarket to purchase the supplies you need to collect and submit them.

2. **Avoid Damp or Wet Surfaces**: Ensure surfaces are dry before wiping, as moisture can interfere with the collection process and contaminate the sample.

3. **Wipe Properly**: Perform a single, firm swipe over the surface to collect dust effectively. Avoid scrubbing or repeated motions, as the first wipe gathers the sample, and additional passes may break up the collected materials into very fine particles that are more difficult for the lab to remove from the wipe in order to analyze the dust in the collected material.

4. **Determine Dust Quantity**: Ensure sufficient dust collection. Ideally, the dust should visibly cover one complete side of the Swiffer wipe (approximately 25–50 mg). It doesn't matter which side you wipe with as long as the combined total equals the necessary amount of dust. Some labs will run the sample with less dust than what EPA has indicated is needed but be aware that insufficient dust can skew the results. EPA research was performed by analyzing only samples with at least 5 mg of sample, but having at least 25 mg can help. The lab will have extra in case something goes wrong with the analysis. (for example, if the power fails in the middle of an analysis run. That sample would be ruined and need to be recollected). Collecting sufficient dust will assist in case unforeseen circumstances result in a reporting issue. Most labs will save the unused dust for a few days, which can then be submitted for additional types of analysis, such as culture if sufficient dust has been collected.

   If the collected amount is insufficient, wait for additional dust to settle before gathering more. Ensure you collect the additional dust before the next cleaning, as cleaning eliminates the dust needed for sampling. Typically, sufficient dust takes around six weeks to accumulate, but waiting this long in a problem building may worsen health risks. To address this, you can collect and clean in repeated steps, using sequential Swiffer wipes to gather the needed dust over time without allowing harmful levels of accumulation. When using this method, remember to collect dry dust without HEPA vacuuming the surface beforehand.

5. **Take a Picture of the Sample**: Photograph the collected wipe, ensuring it is labeled, to document the amount of dust present in case the laboratory will not provide quality control details.

6. **Package and Label**: Place the used wipe into a clean, resealable plastic bag, label it with the sample location, date, and address, and then seal it. Double-bag the sample for extra protection.

7. **Submit for Analysis**: Include a completed Chain of Custody form and follow lab submission instructions.

❏ **Vacuum Dust Sampling**

Vacuum dust collection is ideal for gathering samples from soft, upholstered, or carpeted surfaces. It provides insights into particulate contaminants embedded in textiles or carpets, complementing surface wipe data. You will need to get a special disposable collection canister and specific instructions from the consultant or laboratory you are working with.

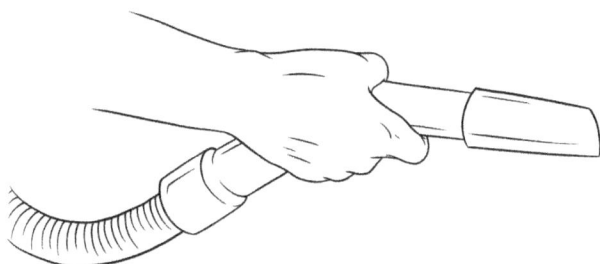

Figure 5-38: Vacuum Dust Collection is performed with a special adapter that contains a filter to collect dust and remove it from the air stream before it enters the vacuum cleaner nozzle. This keeps the collected dust separate from contamination inside the vacuum cleaner or its hose. The nozzle should always be pointed upward after the dust collection until it has been capped to prevent the dust from spilling from the cartridge. Each collection requires a separate adapter.

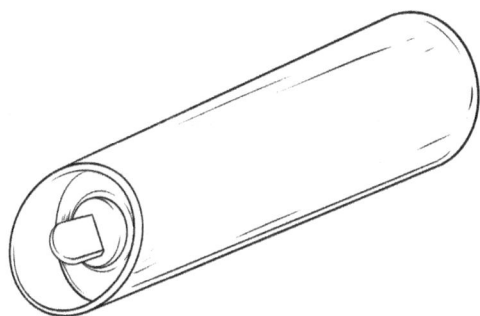

Figure 5-39: The Vacuum Dust Collection Nozzle is designed to fit on a standard vacuum cleaner hose. The collection device contains a filter that collects dust. The collector is capped to contain the collected dust inside the adapter. After collection, each nozzle should be kept upright and bagged separately to prevent dust from different samples from cross-contamination.

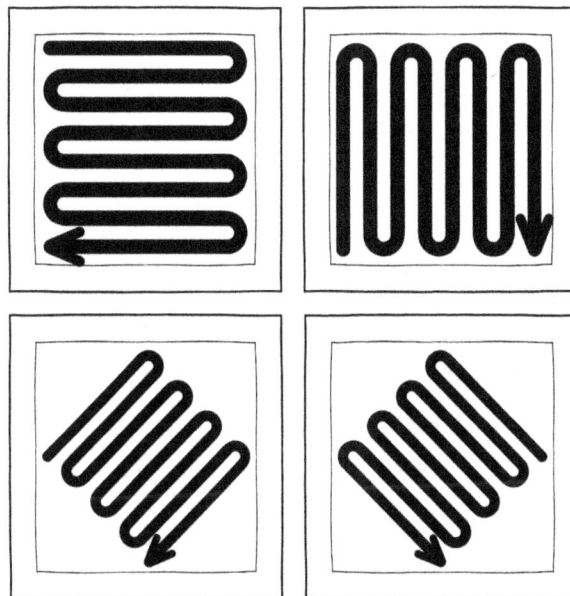

Figure 5-40: The vacuum dust should be collected deeply by vacuuming the carpet, upholstered furniture, or other soft materials using a scraping motion with the tip of the nozzle. Keep the nozzle at a slight angle so it can be moved across the surface while vacuuming in all possible directions.

Instructions for Vacuum Collection

1. **Use Proper Equipment**: Attach a specialized dust collection nozzle or adapter provided by the lab to a vacuum cleaner. Use a separate collection canister to represent the specific area being tested.

2. **Label the Bag**: Prepare a resealable plastic bag with your name, address, sample location, and date before starting collection.

3. **Choose Sampling Areas**: Focus on soft surfaces like carpets, upholstered furniture, or mattress covers. Multiple square feet can be sampled, covering up to 500 square feet for one collection. Similar types of items, such as a set of dining room chairs, can be sampled together.

4. **Vacuum Thoroughly**: Use deep, overlapping motions across the sampling area, starting with visible dust levels as a guide. Sampling a smaller surface (e.g., 4 square feet) may suffice for heavily dust-filled areas, while lighter dust levels may require covering a larger area (up to 20 square feet). Multiple areas can be tested to represent the entire space, ensuring thorough coverage and enough fine dust is collected for analysis. Repeat in multiple directions (horizontal, vertical, and diagonal) for thorough collection.

5. **Determine Dust Quantity**: Ensure at least one table-spoon (approximately 15 ml) of fine dust is collected. Large debris, like hair or fibers, can remain but does not count as fine dust. If insufficient fine dust is collected, continue sampling from additional areas sequentially.

6. **Take a Picture of the Sample**: Photograph the collected sample, ensuring it is labeled, to document its condition and quantity for both Swiffer and vacuum dust samples. This step is especially important if the laboratory does not provide quality control details, as it ensures proper documentation and supports accuracy in case of disputes or incomplete reporting.

7. **Seal and Double-Bag**: Carefully remove the sampling nozzle, seal both ends with the provided plugs, or, according to the instructions provided with the collection cartridge, place it into the labeled resealable bag. Do not include more than one sample per bag. Sometimes, the sampling apparatus may disassemble during shipping, allowing the dust from multiple samples to mix. Double-bagging the samples separately for transport will protect against the sample being lost in such accidents.

8. **Submit for Analysis**: Send the bagged sample to the designated lab with a completed Chain of Custody form and follow all submission guidelines

• **Additional Types of Samples**: Many types of additional sample methods are always being developed. Most of these are worthless, unnecessary, or too complicated and require specialized equipment for the collection to be worth doing yourself. If additional samples are needed or desired, they should generally be performed after consulting a qualified indoor environmental professional.

• **Exposure Assessments**: Air sampling requires specialized expertise, particularly for legal or medically significant cases. Short-term spore trap methods may not provide sufficient data for exposure assessments. For reliable results, professional-grade equipment and long-term sampling techniques are essential.

• **Legal Cases**: Accurate sampling and interpretation by a certified professional are required for supporting legal claims. Surface and air samples must meet evidentiary standards.

• **Medically Important Assessments**: Consult your physician to determine if special testing assistance is required, especially for individuals with compromised immune systems, such as those undergoing chemotherapy, taking anti-rejection drugs, or having other immune-compromising conditions. Physicians can guide testing priorities based on specific health risks, such as allergens or exposure thresholds relevant to the patient's condition. If there are concerns about specific allergens or health issues related to the indoor environment, your physician should provide guidance on what needs to be tested. Collaboration between healthcare providers and environmental professionals is essential to ensure that these more complex testing strategies address the unique health requirements of the occupants.

Choosing the Right Rooms and Areas to Vacuum for Dust Collection Sampling

When the EPA conducted its initial studies of 1,097 homes across the U.S., their protocol focused on two rooms where people typically spent the most time: the bedroom and the living or family room. This approach made sense for a broad population study, emphasizing areas most likely to reflect personal exposure. However, this method has limitations for mold investigations attempting to target specific problems in a home.

For example, if dust samples are collected from two rooms far apart, like an upstairs bedroom and a downstairs family room, and combined into a single analysis, the results might mask the true problem areas. Based on thousands of samples and common sense, proximity to a mold growth site typically results in higher contamination levels. Therefore, dividing the home into logical areas of 500 to 750 square feet ensures a more targeted and actionable approach.

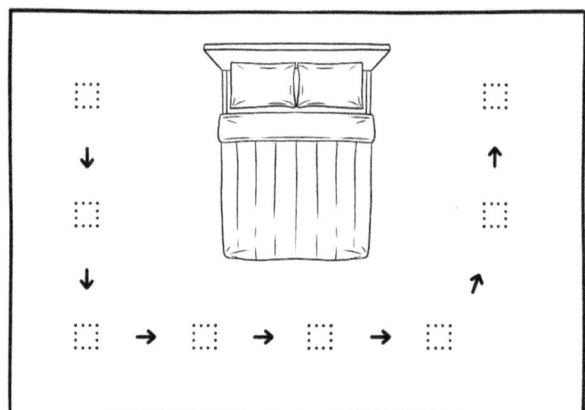

Figure 5-41: Be sure to collect sufficient dust from multiple locations within each sampled area. Dust does not settle evenly in rooms. Try to avoid high-traffic areas close to entry points from the outdoors.

In a 2,000-square-foot, three-bedroom, two-story home, for example, the house might be divided as follows:

1. **Upstairs Primary Bedroom**: Especially if this is occupied by someone suspected of mold illness.

2. **Two Adjacent Upstairs Bedrooms**: Typically grouped, possibly including a shared bathroom.

3. **Downstairs Great Room**: A common area combining kitchen, dining, and living spaces.

4. **Other Downstairs Rooms**: Grouped, such as an office or guest bedroom.

Additional samples might include:

- **Basement**: One for an unfinished basement or split into two samples if areas are finished and unfinished.

- **Attached Garage**: Sampled separately.

- **Outdoor Dust**: Sometimes collected to assess baseline mold levels from outside sources.

In this example, a 2,000-square-foot home would need four samples to assess the living space but might require six or seven samples at several hundred dollars per sample. While this may seem expensive, thorough diagnostics is often a fraction of the expense of remediation. Sampling also helps pinpoint specific problem areas, making remediation efforts more focused and cost-effective.

Frustration can arise when less experienced consultants want to rely on less expensive air samples for medically important cases. This often fails to represent the true nature of mold contamination in a home. Declaring the home "fine" based on incomplete data can expose occupants unnecessarily to harmful conditions, especially those with sensitivities. Comprehensive sampling of settled dust provides a clearer, more reliable picture of where mold problems are concentrated, helping to address the root cause effectively.

Sampling Every Room vs. Targeted Testing

While some people prefer to sample every room in their home to ensure no issues are missed, this expensive approach can sometimes encounter a surprising challenge: individual rooms, especially those that are well-maintained and frequently cleaned, may not have enough dust to complete the analysis. Insufficient dust makes it difficult to gather meaningful results, leaving gaps in the investigation.

In such cases, Pathways™ sampling, discussed in Step 5, can be a more practical and effective method. Pathways™ Testing measures protein and peptide bond residues, objectively identifying suspect problem areas without relying solely on visible dust accumulation. By combining Pathways™ results with strategic sampling of settled dust, homeowners can focus on areas showing signs of contamination while avoiding unnecessary testing in spaces unlikely to contribute valuable insights. This balanced approach allows for a more efficient and targeted investigation, reducing costs and improving diagnostic accuracy.

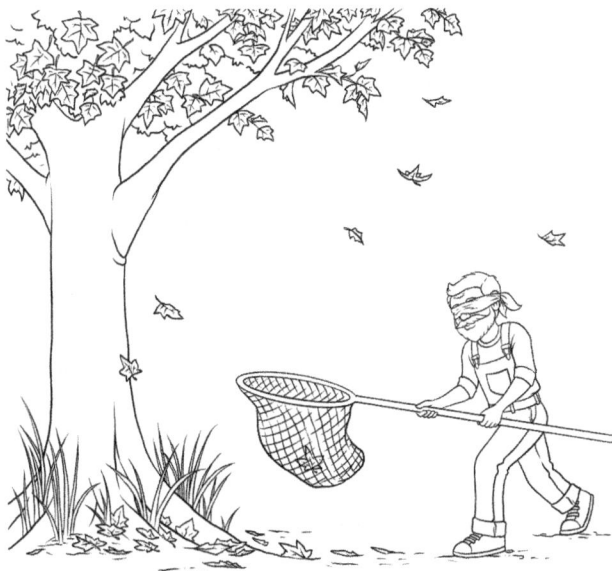

Figure 5-42: Air Sampling for mold is like collecting leaves falling from a tree in autumn in a butterfly net while blindfolded. You might collect some leaves, But only if you get lucky.

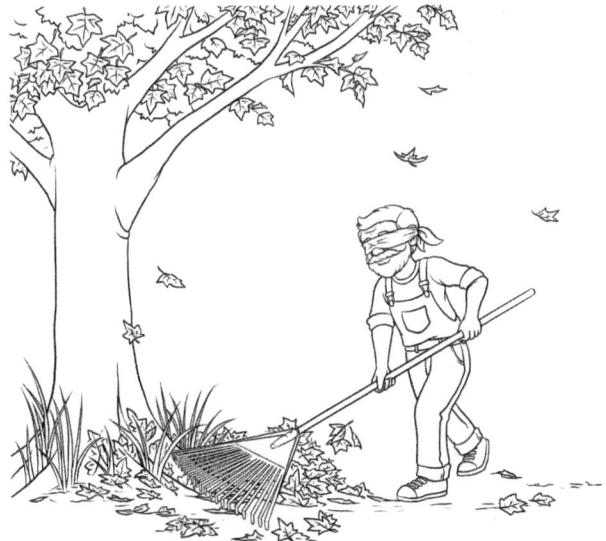

Figure 5-43: Raking leaves while blindfolded is much more efficient. Likewise, surface dust sampling for mold is more efficient at identifying a problem than air sampling.

Mycotoxin Testing of Buildings

Mycotoxin testing of settled dust or from HVAC filters in buildings is often marketed as a definitive method for identifying mold-related problems. However, I find this method problematic, and it should be carefully considered before being used as a diagnostic tool for buildings.

Highly Diverse

It has been estimated that over 2,000 different types of biotoxins can be produced by organisms associated with water damage. *Stachybotrys* alone is believed to produce over 200 different types. Mold does not automatically produce toxins; in many cases, toxin production requires specific stresses to activate the production of toxins. One such stress is spraying mold growth with a biocide to attempt to kill the mold, which can result in an environment containing toxins from both the biocide and the organism—creating a double whammy. Furthermore, some toxins are produced by multiple organisms, making it difficult to match specific toxin levels to particular species. For example, ochratoxin has been documented to be produced by more than 25 species of mold, many of which are food-related and do not occur in water-damaged environments.

Commercially available testing for toxins is usually limited to about two dozen types. It will likely be a long time before we fully understand the full spectrum of mycotoxins, the problems that result, and the conditions that cause their production. This is one reason for focusing on water damage and microbial growth rather than the toxin type. A promising new method under development in Europe involves using human cell cultures to test house dust for toxicity. This approach may help identify conditions where house dust toxicity is adversely affecting occupants, targeting both the human impact and the fungal ecology necessary for maintaining a balanced environment.

Environmental Complexity

Mycotoxins are secondary metabolites produced by certain molds, but their presence in a building does not always correlate with active or historical mold growth or specific contamination issues. These toxins can travel on particles like dust and settle in areas far from their origin, leading to results that may not accurately reflect current mold conditions. This can result in misleading conclusions about the source and extent of contamination.

Cost vs. Benefit

Mycotoxin testing of the building is often expensive, with costs that may not provide proportional benefits in guiding remediation efforts. In many cases, other diagnostic methods—such as dust sampling, moisture mapping, and visual inspections—can provide more actionable information at a fraction of the cost.

Practical Limitations

Collecting samples for mycotoxin testing often requires substantial amounts of settled dust, which may not be available in well-maintained or recently cleaned spaces. This limitation can result in inconclusive findings, necessitating additional tests and increasing costs.

Focus on Root Causes

Rather than testing buildings for mycotoxins, I advocate identifying and addressing the underlying causes of mold contamination, such as water damage and elevated humidity. Targeting the root problems—and confirming their resolution through appropriate diagnostic methods like DNA, culture, and Pathways™ testing—is a more effective and practical approach.

In conclusion, while mycotoxin testing may seem appealing, its limitations often outweigh its usefulness. The more holistic strategy I focus on in this book prioritizes actionable diagnostics and remediation, essential for effectively managing mold-related issues in buildings.

Exercise 4.5: Interpretation of Results

Understanding testing results is necessary for identifying contamination sources, assessing severity, and prioritizing remediation efforts. Interpretation begins with categorizing areas of concern, such as zones with visible mold growth or water staining confirmed through tape lifts, and considering other factors like Actinobacteria and Gram-negative endotoxins. These elements help break down the investigation into actionable segments, ensuring a structured approach to remediation.

Tape lift samples analyzed through direct microscopic evaluation provide valuable insights into visible mold growth. These samples can identify mold at the genus level if growth structures, such as conidiophores, are present. For samples lacking visible growth, hyphae or growth structures may indicate nearby sources requiring additional investigation.

Penicillium/Aspergillus-level identification for sub-visible contamination may be inadequate to determine if the tested dust is from an indoor water damage source. Tape lifts are particularly useful for assessing lumber yard mold, offering a means to determine if rewetting has led to additional growth in affected areas. However, it is important to note that tape lifts cannot distinguish between active, dead, or dormant mold. Active growth may be inferred if the mold appears wet. However, determining dormancy or viability requires culture sampling, which is rarely necessary and should only be pursued after consulting with a qualified IEP.

Interpreting tape lift results involves evaluating spore concentrations. Dense growth typically shows hyphae and growth structures, while lower densities might indicate settled spores or early stages of growth. Tape lifts are limited to assessing the specific surface tested, and their results must always be interpreted within the broader context of the water damage causing the contamination. A common challenge is the misinterpretation of low-density results as "safe." Tape lifts generally do not provide information that can be used for that level of interpretation without other data. It is common for tape lifts to be unable to quantify surfaces with less than 1,000 CFU/in². Culture or MSQPCR methods may be more appropriate if lower densities or quantities are needed. However, due to differing collection requirements, tape lifts cannot be used for culture or PCR analysis.

Despite these limitations, tape lift samples offer actionable insights. They can pinpoint hotspots that provide a starting point for effective remediation strategies. By understanding the context of contamination revealed through tape lifts, homeowners and professionals can take informed steps to address mold issues comprehensively.

Swiffer™ Wipe and Vacuum Dust Samples (MSQPCR Analysis) Interpretation

❑ When collecting vacuum dust samples, focusing on areas outside of high-traffic zones is often beneficial to avoid the influence of foot traffic patterns. Sampling around the perimeters of rooms or in areas with nearby filtration soiling can reveal whether specific organisms are entering from wall cavities, basements, or crawlspaces. This approach ensures that the samples provide a representative picture of contamination beyond surface-level disturbances.

❑ Samples analyzed using MSQPCR provide a historical and current record of spore accumulation. Vacuum samples are primarily useful for soft materials such as carpets, area rugs, and upholstered furnishings. Swiffer wipe samples are primarily used for hard surfaces. The MSQPCR method quantitatively identifies mold DNA, offering a detailed look at the species present and their concentrations. It is especially useful for detecting water-damage indicator species such as *Stachybotrys* and *Chaetomium* as well as other organisms to be identified to a species level, associated with varying moisture levels and nutrient sources. The commonly available MSQPCR molds available are identified in the Mold Gallery on page 73.

❑ Key metrics in vacuum or Swiffer Dust samples include the total mold load, measured in spores per milligram, and the presence of water-damage indicator species and common outdoor molds. Interpretation of these results can be guided by the EPA's geometric mean framework, which classifies contamination levels as follows:

› 0 to 10 times the geometric mean: Normal levels.
› 10 to 100 times the geometric mean: Elevated levels.
› 100 to 1,000 times the geometric mean: Strongly indicative of a nearby growth source.

❑ Additionally, the relative concentrations of mold DNA for either type of collection can be ranked across sampled areas, revealing contamination gradients. Proximity to a growth site typically results in higher spore loads, while more distant areas show a decline. Temporal variability should also be considered; sampling results are snapshots influenced by recent environmental conditions.

❑ The HERTSMI-2 scoring system, developed by Ritchie Shoemaker, offers another layer of interpretation, particularly for individuals with mold-related illnesses such as Chronic Inflammatory Response Syndrome (CIRS). This metric assesses habitability for sensitive individuals by quantifying specific mold species associated with water-damaged environments. Comparing indoor results with outdoor baseline samples collected using Swiffer wipes can help contextualize findings and identify potential indoor amplification. More information about the interpretation of these results can be found at SurvivingMold.com

While preparing this book, I tried using AI to interpret results and found its ability to do so lacking. I suspect that attempts at such interpretations will become common, but I believe it is important to remain cautious.

Actionable Insights for both Swiffer and Vacuum dust collections

❑ Since MSQPCR is collected from approximately 500 square foot areas to help ensure sufficient dust, it can be used to narrow down areas with issues likely to be present within that 500 square foot area, but is unable to pinpoint areas needing remediation unless visual indications like water staining, buckling, discoloration, or musty odors lead to the determination.

• Pathway™ sampling can help to delineate further where to look for growth sources versus areas with elevated levels of contamination or those needing cleaning to address other protein-based contaminants or building memory (See Step 5).

• MSQPCR is very sensitive and may lead to an understanding that problems are present for hypersensitive people when visual evidence is lacking and not able to provide evidence of hidden growth. It is important to not confuse elevations due to settled spores and building memory with elevations from growth sites.

• The use of MSQPCR and Pathways™ in tandem is more likely to be able to narrow down decisions regarding actual growth versus settled spores and building memory when the testing methods are used together. DNA analysis identifies the organisms to a species level regardless of viability. Pathways™ identifies areas where there are a buildup of peptide bonds and proteins. Cleaning and Pathways™ Testing helps demonstrate areas where cleaning has been adequately performed and successful. Timed testing after cleaning helps demonstrate how quickly contaminants return and can be helpful in determining if an area can be maintained by routine cleaning or if remediation is needed.

References

Pitkäranta, M., Meklin, T., Hyvärinen, A., Paulin, L., Auvinen, P., Nevalainen, A., & Rintala, H. (2011). Molecular profiling of fungal communities in moisture-damaged buildings before and after remediation—a comparison of culture-dependent and culture-independent methods. *BMC Microbiology, 11*(1), 235. https://doi.org/10.1186/1471-2180-11-235

Pietarinen, V.-M., Rintala, H., Hyvärinen, A., Lignell, U., Kärkkäinen, P., & Nevalainen, A. (2008). Quantitative PCR analysis of fungi and bacteria in building materials and comparison to culture-based analysis. *Journal of Environmental Monitoring.* Advance online publication. https://www.rsc.org/jem

Stage Two: Develop a Strategy, Team Assembly, and Locating Hidden Problems

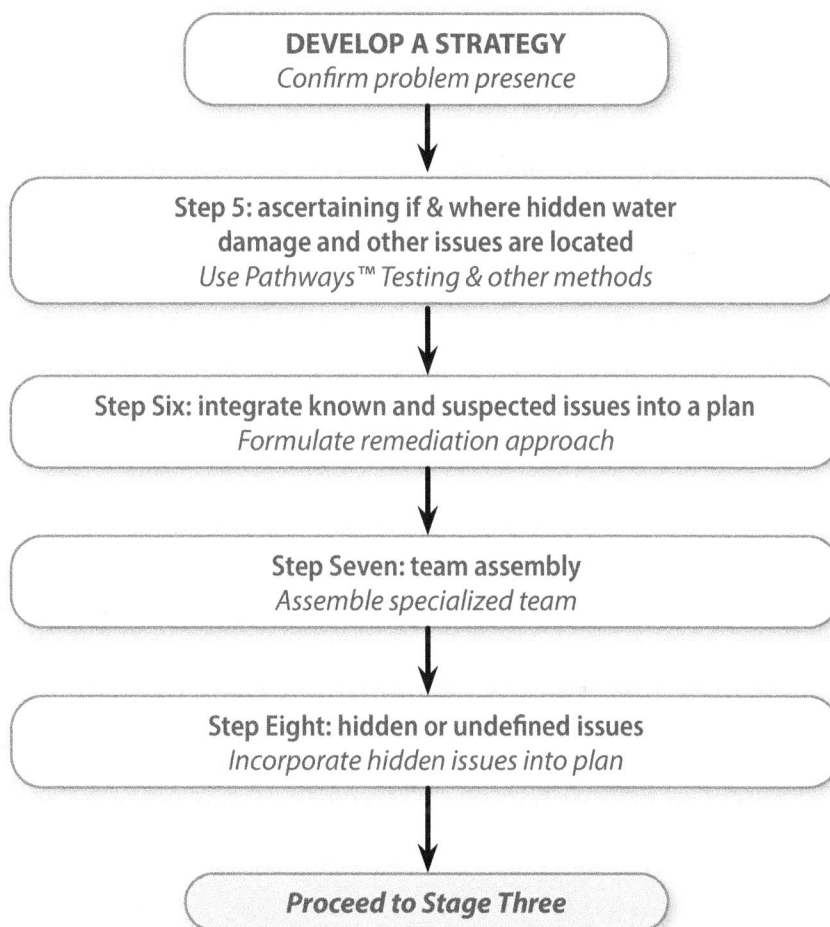

DEVELOP A STRATEGY
Confirm problem presence

↓

Step 5: ascertaining if & where hidden water damage and other issues are located
Use Pathways™ Testing & other methods

↓

Step Six: integrate known and suspected issues into a plan
Formulate remediation approach

↓

Step Seven: team assembly
Assemble specialized team

↓

Step Eight: hidden or undefined issues
Incorporate hidden issues into plan

↓

Proceed to Stage Three

Navigating Remediation Planning with Focused Foresight

Having confirmed the abnormal presence of mold or water damage in your home, Stage Two is dedicated to crafting a targeted remediation strategy. This stage involves a detailed screening for hidden hot spots that eluded initial detection, devising a strategic plan for remediation, and assembling a team with expertise in health-sensitive practices. The aim is to refine preliminary assessments into a well-defined plan that addresses visible issues and uncovers and tackles potential concealed problems. It's a pivotal phase in synthesizing data and observations into a strategy for evident and latent concerns. Selecting a team cognizant of mold hypersensitivity and multiple chemical sensitivities (MCS) is crucial, as it ensures the remediation process is both thorough and mindful of health implications. By establishing a robust foundation for focused remediation, this stage marries scientific analysis with practical application to foster a safer home environment. Here, your initial findings evolve into a clear remediation roadmap, including personal belongings decisions. For individuals with mold sensitivities, these decisions are vital. They are comprehensively addressed in this book's 'Contents and Personal Possessions' section to support a holistic approach to home health restoration.

Goals for Stage Two

By the time you have completed this stage, you should have the necessary information to be able to answer these questions:

- What are your needs for Medically Important Investigations and standard mold investigations for insurance, real estate, or legal purposes?

- What factors should be considered when choosing a team for your home's remediation, cleaning, or reconstruction?

- Do you need to develop a strategy for relocating the members of your household to better housing?

- If occupants are experiencing sensitivity reactions due to mold or water damage, yet immediate remediation isn't feasible due to financial constraints or other barriers, what steps do you need to take to significantly mitigate exposure and improve conditions for staying in the home?

- How can baseline, post-cleaning, and follow-up Pathways™ Testing help uncover hidden problems and provide you the feedback that you need to address issues adequately?

Step 5: Screening for Hidden Sources of Contamination

Revealing Your Home's Hidden Contamination Routes.

When mold is visible on surfaces, it's clear that action is needed. However, mold often grows in places we can't see, like walls, ceilings, or floor cavities. If water damage is only partially dried, these hidden areas can remain damp, allowing mold to thrive unnoticed. Even when the mold dries out and becomes dormant, it can still release tiny particles, such as spores and fragments, into your home through cracks and openings. Surface cleaning cannot address these inaccessible spaces, leaving hidden growth that impacts indoor environmental quality for the life of the house. A big challenge is determining what represents hidden contamination that is likely to affect the living space and warrants remediation versus slightly elevated levels that can be controlled by routine effective cleaning.

Particles travel from hidden spaces into living areas, carried by airflows or pressure changes. Cracks as small as a human hair provide the pathway and allow particles to escape. Even well-sealed homes may develop new openings rapidly from major forces such as strong winds and earthquakes, but also over time due to ongoing expansion, contraction, or settling.

This step introduces various screening methods, weighing the pros and cons of destructive investigation, wall-cavity sampling, mold dogs, and non-invasive Pathways™ Testing.

Minimally Invasive and Destructive Investigations for Hidden Mold

In the early years of mold investigations, destructive techniques, such as cutting observation holes in walls, ceilings, or other interior cladding, were often used to uncover hidden mold. These methods were often performed without containment measures or air filtration systems necessary to limit the release of dust and contamination. If you couldn't see it, it wasn't worth consideration. Negative air filtration controls, now standard in professional remediation, were rarely used, allowing particles to spread freely throughout the home during the investigation process.

Early guidance documents, such as the New York City Guidelines (NYC 1993), classified visible mold growth smaller than 10 square feet as routine maintenance. This classification did not call for significant control measures, leading to the common practice of cutting multiple exploratory openings in suspect walls until 10 square feet of visible mold growth was uncovered. Unfortunately, what initially seemed to be minimal mold growth frequently became extensive once hidden areas were exposed. By the time ten square feet were uncovered, significant spores and fragments had already been released, contaminating large portions of the home. As destructive investigation methods evolved and revealed limitations, minimally invasive techniques like borescopes and wall cavity air sampling began to be introduced. These approaches were intended to reduce the impact on the building structure and limit contamination spread, but they also presented significant challenges in practice.

- Landlords were often reluctant to permit even small holes to be drilled or cut.

- Buildings constructed before 1979 frequently contained lead or asbestos in the gypsum or joint compound. Due to health risks, any disturbance of these materials is heavily regulated, further complicating the use of these techniques.

- Subvisible mold levels due to humidity within wall cavities can develop due to condensation moisture that cannot be visualized with a borescope. Borescopes, designed to provide visual access inside wall cavities, often failed to determine issues, as shadows and obstructions make mold challenging to identify accurately.

- Wall-cavity sampling was too expensive to test every potential space.

- Excessive dust in wall cavities could obscure tiny mold spores. Drilling into walls for sample collection generated high dust levels, obscuring smaller mold spores and fragments.

- Wall cavity air sampling frequently failed to detect hidden mold because the spores or fragments in these spaces were not sufficiently disturbed to become airborne, leading to misleadingly low or negative results.

- Particles and fragments from degraded mold were still allergenic; some types contained biotoxins. Estimates showed that unidentifiable fragments and particles of mold often exceeded the spore count by 300–500 times.

- It was also challenging to determine what level of identifiable spores in a wall or other cavity should trigger remediation or further action.

While these minimally invasive techniques attempted to reduce disruption, they were often insufficient for reliably locating hidden mold.

Mold Dogs

A dog's sense of smell is extraordinary, capable of identifying and differentiating a vast array of odors. While humans might perceive the general aroma of beef stew, a dog detects every ingredient separately. This remarkable ability has been applied to numerous tasks, from locating missing persons to detecting explosives and cancer. It's no surprise that dogs can also be trained to detect mold. Intrigued, my wife, Tricia, and I explored the possibility of training our Labrador mix, Dax, for this specialized work.

Dax had already demonstrated her keen nose, occasionally digging up rotten truffles during family camping trips. With guidance from trainers experienced in disaster recovery, including teams who used dogs to locate victims from the 9/11 tragedy, we began to understand how to channel her natural abilities into mold detection. These trainers emphasized kindness, rewards, and clear communication, a methodology that shaped Dax's training process.

The training focused on building a consistent behavior-response system. Using a clicker to mark correct actions and provide rewards, we taught Dax to recognize mold scents from carefully prepared samples. Over about six months, we refined her training to distinguish mold from other common odors, such as food or lumber-yard fungi, ensuring she only alerted on target materials. This process required discipline not just from Dax but from us as handlers.

Dax became a valuable supplement to my mold investigations. Her ability to pinpoint potential mold "hot spots" was unparalleled, complementing traditional methods like moisture meters, air sampling, and thermal imaging. However, it became clear that the success of mold detection dogs depends more specifically on their handlers. Many handlers lack the rigorous training to set clear expectations about what their dogs will and won't detect. The dog's capacity to detect mold isn't in question, but the human-animal communication gap can lead to misunderstandings, limiting the dog's effectiveness as a diagnostic tool.

Dogs should only serve as indicators, pointing to areas that require further investigation. Without proper calibration and clarity about the levels and types of mold a dog is trained to find, their alerts may be inconsistent or easily misinterpreted.

Despite Dax's success, her health eventually took priority. During some investigations, after about six months of fieldwork, she began showing signs of respiratory distress, likely from repeated exposure to moldy environments. Recognizing the risk to her well-being, we retired her from mold detection. This decision underscored the need to consider canine safety alongside their impressive capabilities.

While Dax no longer worked as a mold dog, her training profoundly influenced my investigation approach. Her instant feedback helped me sharpen my observational skills and identify subtle clues I might have otherwise missed. Though mold detection dogs have limitations, they remain a fascinating testament to the bond and teamwork between humans and dogs.

Establishing a Mold Dog Certification Process

An independent Mold Dog Certification process should be developed to ensure credibility and consistency in mold detection. This certification would help demonstrate proficiency and standardize training and testing parameters, providing a clear framework to evaluate the capabilities and limitations of the dog and the trainer/handler. A robust certification process could include the following elements:

1. **Standardized Mold Panels for Testing Proficiency:** Certification testing would involve sampling for molds from the original 26 ERMI panel Group One organisms, ensuring the dog can detect a wide range of common indoor molds. In addition, the dog would be tested on dry rot, wet rot, the Ceratocystis Ophiostoma group, ethanol (vodka), and fresh meat such as chicken or beef. The dog would be evaluated on its ability to discern distractors from problem molds and ignore blanks and distractors that are not mold-based.

2. **Sensitivity Calibration:** The testing process would include varying concentrations of mold growth, from minor localized patches to more spotty distributions across larger areas. This would help assess the dog's sensitivity and clarify its minimum detection thresholds.

3. **Control Samples:** Non-moldy materials that mimic typical environmental odors—such as wood, cardboard, clean

gypsum board, or food-related substances—would be included to ensure the dog can discriminate between mold and other non-target scents.

4. **Alert Evaluation**: Dogs are trained to demonstrate either passive or aggressive alerts in response to mold samples. I believe only passive behaviors that minimize contamination risk should be allowed. It is inappropriate for a dog to attack the wall where mold is suspected. The handler's ability to recognize and respond to passive alerts would also be assessed.

5. **Scenario-Based Testing**: Certification would include practical scenarios, such as detecting mold behind walls, ceiling cavities, under flooring, and complex environments like crawlspaces or attics. This ensures real-world applicability.

6. **Handler Proficiency**: At least half of the certification process would focus on the handler's skills. This includes their ability to:

- Interpret the dog's alerts accurately.
- Avoid influencing the dog's behavior (e.g., via unintentional cues).
- Communicate the dog's findings to clients.
- Understand construction and how mold impacts buildings.

7. **Ongoing Recalibration**: Annual recertification would ensure the dog and handler remain proficient, maintain calibration to detection thresholds, and adapt to evolving best practices in mold inspection.

By implementing a standardized certification program, mold detection dogs/handler teams could gain independent credentials, bolstering their credibility and establishing their role as valuable tools for identifying potential mold concerns. A well-designed process would benefit homeowners, environmental consultants, and remediation professionals by ensuring reliable results from these highly trained canines.

INTRODUCTION TO PATHWAYS™ TESTING

Pathways™ Testing is a method I developed during the early months of the COVID-19 crisis to address the challenge of identifying hidden contamination in homes without causing unnecessary damage. It started as a personal experiment when my wife and I knowingly purchased a moldy house. Because of Trisha's mold sensitivities, I originally wanted to buy a home without issues. After looking at over 50 homes over three months, we resigned ourselves to buying a moldy fixer-upper and approached the situation as a make-or-break experiment. As our real estate agent put it, it was time for me to "put my money where my mouth was," using everything I had learned about mold, contamination, and indoor environmental quality, I was able to restore that house into a healthful living space that did not trigger Trisha's sensitivities.

Over the years, I have relied on many traditional methods to locate hidden mold and contamination. However, these approaches were often too invasive, expensive, or ineffective, frequently missing key issues for sensitive clients or causing unnecessary disruption. I needed a better approach that could non-destructively reveal where contamination was traveling from hidden locations into living spaces without compromising the home's integrity. I recognized that developing such a system was needed not only for my wife but also for my clients.

Development of Pathways™ Testing

Pathways™ Testing was created to identify the pathway where contamination escapes from hidden spaces. The idea was to trace the path that particles, like mold spores and fragments, follow to travel through a home. By understanding these routes, I could determine where the contamination originated and focus remediation efforts in the right areas.

The Pathways™ method builds on something I learned over 50 years ago in high school physiology: testing for proteins by detecting peptide bonds. Back in the 1970s, nutrition labels didn't exist. My teacher, who had a keen interest in nutrition, assigned several students special projects to analyze food for nutritional content, which we then demonstrated to the class. It was fascinating to see how simple tests could yield valuable insights. I was struck by how easily food manufacturers could apply these methods to help consumers better understand their food. That idea left a lasting impression on me. Fast forwarding to 2019, I found research showing that mold's cellular structure was largely protein-based. The study also revealed that all enzymes are proteins, meaning the same would be true for the enzymes mold exudes to digest building materials.

As I contemplated buying the fixer-upper, I reflected on the risks involved. Trisha would need to live elsewhere during the remediation, and I would have to find creative ways to address the contamination at a time when safety equipment—like respirator cartridges and protective suits—was in short supply due to the COVID-19 pandemic. The scarcity added to the challenges, but it also sparked an idea. The protein research I learned about in high school resurfaced, and I realized I could use protein markers to identify contamination and track its migration through our new home. It was a calculated risk, but one I felt was worth taking.

It felt as though every challenge we faced, the COVID crisis causing us to sell our wonderful home, months of squatting with relatives while failing to find a suitable house, and the daunting prospect of buying a fixer-upper—was puzzle pieces falling into place guided by a series of seemingly unrelated events: a high school teacher ahead of her time, a study on the protein structure of mold, and the convergence of my life experiences, all aligning to spark the creation of Pathways™ Testing.

Practical Applications

Purchasing a moldy home became an opportunity to refine and develop a practical application for the connection between mold and protein-based contamination. I knew I understood what it would take to remediate and remodel the home. I didn't know if I would have the time or money to make it all work using the conventional trial-and-error process of finding and fixing mold. My goal was clear: create a healthy living space that would not trigger Trisha's sensitivities. I was not the first to think of using protein testing to identify potential mold contamination. There are do-it-yourself protein detection swabs, but they are primarily qualitative and do not have sufficient quantitative sensitivity for detecting proteins at a level necessary for people with sensitivities. The Biuret system was what I had learned about in high school, and it became clear that it would not function properly in the presence of soaps or detergent surfactants. Intellectual curiosity, desperation, and inspiration led to solving each problem.

Mold spores and fragments have long presented confounding challenges in testing and identification. Their outer surfaces are coated with fatty substances, which make them water-repellent. This coating delays germination in nature, as moisture must penetrate the coating before the spore can absorb enough water to germinate, typically requiring a minimum of about two days. This same water repellency has much to do with why the chemical biocides and antimicrobials being touted to kill mold have become so problematic.

The breakthrough in Pathways™ Testing came when I replaced the Biuret reaction I learned in high school with a modified set of reagents using bicinchoninic acid in an alkaline medium. This modification significantly sped up the chemical reaction from days to an hour or two. The alkalinity breaks down the fatty coating on mold spores more quickly, allowing the reagents to interact more effectively with the proteins inside. This improvement made the test much faster and more reliable than do-it-yourself swabs, which cannot penetrate the fatty coating effectively. However, while this controlled use of an alkaline medium enhances testing in a laboratory setting, using alkaline solutions in a home environment is a bad idea. Such

solutions can damage personal possessions, degrade building materials, and pose safety risks to occupants, further complicating an already challenging situation.

Because the highly alkaline reagents cannot be safely handled outside a laboratory, the samples are collected and shipped to the laboratory, where trained technicians perform the testing in a laboratory setting. A spectrophotometer is used for the analysis, which is far more precise than visually detecting color changes. This method increased the maximum detection sensitivity from approximately 100 micrograms of protein to 600 micrograms, greatly improving the range of information provided.

Another key breakthrough came when I discovered microfiber swabs. Originally developed for clean room environments, these swabs are designed to pick up and tightly hold fine particles. Switching to microfiber swabs increased the surface area that could be effectively sampled with a single test threefold—from 16 linear inches for conventional swabs to 48 linear inches. This advancement allowed for more comprehensive testing with fewer resources, further enhancing the efficacy of Pathways™ Testing.

Over time, Pathways™ Testing has proven invaluable, not only for identifying hidden sources of proteins—often mold-based—but also as a powerful screening tool. Because it focuses on protein detection rather than specifically identifying mold species, the testing is more cost-effective, making it an accessible option for routine monitoring. It enables the evaluation of cleaning efforts and provides a way to monitor how quickly protein-based contaminants re-enter home environments. This insight has been instrumental in establishing criteria for determining how often a home requires cleaning to maintain low protein levels, which serve as a surrogate indicator that mold and other water-damage organisms are under control.

Pathways™ Testing is also a valuable resource for restoration contractors. It serves as an internal quality control tool to verify the effectiveness of their cleaning processes. Contractors can use the method to satisfy the ANSI/IICRC S520 requirement for verifying work prior to turning the project over for a third-party assessment. Additionally, it functions as a practical training tool for new technicians, providing them with the necessary feedback to help them understand the higher degree of performance necessary to develop the skills necessary to meet Medically Important Remediation requirements.

By pinpointing areas where proteins and peptide bonds are entering living spaces, Pathways™ Testing helps prioritize locations requiring frequent cleaning versus those needing only occasional maintenance. This targeted approach ensures that contamination levels remain manageable, offering a practical, actionable strategy for maintaining a healthy home environment.

Beyond Mold

Pathways™ Testing doesn't just detect mold; it also screens for other protein-based contaminants such as rodent feces, cockroach frass, dust mites, and pollens—substances no one wants in their home. Establishing baseline and follow-up contamination levels makes it easier to determine whether a home is affected by active mold growth or spores and fragments migrating from elsewhere. Understanding these distinctions helps target remediation and maintain a clean, healthful environment.

Transitional Spaces

Beyond identifying contamination, Pathways™ Testing has been instrumental in creating healthful sanctuaries during transitional periods. Whether moving into a new home or living in one part of a house while remediating another, this method helps monitor and maintain safe environments. It provides a clear framework for controlling protein-based contaminants, ensuring that even temporary spaces remain as healthful as possible.

The system focuses on areas where airflow slows, allowing particles to settle and accumulate. Common sampling locations include wall-floor cracks, outlet boxes, plumbing and HVAC penetrations, recessed lighting, and other points where contamination might escape from hidden spaces. By targeting these areas, Pathways™ Testing delivers actionable insights that support more effective control, cleaning, and remediation strategies.

Lessons Learned

Pathways™ Testing is not a one-size-fits-all solution, nor does it provide a complete picture. Like any method, it has its limits. It doesn't identify the specific type of mold or the exact origins of the proteins measured. Instead, it is a strategic tool to flag areas of concern and monitor changes over time. Combined with other diagnostic and investigative methods, it offers a robust approach for identifying,

remediating, and maintaining control over contamination that might otherwise go unnoticed.

For my wife and me, Pathways™ Testing was a lifeline—a way to transform a moldy house into a healthful home. For anyone facing similar challenges, this method provides the tools and insights to regain control of their indoor environment and create a safe, healthful living space.

WHY IT WORKS

Pathways™ Testing identifies tiny particles, such as proteins and peptide bonds, linked to mold, bacteria, and other contaminants commonly associated with water damage. These particles can migrate from hidden areas, like wall cavities or beneath floors, into living spaces through small openings such as cracks, gaps, or joints. Pathways™ Testing works by collecting fine dust from surfaces near these potential routes and analyzing it to determine contamination levels.

The system's effectiveness relies on understanding how particles behave. Tiny particles like mold spores or fragments are often carried by airflow and settle onto surfaces where airflow slows. Smooth surfaces—such as baseboards or flooring near cracks—attract and hold these particles because of molecular forces, including Van der Waals interactions and electrostatic charges. These forces make particles cling tightly to surfaces, causing dust to build up in measurable patterns. The closer a surface is to a source of contamination, the more particles accumulate over time. By analyzing these patterns, Pathways™ Testing can pinpoint areas where contamination is escaping from hidden locations.

Advances from industries like clean room manufacturing have influenced the effectiveness of Pathways™ Testing. These industries, which demand nearly particle-free environments for pharmaceuticals, electronics, and biotechnology, have invested heavily in research on removing even the smallest particles. By applying techniques and tools developed in these fields, the mold remediation industry has improved cleaning standards and achieved more healthful environments, especially for sensitive individuals.

||

How Pathways™ Testing Works: A Technical Explanation

Pathways™ Testing uses spectrographic analysis to semi-quantitatively detect compounds associated with mold, actinomycetes, gram-negative bacteria, and other peptide bond- and protein-based particles found in damp or water-damaged environments. The method employs a modified Biuret reaction with bicinchoninic acid in an alkaline medium. This reaction reduces copper ions (Cu^{2+}

to Cu^{1+}) in the presence of peptide bonds, characteristic of proteins. The reaction is measured spectrographically at a wavelength of 562 nm, allowing for precise identification of proteins and peptide bonds on sampled surfaces.

Peptide Bonds and Proteins: Peptide bonds are the chemical links between amino acids that form polypeptides and proteins. Proteins synthesized via peptide bonds are essential for many biological functions. In mold, proteins play critical roles in survival and digestion. Mold enzymes, which are proteins, facilitate digestion by breaking down building materials to extract nutrients.

The role of moisture is key in this process. Mold enzymes require a specific moisture balance to function effectively: too much moisture dilutes the enzymes, while too little moisture prevents their activation. Each mold species thrives within a particular moisture range, highlighting the importance of managing indoor moisture levels to control mold growth.

Key Advancements: Pathways™ Testing leverages clean room technology, including microfiber swabs, to collect fine dust from surfaces. Microfiber swabs, originally developed for industries requiring ultra-clean environments, dramatically increase sampling efficiency. Detecting proteins and peptide bonds helps assess contamination levels and evaluate the success of cleaning efforts, effectively maintaining a cleaner, healthier living space.

COLLECTING PATHWAYS™ SAMPLES

Pathways™ sample collection uses a standardized method to gather fine dust from surfaces near openings where contaminants may emerge from wall cavities or hidden spaces. This process ensures consistency and comparability across samples, providing reliable data for analysis.

Materials Needed:

- 3.5 mm microfiber swabs
- Protective cellophane sleeves
- Unique identifier labels
- Floor plan for mapping sample locations
- Chain of custody documentation

Step-by-Step Procedure

- **Preparation**: Identify and map the area of the home that will be investigated. The concept is to collect dust that accumulates immediately adjacent to openings where contaminants are likely to settle as they exit small openings. These include cracks, gaps, or joints in walls, floors, or ceilings. The protective cellophane sleeves are labeled with unique identifiers corresponding to the floor plan's mapped locations.

- **Precautions and Limitations**: Avoid using enzyme-based cleaners, as enzymes are proteins that will interfere with the testing process. Essential oil-based products, antimicrobials, and biocides may also compromise testing results.

  › A recommended cleaner is **Branch Basics All-Purpose Detergent**, which has proven effective for individuals with sensitivities and does not interfere with Pathways™ or MSQPCR testing. If another cleaning agent is being contemplated, consult with RestCon Environmental to see if the desired product has been evaluated for enzyme content. If the product has enzymes listed on the label, it will not be appropriate for use. A sample of the cleaner can also be submitted to RestCon Environmental to determine if it is compatible with the Pathways™ Testing System.

- **Swabbing**: Use a 3.5 mm microfiber swab to collect dust. Avoid touching the microfiber sampling tip.

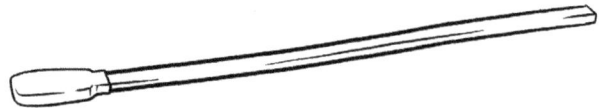

Figure 5-44: The swab used for collecting the Pathways™ test was developed for cleaning in clean rooms. They do a good job of collecting small particles and tend not to pick up larger particles like grains of sand or dust bunnies. This makes them well suited for collecting microorganisms, but they tend to reject rodent feces, insect body parts, and other large proteins like dropped food.

- Collect dust over a 48 linear-inch path:

  › Swab the first 24 contiguous linear inches using one side of the swab with a single, firm swipe.
  › Flip the swab and collect dust from the remaining 24 contiguous linear inches.

- Collecting the sample immediately next to cracks or openings helps determine if it is a pathway for protein-based contaminants working their way from a hidden location through the opening or crack.

- Collecting the sample on other surfaces helps determine how much protein-based contaminant has developed or settled onto the tested surface.

- Apply a consistent, firm pressure to ensure even dust collection.

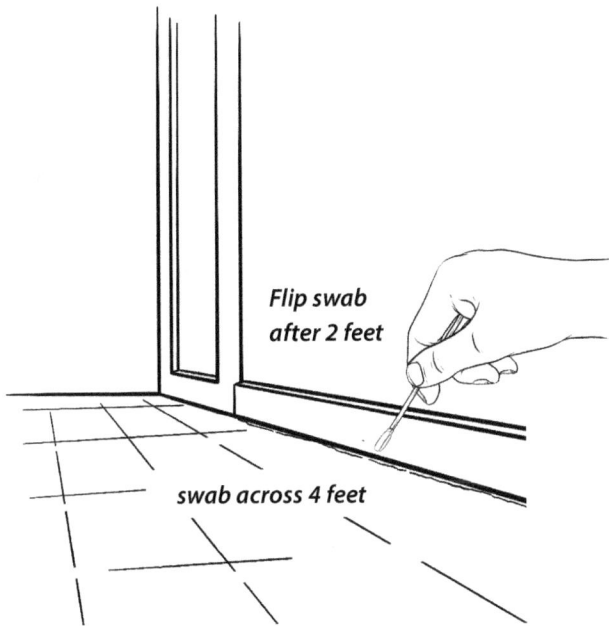

Figure 5-45: Swab a 4-foot-long sample

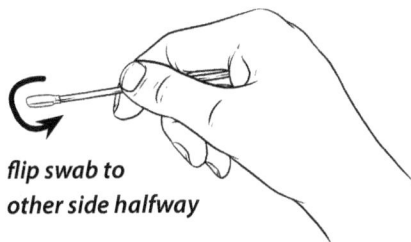

Figure 5-46: Flip swab halfway to use both sides. Hand collection of microfiber swabs for Pathways™ Testing uses a consistent four linear feet (flip after two feet so the collected dust is more evenly distributed over both sides of the swab).

- **Storage**: After collecting the sample, place the swab in a protective cellophane sleeve and seal it properly to prevent contamination. Store the samples at room temperature, avoiding excessively high or low temperatures. If kept dry, samples can be stored for weeks or months without noticeable degradation. If there is a risk of moisture accumulation, then a silica gel packet can be included in the packaging.

- **Documentation**: Mark each protective sleeve with its unique identifier. Record the sample location on the floor plan to correlate it with the specific collection area. Include the sample in the chain of custody documentation to maintain integrity and traceability throughout the process.

- **Shipping**: Ship the collected samples to the laboratory for analysis. Package them carefully to prevent any damage or contamination during transit.

Key Points for Consistency

The total surface swabbed for each sample is always 48 linear inches, with 24 inches swabbed using one side of the swab and the remaining 24 inches swabbed using the other side. Consistent, firm swipes ensure even dust collection across the entire path. Following the same procedure for each sample maintains consistency and comparability, while proper documentation and labeling ensure accurate tracking and analysis.

By following this standardized method, Pathways™ Testing provides a reliable representation of dust contaminants near openings in wall cavities or hidden spaces. This ensures accurate analysis and interpretation by the laboratory, facilitating targeted remediation efforts.

CHOOSING SAMPLE LOCATIONS

Pathways™ Testing requires careful selection of sample locations to characterize where protein-laden dust has settled effectively. Different sampling patterns can be employed based on the goal of the testing, whether it's identifying specific contamination sources, monitoring cleaning effectiveness, or screening for general conditions in the home.

Floor-Level Testing Pattern

One of the most effective testing patterns involves collecting samples every four feet around room perimeters, particularly along baseboards. This dense sampling approach is ideal for identifying hidden water damage that may have led to mold or bacterial growth near the base of walls.

For contamination to migrate into the occupiable space, three conditions must be met:

1. The presence of mold, bacteria, or another protein source.
2. A crack or opening that creates a pathway for contaminants to escape hidden spaces.
3. Airflow or a pressure differential to push or pull contamination along the pathway into the living space.

The perimeter of exterior walls is particularly informative, as protein levels can indicate migration from:

- The crawlspace or levels below.
- The ceiling or attic, particularly when water damage is near the perimeter walls.
- Outside the home, when soil, leaves, or other debris has accumulated above the concrete stem wall or slab foundation.

Interior walls may also show contamination patterns, particularly in areas affected by extensive flooding or where there is a water fixture or plumbing source on the other side of the wall. In these cases, water damage may have created conditions for microbial growth inside the wall cavity, allowing protein-based contaminants to migrate into the living space. This is especially common in areas near bathrooms, kitchens, laundry rooms, or other locations with water fixtures or appliances.

Samples are typically collected every four feet around the room perimeter to compare protein levels between potentially contaminated surfaces and well-cleaned surfaces. This method reduces the likelihood of missing hidden contamination and provides valuable insights into potential sources of protein-laden dust.

Addressing Contamination

If no apparent source of contamination is identified, additional rounds of Pathways™ Testing can help isolate problem areas:

- **Effective Cleaning and Immediate Testing:** Perform detailed, effective cleaning followed by Pathways™ Testing to assess the efficacy of the cleaning. If protein levels remain elevated, the issue could stem from insufficient cleaning or a hidden contamination source releasing proteins faster than they can be cleaned.

- **Follow-Up Testing:** If cleaning appears successful, wait 1.5 to two weeks before conducting follow-up Pathways™ Testing. This can check for signs of contamination resurgence, potentially indicating a migrating protein source from an adjacent or interior wall cavity. Increasing cleaning frequency and improved cleaning techniques may help maintain the living space in such cases.

By systematically collecting samples and evaluating results, this testing pattern provides actionable insights into hidden contamination sources, including exterior and interior wall issues, and helps guide remediation and cleaning efforts.

SCREENING-LEVEL TESTING PATTERN

A screening-level testing pattern provides a general overview of the home's conditions by using fewer strategically collected samples. This approach is helpful for a preliminary assessment but often leads to a need for further testing to help pinpoint specific "hot spots" and contamination sources.

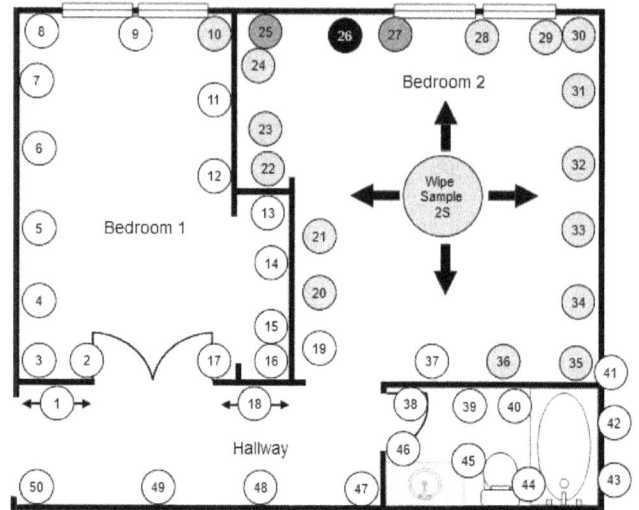

Figure 5-47: A dense testing pattern may reveal a recently developed area of mold growth when a single source is present. It is common for multiple issues and other actions that disturb mold growth without physically removing it under appropriate controls to make such a clear pattern unrecognizable.

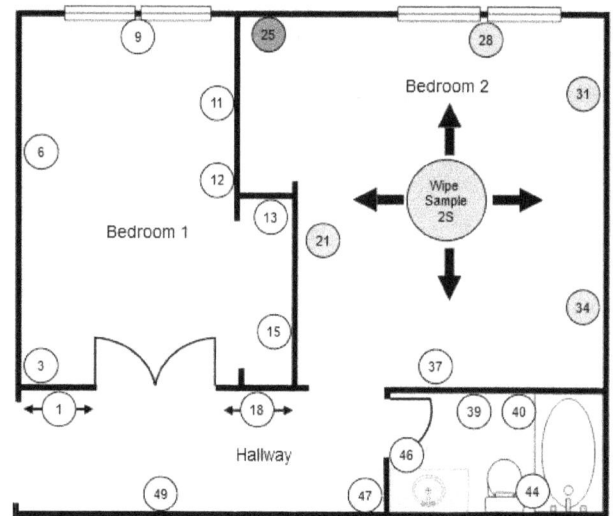

Figure 5-48: A screening pattern may help save money by identifying areas that do not have a major source but will often miss the specific "hot spots."

Hypothesis Testing Using Pathways™ Testing

Not all water damage occurs at floor level. When MSQPCR or other testing methods indicate elevated contamination levels in the living space, hypothesis testing can help identify potential pathways through which contaminants migrate into occupiable areas. This approach uses environmental history, odors, and visible evidence to form a hypothesis—essentially an educated guess about the source of contamination.

In addition to environmental history and visible evidence, potential pathways may include cracks around windows, plumbing penetrations, electrical outlets, and other penetrations for switches and fixtures. Plumbing systems for water and gas, fireplaces, saunas, hot tubs, and pools can also serve as potential contamination routes. Cracks, gaps, and other openings in walls or flooring are often overlooked but may play a role in allowing contaminants to escape hidden areas. Even furnishings adjacent to contaminated spaces can accumulate and spread protein-based particles if not addressed. Currently, Pathways™ Testing is for hard, non-porous, or semi-porous surfaces and not for upholstered materials or soft, porous materials.

By focusing on suspect areas, Pathways™ Testing makes the investigation process more refined, allowing for inexpensive targeted sampling and actionable insights. This method not only helps confirm contamination sources but also supports the development of effective remediation strategies tailored to the home's specific conditions.

Additional Sampling Considerations

- Effective Pathways™ Testing based on thoughtful timing and consistency in sampling can help answer additional questions and provide valuable insights into the home's condition and the effectiveness of cleaning or remediation efforts.

- If elevated levels of peptide bonds and proteins are found, detailed cleaning is performed, followed by Pathways™ Testing immediately to assess cleaning efficacy helps identify surfaces where cleaning was unsuccessful. Ideally, this cleanliness round of testing will be performed the same day after the cleaning and not more than 24 hours later. Surfaces must be allowed to dry before swabbing.

  › If elevated levels remain after cleaning, either the level of cleaning was not adequate or an area of elevated levels of peptide bonds and proteins remains due to a nearby source.
  › Reclean the area in question and collect another Pathways™ Swab immediately to determine if the additional cleaning was sufficient.
  › If the additional rounds of cleaning are unable to reduce the levels, there is a good chance that a nearby source is present.

- After 1.5 to two weeks, after successful cleaning, follow-up testing can check for signs of contamination resurgence, which can indicate:

  › A building memory issue might require more frequent cleaning of that area. Additional timed rounds of testing after cleaning can help determine the necessary cleaning frequency.
  › Actual protein and peptide bond contamination at a level that may require remediation to determine the source of the elevated levels that cannot be resolved by effective cleaning.

Baseline or Initial Sampling

Baseline or initial sampling is conducted to establish a reference point for the home's condition. These results are a foundation for tracking changes over time, evaluating cleaning effectiveness, and identifying potential contamination sources as they develop or persist. By testing immediately before your next scheduled cleaning, a baseline is established.

Sampling Immediately After Cleaning

Sampling immediately after cleaning assesses the efficacy of the cleaning methods and products. The results indicate whether contamination has been effectively removed or if adjustments to cleaning techniques are necessary to improve outcomes.

Contamination Resurgence Testing

Pathways™ Testing can be valuable for identifying contamination resurgence after cleaning efforts. Ideally, this testing is performed between 1.5 and two weeks following an effective cleaning that reduces protein and peptide bond levels to a known quantity. This follow-up testing helps determine whether contamination re-enters the living space from hidden sources or pathways.

Performing a round of testing immediately after cleaning is critical to establish a Clean Standard. Without this baseline, it becomes impossible to compare subsequent results and identify whether elevated levels stem from insufficient cleaning or a resurgence of contamination. If a post-cleaning round is skipped, and later testing reveals high levels, it's unclear whether the cause is a failure to clean effectively or contamination re-migrating from hidden areas.

When contamination resurgence testing is conducted correctly, it provides actionable insights into the home's condition. Elevated levels detected during this round may indicate:

- **Building Memory:** Contaminants are migrating from hidden sources slowly enough that they can likely be managed with more frequent cleaning.

- **Hidden Sources:** Proteins and contaminants are re-emerging from wall cavities, cracks, or other concealed pathways at a faster-than-manageable rate that may require additional remediation.

By analyzing the results of follow-up testing, homeowners and professionals can adjust cleaning frequencies or revisit specific areas for targeted remediation. This strategic approach helps ensure that contamination levels remain manageable and that the environment continues to meet healthful standards.

Pathways™ Testing's ability to track contamination over time makes it an invaluable tool for monitoring and maintaining a clean indoor environment, especially in sensitive settings. When paired with a well-established baseline from initial testing, resurgence testing becomes a cornerstone for effective long-term contamination management.

Establishing the Sample Timing

The timing of sample collection should align with routine cleaning schedules to allow for a typical level of contaminant build-up. Significant environmental changes or specific events, such as after severe weather or major activities within the home, must be considered to adjust the schedule if necessary. Consistent timing ensures meaningful comparisons across test results, providing reliable data to assess ongoing conditions and the effectiveness of interventions.

Myth: If You Can't See Mold, You Don't Have a Mold Problem.
Fact: Mold can grow in hidden places, such as behind walls, under floors, or inside ventilation systems. A lack of visible mold doesn't necessarily mean no problem; musty odors or unexplained health symptoms can indicate hidden mold.

Essay: My Pathways™ Testing Experience
by Alex Kessler

I'm a translational scientist in personalized cancer treatment. I became interested in mold and indoor air quality when I developed some uncomfortable chronic symptoms (full-body eczema with painful itching, nasal allergies, digestive issues, weight loss, and countless food intolerances) after living in a string of homes with mold and bacteria. I have experienced the aforementioned symptoms to varying degrees since 2017.

Through these challenging years, as I learned more about my condition and researched solutions, I discovered a significant gap in accessible, practical guidance for people struggling with chronic illness and poor indoor air quality, especially renters. Questions kept arising: How does one ventilate properly when it's humid, cold, or hot outside? How does one select the right air purifier and dehumidifier, and how can their efficacy be verified?

Driven by my scientific background and my tendency to meticulously test strategies for improving my own health, I realized this was a problem I could help solve. That's why I started *Healthy Home Guide*, my YouTube channel, to turn what happened to me into something good, something that could help others who are asking the same questions.

During this journey, I discovered John Banta's microfiber cleaning protocol. It had a dramatic impact on reducing my symptoms. Inspired by its simplicity, safety, and effectiveness, I reached out to John for an interview, resulting in the video titled "Microfiber Cleaning Removes Pollutants That Air Purifiers Miss." This video has since become an invaluable resource for my audience. John and I both believe that together, we can tell an important story, one that challenges the overuse of disinfectants and chemical cleaners, which not only overcomplicate the process but can also create a more toxic environment. John's saying, "Soap and water is the ultimate," is forever etched into my memory.

Around five months ago, I moved into a small (890 sq ft) rental home in western Washington State built in 2018. My fiancé and I chose this home because it seemed to lack the visible water damage indicators (staining, bubbling, etc.) that we had seen in abundance in other rentals in the area. Over the course of my time here, I was surprised to find my symptoms began to return. I have developed increasingly severe digestive issues and weight loss. I eventually also developed symptoms I had not experienced before: dizziness and brain fog.

Naturally, I began to suspect hidden water damage organisms might be the cause. Months earlier, during a conversation with John Banta about the dangers of bleach, I had mentioned that I wanted to ensure that my next home would be supportive of my health. After listening, John suggested this could be a good opportunity to try out Pathways™ Testing for peptide bonds and proteins as a surrogate marker for potential mold. I decided to move forward with it to see how it worked firsthand.

To collect the samples, I used a microfiber swab and ran it along key pathways where mold and bacteria tend to enter the living space. I focused primarily on the gap where the baseboards meet the floor, testing in consistent 4-foot increments throughout the home to ensure accurate comparisons between samples. I also swabbed other potential pathways, like windows, inside vanities, and areas around appliances through which water moves.

The goal of Pathways™ is to test the first-place contamination builds up, right at these entrances to the conditioned space, since John Banta's research shows it accumulates there before becoming airborne. Round One of Pathways™ Testing is conducted when surfaces are dirty to establish a baseline used to determine initial levels of protein and peptide bonds.

Round One of Pathways™ Testing revealed elevated peptide bond and protein levels throughout my home, which was unsettling to me since I had done a few deep cleans during the months I had been living there. However, these results made sense since I had refrained from cleaning for a few weeks before Round One to allow any potential hotspots to build up.

Round One: Baseline

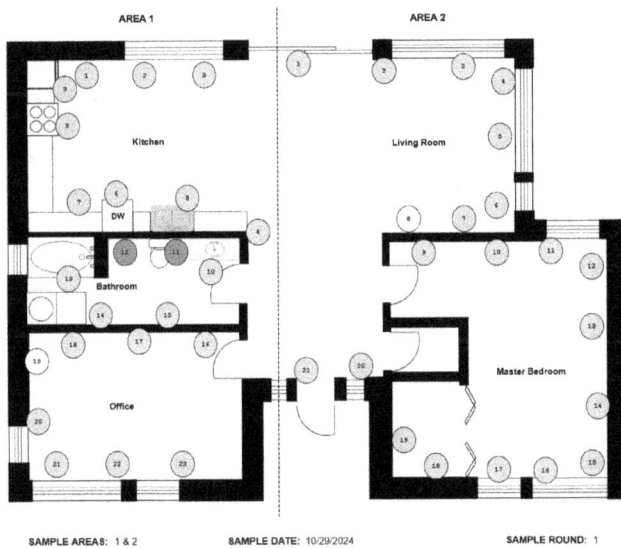

Figure 5-49: Baseline Initial Testing Showed Few Clean Areas.

As I reviewed my initial colorized report, I saw that levels were mostly yellow, with a couple of orange spots below the baseboard behind the toilet. There being water damage organisms behind the toilet made sense. Right when I moved in, I noticed a very slow leak where the toilet supply valve connected to the toilet. I quickly repaired it, but it could have gone on long before I moved in. There was also evidence of some slight separation of the top of that baseboard from the wall. It was subtle, though, and I've seen much worse. Here is a gray-scale diagram of my colorized report:

No Shading (green) = low levels of peptide bonds and proteins.

Light Gray (yellow) = levels of peptide bonds and proteins suggesting that surfaces were not clean.

Dark Gray (orange) = elevated levels of peptide bonds and proteins suggesting a nearby source or a low level of growth.

Black = very elevated levels of a sub-visible or hidden protein-based contamination.

After discussing these results with John, I realized that there could be a mold issue in my home and that further testing would be necessary.

Before Round Two, I cleaned using a microfiber mop slightly dampened with water and a fragrance-free surfactant. I paid close attention while edge-cleaning, as those were the areas I tested in Round One, and I wanted consistency across testing locations. The reason for cleaning is this: imagine an egg had been spilled on the floor some time ago. Round One might detect the proteins from that spill, but after cleaning before Round Two, those proteins would be removed. Unlike proteins from a spill, mold and bacteria from water damage would continue to build up after that cleaning and would be revealed in subsequent rounds of testing.

Within 30 minutes of completing the cleaning, I then conducted Round Two of Pathways™ Testing. The results indicated that I had successfully brought all levels back into the green, confirming the effectiveness of the cleaning. Based on the first and second rounds of testing, it seemed clear that there had been one or more sources contributing to the elevated results.

Round Two: Post Effective Cleaning, Hitting the Reset Button

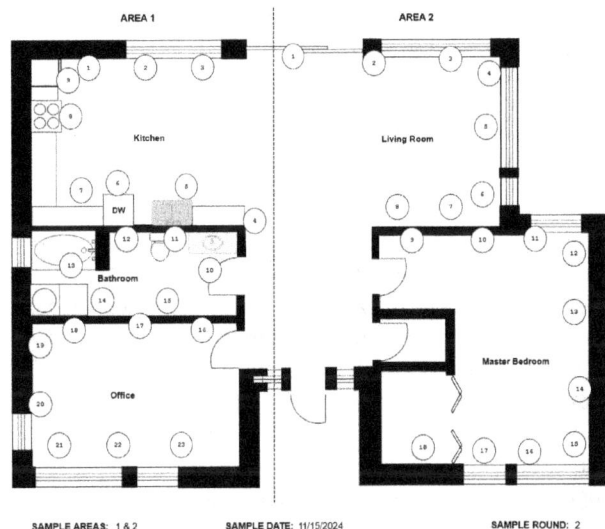

Figure 5-50: After Effective Cleaning, all areas tested with Pathways™ showed low levels of peptide bonds and proteins. The cleaning was successful!

Then, I waited 1.5 weeks and conducted Round Three of Pathways™ Testing. Why did I wait? As I mentioned earlier, waiting reveals which locations become dirty again, highlighting hotspots that may benefit from more frequent cleaning or further investigation. In other words, most non-problem or minor problem areas will stay clean for two weeks, and conversely, problem areas will become dirty again.

Unfortunately, the results showed that much of my space had, in fact, crept back into the yellow. The kitchen, bathroom, and master bedroom all contained elevated results, which seemed to be clustered around appliances through which water moves in the kitchen and bathroom, but it was not a clear pattern. These results are indicative of a home that suggests substantial hidden water damage and are concerning. Only my office remained clean.

Round Three: Potential Hidden Issues Remerge

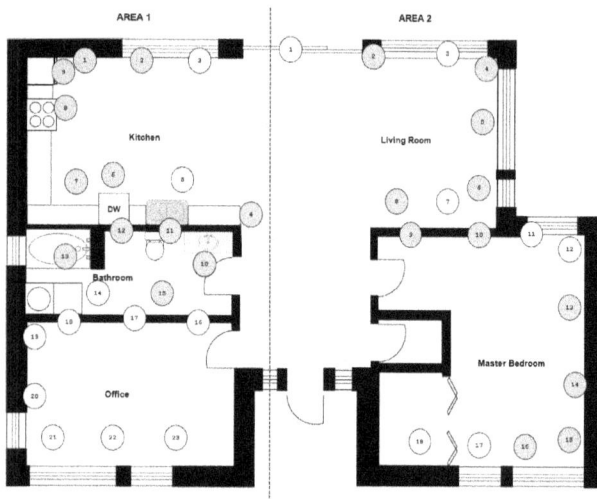

SAMPLE AREAS: 1 & 2   SAMPLE DATE: 11/25/24   SAMPLE ROUND: 3

Figure 5-51: The levels of peptide bonds and proteins are beginning to reaccumulate in potential problem areas ten days to two weeks after successful cleaning. Only the office has been able to maintain its levels of post-cleaning cleanliness. The second round of testing shows if cleaning was successful. The third round of testing helps determine if there is unacceptable building memory or if additional hidden growth is working its way into the living space.

I then conducted an MSQPCR dust test on surfaces I had not cleaned recently to get an overall snapshot of which mold species may be present in the space. The results showed that the geometric means for numerous problem organisms were elevated, and the HERTSMI score was 14, which confirmed that mold is an issue in this building. Of note, *Penicillium brevicompactum* was detected at 511 SE/mg. With these results in mind, it is interesting to note that my eczema hasn't been triggered to a significant degree, but my digestive issues have.

Continuing with our building diagnosis, I turned my attention to another area of interest: the extremely large windows in my kitchen and living room. Window condensation is particularly common here in Western Washington, but I saw no sign of it around these windows, possibly because they're robust and double-pane. Fortunately, massive overhangs shield them from precipitation, making leaks unlikely. The windows, therefore, remain inconclusive.

Interestingly, I've been watching a house be built right outside of our window since we moved in. The structural components like the framing, sheathing, and subfloors have been continuously soaked for months, given that it lightly rains virtually every day in western Washington for almost half the year. Outdoor surfaces never fully dry until the summer. When houses are finished, that moisture can get sealed in. So, that could have occurred with my rental. There could be mold in all of the wall cavities that get drawn into the living

space with negative pressure. For example, when we use our kitchen exhaust hood, drier, or bathroom exhaust fan, which is unfortunately programmed to run automatically throughout the day. Anytime lots of air is sucked out of the house, more air rushes into the house to replace it, and unless you have a dedicated makeup air system, it will probably come through the wall cavities. Given that this space is so small, this likely happens even more readily. What further compounds the issue is that there is a massive gap between the baseboards and the floor, so a wide pathway for moldy dust to come in. Gravity carries water from leaks downward, so the most mold is typically found at the bottom of the drywall. If there's a huge gap right there, through which air flows in, that's not optimal.

What else could be causing my symptoms? Of note, there has been an earthy, fecal smell in the bathroom since we moved in. It seems to be coming from the bathroom sink, possibly from a buildup in the p-trap. There is also a similar odor coming from the washing machine. These are potential sources of exposure to bacterial endotoxins (lipopolysaccharides) or exotoxins.

So, what have I been doing about these potential issues? Throughout my journey with chronic illness, maintaining a clean diet has been a cornerstone of my health. While it hasn't cured my condition, it has played a critical role in keeping my symptoms from becoming completely debilitating. For me, the Medical Medium protocol has been most helpful; eating a plant-based diet with whole, unprocessed foods and avoiding triggers like gluten and dairy has helped me maintain enough stability to work on improving my living space in the following ways:

First, I have installed an energy recovery ventilator (ERV) in my bedroom window. This delivers filtered fresh air to dilute the concentrations of pollutants in the air and ensures the fresh air isn't too cold, hot, humid, or dry. I've also set up three air purifiers with sufficient clean air delivery rate (CADR) to reduce the particle count in my space by 90%. In addition, I dehumidify to ensure that indoor dew point stays below 60F, ASHRAE's threshold above which conditions of indoor dampness can occur.

After testing, I began cleaning every couple of days because I was feeling anxious about all the elevated results. I saw an improvement in my digestive symptoms, but still felt dizzy occasionally. John Banta has been helpful and kind through this process. He has advised me to use removable tape to block the large gap between the baseboards and floor, so I've done that. I've also installed outlet covers, because that's an infiltration route as well. Since blocking these gaps, I've noticed that when I damp wipe, there is less dust on the microfiber pads. Next, I began cracking open a window while using the kitchen exhaust hood and the clothes drier so more air comes through there instead of through the wall cavities.

I have also used enzymatic drain cleaner daily in the bathroom sink to remove the bacterial odor. The odor has reduced, and my symptoms have improved further. In a wildly synchronous turn of events, my washing machine stopped working completely. I don't want to say I'm happy it died, but I'm happy it died. My landlord replaced it, and the odor is gone.

It's essential to mention the importance of daily relaxation in this process. Stress can intensify chronic illness, leaving my mind and body feeling unsettled, like a shaken snow globe. Taking 10 minutes each day to sit quietly and do absolutely nothing is the best thing for allowing that overstimulated, swirling chaos to settle, letting everything gently fall back into place.

Diagnosing this home is not straightforward, especially given that it is a rental. As of yet, there are no airtight explanations for why the peptide bond and protein levels demonstrated by the Pathways™ test show so many elevated results throughout the space. This scenario illustrates that signs of mold aren't always visible and that newer homes can harbor mold issues, too. Pathways™ Testing revealed that there is a significant migration of questionable material into my living space and painted a picture of what I would have to do to keep that migration at bay. As I've sealed the gaps in the building envelope, mitigated negative pressure, and cleaned more thoroughly and consistently, my symptoms have lessened to a degree that I can likely manage living here until my lease runs out. You can continue following my journey by subscribing to the *Healthy*

Home Guide channel on YouTube or visiting my website at healthyhomeguide.com.

It is important to note that pinpointing which factor primarily caused my symptoms and which alleviated them is challenging. Most complex illnesses arise from a constellation of overlapping physiological insults rather than a single cause. Consequently, healing often requires a multimodal approach, combining a healthy diet, a clean environment, and other supportive strategies.

Explore Alex's Resources:

How to Clean Properly: https://youtu.be/3gsuUxqxLbg

Why Most HEPA Air Purifiers Are a Scam: https://youtu.be/gaQTYrisieA

How to Install Your Own Energy Recovery Ventilator (ERV): https://youtu.be/CnLwJxCbxfM

How to Build Your Own Air Purifier: https://youtu.be/KxPk8yOH-z4

How to Set Up and Use a High-Quality Dehumidifier: https://youtu.be/JOZ5TZ-oaP8

How to Do Your Own Water Damage Inspections: https://youtu.be/Dt7qnePPinQ

Exercise 5.1: Pathways™ Determine Collection Patterns

In indoor environmental quality assessment and remediation, the unseen is often as critical as the visible. Hidden conditions lurking beneath the surface of walls, ceilings, and floors can silently contribute to a building's health, deterioration, and structural problems. To unveil the hidden conditions, it is necessary to grasp the fundamental elements at play—a hidden water damage or mold condition, a pathway or conduit to travel into the occupied space, and the vital role of airflow and pressure that draws out the contaminants. This section delves into the science and methodology behind Pathways™ sampling, shedding light on the invisible and making the unseen visible.

- Room Perimeters
- Windows
- Plumbing walls
- Electrical Outlets, Penetrations (Switches and Fixtures)
- Plumbing Pipe Penetrations (Water and Gas)
- Heating Ventilation and Air Conditioning System and Ducts
- Fireplaces
- Saunas, Hot Tubs, Pools, Wine Cellars
- Furnishings
- Other Penetrations, Crack, Openings

Exercise 5.2: Pathways™ Determine Collection Density

Determining the collection density is crucial for identifying elevated peptide bonds and protein patterns, which may point to hidden or sub-visible contamination sources. This exercise guides the selection of the appropriate density pattern for testing, tailored to specific areas of concern.

Choose the Density Pattern for Floor Testing

❑ **Dense Collection Pattern**: A higher sampling density, such as samples taken every four feet along room perimeters, to thoroughly investigate potential contamination sources. This helps ensure that every junction where cracks are present between the top of the floor and the bottom edge of the baseboard has been addressed.

❑ **Screening Collection Pattern**: A screening pattern where four samples are collected from each normal-sized room can help determine which areas are generally clean. If higher-than-expected levels of proteins are discovered, then a dense testing pattern can be used to help determine the pathway contributing to the sources.

❑ **Supplemental Pathways™ Tests Collection:**

Determine how many additional tests will be performed in specific areas of interest, such as HVAC systems. Examples include:

- Testing inside the supply registers can help determine if a duct is distributing protein-based contamination. By testing every duct, you can determine whether the contamination is widespread or limited to specific areas.

- Testing the register grill cover will tell you if condensation moisture accumulates on the grill.

- Testing around the plenum insert, where it penetrates through the ceiling floor or wall, indicates what is coming from the attic, wall, or area below that the duct passes through.

Collection for Other Determinations

- Identify other areas where testing is needed to address unique conditions or potential contamination sources. This could include specific hard-surfaced furnishings, window sills, or other penetration points within the home.

- By selecting and implementing an appropriate collection density, this exercise ensures that sampling captures a comprehensive picture of contamination patterns, supporting targeted remediation and cleaning efforts.

- Count the areas you will be sampling and order an appropriate number of swabs. Since you could be doing multiple rounds, you may want to order extra swabs to have them on hand for the additional testing.

Exercise 5.3 Prepare a Floor Plan Diagram of the Home

Creating a floor plan doesn't require expert drawing skills; it's about translating the layout of your home onto paper.

❑ Here's a simple way to draw a basic floor plan:

- **Gather Materials:** You will need a pencil, a ruler, and graph paper. Graph paper is helpful because the squares can represent a set measurement (e.g., 1 square = 1 foot).

- **Measure Your Space:** Take a tape measure and record the length and width of each room.

- **Outline the Perimeter:** On your graph paper, decide on a scale (1 square = 1 foot), and draw the outer walls of your home according to this scale.

- **Plot the Rooms:** Draw the walls of each room using your scale within the outline of the perimeter. If a wall is 10 feet long and your scale is 1 square = 1 foot, that wall should take up 10 squares on the graph paper.

- **Add Doors and Windows:** Indicate where doors and windows are on your plan. For doors, draw a straight line where the door starts and an arc to show its opening. For windows, just a simple line or double line will suffice to represent the glass.

- **Label Each Room:** Write the name of each room (e.g., kitchen, bedroom) in its respective space.

- **Review and Revise:** Look over your floor plan. Does it look like your home's layout? If something seems off, measure and draw it again.

Exercise 5.4 Collecting Pathway Samples

As mold spores and fragments migrate through tiny pathways—such as the crack between the top of the floor and the bottom edge of the baseboard—they adhere to the floor due to electrostatic charges and molecular forces like Van der Waals forces. Over time, these particles accumulate along the floor until the surface becomes saturated, allowing particles to migrate further or become airborne. Removing these particles from surfaces reduces contamination in the indoor environment by preventing them from recirculating into the air and spreading further until they are so loaded that the contaminants can no longer build up in that area.

Follow these steps to collect Pathways™ samples:

❑ **Prepare for Sampling:**

› Ensure you have all necessary materials: 3.5 mm microfiber swabs, labeled protective sleeves, a floor plan for mapping, and chain of custody documentation.

› Consider using a different chain of custody and diagram for each different type of collection pattern. For example, if you have ten HVAC supply registers that you will be sampling inside, then use a different recording sheet and diagram to show the location of those ten collections.

› You may want to Identify and mark each sampling location with quick-release tape with the sample number to show the center mark for where each swab was collected. Labeling the baseboard-floor junction, HVAC vents, electrical outlets, or any visible cracks and openings separately will make it easier to locate them for retesting or consideration when the results are back.

❑ **Collect the Sample:**

› Use the microfiber swab to collect dust along a 48-linear-inch path.

› Swab the first 24 inches using one side of the swab in a single, firm swipe. Don't scrub back and forth.

› Flip the swab and collect dust from the remaining 24 inches.

› Apply consistent pressure to ensure even dust collection across the entire length.

❑ **Store the Sample Properly:**

› Place the swab in a labeled protective sleeve. Ensure the sleeve is sealed to prevent contamination.

› Record the sample location on your floor plan to ensure traceability and double-check the number on the quick-release tape.

❑ **Document the Process:**

› Complete the chain of custody documentation, including the unique identifier for each sample, the specific collection area, and the date.

❏ **Send for Analysis:**

› Ship the samples to the RestCon Environmental for Pathways™ analysis at the address listed on the chain of custody, ensuring proper handling to maintain sample integrity during transit.
RestCon Environmental
RestConEnvironmental.com
info@RestConEnviro.com
916-736-1100

Exercise 5.5 Pathways™ Interpretation of Baseline Samples

The interpretation of your Pathways™ peptide bonds and protein results depends on the conditions present at the time of sample collection and the timing of the samples for effective cleaning. This section outlines baseline interpretations for Pathways™ Testing. Different criteria are applied for cleanliness testing and assessing the accumulation rate of peptide bonds and proteins. This interpretation framework is integral to understanding the

test results from the Pathways™ method, guiding decisions on investigation intensity, remediation scope, and cleaning necessities. It provides a nuanced understanding of the contamination levels and potential sources, ensuring a comprehensive approach to addressing indoor environmental quality concerns.

❏ **Pathways™ Results Interpretation**

› As you review your Pathways™, keep notes in your diary about aspects you don't understand or have questions about. Interpreting Pathways™ Testing results involves analyzing the presence and concentration of peptide bonds and proteins detected in samples and observing how these values change over time and under different conditions. By comparing these results to baseline data and understanding the historical cleaning methods used, you can assess the cleanliness and stability of various areas in the home.

› Contact your provider or RestCon Environmental with any questions you may have.

Key Factors in Peptide Bond and Protein Results Interpretation

The concentration of peptide bonds and proteins indicates the level of biological contamination that may be present in a specific area. High levels suggest the presence of mold, bacteria, or other protein-based contaminants, while low levels point to effective cleaning or a naturally stable environment.

Changing Values Over Time:
Comparing test results from different time points helps identify trends.

- Decreasing protein levels indicates improved cleaning or environmental stabilization.
- Increasing protein levels suggest potential contamination sources or ineffective maintenance.
- Historical Cleaning Methods Used:
- Understanding past cleaning practices, including frequency, methods, and products, provides context for interpreting results. Persistent contamination may point to a source of contamination or insufficient or inappropriate cleaning strategies.

Stability Classifications
Stability areas represent a framework for understanding contamination levels and their changes over time, offering valuable insights into the effectiveness of cleaning and maintenance efforts.

- **Stable Areas:** Locations that consistently show low levels of protein-based contaminants. Stability is determined by

repeated low readings across multiple testing intervals, even in areas prone to moisture or traffic.

- **Areas Trending Toward Stability:** Areas with decreasing contamination levels over time suggest that improved cleaning efforts are successfully reducing the contamination trend. Continued monitoring is essential to confirm long-term stability.
- **Areas Trending Toward Instability:** Areas with increasing levels of peptide bonds and proteins indicate emerging issues or lapses in maintenance. Investigating potential contamination sources, such as hidden leaks, is critical.
- **Unstable Areas:** Locations that consistently exhibit high protein levels, regardless of cleaning efforts. These areas may require intensive intervention, such as addressing hidden moisture sources or reevaluating cleaning strategies.

Color-Coded Areas on Diagrams

- **Red Areas:** High peptide bond levels can indicate mold or bacterial growth due to dampness or water damage nearby. Still, it could indicate another protein source, such as a spilled egg or the family dog drooling on the floor just before feeding. These areas may require additional investigation to determine the cause and whether remediation is warranted.
- **Orange Areas:** Show somewhat elevated peptide bonds, indicating potential microbial growth. Orange regions near red areas typically need to be included in broader

remediation efforts if the area is determined to have unresolvable levels of peptide bonds and proteins.

- **Yellow Areas:** Elevated peptide bonds reflect settled spores or fragments, which are less likely to indicate actual growth but suggest contamination that has spread from a nearby source. Cleaning is often the recommended course of action.

- **Green Areas:** Indicate clean surfaces with insignificant peptide bond levels. Any microbial growth is likely contained or has not migrated into the tested area.

Exercise 5.6 Additional uses of Pathways™ Testing

The following steps in this 25 Step guide offer additional suggestions for utilizing Pathways™ Testing to gain a deeper understanding of potential contamination issues in your home. These strategies are designed to help identify problem areas, monitor cleaning effectiveness, and track contamination trends over time, providing valuable insights for maintaining a healthful living environment.

❑ **Please see the following for additional Pathways™ Testing method information:**

Step 6: Integrate Known and Suspected Issues into a Plan: In this step, Pathways™ testing results are tailored to fit your remediation plan.

Step 17: Progress Monitoring with Pathways™ Testing: This step uses Pathways™ to monitor the remediation and cleaning process progress.

Step 19: Confirmation of Remediation Success: This step uses Pathways™ Testing to confirm reduced mold levels on framing and remaining gypsum wallboard prior to reconstruction to establish a maintenance testing schedule for early detection of new issues.

Step 22: Establish a Routine Clean Schedule: This Step shows how to use Pathways™ Testing to establish a cleaning schedule for long-term mold control of building memory and to maintain a safe, healthy building environment.

Additional Tips

- Please notify your consultant if you have been using products with enzymes.

- Prior to your inspection, furniture and other personal belongings should be moved at least 2 feet away from walls to provide access to otherwise inaccessible areas. If you are unable to move the furniture yourself, please consider hiring your restoration professional to help

- Remove personal belongings from vanities and cabinets under sinks to provide access.

- Do not schedule indoor maintenance or cleaning service or perform cleaning activities that will interfere with the timing of inspection and testing. Please discuss with your consultant how much time between cleaning and testing should elapse.

Step 6: Integrate Known and Suspected Issues into a Draft Plan

Formulating a Tailored Remediation Plan

This step is where you will combine all the information gathered so far to determine how to continue. Additional rounds of Pathways™ Testing can help determine the extent to which effective cleaning can be used to keep exposures under control, creating a sanctuary versus the degree of remediation needed. Often, a hybrid approach can be practical. This is where the information is gathered, and the previous steps will be assembled into a preliminary action plan to guide the remediation process. This involves mapping out confirmed and suspected mold and moisture damage areas based on Steps 3 through 5 results. By visualizing the distribution of these issues, you can develop a structured, room-by-room remediation strategy.

This step marks the transition from assessment to action. Here, you begin to see a clear path forward, supported by a strategy aligned with your situation's realities. The draft plan you develop will serve as an initial roadmap for whether you get busy with cleaning, the remediation process, or a hybrid approach.

Practical Applications

Not everyone can remediate their home. Renters are often at the mercy of landlords, and homeowners may need time to save for the high remediation costs. Even with sufficient funds, remediation takes time and can require finding temporary housing or carefully staging the process to allow one section of the home to serve as a sanctuary while other areas are being addressed.

Pathways™ Testing can be a valuable tool in these situations. It helps determine whether staying in the home is practical or if contamination levels are too high to remain safe. It can also evaluate whether cleaning methods or practices have been effective and provide insight into the extent of contamination. For those unable to fully remediate, Pathways™ Testing offers a way to prioritize efforts and make informed decisions about managing contamination and maintaining a safer living environment.

Not everyone can remediate their home. Renters are often at the mercy of landlords, while homeowners may

need time to save for the high remediation costs. Even with the necessary funds, the process can result in logistical challenges, such as finding temporary housing during remediation or determining how to stage the process so that one area of the home serves as a sanctuary while the other areas are worked on.

How Pathways™ Testing Helps

Pathways™ Testing can help navigate these challenges by providing insights into contamination levels and the practicality of staying in the home during remediation. It can:

- Help determine if contamination levels make it impractical to remain in the home.
- Assess whether cleaning methods or practices have been effective.
- Identify areas of the home that need prioritized remediation or more frequent cleaning.
- Provide actionable data to guide decision-making for those who cannot immediately afford full remediation.

By using Pathways™ Testing, homeowners and renters can better understand their options, plan their remediation efforts, and take steps to manage contamination even under difficult circumstances.

Exercise 6.1: Strategy for Compiling Data for Known Issues

Consolidate the confirmed mold, moisture, and water damage areas identified in Steps 3, 4, and 5.

❑ **Gathering data** for visible or known mold growth, water intrusion, and elevated moisture. Draft diagrams may be used to map these findings in preliminary form.

› Begin by listing areas with visible or known mold growth. Document the location, quantity, and pattern of growth, and specify how each area was confirmed as an issue. This information will provide a foundation for addressing urgent areas requiring controlled and effective remediation.

› Next, record data for any suspected hidden growth areas. Note locations where you suspect mold but lack visible confirmation, describing the quantity of suspected growth and your strategy for verifying these issues. Listing these areas ensures no potential problems are overlooked in your remediation plan.

› Include details for all instances of active water intrusion or high moisture levels, using findings from moisture measurements and thermal imaging. Describe the location, evidence of moisture, pattern (if relevant), and methods of confirmation. These findings will be critical in addressing underlying causes and preventing future mold growth.

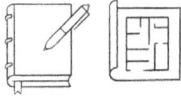

Exercise 6.2: Identifying Suspected Area Identification

Highlight areas where mold growth or moisture issues are suspected but not confirmed. These might be hard-to-access locations or places with indirect indicators of mold. Draft diagrams can also be created here for preliminary mapping.

❑ **Focus on suspected areas** by listing locations and suspected patterns of growth. Because water flows across surfaces and downward, think about where each area of damage may have traveled. Now extend at least one study bay (16 to 24 inches) beyond the area with the last visual indications of visible mold, water staining, or rusty fastener heads. This means you should consider the backside of each wall affected, adjacent rooms, and spaces below. Describe your approach to confirming the issue for each area, whether through additional testing, inspection, or sampling. Including these locations in your preliminary plan will help ensure the greatest possible anticipation of potentially problematic areas are documented for further exploration.

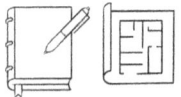

Exercise 6.3: Mapping Draft of Historical Water Intrusion and Moisture Findings

Draft map areas that show evidence of water intrusion or moisture to clarify the extent and source of these issues. This exercise allows you to begin visualizing these findings.

❑ **List each area** exhibiting water intrusion or elevated moisture using your data from thermal imaging and moisture readings. Detail the location, growth pattern (if applicable), and confirmation method. Identifying these areas helps address any causes of water intrusion, preventing future water damage or mold growth.

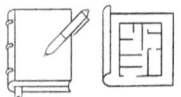

Exercise 6.4: Musty Odor and Staining Identification

Identify spaces with musty odors or water stains. Musty odors indicate active growth caused by damp conditions. Water stains often indicate hidden (and possibly sub-visible) mold or ongoing moisture problems. Draft diagrams can be used here to capture preliminary observations.

❑ **Note locations** with musty odors or visible water stains and describe the observed odor or staining patterns. Tracking these indicators helps identify potential hidden mold and prioritize areas for further exploration.

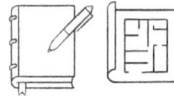

Exercise 6.5: Combine Your Draft Diagrams

After consolidating data from the previous exercises, transfer all identified issues into a composite diagram. This final diagram will visually represent all known and suspected problems, allowing you to compare areas with odors against visual or test results. If musty areas don't correspond to known data, another problem area may be present and will need to be identified.

❑ **Plot each identified or suspected problem area** using the lists you compiled on your home diagram. If the diagrams appear to be complicated, you may want to use transparent overlays to help with visualization. Assign symbols or colors to different issues (e.g., mold growth, water intrusion) and clearly label each area with relevant details. This visual map will explain where mold and moisture problems are concentrated and help identify patterns or sources contributing to these issues.

Exercise 6.6: Material Assessment and Remediation Plan

Evaluate affected materials and determine which should be removed, cleaned, or further investigated, guiding your decisions for each area in your remediation plan.

❑ **List the materials in each room based on their type**: porous, semi-porous, or non-porous. For each affected material, record whether it will need removal (for porous materials) or abrasive cleaning (for semi-porous materials) or cleaning (for non-porous items). Create a Scope of Work document that includes your decisions and the reasoning behind each choice. This will provide a clear plan for addressing each material in the remediation process.

Exercise 6.7: Review and Reflect

With all issues mapped and materials assessed, reflect on how these findings interconnect to complete a comprehensive, prioritized plan.

❑ **Review your completed diagram** and materials assessments, noting any correlations between water intrusion areas and mold growth. Consider how these connections can influence your remediation priorities, ensuring the most urgent issues are addressed first. This reflection will help refine your remediation roadmap and prepare you for productive discussions with remediation professionals.

Step 7: Team Assembly

Building a Team for Medically Important Remediation

Not every remediation firm is qualified or trained to address homes where water damage results in medical issues. This step guides assembling a mold remediation team attuned to health concerns to ensure expert and health-conscious remediation. This step is dedicated to assembling a mold remediation team that possesses expert skills in mold remediation and demonstrates a keen sensitivity to health concerns, particularly those related to hypersensitivity to water-damage organisms and multiple chemical sensitivities. Utilizing data from your initial assessments and Pathways™ testing results, this phase is about developing a holistic remediation plan. It entails a detailed analysis of the extent of mold and water damage and creating a strategy specifically tailored to your home's unique conditions and your health requirements.

In this step, you will be guided on identifying and selecting team members with the necessary expertise in mold remediation and a conscientious approach to health-conscious practices. This includes understanding their experience with environmentally sensitive remediation techniques and their ability to work collaboratively with your Indoor Environmental Professional (IEP) and other stakeholders involved. The goal is to create a team that addresses the physical aspects of mold and water damage and respects and accommodates the health implications for you and your family.

In this crucial step, you will be guided on how to identify and select team members who have the necessary expertise in mold remediation and demonstrate a conscientious approach to health-conscious practices. This involves understanding their experience with environmentally sensitive remediation techniques and their ability to work collaboratively with your Indoor Environmental Professional (IEP) and other stakeholders. The objective is to form a team that effectively addresses the physical aspects of mold and water damage while being acutely aware of and accommodating any health implications for you and your family.

Assembling your remediation team is a pivotal component of this stage. The overall success of the remediation hinges on having the right team in place—professionals who are adept in mold remediation and attuned to the specific needs of your home, particularly concerning health sensitivities that you or your family members might have.

Special consideration should be given to hypersensitivity to mold and multiple chemical sensitivities (MCS). It's essential that your chosen team not only possesses the necessary expertise but also exhibits a willingness to learn and adapt Medically Important Remediation Methods. This ensures that the remediation process is effective in addressing mold issues and conducted in a manner that is safe and respectful of the health needs of all occupants.

In addition, it's important to recognize that not every company may initially possess the full spectrum of skills or understanding required for these specialized remediation projects. Therefore, a key factor in your selection process will be discerning a team's openness to learning and adapting their methods. Many companies might believe they are fully knowledgeable in mold remediation yet may not be prepared to handle your job's unique requirements differently. The following exercise will assist you in evaluating potential remediation companies and their personnel to determine if they are well-qualified or show the necessary flexibility and eagerness to learn.

In this section, you will find guidance and resources to help you in the selection process. This involves assessing potential team members' experience, their grasp of health-related sensitivities, and their readiness to embrace remediation methods that prioritize health and safety. This step goes beyond technical expertise; it's about ensuring a remediation approach that aligns with your specific health needs and the overall wellness goals for your home.

Exercise 7.1: Finding Potential Remediation or Restoration Companies

The goal of this exercise is to guide you through the process of selecting a competent and health-conscious remediation or restoration company. You'll learn how to evaluate potential companies for their expertise, experience, and willingness to adapt to medically important remediation methods, especially for households with sensitivities to mold and chemical exposures.

❑ **Identify a Trusted Water Damage Restoration Company:**

- **Accessibility:** You may find the same company you have already vetted in the Section on Emergency Water Damage is also performing mold remediation. If they are willing to handle your water damage cleanup without using antimicrobials and biocides, they may also be willing to perform the same way for mold. Keep the contact details of your reliable mold remediation company handy. Remember, not all companies are equipped to handle emergencies or are sensitive to medical issues related to mold and water damage.

- **IICRC Certification:** In addition to the Master Restorer designation that was discussed in the Emergency Water Damage section, the Institute of Inspection Cleaning and Restoration Certification (IICRC) is the leading organization that certifies technicians in contaminated water and mold remediation, with over 49,000 certified technicians. As an IICRC-approved instructor in Applied Microbial Remediation Training for two decades, I suggest using the 'Locate A Certified Pro' feature at IICRC's website for assistance. Not every company is equipped to help with special medically important needs, so do your best to vet companies before you need them—then keep them on speed dial!

||||||||||||||||||||||||||||||||||||||||||||||||||||||||||||||||||||||||||||||||||||||||||||||||||||||||||||||||||||||||||||||||||||||||||||||||||||

Questions When Vetting a Water Damage Restoration Company

The Institute of Inspection, Cleaning, and Restoration Certification (IICRC) IICRC.org is a well-known organization that sets industry standards for cleaning and restoration professionals. To become a registered certified firm with the IICRC, restoration contractors must meet certain requirements and follow specific procedures. This form will help you interview each firm you are considering:

Key requirements: For a restoration firm to be registered as a certified firm by the IICRC, they must comply with the following:

- **Employee Certification:** Restoration firms must employ at least one technician with individual IICRC certifications in relevant areas of expertise. Technicians typically earn these certifications through training and passing exams in water damage restoration, mold remediation, fire and smoke restoration, carpet cleaning, and more.

- **Insurance:** Registered firms must carry the appropriate insurance coverage, including liability and workers' compensation insurance, as local regulations and IICRC standards require.

- **Code of Ethics:** Firms must agree to abide by the IICRC's Code of Ethics, which outlines the principles of honesty, integrity, and professionalism in the industry.

- **Written Contracts:** Firms are required to use written contracts that clearly define the scope of work, pricing, and other terms and conditions of the restoration services provided to clients.

- **Compliance with Standards:** Certified firms must adhere to the IICRC's industry standards and best practices for restoration and cleaning services. These standards provide guidelines for performing work to industry-accepted quality levels.

- **Continuing Education:** The IICRC encourages ongoing education and training for technicians and firm owners to stay current with industry advancements and best practices.

- **Inspection:** The IICRC may conduct inspections or audits to ensure that registered firms comply with the organization's standards and requirements.

By meeting these requirements, restoration contractors can become registered as certified firms with the IICRC. This certification is a valuable credential that demonstrates a commitment to professionalism and industry standards in cleaning and restoration services.

||||||||||||||||||||||||||||||||||||||||||||||||||||||||||||||||||||||||||||||||||||||||||||||||||||||||||||||||||||||||||||||||||||||||||||||||||||

PROFESSIONAL MOLD REMEDIATION STANDARD OF CARE

The *ANSI/IICRC S500 Standard for Professional Water Damage Restoration* and *ANSI/IICRC S520 Standard for Professional Mold Remediation* provides comprehensive guidelines and standards for professional water damage and mold remediation in various commercial and residential buildings. The guidelines also include recommended measures that are advised or suggested but not considered the standard of care. These additional recommended measures are typically essential for remediation performed in homes with people who have medical needs.

In environments requiring meticulous care, such as homes of individuals diagnosed with mold sensitivities, the approach to water damage and mold remediation needs to be more tailored to the occupants' specific health needs. While the IICRC S520 offers a solid foundation of standards and guidelines for mold remediation, additional considerations are essential for these sensitive environments.

MEDICALLY IMPORTANT REMEDIATION MIR 101

For homes of individuals with mold sensitivities, a meticulous approach involves a thorough assessment to identify all mold growth sources. This includes employing stringent remediation protocols with enhanced containment measures and confirming HEPA filtration is functioning properly to minimize cross-contamination and exposure. In addition to the standard of care practices, it is also important to implement recommended practices to avoid the use of antimicrobials or biocides, including natural ones such as essential oils, and to avoid the use of sealants intended to encapsulate mold in place, as these measures can introduce additional risks and are not aligned with best practices for sensitive environments. Post-remediation, thorough cleaning, and verification surface testing are crucial to ensure complete mold growth removal, and continued effective cleaning is necessary to address building memory. Collaborating with healthcare professionals can help tailor the remediation to the individual's specific health needs. Additionally, ongoing moisture control and regular home inspections are vital to prevent mold recurrence, emphasizing the importance of maintaining a mold-controlled environment for the health and well-being of sensitive individuals. By integrating these recommended measures into the standard remediation protocols, the remediation process can be tailored to meet the specific needs of medically sensitive individuals, ensuring a safer and healthier living environment for those with specific needs.

Mold remediation does not include the automatic use of antimicrobial disinfectants. —IICRC, 2024

Additional specialized training is crucial to ensure effective mold remediation, especially in environments housing individuals with mold sensitivities or Chronic Inflammatory Response Syndrome (CIRS). The IICRC S500 and S520 standards provide a solid foundation for general water damage and mold remediation. However, these guidelines alone may not be sufficient for medically sensitive environments. (IICRC, 2024)

❑ Medically Important Remediation Training, such as the MIR101 course offered by CIRSx, is highly recommended. This comprehensive 16-hour course qualifies for IICRC Continuing Education Credits (CEC). It is designed for indoor environmental professionals, remediators, and restorers aiming to understand and implement advanced remediation techniques tailored to medically sensitive environments. The training covers advanced microbial remediation techniques, the significance of interdisciplinary collaboration with healthcare providers, and specific medical considerations in remediation. (CIRSx Institute, 2024)

Several contributors to this book, including me, prepared and are instructors for the MIR101 self-paced online course, ensuring that the curriculum is both practical and informed by extensive experience. By completing this course, professionals gain valuable insights into creating safer environments for sensitive individuals. This training emphasizes the importance of avoiding antimicrobials, biocides, and encapsulants, aligning with the principles of ALARA (As Low As Reasonably Achievable) and the precautionary principle. This ensures that the remediation process supports patient recovery without introducing additional risks.

If the technicians for the remediation firms you are considering have not already taken this training, I recommend you encourage the companies you are considering to enroll and complete this course prior to beginning work on your medically important remediation. For more detailed information and to enroll in the MIR101 course, you can visit the CIRSx Institute website. https://institute.cirsx.com/p/medically-important-remediation-101

||||||||||||||||||||||||||||||||||||||||||||||||||||||||||||||||||||||||||||||||||||||||||||||||||||||||||||||||||||||||||||||||||||||||||||||

Essay: Understanding the Difference Between a Bid, Quote, and Estimate
by Bill Weber

Once the indoor environmental assessment is completed, many look to a professional mold remediation company to help them perform controlled removals, remediation, and even small particle cleaning. Meeting with contractors can be daunting, especially when these types of services are so foreign to you, and the costs are

often higher than what you might have expected. Words used by contractors can be confusing because the scope of the work is usually not clear-cut. In other words, we fight an enemy that we cannot see in buildings that have hidden, unforeseen, and unexpected findings. Understanding the differences between bids, quotes, and estimates will help you make good decisions, plan financial resources, and, hopefully, reduce the strain associated with the remediation process.

Remediation Bids

Remediation bids are often confused with similar construction documents like remediation proposals, remediation quotes, and remediation estimates. Remediation bids are generated and used only when the project is well-defined. Usually, a qualified indoor environmental professional (IEP) has written the scope of work and supplied specifications and documents that are site-specific. The sampling and testing of potentially regulated hazardous materials have already been completed. Researching the local jurisdiction for licensing and permitting requirements has been performed. The written scope of work outlines where the containments will be installed, how many machines are needed and where they will be exhausted, where the fresh air will be drawn from, what materials are being removed, and more. The detailing is exhaustive, but the price and timeframe are clearly defined. Competitive bidding can help you select the most qualified remediation contractor since the bids will be based on a submittal package from a third party that will even the playing field.

Remediation Quote

Remediation quotes provide an estimate or budget for a specific task, a portion of a project, or the entire job. The quote is generally valid for a specific time frame ("good for 30 days"). For example, you might get a quote from an HVAC contractor separately from the remediation contractor. But since you don't know exactly when the HVAC contractor will need to clean your air handler(s) or even if the system is salvageable, the HVAC contractor will probably give you a quote that will later turn into a proposal once the project becomes more defined.

Remediation Estimate

A bid is actually an estimate, but they aren't exactly the same thing. Typically, the estimate is literally a guestimate or a projected time and materials price for what they think the work, hopefully to the best of their ability and foresight, will cost. Sometimes, it will include a timeframe, but without knowing what they are getting into, the remediation contractor will need to guess at that as well. With the additional information that is supplied by the IEP and any other needed or required contractor or design professional, the estimate can be turned into a bid.

When you have accepted the bid, quote, or estimate and moved into a contract, consider the following contractor licensing requirements for home improvement contracts in the city, county, or state that has jurisdiction over the work that is being performed in your home. Make sure that you have listed your verbal expectations and agreements in the contract that you sign to affirm there are no misunderstandings. Clear communication is always key in any relationship, especially one that involves work on your castle. Here are a few tips for what you want in a contract:

- A complete listing of contractor contact information and the contractor's license number if they have one and it is needed for the work being performed.

- Your contact information.

- Defines who will be responsible for obtaining local building permits and associated fees (contractors generally pull the building permits).

- Warranties from the contractor for labor and materials, specifying which part of the work is covered and the length of the warranty, and manufacturer warranties, if applicable.

- Detailed costs, including the agreed-upon down payment amount (In California, the legal down payment is $1,000 or 10% of the contract price, whichever is less, and a detailed payment schedule).

- Realistic timelines to complete the job that includes an adjustment for unforeseeable delays.

- Who is responsible for debris removal?

- Special requests by the homeowner, such as saving lumber for firewood or saving certain materials or appliances.

- Be sure to confirm that the remediation contractor has the proper insurance. According to the ANSI/IICRC S520 (2024): "Remediators should carry adequate amounts of commercial general liability, automobile liability, and contractors' pollution liability insurance coverage. When required by statute, remediators shall have workers' compensation insurance coverage."

Every step in the remediation process is important. From the beginning, clear communication could make the difference between a disaster and a success. Bids, quotes, and estimates have nuances, as each one creates similar but different paths. Clarity, preparation, and setting clear expectations before the actual work starts will hopefully put your team on the right path.

	Bid	Estimate	Quote
Definition	A formal proposal with a fixed price is submitted to win a project, often in competitive situations.	An approximate calculation of costs is provided as a rough idea, not binding.	A detailed, fixed-price offer provided for a specific project or service is often binding.
Purpose	To secure a project by outlining the proposed cost, terms, and scope of work.	To give the client an idea of what the project might cost before details are finalized.	To provide a precise and agreed-upon price for a project or service.
Level of Detail	Highly detailed, including costs, timelines, and terms, often customized for a competitive edge.	General and approximate, less detailed, based on preliminary information.	Precise, with clear breakdowns of costs, scope, and timelines.
Binding Nature	Binding if accepted; any changes require renegotiation.	It is not binding and is subject to change as more information is gathered.	A binding agreement once it is accepted unless the scope or terms change.
Use Case	For competitive contracts or formal project proposals.	For early-stage discussions when details are unclear.	For finalizing agreements on clearly defined projects or services.
When to Use	When competing with others to win a project where precision is required.	When providing a rough idea of costs based on limited details.	When the client requests a firm, fixed price for a clearly defined scope.
Examples	Submitting a bid to a government contract or construction project.	Estimating the cost of remodeling a kitchen before finalizing details.	Providing a quote to paint a house after inspecting it and agreeing on requirements.

Exercise 7.2: Vetting the Potential Remediation or Restoration Companies

Research Potential Companies: Start by compiling a list of local remediation and restoration companies. Use online resources, recommendations from your Indoor Environmental Professional (IEP), and referrals from trusted sources.

Initial Screening: Visit each company's website or contact them directly to gather preliminary information. Look for any mention of experience with environmentally-sensitive remediation or working in homes with health sensitivities.

Develop a set of questions to assess each company's suitability. Include questions about their experience with mold remediation, understanding of multiple chemical sensitivities (MCS), and willingness to learn about and implement medically important remediation methods.

❑ **Sample Questions and Considerations:**

- Describe your experience with mold remediation in homes where occupants have health sensitivities.

- How do you adapt your remediation techniques for clients with MCS or similar conditions?

- Are you open to learning and applying medically important remediation methods specific to our needs?

- Conduct Interviews: Arrange meetings or calls with the companies. During these interactions, ask your prepared questions and gauge their responses. Pay attention to not just what they say but also how willing they seem to accommodate your specific health requirements.

- Check References and Reviews: Ask for references from past projects, especially those involving health-sensitive environments. Additionally, look for online reviews or testimonials to get a sense of their reputation and customer satisfaction.

- Evaluate Willingness to Collaborate: Assess their readiness to work with your IEP and other health professionals. A collaborative approach is crucial for a successful remediation process.

- Document Your Findings: Keep detailed notes on each company's responses and your impressions. This will help compare and make an informed decision.

- **HIPAA Compliance and Confidentiality**
  Since the investigation and remediation of this home involve sensitive health conditions, HIPAA regulations for confidentiality must be strictly observed. Your company should have a comprehensive policy for client confidentiality that is binding on all staff members involved in this project.

- **Document Handling and Staff Training**
  It is imperative that documents related to this case are not sent to staff members unless they have been instructed on your company's HIPAA compliance policy. All staff should be fully trained and aware of their responsibilities under HIPAA, ensuring that any information related to the client's health and remediation process is handled with the utmost care and confidentiality.

- **Suggested Language for HIPAA Compliance**
  To ensure compliance with HIPAA regulations, we suggest including the following language in your company's confidentiality agreements and policies: "All information about clients and their homes, including health-related

data, must be treated as confidential and protected under HIPAA. No documents or communications containing such information are to be shared with unauthorized personnel, and all staff must adhere to strict confidentiality protocols."

- **Handling Complex Situations**
  In cases where contamination from adjoining units or shared walls may complicate remediation efforts, it is essential to document these complexities in writing. (S520 8.6) The IICRC S520 suggests this approach but does not offer specific guidance on managing cross-contamination that may impact Medically Important Remediation. For medically sensitive individuals, ongoing monitoring and cleaning may be required, though these measures may not provide a long-term solution. The selected professionals must acknowledge and address these complexities and communications with materially interested parties to provide informed consent and help mitigate ongoing health risks.

- **Post-Remediation Verification (PRV)**
  The IICRC S520 assigns responsibility for establishing PRV to the Indoor Environmental Professional (IEP) (S520 11.7). For medically important cases, careful coordination is required to avoid interference with advanced DNA analysis techniques, such as MSQPCR. PRV testing should be conducted in consultation with the patient's physician to ensure that the results meet the patient's medical needs.

- **Chemical Interference with Testing**
  The IICRC S520 does not specifically address the potential interference of certain chemicals with DNA-based testing methods like MSQPCR. However, for patients with CIRS or MCS, chemicals such as phenol, chlorine-based antimicrobials, and metal oxide coatings should be avoided, as they can interfere with these testing methods.

- **Handling of Stains and Mold Growth**
  Chemical stain removers, permitted by the IICRC S520, can bleach or remove pigments, potentially hiding residual mold growth. (S520 2.1.1) For medically sensitive individuals, the use of such products should be discouraged, as they can obscure the verification of mold removal and may cause adverse reactions. Physical removal of mold is preferred to ensure thorough remediation.

- **Third-Party PRV Testing**
  The IICRC S520 suggests hiring a third-party IEP for PRV testing but does not provide specific guidance for medically sensitive cases. It is vital that the selected IEP, the patient, and the healthcare provider clearly communicate and agree on PRV criteria to ensure the testing meets the patient's medical needs. This collaboration is crucial for ensuring a safe living environment.

- **Avoid Fogging or Misting Chemicals intended to Kill, Encapsulate or Seal.**
  While the IICRC S520 does not prohibit the use of fogging or misting as part of the remediation process, it acknowledges the potential risks involved. For patients with CIRS or MCS, fogging or misting chemicals intended to kill, encapsulate, or seal contamination should be strictly avoided. These methods can cause consequential damage and adverse health reactions in hypersensitive individuals. The chosen remediators must adhere to this guideline to protect the patient's health.

- **Avoid Using Antimicrobials or Biocides**
  The IICRC S520 allows the use of antimicrobials and biocides in the remediation process. However, for patients with chemical sensitivities or MCS, the use of these agents should generally be avoided. Any decisions regarding their use should be made by the occupants and their healthcare providers, with remediators acting only under explicit permission. It is essential that the remediation process prioritizes the health and safety of the patient.

- **Avoid Using Ozone or Photo-Catalytic Oxidation Treatments**
  Both the IICRC S520 and CIRSx recognize that certain treatments, such as ozone or photo-catalytic oxidation, might be deemed appropriate by a physician in specific cases. However, the IICRC S520 advises that ozone and biocides delivered as gas or vapor should not be used to kill mold as part of the remediation process and should not substitute for source removal. This includes the use of hydroxyl radical generators, UV lights, photo-catalytic oxidation, fogging of enzymes, diffusion of essential oils, or similar technologies as alternatives to the physical removal of fungal material. CIRSx aligns with this perspective, emphasizing that while a physician may recommend such treatments in particular cases, these technologies should not replace remediation efforts, and remediators should not employ them as part of their standard practice. The use of such treatments remains a medical decision that should be made in consultation with the affected individuals and their healthcare providers, ensuring that the patient's specific needs are addressed without compromising the integrity of the remediation process. (S520 9.1.7)

Ozone and biocides intended for use and delivery as a gas or vapor should not be used to attempt to kill mold as part of the remediation process and should not be used as a substitute for source removal. This includes utilizing a variety of chemicals and technology as a stand-alone remediation process, including hydroxyl radical generators, UV lights, photocatalytic oxidation, fogging of enzymes, diffusion of essential oils, or other techniques employed as an alternative to physical removal of the fungal material. —IICRC, 2024

Exercise 7.3: Selecting the Remediation or Restoration Company

Decision Time: Based on your research and evaluations, choose the company that best aligns with your needs, demonstrates the necessary expertise, and shows a commitment to adapting their methods for health-conscious remediation.

- If you are unable to identify a suitable remediation company, you may need to assemble suitable resources and personnel yourself to oversee the remediation. In this case, I highly recommend you enlist someone you trust who is not hypersensitive to mold and other water damage exposures to oversee the project. Additionally, you may find the CIRSx

Medically Important Remediation (MIR100) self-paced online learning program helpful, alongside this book, to aid you in learning to oversee the remediation process effectively. The MIR100 course covers the same material as the MIR101 but does not include Continuing Education Credits or a CIRSx Certification of Completion badge. This means you can learn the material without needing to comply with CEC requirements, such as completing the course sequentially and passing an exam for each module before moving on. This flexible approach allows you to gain the necessary knowledge and skills to manage and supervise the remediation process, ensuring the environment's health and safety for those sensitive to mold and other water-damage organisms.

Company Code of Ethics: *Medically Important Remediation*

Objective: This code sets forth the ethical principles and standards that guide restoration contractors engaged in Medically Important Remediation, ensuring that they conduct themselves with integrity, professionalism, and respect for health and property. These standards are essential to protecting the health and well-being of hypersensitive individuals affected by water damage, mold, and bacteria.

Rules of Conduct:

1. **Adherence to Industry Standards:** Restoration Firms must adhere to the industry's highest standards, strictly following accepted protocols and guidelines as outlined in the ANSI/IICRC S500 Standard for Professional Water Damage Restoration and S520 Standard for Professional Mold Remediation (2024), CIRSx Medically Important Remediation guidance, and relevant federal and state regulations.

2. **Truth in Representation:** The Firm must accurately represent the credentials, certifications, training, and experience of the involved parties. Misrepresentation in any form, whether intentional or not, undermines trust and compromises the safety and well-being of those impacted by their work.

3. **Health-Centered Decision-Making:** Contractors must prioritize health, recognizing that medically important remediation involves unique risks for individuals with sensitivities to mold and other contaminants. All recommendations must be made carefully considering the potential health impact on occupants. Making health-centered decisions may require guidance from physicians and/or indoor environmental professionals involved with the patient or client or their home.

4. **Transparency and Responsibility:** Firm management must clearly communicate all findings, remediation plans, and potential risks to both property and health. They are also responsible for providing clear guidance on the necessity of each intervention, supported by the best available scientific evidence and industry standards. This ensures that every recommended action is based on proven methods, balancing effectiveness with safety. All communication should be transparent, allowing clients to understand each intervention's reasoning and expected impact.

5. **Confidentiality:** All personal and business information gathered during remediation must be kept confidential per HIPAA regulations and industry confidentiality standards. Exceptions to this rule apply only when overriding legal obligations or imminent health concerns arise or when authorized in writing by the Patient Client.

6. **Conflict of Interest:** Firms must avoid conflicts of interest that could compromise the integrity of their professional judgment or their commitment to the Patient Client's health. They must disclose any situation that might lead to a conflict and remove themselves from situations where they cannot act impartially.

7. **Non-Chemical Remediation:** Medically Important Remediation emphasizes non-toxic, non-chemical methods. Firms must avoid using toxic treatments, including antimicrobials, biocides, fogging or misting agents, and containing harsh/harmful chemicals. Encapsulant sealants and other chemical agents unless explicitly required and agreed upon after a thorough risk assessment and consultation with the Patient Client and their environmental and/or physician representatives.

8. **Respect for the Patient Client and Their Home:** The occupants, the home, and their personal properties must be treated respectfully. The Firm and its employees must understand the emotional and physical strain that water damage, bacteria, and mold problems impose on affected individuals, particularly those with health conditions. They must perform their duties with empathy and care, aiming for minimal disruption and maximum health protection.

9. **Continuous Education and Compliance:** Firms are expected to stay informed of the latest developments in remediation technologies, health protocols, and

environmental safety standards and convey this important information to their employees. Ongoing education and certification renewals for employees are important to ensure the Firm's practices remain compliant and effective. Examples of continuing education would include programs offered or approved by CIRSx and/or IICRC emphasizing the latest developments in medically important remediation and maintenance.

10. **Integrity and Accountability:** Every person representing the Firm must act with the highest level of integrity, ensuring that their actions uphold the professional standards of the CIRSx endorsement and reflect positively on the field of Medically Important Remediation. Any conduct that compromises this trust is grounds for corrective action.

|||||||||||||||||||||||||||||||||||||||||||||||||||||||||||||||||||||||||||||||||||||||||||||||||||||||||||||||||||||||||||||||||||||||||||||||||||||||||||||||

Technician Code of Ethics: Medically Important Remediation

Objective: This code outlines the ethical responsibilities of technicians involved in medically important remediation, ensuring they perform their duties with integrity, diligence, and a commitment to protecting the health of hypersensitive individuals and others impacted by water damage, bacteria, and mold contamination.

Obligations:

1. **Commitment to Health and Safety:** Technicians must prioritize the health and safety of all individuals affected by water damage, bacteria, and mold, with particular attention to those with medical sensitivities. They are responsible for carrying out remediation tasks that minimize risks to occupants' health.

2. **Adherence to Protocols:** Technicians must strictly follow the remediation protocols established by Indoor Environmental Professionals per CIRSx standards. All actions should prioritize health-centered, non-toxic methods, focusing on physical removal and cleaning rather than using harmful chemicals. It is important to note that while some cleaning agents, such as detergents, may be used to break down and remove contaminants, the use of biocides, antimicrobials, and other harsh chemicals that pose health risks or leave toxic residues must be avoided to prevent further contamination or exposure to harmful substances.

3. **Professional Competence:** Technicians must maintain the highest level of skill in their work. This includes ongoing education, training, and adherence to the latest techniques and tools that meet the requirements of medically important remediation.

4. **Truthful Communication:** Technicians must communicate honestly with both their team and the property owner by following company policies and procedures and the chain of command. They must accurately report all findings, methods, and concerns, never misrepresenting the situation to either downplay or exaggerate the risks.

5. **Respect for Personal and Property Privacy:** Technicians must respect the confidentiality of all personal, medical, and property-related information encountered during the remediation process. This includes compliance with HIPAA regulations and any applicable industry confidentiality standards.

6. **Use of Safe and Clean Equipment:** Technicians must ensure that all equipment brought into a home is clean and free of contaminants. They must adhere to rigorous standards of cleanliness and maintenance to avoid introducing new risks into an already compromised environment.

7. **No Conflicts of Interest:** Technicians must disclose any potential conflicts of interest that may arise during a project and avoid any situation that compromises their ability to act in the best interest of the Patient Client's health and the integrity of the remediation process.

8. **Non-Toxic Remediation Practices:** In medically important remediation, using non-toxic, non-chemical cleaning methods is a basic principle. In this context, "non-chemical" refers to avoiding harmful substances such as biocides, antimicrobials, or encapsulants that may pose health risks while recognizing that some cleaning agents, like detergents or soaps, may still be used for their ability to break down and remove contaminants safely. "Non-toxic" refers to methods and products that do not introduce harmful or reactive chemicals into the environment, prioritizing the health of occupants. Technicians must avoid using any substances that could aggravate health conditions unless specifically directed by a certified professional and only with the client's informed written consent.

9. **Diligence and Precision:** Technicians must be thorough and precise. Every step, from containment to cleaning, should be carried out meticulously to ensure a safe environment for occupants, particularly those with compromised immune systems or chemical sensitivities.

10. **Upholding Professional Integrity:** Technicians must conduct themselves with professionalism and integrity, representing the firm's values and the standards of the CIRSx certification. They must avoid any behavior that could reflect poorly on the remediation process, the Firm, or the industry.

|||||||||||||||||||||||||||||||||||||||||||||||||||||||||||||||||||||||||||||||||||||||||||||||||||||||||||||||||||||||||||

Top 10 CIRSx Considerations for Medically Important Remediation Technicians

1. **Do Prioritize Health and Safety:** Always prioritize the health and safety of occupants, especially those with medical sensitivities. Take extra care to minimize exposure to contaminants, bacteria, mold, and chemicals.

2. **Do Follow Established Protocols:** Strictly adhere to the remediation protocols and product guidelines provided by certified professionals, ensuring no deviations that could compromise health or safety.

3. **Do Use Non-Toxic, Approved Products:** Only use products explicitly approved for medically important remediation. Substituting products without prior approval may introduce harmful chemicals or fragrances that could negatively impact Patient Clients.

4. **Do Maintain a Clean Work Environment:** Ensure all equipment and materials brought into the home are clean and free from contaminants. Regularly clean and maintain tools to avoid cross-contamination.

5. **Do Respect Patient Clients' Sensitivities:** Be mindful of odors and fragrances that may linger in the home. Always use free and clear/unscented hair, body care, and deodorant products, ensuring you don't introduce any unnecessary irritants into the environment.

6. **Do Communicate Clearly and Honestly:** Provide accurate updates on progress, issues, and next steps. Transparency builds trust with the Patient Client, ensuring they are informed and comfortable with the remediation process.

7. **Do Contain Work Areas Properly:** Properly set up containment and negative air systems to prevent contaminants from spreading to other parts of the home. Always ensure containment is secure before beginning work.

8. **Do Use Personal Protective Equipment (PPE):** Always wear appropriate PPE and ensure it is clean and properly maintained. Proper PPE use protects both the technician and the Patient Client from exposure to harmful particles.

9. **Do Take Detailed Notes and Document Work:** Keep thorough records of all work performed, products used, and any notable observations. This documentation is crucial for quality control and future reference. Photographs throughout the process can provide much-needed information and can assist in understanding the cause and extent of the water-damaged area(s).

10. **Do Seek Guidance When Needed:** If you encounter a situation you are unsure about, seek advice from a certified professional rather than guessing. It's essential to follow best practices at all times.

|||||||||||||||||||||||||||||||||||||||||||||||||||||||||||||||||||||||||||||||||||||||||||||||||||||||||||||||||||||||||||

Top 10 CIRSx Don'ts for Medically Important Remediation Technicians

1. **Don't Use Fragranced or Perfumed Products:** Avoid wearing scented shampoos, deodorants, or other body care products that could introduce strong or lingering odors into the remediation environment. A no-smoking policy is crucial because secondhand smoke and odors can be transferred and remain on the property, adversely affecting sensitive people.

2. **Don't Substitute Specified Products:** Never substitute products for those specified in the remediation plan. Using unapproved cleaners or chemicals can jeopardize the health of sensitive individuals.

3. **Don't Rush Through Containment Setup:** Do not skip or rush the process of setting up containment barriers, air Filtration Devices, or other appropriate controls. A properly set-up and sealed work area is critical for prohibiting cross-contamination.

4. **Don't Use Toxic Chemicals or Biocides:** Avoid using harsh chemicals, antimicrobials, or biocides unless approved by a certified professional and the Patient Client. Medically important remediation focuses on non-toxic solutions.

5. **Don't Use Products with Unclear Ingredients:** Avoid using any cleaning or remediation product without clearly understanding its ingredients. Fragrance-free, non-toxic, and approved products are essential in medically important settings.

6. **Don't Ignore Client Feedback:** Always listen carefully to Patient Clients' concerns, especially if they mention experiencing adverse reactions to odors or materials used. Their feedback can provide essential insights into sensitivities you may need to adjust for them and future projects.

7. **Don't Enter a Home Without Proper PPE:** Never enter a remediation environment without wearing appropriate personal protective equipment, as this can introduce contaminants and compromise the health of occupants.

8. **Don't Leave Equipment Dirty:** Do not bring dirty equipment or tools into the remediation environment. Always clean and sanitize equipment before and after use to prevent contamination.

9. **Don't Assume All Clients Are the Same:** Be mindful that every Patient Client's sensitivities and needs differ. What works in one home or building may not work in another, so constantly tailor your approach based on the Patient Client's medical requirements.

10. **Don't Compromise on Quality Control:** Don't cut corners or skip steps in the remediation process. Every detail matters when protecting the health of individuals in medically important remediation settings.

Step 8: Hidden or Unidentified Issues: Attics, Crawlspaces and Basements

Remediation's Hidden Challenges

This step adopts a detective-like approach to uncovering and incorporating hidden or unforeseen issues into your remediation plan and developing contingency strategies. It focuses on uncovering hidden or unidentified issues, particularly in non-occupied and hard-to-access areas, and preparing contingency plans for unexpected discoveries during remediation. This step ensures a comprehensive, adaptable approach by examining areas like attics, crawlspaces, and basements that may harbor concealed problems and considering external factors that could impact remediation success.

In this step, you'll refine your remediation plan by incorporating possible hidden or unidentified mold and moisture concerns, especially those in non-occupied spaces. Using a detective-like approach, this step combines all previously gathered information to target concealed issues and guide further investigations where necessary. Contingency plans will be developed for potential surprises that may arise during remediation. The exercises include focusing on reviewing data, inspecting overlooked spaces, and creating a comprehensive plan that prepares for any unexpected issues, ensuring smooth and effective remediation progress.

Exercise 8.1: Safety First, Investigative Review of Collected Data

The objective of this exercise is to safely perform a detailed analysis of all collected data for indications of potential hidden or unidentified issues, with an emphasis on identifying concealed concerns in challenging areas such as attics, crawlspaces, and basements.

❏ **Prioritize Safety in Non-Occupied Spaces:**
Begin by ensuring that any inspections in attics, crawlspaces, or unfinished basements prioritize safety. These spaces often pose unique risks, such as weak or compromised attic structures, hazardous debris in crawlspaces, and poor air quality or contaminants. Unless you have specialized training and appropriate personal

protective equipment, inspections in these areas are best left to trained professionals.

❏ **Data Analysis and Identification of Potential Hidden Issues:**
Review the data and observations from previous steps carefully, paying close attention to inconsistencies, unexplained findings, or patterns that might hint at concealed issues. Look for any unexplained areas of elevated moisture, musty odors, or irregularities that may indicate hidden mold. From this analysis, create a list of areas or components in the home that could harbor concealed mold or water damage. For example, if one window, wall, or structure shows signs of water intrusion, consider extending scrutiny to similar locations throughout the home to ensure no potential issues are overlooked.

❏ **Engage the Remediation Contractor for a Preliminary Inspection:**
Now is the time to actively involve your remediation contractor by having them conduct an on-site inspection specifically to identify discrepancies or hidden challenges. According to the S520 Standard, restoration contractors are required to perform a preliminary assessment and bring up any issues they observe. This inspection process is crucial for developing an accurate estimate, as fixed bids are often impractical in mold remediation due to its complexity. Instead, plan on paying for the Preliminary Determination and an estimate that outlines the scope of work and possible limitations. By hiring the remediator to perform this Preliminary Determination and provide an estimate before approving the job scope, you can evaluate how thorough and careful the firm is, as well as their understanding of Medically Important Remediation. This step will allow you to screen the company more effectively, helping to ensure that unforeseen issues are minimized once the project begins.

Exercise 8.2: Conducting the Inspection of Non-Occupied Areas and External Factors with the Remediation Contractor

To involve the remediation contractor's key personnel in reviewing the collected information from you and your Indoor Environmental Professional (IEP). This ensures they have a thorough understanding of the conditions, can assess whether an expansion of the scope may be needed, and are aligned on the Medically Important Objectives and Approach for the project.

❑ **Reviewing Information with the Contractor's Key Personnel:**
Request that both the project manager and crew chief that will be involved with your project participate in the inspection and review of the data and findings collected by you and your IEP. This includes observations, test results, and specific conditions of concern in non-occupied spaces such as attics, crawlspaces, and basements. If the company has a separate estimator, having the project manager and crew chief involved, rather than someone solely focused on sales and estimating, ensures that the on-the-ground team fully understands the project's health-focused objectives and unique requirements.

❑ **Preliminary Determination and Scope Assessment:**
With the gathered information, the contractor's team should conduct the inspection and preliminary determination of the site to provide their estimate and considerations or concerns about the conditions. During this assessment, they should identify areas where they recommend expanding the scope of work due to additional findings or concerns not apparent in the initial data. This collaborative process allows them to specify any additional inspection or testing they believe may be necessary to address all areas comprehensively.

❑ **Clarifying Medically Important Objectives and Approach:**
Work with the team to clarify the Medically Important Objectives and Approach, ensuring they are fully aware of the health-focused goals of the remediation. This will allow you to observe if they arrive with any strong, potentially unacceptable personal or other odors that could impact your acceptance of the completed project. Discuss any specific sensitivities or high standards crucial for the project, such as avoiding antimicrobial, encapsulant, or other chemical use, employing HEPA-rated equipment, and adhering to strict containment protocols. This shared understanding helps align the remediation team's work with the project's overall health objectives, ensuring thorough efforts are tailored to medically sensitive needs.

❑ **Document and Confirm Findings and Recommendations:**
Document the findings, recommendations, and any scope adjustments suggested by the project manager and crew chief during this preliminary inspection. Ensure that any additional suggestions or potential modifications are clearly outlined in the scope of work. This documentation establishes a clear foundation for moving forward with a remediation plan that is both robust and adaptable to new findings.

Exercise 8.3: Development of Contingency Plans

Creating adaptable plans that address unexpected findings during the remediation process, ensures minimal disruption to the workflow.

❑ This is the time to clarify which contingencies are already built into the scope of work, to avoid a contract where you may be excessively charged for minor adjustments, and to understand what additional change orders might be anticipated.

• **Identify Potential Scenarios:**
Consider various situations where new issues might surface, such as during demolition or deep cleaning, when hidden mold or structural damage could be revealed. Anticipate the steps that may be necessary if these issues are discovered, including potential work adjustments or additional testing.

• **Draft Contingency Plans:**
For each identified scenario, outline a course of action to address unexpected findings without significantly impacting the project timeline. Contingency plans might involve a temporary halt to evaluate the new issue, a decision-making framework for immediate remediation steps, or strategies for adjusting the broader remediation plan if needed.

• **Collaborate with the Remediation Team and IEP:**
Work closely with your Indoor Environmental Professional (IEP) and remediation team to develop practical and realistic contingency plans. Each plan should include steps for assessing unexpected findings, deciding if additional testing (such as Pathways™ testing or invasive techniques) is warranted, and determining immediate actions.

• **Review and Refine Plans for Integration:**
Collaborate with your team to refine each contingency plan, ensuring they can seamlessly integrate into the workflow. Confirm the plans are flexible enough to handle unexpected discoveries without causing costly delays or interruptions. This collaborative review process ensures that contingency plans are actionable and aligned with project goals.

Stage Three: Remediation Planning and Execution

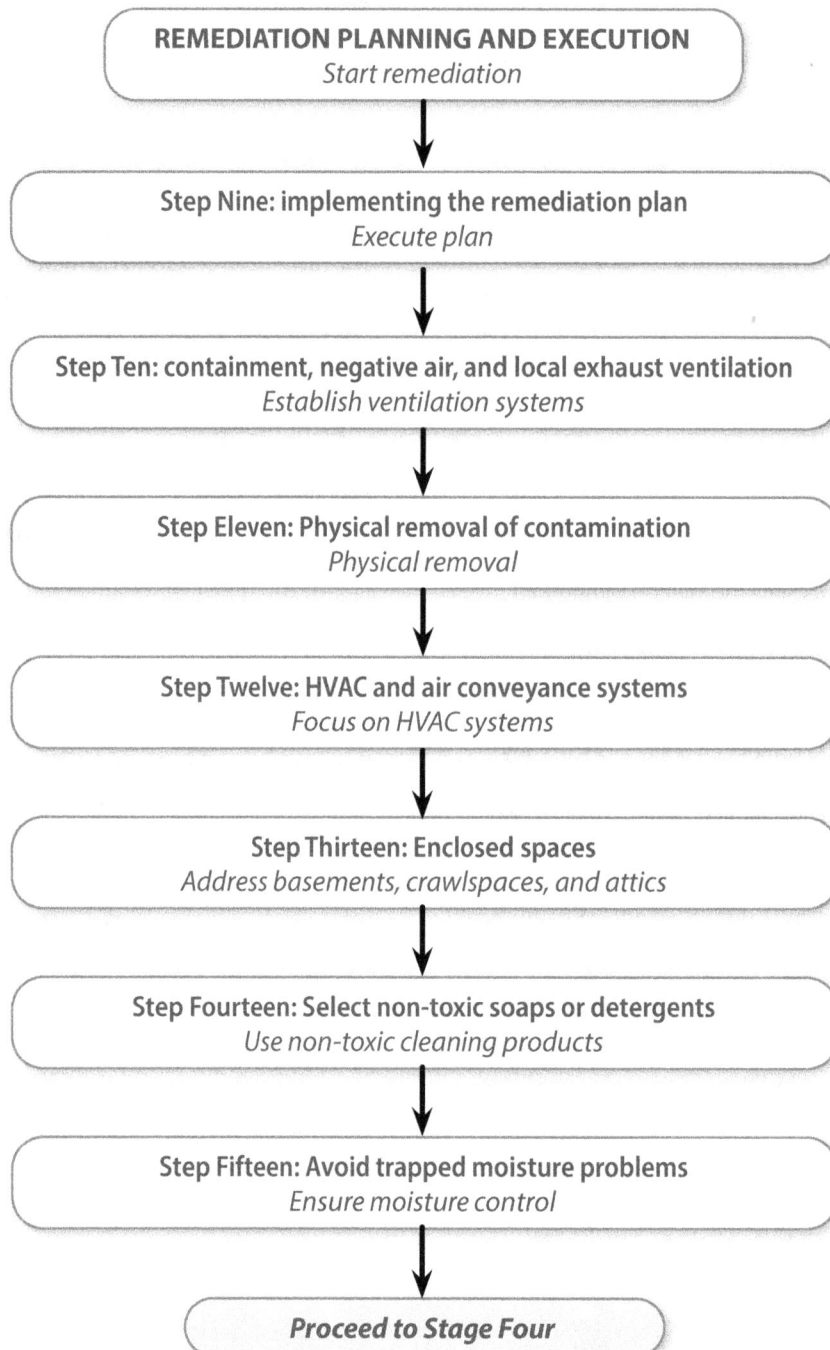

REMEDIATION PLANNING AND EXECUTION
Start remediation

Step Nine: implementing the remediation plan
Execute plan

Step Ten: containment, negative air, and local exhaust ventilation
Establish ventilation systems

Step Eleven: Physical removal of contamination
Physical removal

Step Twelve: HVAC and air conveyance systems
Focus on HVAC systems

Step Thirteen: Enclosed spaces
Address basements, crawlspaces, and attics

Step Fourteen: Select non-toxic soaps or detergents
Use non-toxic cleaning products

Step Fifteen: Avoid trapped moisture problems
Ensure moisture control

Proceed to Stage Four

Effective Remediation: Translating
Plans into Practical Action

Stage Three is the juncture where plans become actions in the remediation of mold and water damage, specifically tailored to protect those sensitive to mold and enhance living conditions for all. In this phase, careful execution of the remediation plan involves meticulous contamination removal, establishing robust containment zones, and using local exhaust ventilation to curb mold spore spread. This stage demands special attention to HVAC systems and enclosed spaces to prevent them from becoming mold propagation points. By focusing on safe, non-toxic cleaning methods and steering clear of moisture-trapping sealants and encapsulants, the process not only benefits individuals with sensitivities but also contributes to a healthier living environment for everyone. Stage Three synergizes detailed, health-focused remediation with proactive strategies, laying a solid groundwork for the subsequent evaluation and maintenance stages, thereby ensuring a safer and healthier home environment.

Goals for Stage Three

By the time you have completed this stage, you should have the necessary information to be able to answer these questions:

❑ What are the key objectives of this stage in the mold remediation process, particularly for individuals sensitive to mold?

❑ What do you need to accomplish to review and execute a remediation plan, emphasizing excluding certain types of products?

❑ How do containment zones and local exhaust ventilation systems aid in mold remediation, and what is the role of particle counters in this context?

❑ What is your focus for the non-chemical mold remediation approach regarding materials and techniques used for removing contaminants?

❑ What special attention to HVAC systems and enclosed spaces must you apply for medically important remediation to maintain indoor air quality?

Step 9: Implementing the Remediation Plan

Guiding Healthful, Remediation
& Chemical-Free Cleanup

Step 9 signals the official start of on-site remediation work. This is when the remediation plan transitions from preparation to action, as the team begins addressing mold and water damage. The focus in this step is on executing the plan with strict adherence to health-centered, chemical-free methods, including mechanical removal and approved non-toxic products.

To maintain a safe work environment and ensure effective post-remediation evaluation, the plan excludes anti-microbials, biocides, encapsulants, sealants, and any other potentially toxic chemicals. Ideally, unapproved chemicals should not even be present in workers' vehicles.

Clear communication and a well-defined team hierarchy are essential to keeping the project on track. Understanding the team's chain of command will facilitate efficient communication, issue resolution, and adherence to project goals.

Quality control is fundamental as the remediation work begins. Familiarity with the standards and control measures that will be applied can prevent setbacks and reinforce health-centered practices. However, despite thorough planning, unexpected issues can arise. Ways to address the issues of when things go wrong will also be discussed to provide guidance for managing unforeseen challenges and ensuring quick, effective responses.

Exercise 9.1: Confirming Chemical-Free Protocols with the Team

❑ **Ensure all team members understand** and strictly follow chemical-free protocols as they begin work:

› Review the chemical-free standards and list of prohibited substances with the team before work begins.
› Confirm that unapproved chemicals will not be brought on-site or stored in vehicles.
› Reinforce guidelines with the project manager to ensure compliance throughout the project's duration.

Exercise 9.2: Establishing Clear Communication Channels

❑ **Set up clear communication lines** and understand the team's chain of command for efficient issue resolution as the work progresses.

› Review roles within the team, identifying the project manager and crew chief as primary contacts.
› Set expectations for promptly reporting any issues or deviations from the plan.
› Establish a system for regular updates to track progress and address emerging concerns in real time.

Exercise 9.3: Quality Control and Contingency Preparation

❑ **Verify that quality control measures** are in place and establish contingency plans for unexpected challenges during the work.

› Review the quality standards that will guide each phase of the remediation.
› Discuss contingency protocols for managing unexpected issues, especially accidental use of unapproved substances.
› Confirm that the remediation plan allows for adjustments without compromising quality or health-focused goals.

Essay: When Things Go Wrong (It Will Be Okay)
by Michael Schrantz

The Rule, Not the Exception

It will happen. Trust me. That's the rule. Things go wrong, not because someone is always unaware or lazy, but often because we set our expectations so high that anything less seems like a failure, a dealbreaker, a life-is-over sort of event.

Sure, we are responsible for making grounded decisions and managing our reactions to setbacks. But sometimes, situations are extreme or emotionally charged, making it hard to respond calmly. How many of you have made the mistake of reading about health symptoms online, only to feel more worried? Or have you heard something from a "credible" source that left you anxious about your health or home?

I've worked with thousands of clients, many of whom have felt this way. I've been there too.

Allow me to put a few things on the table:

Mold Is Not Plutonium

Mold is not plutonium—we don't treat it as such. The same mold spores and mycotoxins people worry about indoors also exist outdoors. While elevated indoor mold levels can be a problem, it's important to remember that our reaction often makes things worse. Fear activates our survival instincts—helpful if we're running from a bear but harmful if it leaves us in constant anxiety. Living with ongoing fear can make recovery much harder. There is nothing secret about that.

Normal vs. Elevated Mold vs "Mold-Free"

Did you know that most mold inspections compare indoor mold levels to outdoor levels? The goal isn't to have a completely "mold-free" indoor environment—that's neither practical nor necessary. Instead, the focus is on preventing "mold growth" indoors, except in areas designed to handle moisture, like showers, sink drains, or toilet tanks, where mold is often naturally present.

Mold spores and structures found in your home (air and surface) often originate from the outdoors, even those same species that can grow in water-damaged buildings. After a remediation project, an Indoor Environmental Professional (IEP) might say your home has a "normal fungal ecology." But (ironically), did you know that some of those fungal spores or structures (even mycotoxins) that were identified as "normal" may be "residual" from the indoor source that was previously remediated? That suggests that you don't have to "perfectly remediate or clean" your home that experiences a mold growth event(s). Many people get their home "good enough (for them)" to recover or heal successfully. We see this all the time.

Food for thought: Why does it seem that many people are significantly worried about mold and its byproducts produced indoors (such as in water-damaged buildings) but don't consider their daily exposure to the same mold and byproducts outdoors? Considering indoor and outdoor exposures could provide a clearer understanding of what 'mold exposure' truly means and help us recognize that achieving safety and healing doesn't require an impossible standard of being completely 'mold-free.' Instead, it's about managing our environment in a balanced and practical way.

Our Biggest Obstacle: Ourselves

One of the biggest obstacles to getting better is our own response. Let's explore how we can navigate setbacks without spiraling into fear.

Take, for example, a containment barrier falling during mold remediation. Many might assume the entire house is now contaminated and all contents are ruined. But the truth is, these situations are often manageable. Mistakes don't automatically mean the project has failed. With a proactive response, setbacks can be addressed without significant harm.

Practical Steps When Setbacks Happen

If a containment partially falls, close nearby doors and turn off HVAC systems if possible. Contact the remediation company to fix the issue or hire someone locally. Often, the home already has some level of contamination from the source being addressed, so thorough cleaning will be needed regardless. Mistakes like these are common and usually manageable.

Similarly, if there's a power failure during remediation, remember that setbacks do not mean the project is compromised. Keep containment intact, notify the remediation company, and consider using portable power sources. A short delay is unlikely to make things significantly worse.

If a remediation company doesn't follow the protocol exactly, adjustments can still be made. It's frustrating, but it doesn't mean the entire process is doomed. Involve an IEP if needed to get things back on track, or bring in a second mold remediation company to help provide a voice for you and properly document what has taken place, as well as how to fix it.

Recovery Takes Time

Health recovery after remediation is another area where expectations often need adjusting. Just like surgery recovery, it takes time. The environment can be made safe, but the body may need weeks or even months to heal. Be patient and compassionate with yourself. And while you are on your road to recovery, stay observant, not anxious, about your surroundings. Watch for signs of potential water leaks, such as water stains near windows or on ceilings or leaks under plumbing fixtures like kitchen sinks or bathroom vanities. To proactively address these risks, consider installing moisture alarms in areas where water intrusion is possible (I personally use over 11 of these alarms in my own home!). These devices can provide early warnings and help prevent small issues from becoming larger ones.

Hope Beyond Setbacks

Unfortunately, fear-based messaging is everywhere, including in the media and parts of the medical field. It's easy to feel overwhelmed and alone. However, mold issues can be resolved, and homes can be healthy again. The journey may not be immediate, but it's achievable, and there are people ready to help.

When setbacks happen—whether it's containment issues, power failures, protocol deviations, slow recovery, or feeling overwhelmed—remember that you're not alone. Things are rarely as catastrophic as they seem. This journey is about perseverance, and there is always hope beyond the setbacks. So, bet on the rule, not the exception.

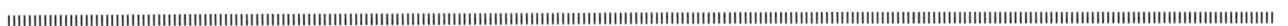

Step 10: Containment, Negative-Air, Local Exhaust Ventilation and Makeup Air

Isolating Water Damage with Strategic Barriers and Airflow Controls

Effective mold remediation and water damage restoration require precision and a scientific approach to control workspaces. In Step 10, we explore the concepts, application, and installation of containment, airflow, and makeup air systems. These are essential to control the dust, debris, and contaminants generated during the remediation process, ensuring its effectiveness and safety while preventing the unintentional spread of contaminants." Containment zones, meticulously maintained under negative pressure, serve as the first line of defense, preventing the escape of mold spores and contaminated particles. These zones work with local exhaust ventilation systems, which capture and remove airborne contaminants. Real-time monitoring using particle counters enhances quality control, providing objective evidence of the controls' effectiveness. This multifaceted approach is essential for creating controlled environments that are necessary for successful remediation.

The Role of Containment in Remediation

Containment barriers are indispensable tools in the mold remediation process, serving multifaceted purposes that are crucial for a successful outcome. Their primary goal is to isolate the affected area from the rest of the home, preventing the spread of mold spores and contaminants. Advantages include:

Isolation: Containment creates a physical barrier that should not trap contaminants but rather facilitate the implementation of isolation. By segregating the areas with issues from those without or with lesser issues, containment minimizes the risk of cross-contamination.

Preventing Cross-Contamination: It ensures that mold spores and contaminants are contained within the remediation zone, reducing the potential for these particles to escape into other non-contaminated or less contaminated areas of the home.

Reducing Hidden Contamination: Containment barriers play a vital role in reducing the development of

contamination in hard-to-reach areas within your home. Contaminants can infiltrate nooks and crannies without proper containment. The less contaminants are controlled during remediation, the greater the building memory that will accumulate in hidden or inaccessible areas. This will increase the amount of time and effort that will be necessary for the building to forget the mold contamination that occurred.

Maintaining Indoor Air Quality: Over time, these contaminants may build up, creating a reservoir that can release particles back into your home, affecting indoor air quality. Containment helps prevent this scenario by confining the contamination to the designated remediation area.

Control of Dust and Moisture: Containment aids in controlling dust and moisture levels within the workspace, making the remediation process more manageable.

Facilitating Cleaning: It also facilitates cleaning, as it confines contaminants to a specific area, allowing for focused and effective cleaning efforts.

Critical Component: Containment, when correctly installed and maintained, is a critical component of mold remediation, ensuring the safety of your home and the success of the restoration process. Containments that are not to be breached or used for entry or exit are often referred to as critical barriers.

Exercise 10.1: Containment Barriers

❏ **The use of containment barriers** helps separate contaminated areas from clean areas or areas of higher contamination from areas of lower contamination. They are helpful in reducing the risk of cross-contamination, thereby reducing the amount of cleaning that is required to remove contaminants that spread between areas. Containment works best when combined with negative air pressure which helps reduce turbulence and work activities from allowing contaminant particles to escape.

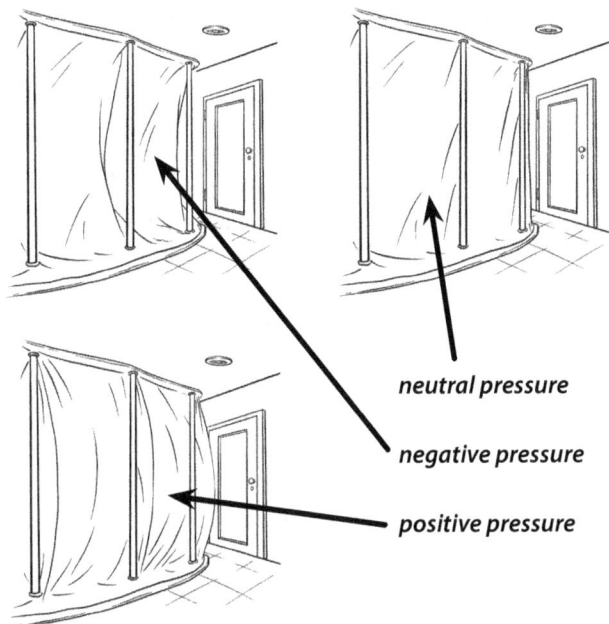

Figure 5-52: Containment behavior under Negative Pressure, Neutral Pressure, and Positive Pressure

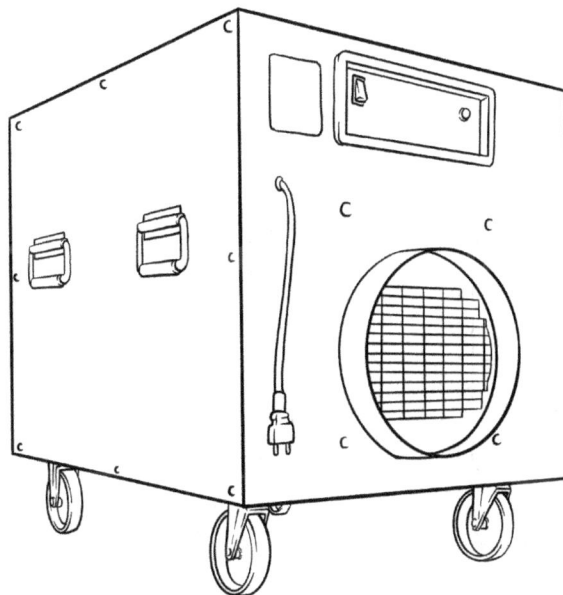

Figure 5-53a: HEPA-filtered Air Filtration Device (AFD)

THE ROLE OF NEGATIVE AIR IN REMEDIATION

Negative Air is a critical component of mold remediation and water damage restoration, playing a central role in preventing the escape of contaminants from containment areas. It involves installing properly sized HEPA-filtered air filtration devices (AFDs) to establish powerful negative pressure within the containment. When used in conjunction with proper containment measures, this negative pressure creates an effective barrier that contaminants cannot breach. Turbulence within containment, often caused by workers' movement, can lead to the inadvertent release of contaminants and dust. Properly installed and maintained Negative Air systems are instrumental in preventing this scenario.

Furthermore, Negative Air actively manages airflow between different areas. By closely monitoring and adjusting the levels of negative air, it becomes possible to ensure that contaminants from other areas, such as attics or crawlspaces, do not infiltrate clean zones. This level of control extends to creating distinct airflow zones within the workspace, with the most contaminated areas maintained under the highest negative air pressure, while cleaner areas are upheld by positive air pressure. The careful orchestration of Negative Air, in conjunction with containment, not only ensures the success of remediation but also safeguards the safety and integrity of your home throughout the remediation process.

Exercise 10.2 Establishing Negative Air— Venting to the Outside

❑ **Exhaust air filtration devices (AFD) to the outside** to establish a negative air pressure in remediation areas, ensuring that contaminated air is captured, filtered, and vented outdoors rather than spreading to unaffected parts of the building. This process minimizes cross-contamination and protects occupant health by drawing clean air into the containment and preventing the escape of mold spores, dust, or other contaminants. When monitoring the efficiency of HEPA AFDs with a particle counter is not feasible, venting the AFD exhaust directly to the outside is a precautionary measure. This approach reduces the risk of indoors recirculating potentially unfiltered or inadequately filtered air. To achieve this, connect a HEPA-filtered AFD to a sealed containment area and attach a flexible duct to its outlet, directing the air to an exterior window, door, or vent. While venting outdoors does not offer the same level of filtration assurance as monitoring with a particle counter, it significantly lowers the risk of mold spore proliferation within the building, ensuring remediation efforts maintain indoor air quality.

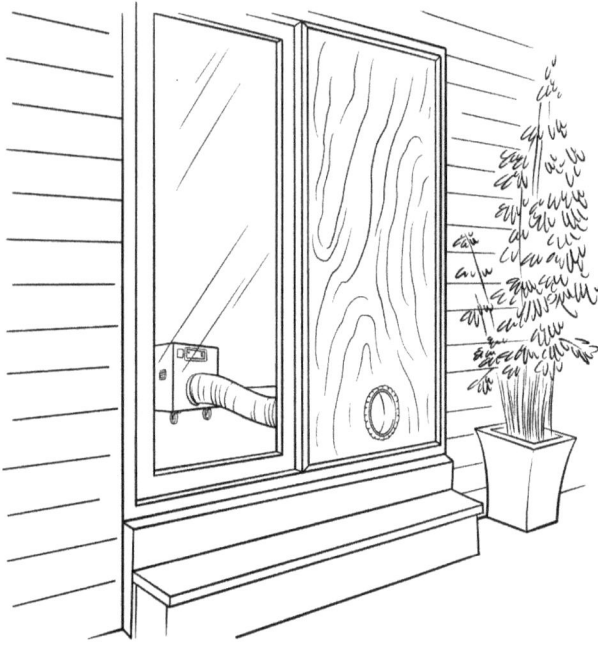

Figure 5-53b: Venting HEPA-filtered equipment to the outdoors from containment is an effective way to prevent contamination created inside the containment from cross-contaminating the home. A properly functioning HEPA Air Filtration Device (AFD) with 99.97% efficiency is remarkably effective at reducing the number of released spores. This significant reduction underscores the vital role of properly maintained and functioning HEPA filtration in controlling mold spore dissemination during remediation. Malfunctioning unit that releases particles around or through holes in the filter. Research has shown that approximately 50% of air filtration devices used on remediation projects are not functioning properly and leak either through holes in the filter, improperly seated gaskets, or damaged equipment. (Brandys, 2012)

Exercise 10.3 Why Local Exhaust Ventilation is So Effective

❑ **Local exhaust ventilation (LEV)** serves as the ultimate control measure to prevent the buildup or inadvertent release of contamination. LEV is designed to capture and remove airborne contaminants at their source, ensuring that they do not disperse into the surrounding environment.

Setting up Local Exhaust Ventilation

- **Identification of Contaminated Sources:** The first step is to identify the sources of contamination within the remediation area. This includes pinpointing areas with visible mold growth, water-damaged materials, or other sources of contamination.

- **Strategic Placement of Equipment:** Units equipped with HEPA filters are strategically placed near these contaminated sources. The placement depends on the specific conditions and the stage of remediation. For

example, if there is active mold growth on a wall, an LEV unit may be positioned to capture airborne spores released during the remediation process.

- **Ducting and Airflow Management:** Ducting is the conduit that connects the path of airflow from the contamination source to the HEPA-filtered AFD to control the local exhaust ventilation. Sometimes, a portable hood assembly can help act as an adjustable collection point. The airflow is carefully managed to ensure that contaminants are effectively captured. Negative air pressure is maintained within the containment area, directing the airflow towards the LEV units, where it is filtered before exhausting to the outside and away from clean areas.

Monitoring and Adjustment

- **Real-time Monitoring:** During the remediation process, particle counters and air quality monitors are employed to provide real-time data on the concentration of airborne particles, including mold spores. This data allows remediation professionals to assess the effectiveness of LEV and make adjustments as needed.

- **Adjusting Airflow Rates:** Depending on the stage of remediation and the level of contamination, the airflow rates of LEV units may be adjusted. For instance, higher airflow rates may be necessary for effective control during the initial stages when contaminants are disturbed and removed. Studies have shown that airborne levels of contamination are commonly 10 to 1000 times higher during active phases of remediation, such as during demolition and aggressive cleaning. As the remediation progresses and the contamination is reduced, airflow rates and paths can be adjusted so that fresh airflow remains from clean to dirty.

- **Visual Inspections:** Regular visual inspections of the containment area and collection systems are conducted to ensure that everything is functioning as intended. Any issues, such as leaks in ducting or a decrease in airflow as filters load, are addressed promptly to maintain the integrity of the containment.

- **Adaptation to Changing Conditions:** Remediation is a dynamic process, and conditions within the containment area can change. LEV systems are adaptable to respond to these changes. For example, if a new source of contamination is discovered, an additional LEV unit may be deployed to address it.

Benefits of Local Exhaust Ventilation

- **Prevents Contaminant Release:** LEV captures contaminants at their source, preventing their release into clean areas or the environment.

- **Reduces Contamination Buildup:** By continuously removing contaminants, LEV minimizes the buildup of contamination within the containment.
- **Enhances Worker Safety:** LEV ensures workers are exposed to lower contaminants, improving their safety.
- **Maintains Clean Areas:** LEV helps prevent a buildup of contaminants in areas where air stratifies or stagnates within a containment work area. Maintain clean zones within the workspace, reducing the risk of cross-contamination.
- **Real-time Control:** Monitoring and adjustment of LEV provide real-time control over the containment environment, optimizing remediation efforts.

In summary, local exhaust ventilation is critical to mold remediation and water damage restoration. It is carefully set up, monitored, and adjusted to effectively capture and remove contaminants at their source, preventing contamination release and ensuring the success of the remediation process.

Exercise 10.4 Establishing and Monitoring Makeup Air

Makeup air is an important component in the control of contaminants within containment areas during remediation. To understand its significance, imagine the action of sucking air through a straw. When you use a straw to draw air, you create airflow from the surroundings into your mouth. This flow is smooth and unrestricted as long as the end of the straw remains open.

Now, picture placing your finger over the end of the straw while trying to suck air. You would immediately notice that the airflow is impeded, and drawing in any more air becomes impossible.

In the context of containment, a tightly sealed containment area with inadequate makeup air will restrict the airflow. Without makeup air, the interior of the containment becomes stagnant, much like when you suck on a straw with the other end covered with your finger. Contaminants accumulate at higher levels, and the effectiveness of containment is compromised.

❑ **Use Makeup Air to Facilitate Successful Remediation:**

› **Facilitating Airflow:** Makeup air is like removing your finger from the end of the straw. It introduces a controlled flow of fresh air into the containment area. This influx of air helps maintain airflow, preventing the buildup of contaminants and ensuring that the containment remains an effective barrier.

› **Preventing Stagnation**: Stagnant air within containment can accumulate contaminants, moisture, and other unwanted elements. Makeup air disrupts this stagnation by introducing a continuous fresh air flow, ensuring the containment remains dynamic and effective.

› **Balancing Air Pressure:** Makeup air also plays a crucial role in balancing air pressure within the containment. Without it, negative air pressure from exhaust systems can create an overly depressurized environment, potentially causing doors to be difficult to open and contaminants to be pulled in from unintended areas. Failure to provide adequate makeup air can also lead to dangerous conditions such as back-drafting of combustion fumes from affected gas furnaces and hot water heaters.

› **Ensuring Worker Comfort:** In addition to contamination control, makeup air contributes to the comfort and safety of workers within the containment area. It ensures that workers have a fresh supply of air to breathe and minimizes the feeling of being in a confined, stuffy space.

Makeup air, when properly designed and implemented, transforms containment areas into dynamic environments. It allows for the continuous exchange of air while preventing the escape of contaminants. This dynamic containment ensures that the remediation process is not hindered by stagnant conditions and that contaminants are effectively controlled.

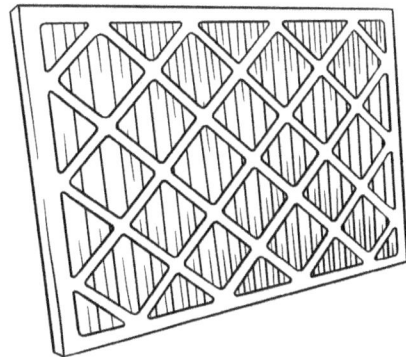

Figure 5-54: A high-rated MERV filter can bring makeup air into the home or the containment.

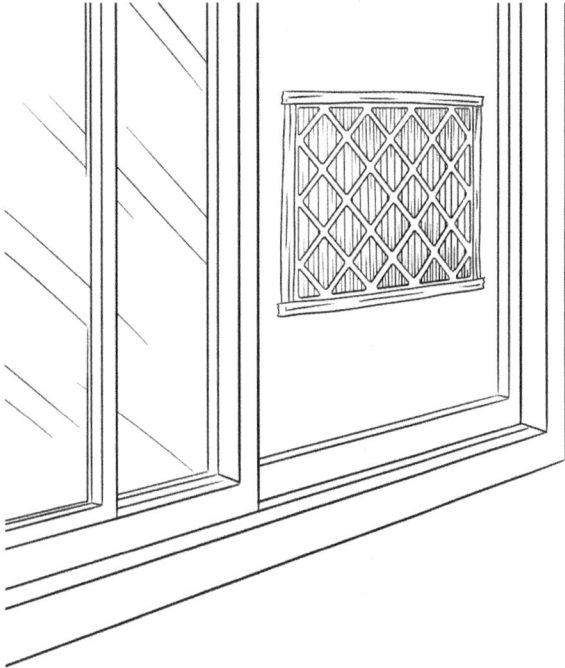

Figure 5-55: Make-up Air installed in an open window using a MERVE filter.

Exercise 10.5: Methods for Establishing Makeup Air

❑ **Creating a Balanced System for Mold Remediation and Contaminated Environment Control**

Mold remediation and the control of contaminated environments require a balanced and strategic approach that combines various elements to ensure effectiveness and safety. In this discussion, we'll explore how containment, HEPA-filtered Air Filtration Devices (AFDs) for negative air, local exhaust ventilation, and makeup air work together to create a harmonious and efficient system for mold remediation and contamination control.

1. **Containment:**
   Containment is the foundational element in this system. It involves the strategic installation of physical barriers to isolate the affected area from the rest of the environment. The primary goal of containment is to prevent the escape of mold spores and contaminants. Containment can vary in size, ranging from small, room-level containment achieved at doorways to medium-sized areas cordoned off for isolation.

2. **Negative Air with HEPA-Filtered AFDs:**
   To enhance containment, negative air pressure is established within the containment area using HEPA-filtered AFDs. These devices create a powerful suction force that draws air and contaminants into the containment, preventing their escape. Negative air is a crucial component as it ensures that any disturbance within the

containment, such as worker movement, does not lead to the release of contaminants.

3. **Local Exhaust Ventilation:**
   Local exhaust ventilation complements containment and negative air by actively managing airflow within the workspace. It involves the use of ventilation systems to capture and remove airborne contaminants. By positioning exhaust systems strategically, contaminants are efficiently captured and directed away from the workspace. This process helps prevent the buildup of contamination, ensuring that the environment remains controlled.

4. **Makeup Air:**
   Makeup air is the final piece of the puzzle. It introduces a controlled flow of clean, fresh air into the containment area. This influx of air prevents the containment from becoming stagnant and ensures that negative air pressure does not hinder the ability to open doors or create discomfort for workers. Makeup air is vital for maintaining a balanced and dynamic containment system.

5. **Balancing the System:**
   Balancing these elements is the key to a successful remediation and contamination control system. Containment provides the first line of defense by physically isolating the affected area. Negative air and local exhaust ventilation work in unison to actively manage airflow and capture contaminants. Makeup air ensures that the containment remains dynamic and functional.

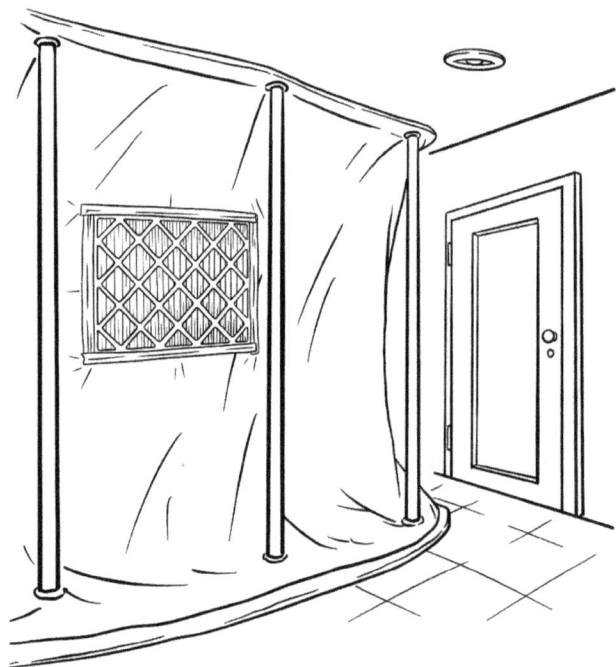

Figure 5-56: If negative air in the containment is too great, it may cause the containment barrier to collapse. Makeup air installed on the side of a containment allows air to pass through a MERV filter, which can be used for negative pressure relief and control.

Benefits of a Balanced System

Effectiveness: By working together, these elements create a highly effective system that prevents the escape of contaminants, controls airflow, and maintains a balanced environment.

Safety: The combination of containment, negative air, local exhaust ventilation, and makeup air ensures the safety of workers and the integrity of the containment area.

Contamination Control: This balanced system minimizes the potential for cross-contamination, ensures that contaminants are confined to the designated area, and prevents the buildup of contamination.

Efficiency: A well-balanced system streamlines the remediation process, allowing for efficient and successful mold remediation and contaminated environment control.

In summary, the synergy of containment, negative air with HEPA-filtered AFDs, local exhaust ventilation, and makeup air creates a balanced and effective system for mold remediation and contaminated environment control. This approach ensures that contaminants are contained, controlled, and prevented from escaping, ultimately leading to a successful remediation process.

The Crucial Role of HEPA Air Filtration in Mold Remediation

In the intricate process of mold remediation, the use of High-Efficiency Particle Air (HEPA) filtration equipment is a cornerstone for ensuring a healthy indoor environment. This equipment, when functioning correctly, minimizes the release of mold spores into the air. The effectiveness of HEPA filters, designed to trap 99.97% of airborne particles, is not just a technical specification but a vital component in preserving indoor air quality, particularly during the disruptive activities of mold removal.

Detailed Explanation:

Efficiency of HEPA Filters: HEPA filters are renowned for their ability to capture minute particles, including mold spores, with an efficacy rate of 99.97%. This exceptional performance is crucial during mold remediation, especially considering that activities like demolition can increase airborne mold levels by 10 to 1000 times. Controlled demolition in a room with a concentration of 25,000 cfu (colony-forming units) per cubic meter of mold spores, for instance, can

still release a significant number of spores even with HEPA filtration. However, this release is markedly lower compared to environments without properly functioning filtration.

Impact of Malfunctioning Equipment: The stark contrast in indoor air quality with malfunctioning HEPA equipment cannot be overstated. A hypothetical scenario where a HEPA device malfunctions, releasing 5% of captured particles, illustrates a dramatic increase in mold spore dissemination. In one hour, such a device could release over 1.5 million spores in a typical 20 by 20-foot room, significantly elevating the risk of mold exposure and cross-contamination to other areas. The aftermath of mold spore release has tangible consequences. For example, in the case of a malfunctioning HEPA unit, the concentration of mold spores settling on the floor can reach upwards of 27 cfu per square inch per hour of release. This highlights the importance of not only airborne spore management but also post-remediation cleaning and decontamination to address any residual contamination. To put this into perspective: In the scenario of controlled demolition in a room with an airborne concentration of 25,000 cfu per cubic meter of mold spores, a properly functioning HEPA Air Filtration Device (AFD) with 99.97% efficiency releases approximately 9,557 spores into the air over the course of an hour.

In contrast, if a HEPA AFD were to malfunction and release 5% of the captured particles, it would release approximately 1,592,820 spores in the same timeframe.

A properly functioning HEPA Air Filtration Device (AFD) with 99.97% efficiency is remarkably more effective, reducing the number of released spores by approximately 99.4% compared to a malfunctioning unit that releases 5% of captured particles. This significant reduction underscores the vital role of properly maintained and functioning HEPA filtration in controlling mold spore dissemination during remediation processes, greatly mitigating the risk of airborne contamination.

Preventive Measures: Ensuring the proper functioning of HEPA filtration units is paramount. Regular maintenance, performance checks, and immediate rectification of any identified issues are essential steps. These measures, coupled with effective containment strategies, significantly mitigate the risks associated with airborne mold spores during remediation efforts.

ENSURING THE EFFICIENCY OF HEPA AIR FILTRATION DEVICES: THE ROLE OF PARTICLE COUNTERS

In the realm of mold remediation, the integrity and performance of HEPA Air Filtration Devices are of paramount importance. Recent studies, such as the one by Bob and Gail Brandies, have highlighted a concerning trend: a significant percentage of HEPA AFDs in use do not perform to their specified standards. This revelation brings to light the crucial need for regular and rigorous testing of these devices. One of the most effective methods for ensuring that a HEPA AFD is functioning correctly is using a particle counter.

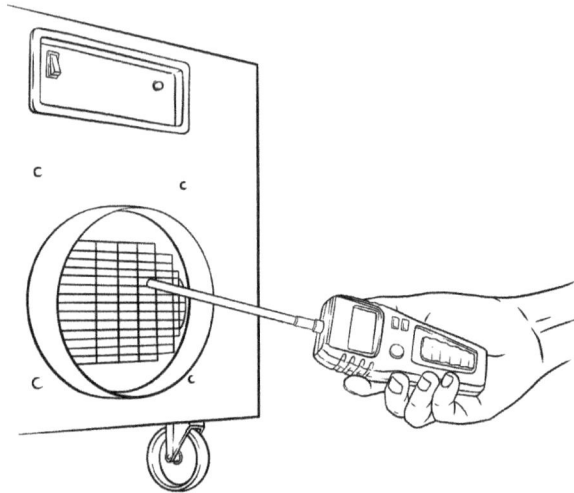

Figure 5-57: The particle counter probe must be placed as close to the exhaust point as possible to prevent room air turbulence from mixing particles into the exhaust stream.

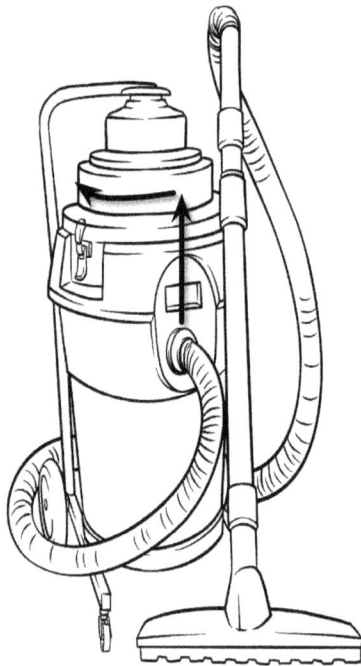

Figure 5-59: The arrow indicates common positions for the HEPA-filtered exhaust air stream. When the filter is located as the final stage for the air to pass through, a particle counter can be used to assess its efficiency. Position the particle counter probe as close as possible to the filter's exhaust to minimize turbulence and prevent mixing with ambient room air, ensuring accurate measurement of the filtered air. I have tested over 200 Shark vacuum cleaners (Navigator and Rotator with complete seal technology). They are my favorite low-cost vacuums.

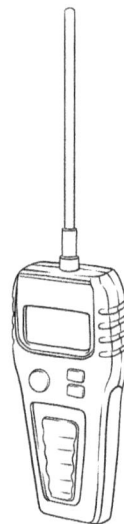

Figure 5-58: Some HEPA vacuums combine the filtered air stream with a cooling air exhaust stream to cool the motor. In this case, a particle counter may not be able to check the operation of the equipment directly. The unit's specifications and technical support may be able to provide recommended methods for checking filter efficiency.

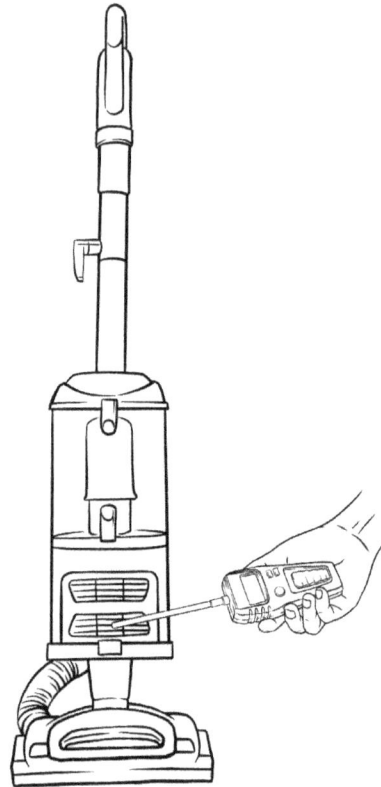

Figure 5-60: A particle counter is an invaluable tool for measuring the concentration of particles, including mold spores, in the air. By assessing the particle count upstream and downstream of the AFD, one can determine the actual efficiency of the filter. The HEPA standard, aimed at capturing 99.97% of particles that are 0.3 microns in diameter, serves as a benchmark for these measurements. If a particle counter indicates that the AFD is not achieving this level of filtration, immediate action is required to either service or replace the unit. This ensures that the remediation process does not inadvertently exacerbate mold issues by releasing inadequately filtered air back into the indoor environment.

Assessing Particle Counter Accuracy

You probably won't spend the money on a professional-grade particle counter, which can cost thousands of dollars. Less expensive consumer-level particle counters are available for a couple of hundred dollars. But how do you know it is providing accurate and helpful information? Professional calibration can cost hundreds of dollars, but there are simple ways to check if your meter is working properly.

Start by ensuring the basics are in order. If readings are erratic, replace the battery, as low power can affect performance. A zero-check filter is another essential tool. Many counters come with one, but you can purchase one for about $50 if needed. The filter removes all particles from the air entering the meter. Attach it, turn on the device, and verify it reads zero across all particle sizes. If it doesn't, cleaning or adjustment may be necessary.

Another option is to compare your device to a known standard. Use a controlled environment, like a cleanroom, or borrow a recently calibrated counter to measure the same location side-by-side. Consistent readings indicate that your counter is functioning properly.

Testing in predictable environments provides further confirmation. Outdoor particle levels are typically higher but vary based on conditions like wind and fog, which make them go up, but after long, gentle rains or snow, airborne particles will go down. Indoors, you can create particles by burning a candle or spraying an aerosol. Your counter should detect a spike and return to baseline once the source is removed.

Regular consistency checks are crucial. Measure the same location multiple times under identical conditions; readings should be somewhat stable. Controlled tests with incense or smoke should show expected gradients as you measure at increasing distances.

When these common-sense accuracy checks line up, you can have more confidence in your particle counter's readings in more specific applications, like inside HVAC ducts, HEPA vacuum cleaners exhaust, and air purification devices. Keeping a log of readings over time helps confirm your device's reliability and ensures accurate insights.

Step 11: Physical Removal of Contaminants

Guiding Concept: Physical Removal for Effective Mold Remediation

Step 11 focuses on the non-chemical remediation of mold by prioritizing the physical removal of mold-affected materials. This process is essential for effectively eliminating mold growth. By emphasizing safe removal and disposal practices, this step underscores techniques that protect the health of individuals, especially those with sensitivities to mold and its by-products.

I strongly emphasize non-chemical mold remediation, physically removing water-damaged, soft, porous materials like insulation and gypsum board. Abrasive cleaning techniques are recommended over chemical treatments for sturdier materials like wood framing. This approach ensures effective mold removal while maintaining the structural integrity of materials and is particularly important for individuals with sensitivities. Throughout the work, measures should be in place to limit the release of contamination, bagging, and disposal of contaminated materials while adhering to medically important remediation practices. Prioritizing physical removal using HEPA-filtered negative air and local exhaust ventilation while abrasive cleaning ensures thorough decontamination of affected areas, safeguarding a healthy environment post-remediation.

Exercise 11.1: Controlled Removal—Avoid "Bash and Trash" Techniques

❏ To effectively remove and dispose of contaminated materials while minimizing contaminants' release.

› **Safe Work Practices**: All workers should wear appropriate personal protective equipment. This not only protects the workers, as required by OSHA but also protects the worksite, which is your home. Workers concerned with Medically Important Remediation are not doing it merely to protect themselves.

› **Work Within Containment Areas:** Containment with HEPA-filtered negative air equipment creates negative pressure, which helps facilitate maintaining the contained environment and keeps airborne contaminants from migrating outside the work zone.

› **Controlled Demolition Approach:** By Using precise removal techniques and avoiding forceful demolition ("bash and trash"), the release and spread of high quantities of mold spores and fragments can be avoided. Careful cutting and control methods, such as employing a razor knife for small areas, can minimize dust production. A Kett™ saw, specially designed for removing gypsum board and simultaneously controlling dust using a HEPA vacuum attachment, is a great way to control dust production for larger jobs. The Kett™ sawblade can be adjusted to match the thickness of the gypsum, allowing any dust generated to be vacuumed up by an attached HEPA vacuum as the cuts are made. This approach removes pieces in manageable segments, minimizing dust and contamination.

› **Handle Hazardous Materials Properly:** If materials contain lead-based paint or asbestos, ensure that all work complies with local, state, and federal regulations. OSHA cites employers if their rules are not followed. If you hire workers directly, you could be cited as an employer and face steep fines if you allow the people working for you to violate these laws.

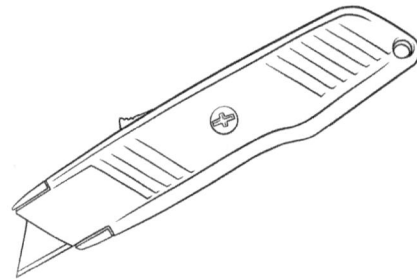

Figure 5-61: When used within the capture zone of a HEPA vacuum, a razor knife is an inexpensive cutting tool that is good for removing small or limited areas of gypsum wallboard.

Exercise 11.2: Safe Removal Techniques for Various Materials

❏ Applying the correct removal methods for each type of material helps ensures contaminants are removed without causing further damage.

› **Bag and Seal Materials:** As soft, porous materials like gypsum board and insulation are removed, they should be placed directly into heavy-duty plastic bags. Each loaded bag should then be double-bagged, and the outside of the bag should be cleaned before being transported out of the work area and through your home for disposal. It is preferable that the bags be loaded from the work area directly to the outside, such as by passing them out of a window. The bags should never be dragged or handled roughly so they do not rupture.

› **For Semi-Porous Materials**: Wood framing and sturdier materials are usually not removed but will require cleaning. If visible mold growth is present on the surface of the wood, then abrasive cleaning, such as wire brushing or sanding, while simultaneously HEPA vacuuming is recommended to remove the surface mold. Work cautiously to preserve the integrity of the material.

› **All Tools and Equipment Should Be Cleaned After Use:** HEPA vacuums should be used to remove any remaining dust and debris from tools. This is followed by damp wiping with the same mild, non-toxic cleaning solution used to clean the building to eliminate residues. If tools are not cleaned before being removed from your home, they should be double-bagged, and the outside of the bag should be cleaned before transporting them through your home.

› **Debris Disposal:** Moldy construction debris should be disposed of following local, state, and federal requirements. Most municipalities allow moldy debris to be disposed of in regular landfills and household waste facilities. Landfills are like retirement communities for mold. Landfills always have high mold levels, so adding more should not be problematic. However, some facilities do not accept construction waste. In addition, only waste disposal facilities licensed and approved for asbestos and lead disposal can handle these hazardous wastes. Understanding your local requirements

for hazardous waste disposal is essential. If asbestos or lead-containing debris is improperly sent to a disposal facility not licensed for that type of waste, you, as the waste owner, can be held legally responsible for the cleanup costs. If the waste originates from your home, you retain ownership—and responsibility—for it indefinitely.

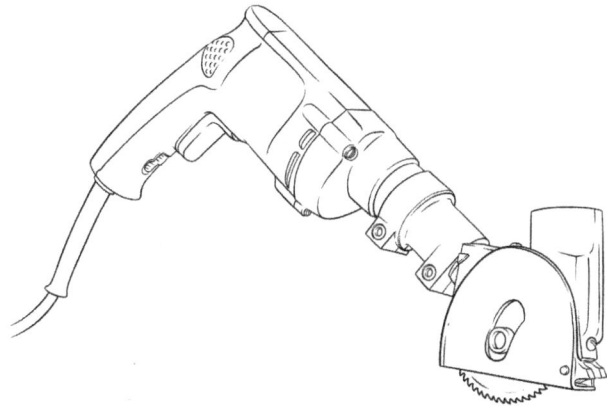

Figure 5-62: When connected to a HEPA vacuum, a Kett saw is a precision cutting tool ideal for removing sections of gypsum board with minimal dust generation. Its compact design allows for controlled, clean cuts, making it especially useful in mold remediation and other applications where dust containment is necessary. Paired with a HEPA vacuum, the Kett saw helps maintain a clean work environment by capturing fine particulates at the source, reducing airborne contamination, and protecting indoor air quality.

Aggressive Abrasive Cleaning of Wood Framing and Structurally Engineered Wood Panels

Aggressive abrasive cleaning plays a crucial role in the remediation of water-damaged buildings, especially for wood framing and engineered wood, such as plywood panels that exhibit water or other types of stains and are not being physically removed from the building. This process typically involves using a HEPA-filtered vacuum-assisted random orbital sander or HEPA vacuuming while using a wire brush or synthetic abrasive scrubbing pads, depending on the nature and severity of the staining.

1. HEPA Filtered Vacuum-Assisted Random Orbital Sander: This tool effectively removes surface-level stains and minor mold growth from wood. Random orbital motion ensures a more uniform abrasion, reducing the wood's risk of damage. The integrated HEPA vacuum feature captures fine dust and mold particles, preventing them from becoming airborne and contaminating the work environment. This method is particularly suitable for larger surfaces and where a smoother finish facilitates the desired cleaning that follows. Typically, the amount of wood removed is no more than 100 microns per sanded surface (the approximate thickness of a dollar bill).

2. Wire Brush Cleaning: A wire brush may be employed for more ingrained stains or heavier mold infestations. This tool provides a more aggressive abrasive action capable of penetrating deeper into the wood's surface. While highly effective, it's essential to use the wire brush judiciously to avoid unnecessary damage to the wood.

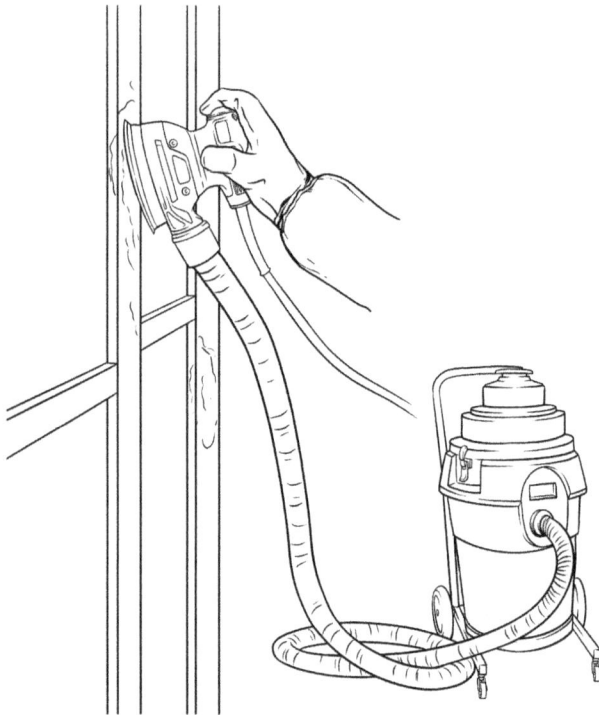

Figure 5-63: Random Orbital Sander with HEPA vacuum attachment.

Workers should wear appropriate personal protective equipment (PPE) to satisfy the employer's State and Federal OSHA requirements. Consider safeguarding against noise levels exceeding 85 decibels and inhaling particulates should be considered.

1. The aggressive abrasive cleaning should be performed systematically, ensuring all affected areas are adequately addressed.

2. After cleaning, the area should be re-inspected to ensure all contamination has been adequately removed. The water stains may have penetrated more deeply than the contamination, so some staining may remain after this step.

3. The wood surfaces should be vacuumed with a HEPA-filtered vacuum during and after the process to control and remove any residual dust and particles.

4. Finally, the abrasively cleaned wood should be moisture tested and allowed to dry completely before any reconstruction or further remediation work.

This aggressive abrasive cleaning method effectively restores wood framing and plywood panels impacted by water damage, ensuring they are clean, free of contaminants, and ready for further restoration.

DRY ICE BLASTING FOR MOLD AND WATER DAMAGE REMEDIATION

Dry ice blasting is a cleaning method that uses compressed air to propel small pellets of solid carbon dioxide (dry ice) at high speed onto contaminated surfaces. The process effectively dislodges mold, soot, and other residues while the dry ice sublimates (transforms from a solid to a gas), leaving no secondary waste. This method is primarily used in mold and water damage remediation for large-scale or severe contamination issues, particularly when adequate ventilation is available. It is rarely cost-effective for small to moderate projects due to its high equipment and operational costs. Moreover, the high-pressure air stream can cause significant cross-contamination to adjacent areas if adequate engineering controls, such as containment barriers and negative air systems, are not implemented. Due to these risks and the potential for asphyxiation if carbon dioxide displaces oxygen and builds up in enclosed spaces, dry ice blasting should only be conducted by trained professionals equipped with the necessary safety measures.

Step 12: Special Attention to HVAC Systems or Air Conveyance Systems

Refining Air Quality through HVAC Care

In medically necessary remediation, Step 12 focuses on thoroughly inspecting and cleaning HVAC systems and ductwork to ensure improved indoor air quality, particularly for sensitive individuals. Using mechanical and chemical-free methods, the objective is to carefully address mold and contaminants in HVAC components, such as cooling coils, ductwork, and other system parts.

HVAC system cleaning involves special protocols, including containment and HEPA-filtered airflow, to capture contaminants during cleaning and prevent their spread. Mechanical cleaning methods like specialized brushes, HEPA vacuuming, and controlled ventilation are emphasized over chemical cleaning agents, which are unsuitable for sensitive individuals. The goal is not just to remove mold but to eliminate particles that can still impact health if left in the system. Additionally, post-cleaning Pathways™ surface sampling serves as evaluation metrics, ensuring that the system is effectively cleaned and maintained to prevent future growth.

Exercise 12.1: Self-Evaluation Checklist for HVAC Ducts and Systems

Use this checklist to inspect your HVAC system and ducts for any visible signs of contamination or issues that may impact indoor air quality. The following inspection of the visible components does not prove that the hidden components are contaminated, but a visual inspection can indicate the system's condition.

❏ **Visible Mold, Moisture, Condensation or Discoloration:**

› Inspect the accessible parts of your HVAC system (ducts, vents, and registers) for visible mold, dark spots, or unusual discoloration. Mold growth may appear in clusters or as patches on interior surfaces. It is especially likely and problematic when ducts have loose fibrous insulation, which collects dirt and serves as a growth site when damp with condensation.

› A particular concern exists when the system was constructed without return air ducting using the building's wall cavities as the return airflow path. This frequently results in wall cavities filling with spore-containing dust, which is practically impossible to clean.

› Visible mold/discoloration on vents, registers, or the ceiling immediately adjacent to them is usually a sign of condensation moisture resulting in growth. It indicates elevated room humidity levels or the system running too cold. This is frequently due to conditions such as an undersized cold air return, an oversized system, or anything restricting airflow, such as dirty filters or furniture partially blocking the cold air return.

❏ **Unusual Odors:**

› Run your HVAC system and note any musty, moldy, or otherwise unusual odors from the vents. Persistent odors can indicate mold or microbial growth within the system or ductwork.

› A musty/moldy odor detected when the HVAC system is running indicates that some surfaces inside the system remain wet. Resist the sales pressure to install UV, ozone, or photocatalytic air filtration systems inside HVAC systems or ductwork. Unusual odors indicate something is going wrong and must be addressed appropriately. Attempting to put your system on life support using expensive treatments can cover up the real issue and result in more significant health problems developing and more costly system replacement costs. It is always essential to determine the source of the issues when they are noted and not just cover them up.

❏ **Accumulated Dust or Debris at Vents:**

› Look at the registers and vent cover for any visible dust buildup or debris. Excessive accumulation can indicate a need for cleaning and may reduce air quality. However, it may also indicate duct leakage, which allows dust infiltration or improper or dirty filters.

❏ **Leaking or Blocked Condensate Pans and Drains:**

› Examine the condensation collection pan and drain lines for any signs of blockages or leaks. All AC systems have a hidden internal condensation pan. Some systems have a visible secondary backup collection pan underneath them. If the secondary pan ever accumulates water, it indicates that the internal collection and drainage system is malfunctioning. Blocked drains can lead to water accumulation and mold growth.

› Battery and hardwired alarm systems can be installed inside the secondary condensate pan. They should be inspected frequently to ensure proper operation. Battery-operated warning systems should have their batteries regularly changed. Plan on doing this every year when you service and change your smoke and carbon monoxide detector batteries.

❑ **Airflow Issues or Hot/Cold Spots:**

› While the system is running, move through different rooms and note any inconsistent airflow temperature variations or changes in operation, as these may indicate issues with ductwork or blockages.

› Regular filter changes are essential because they can help keep the system clean and because clogged filters will result in airflow issues. Restricted airflow can result in system damage and mold growth due to the formation of condensation moisture. MERV 11 to 13 filters are typically adequate for most systems but must be changed when they fill with dirt, or they will restrict airflow. Blocked airflow can damage the system, leading to inadequate airflow, which can lead to condensation and mold growth. System filters are primarily present to help protect the system. They cannot provide uniformly pure air throughout a home. Portable air purification units with HEPA are a better choice. They are portable, easier to clean and maintain, and less expensive to operate. Always remember that clean floors and horizontal surfaces are much better room air purifiers than any filtration system.>

Essay: *Discussion of Air Purification Technologies*
by Michael Schrantz and John Banta

John: One of the most common questions I receive is about using air purification to resolve building mold problems. I'd like you to meet my friend and colleague, Michael Schrantz. Michael and I have spent countless hours discussing ways to tackle mold and improve indoor air quality, especially regarding Photocatalytic Oxidation (PCO) air purifiers. (Zeng, 2021) We don't always agree on everything, but we share the same goal: helping you create a healthier home. Recognizing that there's no one-size-fits-all answer to this issue, we've decided to share our thoughts. We hope to provide you with a well-rounded perspective so you can make the best decision for your situation.

Michael: Thank you, John, for the introduction and for inviting me into this important conversation. First off, I'd like to echo your sentiment that our goal here is to help people create healthier indoor environments. I believe that what unites us is our commitment to empowering people with the information they need to protect their health and well-being in a pragmatic way.

So, let's dive in: Our primary focus here is regarding the use of the purification technology: Photocatalytic Oxidation (PCO) technology. PCO air purifiers have certainly garnered attention as a means of improving indoor air quality, and the science behind them is fascinating. In essence, PCO works by using ultraviolet light to activate a catalyst, which then converts humidity (moisture) into hydroxyl radicals. These oxidizing radicals break down chemical compounds and biological contaminants that come into contact with the coated target surface. The lifespan of a hydroxyl radical is short—milliseconds—meaning most of the reaction occurs on the surface of the catalyst target. While PCO has been used in multiple industries (e.g., water treatment and air purification), the reality of using PCO in our field has prompted me to pause.

We need to be careful not to add another layer of risk when trying to mitigate an existing one.

Understanding PCO (purification technology) vs HEPA (filtration technology)

It's important to recognize that purification technologies like PCO and filtration technologies like HEPA serve different purposes. HEPA filtration is excellent for removing particulate matter, especially smaller particles, and is considered a safe and proven method of reducing smaller particle concentrations in the air. Purification technologies like PCO aim to break down chemical compounds (versus physical removal like the case of HEPA (particles) and carbon (chemical) filters) but don't have the same level of research (in field application). Thus, it is more difficult to say that all related purification technologies have been "proven safe." In short, a combination of HEPA filtration and other purification technologies may offer a superior improvement or their use separately; however, it should not be automatically assumed that all purification technologies are "safe" or reasonable to use in your unique situation.

My main concern lies in the potential byproducts these devices can generate. While PCO units are meant to break down pollutants, they don't always do so completely or consistently, which means there's potential for producing secondary byproducts—some of which can be harmful—that could be released into the air. For instance, certain oxidizing agents and intermediate compounds can form, potentially contributing to new indoor air quality issues. An example of this is the production of formaldehyde and acetaldehyde in certain environments. The complexity of how PCO interacts with the varied mix of chemicals in our homes makes the technology less predictable than one might hope. This is a concern when working with clients suffering from various forms of chronic illness or low-dose environmental exposure concerns. That's why I am encouraged by companies that have moved beyond PCO to develop more effective ways to treat the air.

After years of experience with PCO, some manufacturers have recognized the limitations and potential issues associated with it and have chosen to focus on safer, more reliable technologies that can deliver better outcomes without relying on PCO. As discussed above, these companies now utilize technologies such as HEPA filtration, activated carbon, ultraviolet light, and bipolar ionization, which are designed to provide effective air filtration and purification without the concerns associated with PCO. HEPA filtration is highly efficient at removing particulate matter; activated carbon excels at adsorbing volatile organic compounds (VOCs) and odors.

Ultraviolet light works by generating a certain wavelength (`200–280 nm) of light that can inactivate ("kill") microorganisms by damaging their DNA or RNA and preventing them from replicating. Bipolar ionization works by generating positive and negative ions that help reduce airborne pollutants in a safer and more controlled manner. There are concerns, however, regarding the extent of the claims made by companies that utilize these technologies and whether they "work as marketed." My personal experience is also that it's not just "what" the technology that is being utilized is, but "how" it is being utilized (e.g., how it is being designed and installed in devices and operated in buildings). Another fair question to ask would be this: If the technologies being marketed "don't" produce the level of performance stated, are they still beneficial to the public or some of the public? Forward-thinking companies making this technology should be held accountable for performing third-party testing to validate their claims and address concerns like the production of by-products and exposure to the technology (e.g., PCO, bipolar ionization, UV) itself before making it available to the public. Regardless of the technology, I always recommend a responsible approach for each client, helping weigh the potential risks versus benefits of their unique situation. It truly is a case-by-case situation.

At the end of the day, my perspective on PCO technology is shaped by the principle of "first, do no harm." I want to help ensure that any solution I recommend truly benefits my clients without introducing unintended consequences. And, while PCO might play a role in certain specialized applications, I think it's important to have a clear understanding of its claimed benefits and concerns, especially when we're talking about something as fundamental as the air we breathe.

Check out this technical summary on residential portable air cleaners written by the EPA (focus on the section titled, "Byproduct emissions From Some Air Cleaner *Technologies*"):

www.epa.gov/sites/default/files/2018-07/documents/residential_air_cleaners_-_a_technical_summary_3rd_edition.pdf

The Importance of Dust Cleaning

Another crucial aspect of maintaining indoor environmental quality is regular dust cleaning. Dust can harbor a variety of pollutants, including allergens, microbes, and chemical contaminants, which can affect both air and surface quality. Routine dust removal reduces the load of these pollutants, preventing them from becoming airborne and being inhaled. By combining effective cleaning of the air with consistent surface dust cleaning practices, we can significantly improve the overall indoor environment. Clean air and surfaces not only contribute to better respiratory health but also enhance comfort and well-being within indoor spaces.

Another issue I often see is the misconception that air purification alone can replace source control and remediation when it comes to mold or bacteria (microbes). Microbial problems are fundamentally a moisture issue—and while cleaning the air (and surfaces) might help reduce airborne contaminants temporarily, it does nothing to address the root cause. Without removing moisture and properly remediating the affected materials, you're essentially treating a symptom without tackling the illness itself. In the context of environmentally produced exposures, true microbial remediation means identifying and correcting water issues, removing contaminated materials, and ensuring the environment is stable and dry.

In conclusion, creating a healthier indoor environment involves a multifaceted approach. While advanced air purification technologies have their place, they should be complemented by basic practices like regular dust cleaning and addressing sources of contaminants. By integrating these strategies, we can achieve a more comprehensive improvement in indoor environmental quality.

John: Thank you, Michael. As I suspected, you and I do substantially agree, and I consider it likely that our differences are often more a matter of subtle degree than significant substance. I do have some points I want to make or reiterate. While many people report feeling better when using specific air purification systems, it's essential to consider that some beneficial effects may be temporary or influenced by placebo or masking effects. This temporary relief might provide a false sense of security, leading occupants to believe that the underlying issues are resolved when, in fact, the sources of contaminants are still affecting the building and indoor environment.

Even if one recognizes that the building conditions remain suboptimal, it's crucial to know that every indoor air quality situation is unique. There are numerous potential adverse reactions that can occur due to unknown substances present in the environment, including hundreds of thousands of potential chemicals that have not been thoroughly studied in this context. Essentially, using air purifiers without addressing the root causes can be likened to "robbing Peter to pay Paul"—solving one problem while potentially creating another.

Moreover, if someone doesn't feel well when a unit is running but feels better when it's turned off, they should take heed of this response. I've encountered many situations where clients have been advised that if they sense the problem is worsening, they should use the unit more frequently or at higher settings. This approach can be dangerous, as it may exacerbate the issue rather than resolve it.

It's also important to understand the dangers of masking. Masking occurs when an air purification system temporarily reduces the perception of contaminants without eliminating them at their source. This can lead to prolonged exposure to harmful substances, potentially worsening health outcomes over time. Relying solely on any air purifier may delay necessary interventions, allowing the underlying problems to grow and become more expensive to fix, possibly causing significant damage to the structure. I am also concerned that the use of systems may mask or inhibit the detection of the problem sources when trying to discover them to perform effective remediation.

In summary, while air purification technologies might offer temporary relief, they should not replace comprehensive solutions that address the root causes of indoor air quality issues. Remediation and cleaning are the primary tools to effectively return buildings to a healthy condition. It's essential to approach each situation thoughtfully, consider the potential risks and benefits, and prioritize strategies that ensure a healthy and safe environment.

Exercise 12.2: Evaluating Flex Ducts for Cleaning

This exercise will help you assess the condition of flex ductwork and decide between cleaning or replacement based on the level of contamination, material condition, and potential risks to indoor air quality. This evaluation ensures the ductwork meets health-focused standards for those with chemical or mold sensitivities.

❏ **Inspect Flex Ducts:**

› Begin by thoroughly inspecting the flex ductwork for physical damage, including tears, cracks, or signs of wear that could compromise air quality and duct integrity. Look for signs of extensive contamination, such as visible mold growth, heavy dust accumulation, or odors that indicate microbial growth.

› Move through accessible areas of the ductwork and assess each section. Flex duct is more delicate than metal ductwork and may be prone to damage, so handle it carefully during inspection. If contamination is visible on the duct's surface or if sections feel brittle, consider these areas for replacement.

❏ **Cleaning Options:**

› If the flex ducts are in generally good condition but have some contamination, they may be suitable for cleaning rather than replacement. Mechanical cleaning methods, like soft-bristle brushing and low-pressure HEPA vacuuming, are effective for flex ductwork because they avoid using chemicals that can exacerbate sensitivities. Manual cleaning using disposable microfiber cloths avoids the need for expensive equipment and is gentler and less likely to damage ductwork.

› The mechanical process uses soft-bristle brushes to dislodge contaminants gently, being cautious not to tear or damage the duct's flexible material. A low-pressure HEPA vacuum should follow brushing to capture dislodged particles. The HEPA vacuum's filtration helps prevent particles from being released into the air, an essential step for maintaining indoor air quality. Duct cameras can inspect and evaluate the cleaning as it occurs.

› When flex ductwork is accessible, such as in an attic or crawlspace, it can be manually cleaned by disconnecting one end from the metal plenum collar, allowing the duct to be telescoped for easier access along its entire length. The interior is then HEPA vacuumed using a soft-bristle attachment to safely remove dust, mold, and other contaminants without damaging the flexible material. After vacuuming, a dampened disposable microfiber cloth is used to hand-clean the interior, ensuring a more thorough removal of residual particles. A mild detergent solution (Branch Basics, All Purpose Detergent, five drops in a quart of water) is applied to the cloth for effective, chemical-free cleaning. This process also allows direct access to the plenum boxes and other components, which are vacuumed and wiped clean. Finally, the duct is reconnected securely to the plenum, completing a careful, non-toxic cleaning of the flex ductwork to improve indoor air quality. While this is occurring, it's also an excellent time to inspect and seal plenum boxes, collars, and other components to prevent leaks or the drawing in of contaminants that bypass the filter.

› When a flex duct is inaccessible for telescoping, such as running through a wall cavity or a tight space, it can still be cleaned effectively if both ends are accessible. Begin fishing a heavy-duty washable cord through the duct to a helper on the opposite end. Flexible fiberglass rods, typically used for cleaning dryer ducts, can be connected in short sections to help guide the cord through the ductwork. Once the cord has been fished through, securely tie an appropriately sized bundle of dry disposable microfiber cloths at the cord's midpoint (Using damp microfibers at this point makes mud, so use them dry). Pull the cord back and forth using a coordinated sawing motion, passing the microfiber bundle along the duct's interior to wipe down the surfaces effectively. Start with dry microfiber bundles to remove the bulk of the dust and debris. During this initial phase, a HEPA vacuum can clean the microfiber bundle between passes, allowing it to be reused until the bulk of debris is removed without creating mud.

> After the initial dry wiping, switch to slightly dampened microfiber bundles using the 5-drop detergent solution in a spritzer bottle. These dampened bundles will provide a final, detailed cleaning. Replace the microfiber bundle as it fills with dirt, and repeat the process until a fresh bundle comes out clean after passing through the section. This method allows for effective, non-toxic cleaning of hard-to-reach duct sections, thoroughly capturing dust, mold, and other contaminants while maintaining air quality and avoiding cross-contamination.

> For shorter duct lengths, the flexible rods can be attached to the microfiber bundle and used to "ramrod" clean the duct by pushing the bundle through.

Exercise 12.3: Evaluating Flex Ducts for Replacing

❏ In cases where contamination is extensive, or the flex ducts are old or brittle, replacement may be the safer and more effective option. Flex ductwork is typically more affordable than metal ducting, making replacement a practical choice when contamination is severe or the duct material is deteriorating.

❏ Identify duct sections with heavy contamination, stubborn odors, or visible mold that cleaning alone may not fully address. For older ductwork, replacement ensures that new ducts start free from contaminants, supporting a cleaner indoor environment. Remember that any metal connections, such as connectors or boots, should be thoroughly cleaned or replaced to avoid cross-contamination with the new ductwork.

❏ Evaluate the cost-effectiveness of cleaning versus replacement and decide on replacement if contamination is severe or duct condition is poor.

Exercise 12.4: Post-Cleaning Evaluation

After cleaning, a thorough evaluation is performed to verify that the ductwork has been effectively cleaned. This step ensures that all parts meet acceptable standards for indoor air quality, particularly in homes with sensitive individuals.

Use a camera, manual inspection, or Pathways™ testing to confirm the cleanliness of the cleaned flex duct sections. Camera inspections can reveal any remaining contaminants in hard-to-reach areas, while manual inspections help verify that visible mold and dust have been removed.

Pathways™ surface sampling can provide an objective measure of cleanliness by measuring peptide bonds and proteins as an indicator of contaminant levels.

❏ **Visual Inspection:**

> A thorough visual inspection after cleaning complements surface sampling by directly assessing cleanliness, particularly in hard-to-reach areas that may be difficult to test with sampling alone. This inspection ensures that all visible mold, dust, and debris have been physically removed from the HVAC system's components.

> After cleaning, use a flashlight and mirror or camera with a flexible extension to inspect the interior surfaces of the ducts, coils, fan blades, and other HVAC components. Look for any remaining visible mold, dust, or debris, paying close attention to corners, seams, and other hidden areas where contaminants may still reside. Note any areas that appear insufficiently cleaned and require additional attention.

> After cleaning, the HVAC system should be free of visible contamination. Additional cleaning should be considered to ensure the system meets acceptable standards if mold or debris is observed. Visual inspection is particularly valuable for spotting potential problem areas that might need further cleaning or verifying the thoroughness of previously cleaned sections.

❏ **Pathways™ Surface Sampling:**

> Surface sampling using the Pathways™ method before and after cleaning provides a scientific basis for evaluating mold and contaminant levels on HVAC surfaces. Pre-cleaning samples establish baseline contamination levels, while post-cleaning samples verify that cleaning effectively reduces contaminants to acceptable levels.

> Begin by selecting a representative set of sampling locations within the HVAC system, such as the duct interior, cooling coils, fan components, and areas with visible contamination. Using the Pathways™ surface sampling kit, carefully collect samples from each location before cleaning begins, following the kit's instructions to ensure accurate results. After cleaning, return to the same locations to collect post-cleaning samples for comparison.

> Compare the pre- and post-cleaning sampling results to assess reductions in contaminants. Significant reductions in mold, bacteria, or particulate matter between pre- and post-cleaning samples indicate successful cleaning. Any remaining high levels of pollutants may suggest that further cleaning or additional intervention is needed.

NADCA-ACR 2021: The Standard of Care for Mold and Water Damage in Ducts

The National Air Duct Cleaners Association (NADCA) released the latest edition of their standard, "NADCA-ACR 2021; The NADCA Standard for Assessment, Cleaning, and Restoration of HVAC Systems." This standard is the benchmark for best practices in HVAC cleaning and restoration, providing comprehensive guidelines for residential and commercial duct cleaning.

Adherence to NADCA-ACR 2021 ensures that cleaning and restoration are performed effectively and safely, particularly in mold and water damage cases. For optimal results, it is recommended that duct and system cleaning be conducted without antimicrobials or chemicals by a NADCA-certified firm, following the specifications outlined in this standard. Following NADCA-ACR 2021 offers confidence that work is completed with the highest standards of care, supporting indoor air and system integrity.

Using a Particle Counter for Evaluation

A particle counter is an excellent way to confirm when duct and system cleaning is complete. Pre-cleaning and post-cleaning air samples can be used to verify the reduction of contaminants in the system and ducts.

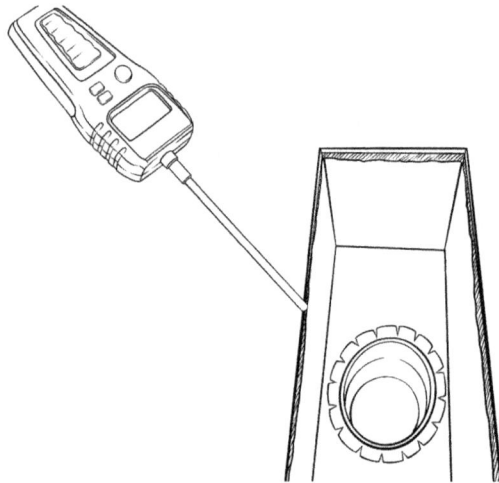

Figure 5-64: Measuring particle counts from cracks or openings around the HVAC supply register can indicate particles passing from the crawlspace or basement below into the living space.

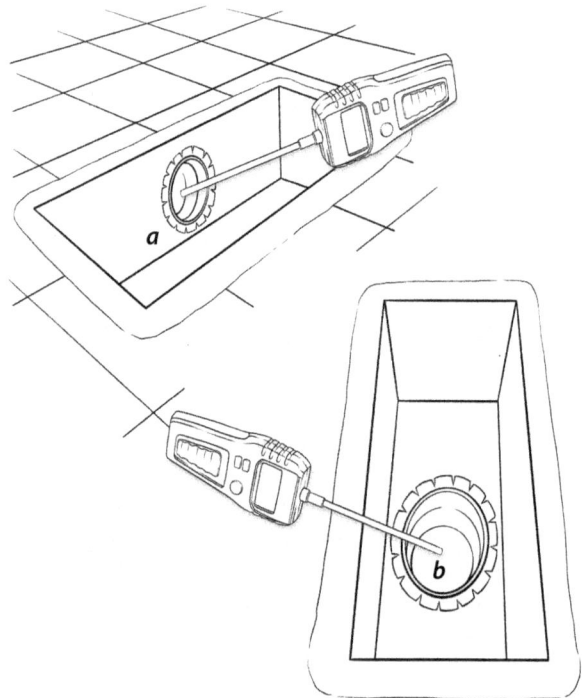

*Figure 5-65: Ductwork entering from (**a**) a few inches higher up the side prevents dirt and contaminants from (**b**) falling deeply into the ductwork and makes cleaning the recess with a HEPA vacuum cleaner easy. This illustration also shows how particle counts inside the ductwork are measured. This measurement can indicate the particles being transported through the system.*

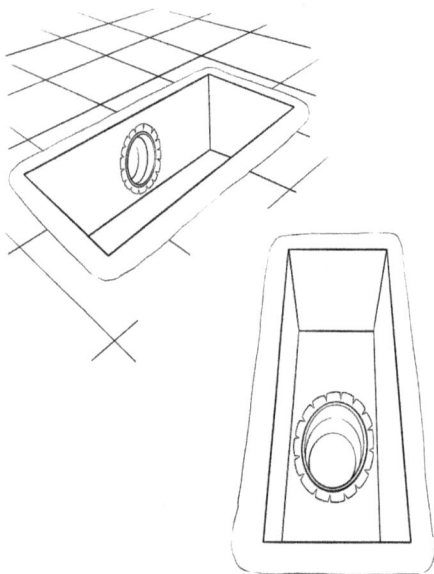

Figure 5-66: Sealing the penetrations with foil tape or mastic can help prevent contaminants from infiltrating from the crawlspace or basement below into the living space.

Step 13: Special Attention to Enclosed Spaces

Prioritizing Special Attention in basements, crawlspaces, and attics

In medically important remediation, it is essential to address mold in enclosed or difficult-to-access spaces such as unfinished basements, crawlspaces, and attics due to their high propensity for mold growth. These spaces often experience limited airflow, higher humidity, and temperature fluctuations, leading to mold spreading into other parts of the home. Additionally, enclosed spaces frequently harbor immediate dangers to life and health (IDLH) due to hazardous conditions, making specialized training and personal protective equipment (PPE) essential for safe entry.

Step 13 focuses on effective inspection and remediation strategies for these often overlooked areas and preventive measures like protective soil membranes, ventilation, and humidity control. These efforts are significant for maintaining indoor air quality in homes where occupants have heightened sensitivities.

In addition to these hazards, contractors who leave materials like cardboard sheets in crawlspaces are often negligent. Left behind, these materials can collect moisture and grow mold, complicating remediation. Step 13 emphasizes thorough safety and remediation practices to ensure a healthy environment, especially for sensitive individuals.

Enclosed spaces, such as attics, crawlspaces, and unfinished basements, often pose significant challenges in the context of medically necessary remediation. Due to their unique propensity for mold growth, higher humidity, and poor airflow, these spaces can significantly impact indoor air quality. For sensitive individuals, however, entering these spaces can introduce serious health risks. The hazards present—including exposure to mold, dust, and potentially toxic or contaminated materials—can worsen symptoms for those with chemical or mold sensitivities, not to mention the physical risks associated with accessing these confined spaces.

While addressing the conditions in these areas as part of a comprehensive remediation plan is essential, this step will not attempt to provide detailed, hands-on instructions for assessing and remediating them. Instead, key considerations and resources are provided to help readers understand the issues and engage trained professionals who can address these spaces safely and effectively.

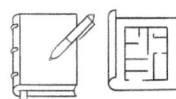

Exercise 13.1: Key Issues in Enclosed Spaces to Address with a Professional

❏ **Mold Growth Due to High Humidity and Limited Ventilation**: Mold thrives in areas with inadequate airflow and moisture management, which are common characteristics of enclosed spaces.

❏ **Standing Water or Flooding**: Enclosed areas, especially basements, are prone to flooding, which can lead to mold growth and structural damage if not properly addressed.

❏ **Insulation and Vapor Barrier Issues**: Old or improperly installed insulation can trap moisture, encouraging mold growth; vapor barriers may need to be added or repaired to mitigate moisture.

❏ **Contaminants Left by Previous Occupants:** Leftover materials or contaminants (e.g., hazardous waste, debris from drug labs, or sewage contamination) require specialized cleanup methods.

❏ **Asbestos and Lead Hazards in Older Homes**: These materials, if present, require professional removal due to serious health risks, particularly when disturbed.

❏ **Structural Integrity Concerns**: Issues like weakened beams or floor joists from previous water damage can make enclosed spaces hazardous to navigate.

❏ **Pest Contamination:** Animal droppings or nests left by rodents or insects can carry pathogens and need safe, professional cleanup.

Essay: Attics

by Bill Weber

"Don't fall through the ceiling, don't fall through the ceiling, don't fall through the ceiling"—a mantra that those inspecting unfinished attics often repeat to themselves. Inspecting attics is just as important as inspecting crawlspaces and interstitial cavities. Whether finished, unfinished, or "inaccessible," the area between the ceiling of the uppermost level and the underside of the roof is a gathering place or accumulation point for the air and airborne particulates that drift or are drawn to the uppermost part of the building. Although there is a plethora of discussion topics related to unfinished attic spaces (and their inhospitable environment), finished attics, and other types of construction for the uppermost areas of the building, there are some basic concepts and places of interest that are key to every attic.

The stack effect is a natural phenomenon that occurs when there are temperature differences between the interior of the building and the exterior. The difference in temperature results in air movement. If it is colder outside, the warm air will rise and exit through the upper parts of the building, drawing in air from the outside through the lower areas of the building (think an open window, crawlspace, and even small openings in the building envelope).

Reverse stack effect generally occurs when it is [significantly] warmer outside and cooler inside. The cooler air sinks to the lowest levels of the home and creates a low-pressure area in the uppermost part of the house, drawing air from the outside into the attic and, eventually, the living space and crawlspace.

Pathways from the crawlspace to the living space and the living space to the attic (and vice versa) differ in size, but they all contribute to the quality of the air inside your home. This is why attention needs to be given to all areas of the building envelope. When there is a significant water damage condition in one area, it can impact all areas of the building.

Inspection of the attic should be included during every home assessment. Due to the numerous potential hazards (exposed nail tips, potential slip/trip/fall, enclosed and hard to get to areas), a qualified indoor environmental professional should be utilized when investigating a potential mold condition. During that inspection, items of interest would include:

Ventilation of the attics: Some attics in the country are finished and used as living areas; others are non-living spaces but sealed and even conditioned or mechanically ventilated;

most attics are unconditioned spaces. When an attic is designed for natural ventilation and has a sloped roof, proper air intake and exhaust are required to maintain airflow. Eave vents, soffit vents, or low-profile shingle vents must remain unobstructed to allow fresh air to enter. Blockages caused by insulation, paint, or construction oversights can significantly hinder airflow. Similarly, the attic air must have an escape route, which can be provided through gable vents, ridge vents, or other ventilation options. Adequate ventilation is essential to prevent moisture accumulation, as excess moisture in the attic can create conditions that support mold growth.

Watertightness of the roof, especially at penetrations. The weakest point for physical water entry is at penetrations like vent pipes, exhaust fans, and chimneys. If water has entered through these openings, there will be evidence of staining or discoloration on the underside of the roof (the roof deck) at or below the penetration, on the pipe, duct, or chimney, and or the insulation and wallboard beneath the leak, supporting mold growth.

Rodents, insects, and even birds like it where it is warm, safe from predators, and where there is a food source. Unfinished attics offer the opportunity for bedding in the insulation, conditioned air in the ductwork, and access to the exterior. But sometimes, they leave a mess, and that mess can support mold and bacteria proliferation.

Leaking HVAC components. Many attics house an air handler and or ductwork. Gaps or openings within these components can allow the unintended consequences of pressurizations and energy loss and can have a direct effect on the interior air quality. Air handlers also have condensate pans, drainpipes, and even pumps to capture and remove excess moisture accumulation. When these components become clogged, sloped incorrectly, or just stop working, the excess moisture can support fungal and bacteria amplification.

Attics are an overlooked part of the building. Difficulty in access, hazards, and extreme temperatures make the attic one of the least inspected areas of the building. That's why thorough and routine inspections are so important—the health of the attic has a direct impact on the health of the living space.

Exercise 13.2: Resources for Addressing Enclosed Space Safety Issues

❑ **American Industrial Hygiene Association (AIHA)**
Website: aiha.org
AIHA provides resources for identifying qualified industrial hygienists and other professionals specializing in indoor environmental quality, hazardous material handling, and mold remediation.

❑ **Occupational Safety and Health Administration (OSHA)**
Website: osha.gov
OSHA offers standards and guidelines for confined spaces and hazardous material handling, which is useful when assessing contractors' adherence to safety standards.

❑ **Environmental Protection Agency (EPA)—Mold and Moisture**
Website: epa.gov/mold
The EPA offers general guidance on mold remediation and indoor air quality, including information on handling mold in hard-to-reach spaces.

❑ **Institute of Inspection, Cleaning and Restoration Certification (IICRC)**
Website: iicrc.org
The IICRC offers certification programs and standards (like the IICRC S520) for mold remediation for the general population. IICRC offers continuing education credit for technician training in Medically Important Remediation through CIRSx.com, offering specialized training for remediators in methods suitable for sensitive individuals.

❑ **National Air Duct Cleaners Association (NADCA) Standards**
Website: nadca.com
NADCA provides guidelines on HVAC system cleaning, which includes ductwork in enclosed spaces. Certified professionals follow the ACR 2021 standard, which is especially important in spaces where ducting may be contaminated.

Exerciese 13.3: Resources for Crawlspace Design, Insulation, and Moisture Control

❑ **The following organizations provide research-based recommendations** and resources that can help homeowners and professionals address crawlspace concerns safely and effectively.

› **Building Science Corporation**
Website: buildingscience.com
Building Science Corporation, a research-based nonprofit, offers resources on crawlspace design, insulation, and moisture control. They advocate for closed crawlspaces with dehumidification or mechanical ventilation to improve air quality and reduce mold risks. They recommend using a continuous polyethylene barrier over the crawlspace soil to reduce moisture and radon infiltration, along with proper sealing and taping around foundation walls and piers.

› **National Center for Healthy Housing (NCHH)**
Website: nchh.org
NCHH provides recommendations for managing moisture and improving indoor air quality in crawlspaces as part of their focus on healthy housing. They highlight strategies like vapor barriers, proper drainage, and air sealing to prevent contamination in crawlspaces.

Exercise: 13.4:Guidelines for Crawlspace Soil Barrier Installation

❑ For crawlspace soil barrier installation, the following organizations provide recommendations and guidelines:

› **The U.S. Department of Energy (DOE)**
Website: energy.gov
The DOE offers guidelines for crawlspace insulation and vapor barrier installation in their resources on energy-efficient building practices. They advocate for soil barriers as part of closed crawlspace systems, detailing materials, installation techniques, and sealing methods to prevent ground moisture from affecting indoor air quality and home efficiency.

› **International Code Council (ICC)—International Residential Code (IRC)**
Website: iccsafe.org
The IRC, part of the ICC, outlines code requirements for vapor barriers in crawlspaces, especially in the sections on moisture control and insulation. They specify materials (typically 6-mil polyethylene or thicker) and installation methods that comply with building codes for residential construction.

› **Advanced Energy—Closed Crawlspaces**
Website: advancedenergy.org/crawl-spaces
Advanced Energy, a nonprofit organization, has a dedicated "Closed Crawlspace" project, offering best practices for crawlspace encapsulation. They provide detailed instructions for installing soil vapor barriers, including recommendations for material thickness, overlap, and proper attachment to foundation walls.

Essay: Crawlspaces
by Bill Weber

Those mysterious and daunting areas between your beautiful floors and the earth below your house can hold the key to the environmental health of your home. Homeowners rarely visit crawlspaces because they are typically small, tight, dirty spaces that don't "require" homeowner maintenance. Guests don't come to your home to gather there; the kids are not playing down there, and there is no "need" to dust or clean since it's not a living space. However, nearly all crawlspaces have a profound effect on the living space.

Air is constantly moving throughout the house. When warm air rises in a building, it creates a Stack Effect. The amount of stack effect depends on the height of the building (stack) and the temperature difference between indoor and outdoor air. Since the warm air is rising and (usually) exiting through the attic or mechanical ventilation, it needs to be displaced with cooler air (usually) found in the crawlspace. Air flows through large and small penetrations, including annular spaces around pipes and wiring and around seismic hold-downs, gaps, and the unsealed areas around ducting boots. The air drawn into the living space via natural or mechanical ventilation is from the same area you rarely go in, if ever. The same area of the home that never gets cleaned or is seldom attended to.

Crawl spaces vary throughout the country and may be fully sealed and insulated (cold climates) or completely open with screening or lattice around the perimeter (hot, humid climates). It may be conditioned, or it may be dehumidified. Regardless of what type or configuration of crawlspace your home has, here are a few questions to consider:

- Is the crawlspace damp or wet? If it is, the organic trash or debris on the soil will support mold and bacteria growth. Condensing moisture can support mold growth on the building materials throughout the house as the moist air migrates from the crawlspace into the living space and makes its way to the attic. A wet crawlspace can also attract insects, spiders, and even rodents.

- Is the HVAC duct work intact? Ducting with holes or gaps will draw air into the airstream and directly into the furnace or home through the supply registers. Holes can develop from rodents, ducts rubbing on sharp surfaces during operation, or tradespeople crawling through. Rodents are attracted to warm ducting during the winter months, often chewing through the liner of the ducting and removing insulation for bedding against the warm air delivery system. Gaps can occur due to adhesion problems with tape, mastic failures, or ducting stresses, causing them to separate.

- Is there an active leak? Every building material has a serviceable life. This includes galvanized, copper, ABS, PVC, and VPVC pipes. It also consists of the drain assemblies, seals, and couplings under tubs, showers, and toilets. An ongoing leak can attract rodents and insects and help support mold and bacteria growth.

- Is your crawlspace accessible? Some homes, due to their age, lack of skilled or knowledgeable contractors, or man-made and natural obstructions (like a 6' diameter stump I found in one crawlspace inspection) can impede the inspection and serviceability of components located in various areas of the crawlspace. If you can't see if there is a problem, how can you fix it?

The crawlspace is one of a house's most important areas. If you are not qualified to inspect it, call a qualified indoor environmental professional. The air in your home will thank you.

Step 14: Using Appropriate Products and Methods for Effective Cleaning

Beyond the Hype

This step emphasizes using approved, non-toxic cleaning products to protect the health of all occupants, especially those with multiple chemical sensitivities (MCS). It guides the selection of gentle yet effective cleaning agents that remove mold and biotoxins without introducing new irritants or toxins, avoiding substances like fragrances and essential oils that can trigger sensitivities or affect post-remediation testing. The focus is on thorough cleaning techniques that address every surface to ensure complete decontamination without compromising air quality or exacerbating health issues. The goal is to restore the environment to a safe, healthy state, free from mold and chemical irritants.

If you are hypersensitive to mold, you may want to talk with your physician about whether it's appropriate for you even to be a part of the cleaning process. Some sensitive people insist on being a part of the cleaning process no matter what! In that case, it is important to realize that even with personal protection, minor lapses in attention to detail may result in exposures that, depending on your sensitivity, can make you feel miserable or worse. Unconsciously wiping the sweat off your forehead with the gloved hand you've been using to handle items with settled spores and fragments may be too much exposure for a sensitive person. It may take extra time to recover or even cause further setbacks in medical treatment. Also, a person suffering from mold-induced brain fog may not make the best decisions or be very effective in their cleaning efforts.

Exercise 14.1: Proper Use and Maintenance of a HEPA Vacuum Cleaner

HEPA vacuums are the first step in detailed, Effective Cleaning. It is important to understand what they can and can't do.

❏ The following information is provided to help understand how HEPA vacuums should be used, cleaned, and maintained to ensure effective use and longevity while preventing cross-contamination and maintaining high filtration standards.

› **HEPA vacuums:** HEPA vacuum cleaners are used to remove gross debris and dust. *(See "Essentials: Choosing and Using a HEPA Vacuum Cleaner" on page 62 for proper selection and use of a HEPA vacuum cleaner).*
› **A combination of HEPA vacuuming and damp-wiping is usually necessary** to effectively clean and capture any residual spores and fragments, ensuring a thoroughly decontaminated space.
› **Fine Particle Cleaning** is also sometimes needed to decontaminate a remediation area.

Exercise 14.2: Effective Cleaning

Effective surface cleaning to remove spores and particulates from surfaces is needed in water damage restoration and mold remediation.

- This process involves using a mild detergent solution and disposable microfiber cloths to ensure thorough cleanliness without damaging the surfaces.
- The cleaning is performed as often as necessary to strip away the layers of contamination that have built up over time.
- Rapid discovery and action soon after water damage and the resulting microorganisms develop take fewer rounds of cleaning than when a problem has built up over time.
- *(See "Essentials: Effective Small Particle Cleaning" on page 65).*

Exercise 14.3: Removing Fine Particles from the Air

Fine and Ultra-fine particles (UFPs) are sub-micron-sized particles that pose unique challenges during remediation. Generated by activities such as abrasive cleaning (e.g., sanding, dry ice blasting) or released from degraded water-damage organism fragments, UFPs remain airborne for extended periods due to their small size and low settling velocity. These particles can bypass natural air currents and filtration systems, making their removal particularly difficult. UFPs are inhaled deeply into the lungs and can cross the lung-blood barrier, posing significant health risks.

Understanding the Challenges

- **Behavior of UFPs**: Unlike larger particles, UFPs do not settle easily and resist removal through general ventilation. Their behavior is governed by Brownian motion, making them highly mobile but less likely to be captured by airflow or filtration systems.

- **Health Risks**: UFPs are inhaled deeply into the lungs, where they can cross the alveoli into the bloodstream, delivering contaminants directly to the circulatory system.

- **Surface Adhesion**: UFPs readily adhere to surfaces due to their high surface-area-to-volume ratio and electrostatic interactions, creating reservoirs of contamination that can re-enter the air if disturbed.

Determining When is Mitigating Ultra-Fine Particle Contamination Necessary

❏ When proper containment, HEPA-filtered negative air systems, and controlled removal techniques (Steps 10–12) are not implemented effectively, large quantities of UFPs may be released into the environment. This exercise provides a second opportunity to mitigate contamination by emphasizing thorough cleaning and air management. A Particle counter that measures 0.3μm can indicate if excessive fine particles are present when the indoor level is significantly greater than the outdoor level. If procedures like dry ice blasting or sanding without HEPA controls, then fine particle cleaning will almost always be needed.

Key Takeaways

- Ultra-fine particles are exceptionally difficult to manage due to their size and behavior.

- Effective mitigation involves encouraging UFPs to settle. They are then removed by thoroughly cleaning the contaminated surfaces.

- Poor containment or ineffective remediation practices necessitate a "clean, clean, clean" approach to remove these particles and restore safe air quality.

- The appropriate use of Aerosolver Pure is an effective way to encourage these ultra-fine particles to settle on surfaces where cleaning is used to remove them from the environment. This process provides a second chance to get the remediated environment back under control.

- *(See "Essentials: Principles for Effective Fine Particle Removal" on page 66).*

By implementing these strategies, this exercise ensures that ultra-fine particles are managed comprehensively, maintaining indoor air quality and safeguarding occupant health.

Fine-Particle Cleaning and Setting the Record Straight

Greg Weatherman

Greg Weatherman is one of the smartest and most resourceful individuals I've had the privilege to work with. He has an exceptional ability to track down authoritative references, often knowing exactly where to look when I'm at a loss. His depth of knowledge and his dedication to accuracy have been invaluable to me over the years.

As readers will notice, I rarely endorse products when it comes to mold. In this case, I am endorsing Greg himself. His Aerosolver Pure is not just a product—it's a carefully developed system for fine-particulate cleaning designed to drop fine particles that tend to remain suspended in the air to the flat surfaces below so they can be cleaned. It requires strict adherence to the detailed instructions Greg provides to achieve its full potential. If you decide to use Aerosolver Pure, it's essential to approach it with the same level of care and commitment that Greg applies to his work.

Greg's contribution to this field is more than what he has developed; he brings a thoughtful system to solving a complex problem. He has set a standard of excellence that is well worth recognizing. The following is excerpted from Aerosolver's technical data. The full information, instructions, safety information, and personal protective equipment are available at aerosolver.com/specs.

AeroSolver Pure: The Evolution of Fine Particle Cleaning

The concept of "fine particle cleaning" has emerged as a response to limitations in the industry's standard methods, which primarily addressed larger particles like dust and mold spores but often missed the smallest fragments that linger in the air. Greg Weatherman developed AeroSolver Pure to fill this gap by creating a mist that captures these fine particles, effectively clearing the air in indoor spaces where traditional HEPA filtration struggled. Over time, the benefits of this approach became apparent as it helped reduce airborne contaminants and was adaptable to real-world conditions, especially for sensitive individuals.

Purpose and Functionality of AeroSolver Pure

- The core purpose of AeroSolver Pure is to target particles that behave like smoke—remaining airborne and resistant to gravitational settling in remediated spaces.

- A second advantage is that other odor-causing particles in the air can mask the distinct smell of hidden mold. By removing small particles that mask their competing background odors, AeroSolver makes it easier to detect hidden mold growth with the nose, an often-underappreciated but effective detection tool.

- The particles physically cleaned from the air may still be infectious, allergenic, inflammatory, carcinogenic, mutagenic, or able to reproduce. But, they have now settled onto the floor or horizontal surface where they can be cleaned using the other product I wholeheartedly recommend—branch basics.

Composition and Mechanism

AeroSolver Pure is formulated with water, glycerol, and sodium borate. This blend promotes coagulation, where tiny airborne particles attach to mist droplets and settle out of the air. Unlike simple water misting, this approach works for the small, airborne particles associated with water-damage organisms and clears the air to make final surface cleaning more manageable.

How to Use AeroSolver Pure in Practical Applications

Using AeroSolver Pure requires the right equipment and technique to achieve its full potential. A ULV fogger (ultra-low volume mister) with adjustable settings should be used to produce a fine mist without over-wetting surfaces. Here are the specific steps to use AeroSolver effectively for mold-sensitive environments:

Preparation

Pre-clean walls, floors, and other surfaces with a HEPA vacuum (if needed for visible dust) and a damp disposable microfiber cloth to remove remaining sub-visible dust.

If sensitive items such as electronics remain, they should be removed or covered. HVAC ducts should be sealed (if they aren't already) for added protection.

Setting the Misting Device

- The appropriate humidity range for using AeroSolver Pure is **between 40% and (higher) relative humidity (RH)** for optimal particle capture and settling:

- **If RH is below 40%**, Start by misting the area with light water mist before applying AeroSolver Pure.

- This pre-misting helps prevent rapid evaporation, allowing the AeroSolver droplets to stay airborne longer for more effective particle capture.

- Use a ULV fogger with a flow rate of around 10 ounces per minute and an adjustable venturi knob to control mist flow (BG, FlexALite 2600 ULV Ultra Low Volume Fogger). Move the misting plume steadily around the room without soaking surfaces.

Mixing the AeroSolver Solution

Prepare a 7:1 water-to-concentrate solution (seven parts water to one part AeroSolver Pure), ensuring the right balance for effective particle settling.

Applying the Mist

Mist the room with AeroSolver for approximately 2 minutes per 100 square feet, moving the device around the room at about an 8-foot height.

If ceilings are higher, adjust the misting time: for 10-foot ceilings, increase to 2.5 minutes; for 12-foot ceilings, use 3 minutes per 100 square feet.

Rinsing with Water Mist

Follow the AeroSolver application with a light water mist to settle any remaining airborne particles. Use the same duration and pattern for this water rinse.

Final Surface Cleaning

After misting, allow particles to settle before wiping surfaces with a new disposable microfiber cloth. For stubborn residues or if the Aerosolver mist dries on the surface before it is wiped up, use a light, soapy solution (seven drops of unscented dish soap in a quart of water) on the cloth, ensuring thorough physical removal without chemical irritants.

Standards Compliance

AeroSolver Pure's use aligns with the ANSI/IICRC S520-2024 (Section 9.1.6) for misting devices. It also aligns with the Surviving Mold 2020 Consensus Statement and the CIRSx Medically Important Remediation (MIR101) training.

In my opinion, AeroSolver Pure is the only misting agent specially designed for people with sensitivities and is a valuable tool for those needing effective, non-biocide, small particle air cleaning adjunct to mold remediation solutions and water-damaged environments. Its role in physical particle removal from the air, when needed, reflects the core theme of this book—achieving a healthier, cleaner space through safe and effective remediation methods.

For more information: Aerosolver.com/specs

Step 15: Avoidance of Trapped Moisture and Problems Caused by Sealants and Encapsulants

*Use Vapor Permeable Materials: Avoid
Using Materials that Trap Moisture*

This step highlights the risks and importance of avoiding products like sealants and encapsulants in ways that could conceal contamination or trap moisture, exacerbating mold growth and compromising building integrity. It introduces methods for creating airtight wall cavity installations that prevent airflow without hindering moisture management. It offers these techniques to help you meet the building's ventilation needs while emphasizing the crucial role of maintaining dry buildings to prevent mold growth and water damage. This approach addresses immediate remediation needs and focuses on the long-term health and stability of the building, integrating effective mold control with moisture control and building preservation.

THE CASE FOR MOISTURE CONTROL OVER ANTIMICROBIAL SEALANTS

Moisture control is the foundation of preventing mold growth in any environment. If materials become and remain wet, mold will grow. Conversely, if materials are kept dry, mold cannot thrive. This simple but crucial principle must be prioritized when addressing mold prevention. Antimicrobial sealants and coatings are often falsely marketed as the ultimate solution for mold growth, but they are not substitutes for moisture control. While these products can inhibit mold growth on their surface, they cannot stop the mold that forms beneath the surface or in trapped moisture. If moisture remains uncontrolled, the potential for mold growth under these products persists, posing a significant risk to the integrity of materials and overall health.

> *Mold-resistant coatings should not be used as 'sealants' or 'encapsulants' to contain or cover mold growth.* —IICRC, 2024

Are Antimicrobial Sealants Ever Useful

In some specific or unusual situations, antimicrobial sealants and encapsulants may serve as a secondary line of defense. For instance, in environments where moisture control is temporarily compromised—such as during a construction project or in high-risk areas like basements or crawlspaces—these products may offer short-term or incomplete solutions by reducing the surface's suitability for supporting mold growth. In contrast, proper moisture control measures are always best. Additionally, in cases where materials have already been contaminated with mold and cannot be immediately removed, sealants might help contain the mold and prevent further spreading, but they will also trap more moisture, impeding drying. If temporary controls are going to be used, I prefer to seal the surface with quick-release tape, which can be easily removed when needed. However, these applications are limited, and the long-term use of such products should be avoided without proper moisture control in place.

Limitations and Risks of Antimicrobial Sealants

While antimicrobial sealants can prevent mold on the coating surface, they have significant limitations. A layer of dirt or organic material on the surface of the sealant can provide nutrients for mold to grow, negating the product's protective benefits. Furthermore, mold can grow underneath the surface if moisture becomes trapped beneath an impermeable sealant, leading to hidden problems. This mold growth may not be visible until structural damage has occurred, and at that point, remediation can be far more complex and costly. Additionally, trapped moisture under the sealant can lead to rot and further material deterioration, compounding the damage.

The Argument Against Antimicrobial Sealants for Hypersensitive Individuals

The risks associated with antimicrobial sealants and encapsulants far outweigh any potential benefits for individuals hypersensitive to mold or chemicals, such as those with CIRS or MCS. People who are highly reactive to even small amounts of mold spores, fragments, and mycotoxins, as well as chemicals, should avoid the use of antimicrobial coatings. The presence of off-gassing from these products can trigger severe health reactions, making them unsuitable for use in environments where sensitive individuals live or work. Furthermore, if moisture becomes trapped beneath a sealant and mold begins to grow, it will deteriorate the material and release contaminants, causing significant health issues for hypersensitive individuals.

> *While antimicrobial sealants and encapsulants may have niche applications, they are not substitutes for moisture control and pose significant risks, especially for hypersensitive individuals. —IICRC, 2024*

THE IMPORTANCE OF NON-TOXIC, MOISTURE-CONTROL-BASED SOLUTIONS

For hypersensitive individuals, the best approach is to focus on comprehensive moisture control and non-toxic cleaning methods. Keeping materials dry is the most reliable and healthful way to prevent mold growth. In these situations, antimicrobial products can introduce additional risks without providing substantial benefits. Instead, ensuring proper ventilation, dehumidification, and regular cleaning with non-toxic products will create a much safer environment for those with sensitivities. Hypersensitive individuals can maintain healthier, safer spaces by addressing moisture at its source and avoiding chemical-based coatings.

Exercise 15.1 Prohibiting the Use of Antimicrobial Sealants on Your Home

❏ Request the technical specifications and Safety Data Sheets (SDS) for any sealants or encapsulants proposed for use on your property. Carefully review these documents and reject products that are unsuitable for your situation, particularly if you have sensitivities to chemicals. Professional remediation companies consistently achieve successful water damage restoration and mold remediation without relying on antimicrobial sealants or encapsulants. If a contractor claims that IICRC standards require these products or are essential for success, know that this is not accurate. IICRC-certified firms are bound by a code of ethics that supports ethical and effective practices. If you encounter a company unfamiliar with medically important

remediation, you should recommend that they seek training through the CIRSx Academy at CIRSx.com. This training, developed by myself and other contributors to this book, offers 16 hours of specialized instruction and is approved by the IICRC for two days of continuing education credits, equipping professionals with the skills to meet the needs of sensitive individuals.

Stage Four: Quality Control and Monitoring

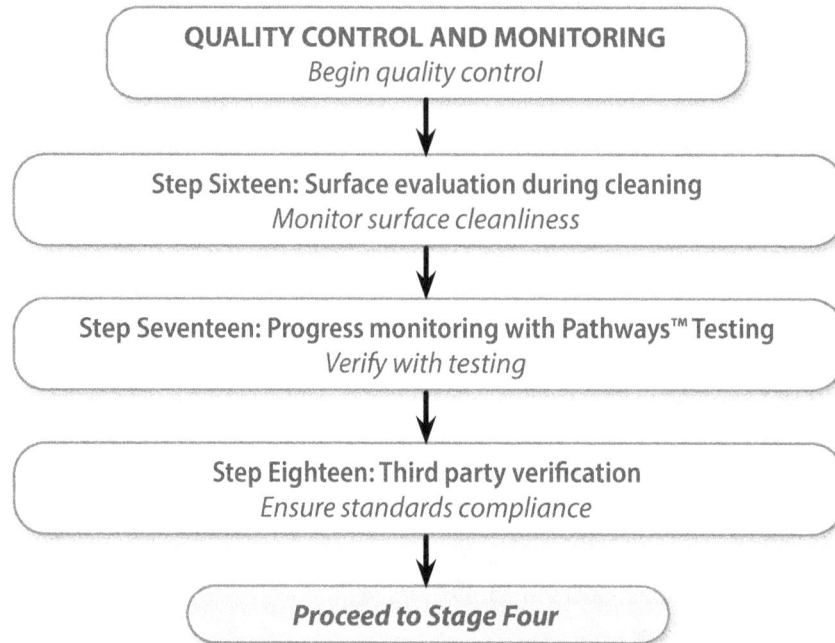

```
┌─────────────────────────────────────────┐
│      QUALITY CONTROL AND MONITORING       │
│           Begin quality control           │
└─────────────────────────────────────────┘
                    │
                    ▼
┌─────────────────────────────────────────┐
│  Step Sixteen: Surface evaluation during  │
│                 cleaning                   │
│          Monitor surface cleanliness       │
└─────────────────────────────────────────┘
                    │
                    ▼
┌─────────────────────────────────────────┐
│ Step Seventeen: Progress monitoring with  │
│            Pathways™ Testing               │
│            Verify with testing             │
└─────────────────────────────────────────┘
                    │
                    ▼
┌─────────────────────────────────────────┐
│   Step Eighteen: Third party verification  │
│         Ensure standards compliance        │
└─────────────────────────────────────────┘
                    │
                    ▼
┌─────────────────────────────────────────┐
│           Proceed to Stage Four            │
└─────────────────────────────────────────┘
```

Measured Mastery: Ensuring Long-Term Excellence in Water Damage Restoration

Stage Four: Quality control methods like visual inspection and testing are reviewed to confirm successful mold growth removal and cleaning. This evaluation helps avoid premature reconstruction that might result in trapped contamination, emphasizing remediation effectiveness, safety, and healthfulness.

Subjective visual inspections usually help confirm the successful removal of mold and are used when household members have normal levels of sensitivity. When sensitive household members cannot rely on their senses to identify continuing issues, objective measures such as Pathways™ testing can help ensure that surfaces are clean to the higher levels necessary to promote healing. This is the phase where the focus shifts to ensuring the longevity and effectiveness of the remediation efforts. This stage is about confirming the immediate success of the remediation and helping ensure its lasting impact. Continuous progress monitoring is integral, allowing for adjustments in remediation tactics. Another aspect of this stage is third-party verification, which balances the health-centric needs of sensitive individuals with the standards of legal, real estate, or insurance contexts. This stage emphasizes that while visual inspections are valuable, they are subjective, and objective measures also assist in assessing cleanliness and maintenance of post-remediation effectiveness. Stage Four prepares for the transition to Stage Five, focusing on long-term maintenance and health of the environment, ensuring that the remediation efforts have a lasting, positive impact on the living space.

Goals for Stage Four

By the time you have completed this stage, you should have the necessary information to be able to answer these questions:

❑ What quality control and monitoring measures do you want to be implemented in your mold remediation process during and after remediation efforts?

❑ How do you want objective methods like Pathways™ testing to contribute to the quality control process in your water damage or mold remediation?

❑ What role or need will third-party verification play, especially when balancing health-centric needs and external legal or commercial standards?

❑ How will you use interim surface evaluation during cleaning to ensure that surfaces meet your cleanliness standards?

Step 16: Visual Surface Evaluation for Cleaning Effectiveness

Assessing Cleanliness

Step 16 involves using visual inspections during and after cleaning to monitor surface cleanliness and identify potential hidden conditions needing further attention. This step is not just a formality but a component of the quality assurance process, ensuring the remediation work has successfully achieved its intended goals. Surfaces that cannot be successfully cleaned usually indicate a nearby hidden condition that may require additional remediation or other measures to control.

Exercise 16.1: Monitoring Progress with Visual Inspections

❑ Visual inspections are an inexpensive tool for tracking progress during the remediation process. Many contractors only perform a final cleaning at the end of the project, but this approach is insufficient for properly managing contamination. Allowing dirt and contaminants to accumulate throughout the remediation increases the risk of these materials migrating into inaccessible spaces, contributing to an extended "building memory" that may impact long-term indoor air quality.

› To limit building memory, routine effective cleaning and inspections should be performed regularly during the remediation and reconstruction. Consistent visual inspections ensure that the remediation is progressing as planned, identifying areas where contaminants may still be present and allowing adjustments to be made promptly. Maintaining cleanliness throughout the process can significantly reduce the dust and contaminants that will require removal after the project is complete.
› Use a flashlight or angled light source to shine light across surfaces at a low angle, highlighting fine particles that may not be visible under direct light.
› Dim ambient lighting, if possible, or conduct inspections during fading daylight to reduce glare. Bright overhead lights can obscure fine details and make dust harder to detect.
› Look closely at flat, horizontal surfaces in finished areas like baseboards, windowsills, shelves, flooring, fan blades, door frames, cabinet tops, and other hard-to-see or less accessible areas where dust accumulates.
› In remediated areas with open wall cavities or exposed materials, focus on horizontal surfaces such as sill plates, fire blocking, and ducts, wiring, or plumbing tops.
› Look for concentrated dust areas, as these may indicate active pathways where contaminants are migrating into the space.
› Pay attention to fine layers of dust that appear denser near cracks, edges, or openings, which could signal ongoing dust infiltration.

Step 17: Progress Monitoring Using Theatrical Fog, Surface and Pathways™ Testing

Progress Monitoring for Success

Step 17 highlights the role of monitoring surface cleanliness throughout the remediation process to ensure that actual growth is physically removed and sources of cross-contamination are identified and effectively addressed. This step enables timely adjustments of cleaning and remediation efforts by consistently tracking progress, ensuring that all actions remain precise and effective. This diligence helps restore a safe and healthy living environment by establishing successful mold remediation.

Key to this step is the use of objective surface cleanliness evaluation methods, such as Pathways™ testing, ATP, and Mycometer™ assessments. These tools validate that cleaned surfaces meet or exceed health and safety needs. At the same time, theatrical fogging helps identify the routes that contaminants can travel from contaminated crawlspaces, cellars, and basements, spreading contamination into occupied spaces. Step 16 was about using visual evaluation first to screen for visually clean surfaces. Step 17 uses testing methods to help ensure the remediation process remains thorough, effective, and aligned with health-centric goals.

Exercise 17.1 Choose the Type(s) of Surface Cleanliness Testing

❏ In water damage remediation where microorganisms are present or formed, validation of surface cleanliness, including those that do not show visible signs of water damage, helps affirm that restoration and remediation work has been completed. Different methods have been developed to test for residual contamination after the surfaces have passed visual confirmation (Step 16). Confirmatory testing for ATP, Mycometer™ Testing for Fungal Enzymes, or Pathways™ Testing for Peptide Bonds and Protein testing can help ensure that affected surfaces are cleaned to remove contaminants. Post-cleaning testing is important for detecting Invisible Contaminants: Even visually clean surfaces can harbor microscopic contaminants, including proteins and peptide bonds, which may indicate biological residues.

ATP Testing: Advantages and Limitations in Evaluating Organic Residues

ATP (Adenosine Triphosphate) is a molecule found in all organic matter, making it a useful indicator of residues left on insufficiently cleaned surfaces. ATP testing is particularly effective for detecting bacterial and organic residues, and I have extensively employed it when evaluating sewage damage, such as municipal backflows. Its efficacy stems from its ability to identify bacterial residues based on the ATP they contain.

While several companies have marketed ATP testing for mold evaluations, I have not found it as effective compared to methods like Mycometer™ and Pathways™. This limitation may be due to the durability of mold spores encased in a resilient hydrophobic coating. Unlike other methods that use caustic chemicals to break down these coatings during analysis, ATP testing relies on gentler processes, which are very effective for bacteria, enabling on-site, immediate analysis. This lack of aggressive chemical penetration may prevent ATP testing from providing accurate readings for mold contamination. Despite this limitation, ATP testing has distinct advantages in scenarios where rapid, on-site analysis is required for bacteria. Its ability to deliver immediate results without introducing potentially hazardous chemicals makes it a valuable tool, particularly in bacterial contamination scenarios. However, more specialized methods are often necessary for thorough mold evaluations to achieve reliable and actionable results.

Mycometer™ Surface Testing for Fungal Enzymes

Mycometer™ Testing is a specialized method for assessing fungal contamination on surfaces by detecting and quantifying fungal enzymes. This approach can provide specific information about mold presence and activity levels, making it an effective tool in post-remediation evaluations. Mycometer™ testing is ideal when fungal-specific contamination needs to be assessed, particularly in environments where mold-sensitive individuals reside or where compliance with stringent remediation standards is required. It is an excellent complement to visual inspections and other surface testing methods, providing a targeted and reliable way to confirm remediation success.

Advantages of Mycometer™ Surface Testing

- **Specificity to Fungi**: Mycometer™ testing is designed to measure fungal enzymes, offering more direct insight into mold activity compared to broader methods like ATP testing, which may detect non-fungal organic material.

- **Quantitative Data**: The results provide numerical values, allowing for comparisons against baseline levels or thresholds to confirm surface cleanliness.

- **Useful for Mold-Related Assessments**: Because it targets fungi specifically, Mycometer™ testing can identify whether remediation efforts have successfully reduced fungal contamination to acceptable levels.

- **Field Usability**: Unlike some laboratory-based tests, Mycometer™ can be conducted on-site, enabling faster decision-making during remediation and cleaning processes.

Disadvantages of Mycometer™ Surface Testing

- **Sample Preparation and Handling**: Proper sample collection and preparation are crucial to ensure accurate results. Mishandling can lead to contamination or variability in the data. Samples collected and stored at room temperature must have their analysis completed within seven days of the collection. Refrigerating or freezing the collected samples can extend the preservation of the collected samples for analysis that cannot be completed within seven days.

- **Technical Expertise**: The analysis requires trained personnel due to the use of **caustic chemicals** in the sample development process. While the sampling itself (e.g., swabbing a surface) can often be done in the field, the subsequent analysis typically needs to be conducted in a controlled laboratory setting.

PATHWAYS™ CLEANLINESS TESTING

This cleanliness testing method detects the presence of peptide bonds and proteins, which are components of bacteria, mold, protein-based organic material, and allergens. These proteins can be residues from microbial contamination or other biological sources. The absence of protein residues is a low-cost screening technique that tests for the cleanliness of a surface. It was discussed in detail in Stage Two, Step 5 on page 211.

When to Use Pathways™ Testing instead of Tape Lifts

Pathways™ testing and tape lifts serve different purposes in assessing contamination, and understanding when to use each is crucial for effective evaluation. Tape lifts are ideal for identifying mold species and assessing mold growth visible on surfaces, as they capture spores and hyphae directly for laboratory analysis. In contrast, Pathways™ Testing does not identify mold. Instead, it measures peptide bonds and proteins, which can indicate the presence of protein-based contaminants such as mold spores, fragments and particles, bacteria, pollen, or other biological residues. Pathways™ Testing is especially useful when evaluating overall surface cleanliness or when assessing environments for individuals sensitive to a broad range of contaminants. This method provides a more generalized view of contamination levels rather than pinpointing specific mold species. Use Pathways™ Testing when the goal is to determine whether cleaning efforts have sufficiently removed protein-based contaminants rather than focusing exclusively on mold identification.

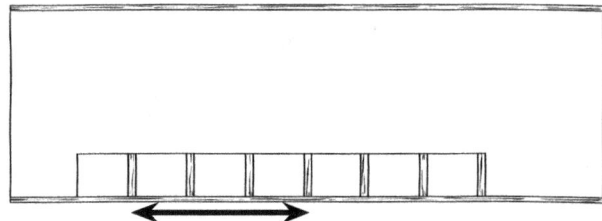

Figure 5-67: This illustration shows the area of the gypsum wallboard removed by the remediator. The solid line shows the area where visible mold growth was observed and remediated. It also represents one 48 linear inch area of wood that can be tested using Pathways™ for cleanliness post-remediation.

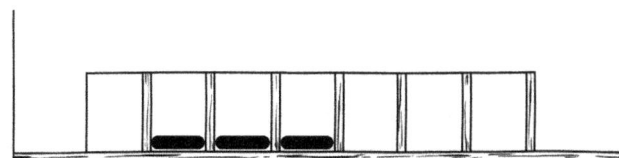

Figure 5-68: This illustration shows the same area. Testing at the line shows the 48 linear inches that will help determine if the back side of the wall (remaining gypsum) needs removal.

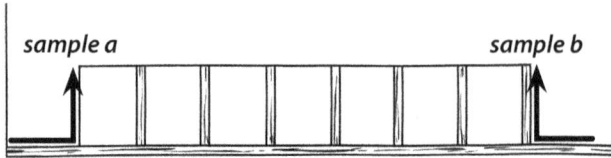

Figure 5-69: Testing the 48" shown on each side of the removed gypsum will help determine if additional material should be removed because sub-visible contamination extends into the remaining wall.

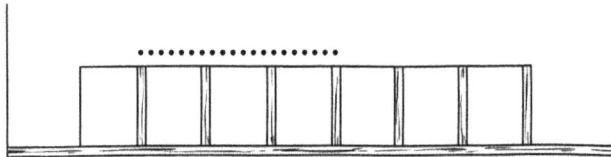

Figure 5-70: Pathways™ Testing the 48" dotted line collected by reaching up into the wall cavity shows if the removed gypsum went high enough to address sub-visible contamination.

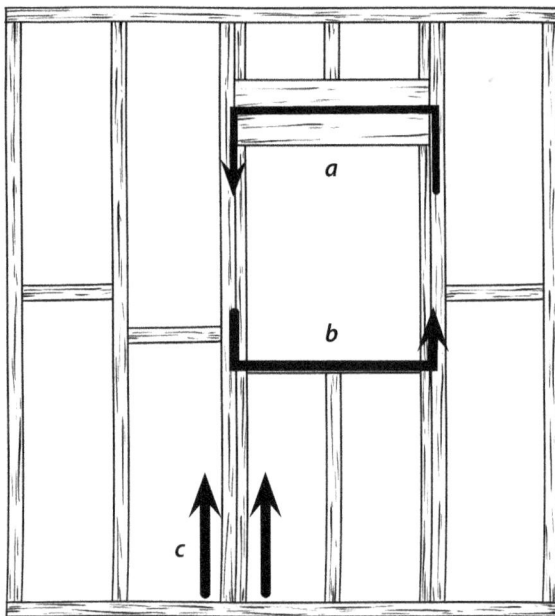

Figure 5-71: Pathways™ Testing 48" at the header location "a" helps determine if water coming from above the window

resulted in growth. Testing 48" at the under window-sill location "b" helps determine if mold caused by water leaking into the sill plate area of wall cavity below the window was addressed. Testing 48" total for both sides of the stud in location "c" shows if the framing in that location was adequately cleaned.

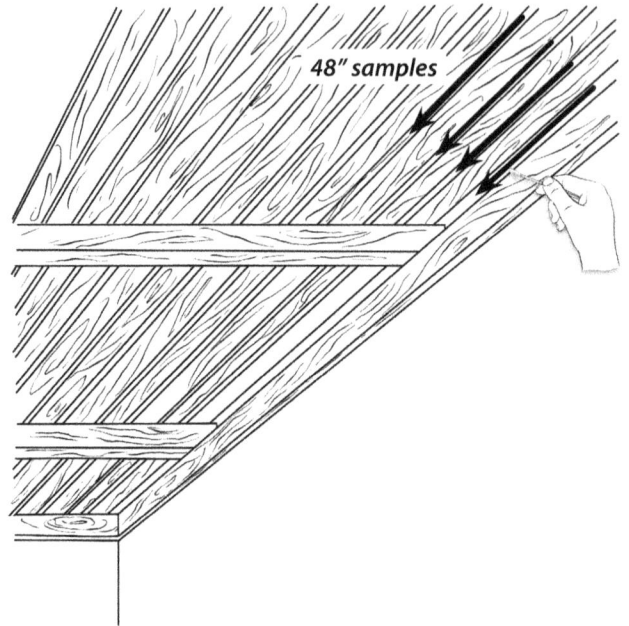

Figure 5-72: Tongue and Groove Ceiling Testing with Pathways™ by collecting multiple 48" swabs for contamination migration between grooves. By swabbing multiple grooves between the tongue and groove planks, it is possible to determine if hidden growth fragments and spores are filtering down from water damage above that section of ceiling.

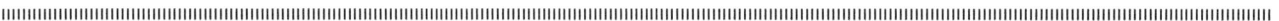

Exercise 17.2: Using Pathways™ Testing to Monitor Cleanliness

Pathways™ Testing can help more than just pathways with hidden contamination. The Pathways™ Testing also helps demonstrate if remediated surfaces are sufficiently clean for reconstruction and provides a semiquantitative measure of the level of contamination that remains on specific surfaces in the structure. This information can then be used to determine if additional remediation or cleaning of the tested and adjoining surfaces is needed.

An elevated level of proteins or peptide bonds on surfaces may mean there is a presence of microbial growth or contamination on the tested surface, or a source located on a nearby surface. All surfaces will have some level of biological material because mold, bacteria, allergens, and other proteins are a part of our natural environment. We cannot keep these natural particles out of our buildings, but we can tell when surfaces have normal or abnormally high levels of target proteins and peptide bonds detected by Pathways™ testing.

❑ In Step 5, the use of three rounds of testing was explained for testing for pathways that would allow hidden mold to migrate from hidden areas into the living space. This would help identify hidden sources of water damage or mold contamination. In this Step, Pathways™ Testing is used to establish cleanliness during or after the completion of remediation.

  › **Post Demolition and Cleaning Quality Control Testing:** Any of the Pathways™ Testing Patterns can be re-checked as many times as necessary after additional remediation or cleaning is performed to determine if the protein levels have been reduced and remain at a level where reconstruction is ready to proceed.

  › **Cleaning Effectiveness Testing:** A dirty surface is cleaned and tested immediately after the cleaning (15 minutes to 24 hours). Surfaces should be allowed to dry before testing but can be tested as soon as they are dry. By testing immediately (within 24 hours) after cleaning, it can be determined if the method of cleaning used was effective. However, the elevated level of proteins may indicate a large amount of contamination working out of a nearby area faster than it can be cleaned. In this case, additional inspection and investigation using other methods are recommended to confirm that unresolvable contamination is, in fact, present. Pathways™ can be repeated as many times as necessary to get the surfaces to a point where they are considered clean. When samples cannot be collected in the usual way because surfaces are rough and will snag the swab, the test can be conducted by dabbing the swab across the surface in a 48 linear-inch line. As you do this, change the angle of the swab so that the sample is collected across the surfaces of the swab to provide sufficient surface contact.

  › **Determining How Often Cleaning is Needed for Mitigation Control:** A surface Is confirmed clean by Testing for Cleaning Effectiveness and can be retested at intervals to determine how long it takes to become re-contaminated with proteins. For example, when tested two weeks later, a clean surface that shows some buildup of proteins would demonstrate that the surface needs to be cleaned at least once a week. If the surface remains clean with only a regular build-up of proteins over two weeks, then the twice-a-month cleaning is typically the minimum that should be considered. By cleaning, waiting, and Pathways™ testing at different intervals, it can be determined what frequency of cleaning is necessary to keep an area clean. An identified pathway may require daily cleaning, whereas the rest of the room may be controlled by weekly cleaning. This determination allows the home to be maintained.

|||||||||||||||||||||||||||||||||||||||||||||||||||||||||||||||||||||||||||||||||||||||||||||||||||||||||||||||||||||||||||||||||||||||||||

Essay: Smoke Testing (Theatrical Fog) for Home and Septic Systems
by Bill Weber

Air pathways are abundant in structures, influenced by pressure differentials that constantly move air and airborne particles from one area to another. This movement can be lateral, from room to room, or vertical, from one story to the next. Crawlspaces, attics, and interstitial spaces all interact with a home's living areas, impacting the movement of air and its contents. In multifamily housing and older commercial buildings, different areas, zones, and units often interact with one another as well. Because air itself is invisible and most airborne particles are less than ten microns in diameter, understanding airflow and currents can be challenging. However, introducing a large quantity of visible particles can help reveal these air patterns.

Smoke pencils have long been valuable tools for identifying small air pathways. HVAC companies regularly use smoke pencils to locate leaks in ductwork, and contractors specializing in building envelope integrity and energy efficiency also rely on smoke pencils to detect leaks.

Sanitary sewer piping, storm sewer piping, and septic systems have been tested for many years using opaque fog. Several leak detection companies have smoke generators that emit fog into a clean-out or vent pipe to test the systems for cracks and openings. This is generally done when occupants detect an irregular sewer odor.

Theatrical fog is an excellent, cost-effective way to visualize air pathways in any building. Commonly used in theater and dance to create an atmospheric effect, it also serves as a valuable tool in forensic applications. A fog generator, equipped with a high- or extra-high-density fog solution, can cost under $150 and offers hours of both entertainment and insight into air movement.

John Banta and I worked on a legal case involving a townhouse where the crawlspace, owned by the Homeowner's Association, had suffered water damage that fostered mold and bacterial growth. Spores, fragments, and secondary metabolites from these contaminants, confirmed through air and dust sampling, entered our client's living space. Despite this evidence, the Homeowner's Association and their experts denied contaminants could travel from the crawlspace into the townhouse interior, leading to years of litigation. However, when theatrical fog was introduced in the crawlspace, it revealed numerous pathways, including gaps around plumbing, unsealed duct boots, and in-floor vents for mechanical combustion appliances. The fog also highlighted airflow patterns, showing the master suite as a low-pressure area. Notably, this room had the highest contaminant levels in the three-bedroom townhouse, as confirmed by analytical tests. Using sampling data, expert testimony, and the results from theatrical fogging, the arbiter ultimately ruled in favor of the unit owner.

In our practice, theatrical fog is primarily used to confirm air exchange between the crawlspace and living space, highlighting specific pathways for targeted air sealing. When financial or access constraints limit immediate mold remediation in attics, crawlspaces, or other interstitial spaces, theatrical fog can guide precise air sealing to block contaminated air from problem areas. It's important to avoid broad application of sealants that could trap moisture—such as encapsulant sealants over large surfaces—as this can exacerbate and trap moisture issues. Proper remediation of environmental hazards remains the preferred approach, and air sealing should only be pursued in consultation with an indoor environmental professional experienced in medically important assessments.

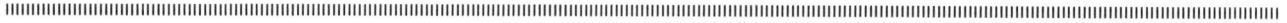

Step 18: Third-Party Verification

Independent Verification in Remediation

An independent third-party assessment after mold remediation ensures that the remediation was completed effectively and that the environment meets agreed-upon standards for cleanliness and safety. This assessment verifies the project's success, protects occupant health, and minimizes liability for all parties involved.

Step 18 differentiates the goals of third-party verification for general populations who may not experience adverse health effects from those requiring medically important assessments due to heightened sensitivities or health risks. It also acknowledges the distinct needs of legal, real estate, or insurance contexts, which can vary dramatically. This step guides balancing health-centric remediation with external obligations, ensuring safety for sensitive individuals while addressing broader legal and public health guidance.

Post-Remediation Assessment for Households Without Mold-Sensitive Occupants

An independent third-party assessment after mold remediation verifies the effectiveness of the remediation process and ensures the property complies with the established standards for occupancy. For households without mold-sensitive occupants, the primary goals of this assessment include confirming that all visible mold growth has been removed and that moisture issues contributing to mold growth have been resolved. Contaminated materials should be appropriately cleaned or removed, and the assessment addresses these tasks to determine if they have been completed.

Airborne and surface testing may also measure mold spore and particle levels, comparing the results to baseline data or acceptable industry standards. These criteria may help serve most occupants but are usually inadequate to confirm they will be acceptable for those with sensitivities. Additionally, the inspection may include checks for hidden mold in areas not addressed during remediation. Tools such as infrared cameras, moisture meters, or bore scopes can be employed to assess concealed spaces.

To ensure compliance, the assessment verifies that the remediation adhered to industry standards, such as the IICRC S520 Standard, and that the contractor followed the agreed-upon scope of work and methods. This step helps protect the public health of occupants.

Public health criteria are state or local criteria, or industry-specific standardized guidelines designed to protect the general population, establishing thresholds and methods considered safe for most people. In contrast, personal medically based criteria are tailored to individuals with specific health needs, often requiring stricter standards and customized approaches. While public health criteria provide a general baseline, personal criteria address unique vulnerabilities to ensure individual safety and well-being.

Finally, the independent assessor provides a detailed report documenting the findings, including testing results, observations, and conclusions. This documentation serves as a valuable record for property owners, tenants, and contractors, offering documentation in case of future real estate transactions or disputes. By using an independent third party, the assessment eliminates conflicts of interest to provide unbiased verification of the remediation's quality and enhance the credibility of the process.

Exercise 18.1 Determine the Type Third Party Assessment Needed

Indoor Environmental Professionals (IEPs) identified and possibly engaged during Step 4 may be suitable for verifying the success of remediation efforts, especially if their expertise aligns with both general public health standards and medically important cases involving sensitive individuals. The selected IEP should have specialized knowledge and experience in addressing health-centric criteria, as their verification process often requires stricter standards and tailored methodologies to ensure the environment is acceptable. In cases where it has been determined that the home is not suitable for occupancy by those with sensitivities, then any Independent third-party inspections and seller or landlord disclosures accompanying the rental or sale of the house should comply with the laws of that state. These are discussed in more detail in the Section of this book on looking for a home to rent or own.

❑ **Determine How Occupant Sensitivities Impact the Post-Remediation Assessment:**

› Review occupant sensitivities, chronic health conditions, or risk of adverse effects from exposure to water-damage organisms. This determines whether the evaluation should meet public health criteria or stricter, medically important standards.

› **Consider Future Occupants:** For rental or resale properties, consider the potential for sensitive individuals to occupy the home in the future. This may influence the decision to pursue more rigorous assessments.

Exercise 18.2: Select the Appropriate Assessment Criteria

❑ **For General Occupants (Public Health Criteria):**

› Follow state or local regulations, IICRC S520 standards, or other applicable industry guidelines.
› Verify that remediation successfully addressed visible mold, moisture sources, and contamination removal.
› Include airborne and surface mold testing as appropriate, comparing results to established public health benchmarks.

❑ **For Sensitive Occupants (Medically Important Criteria):**

› Engage an IEP with expertise in medically important remediation.
› Employ stricter testing protocols, such as MSQPCR or Pathways™ testing, to evaluate residual contaminants.
› Include physiological response considerations, such as Sequential Activation of Innate Immune Effects (SAIIE), if necessary.
› Ensure assessments account for individual-specific tolerances and vulnerabilities.

Exercise 18.3: Evaluate Legal and Documentation Needs

❑ **Comply with Legal and Disclosure Requirements:**

› Research state and local disclosure laws for real estate or rental transactions. Ensure that these third-party findings are documented and communicated appropriately.
› Choose an independent assessor to provide unbiased verification. Ensure their documentation is thorough and includes detailed findings, testing results, and compliance with standards.

Exercise 18.4: Engage the Right Professional

❑ **Select a Qualified IEP:**

› For general criteria, choose an IEP experienced in public health-oriented mold assessments.
› For medically important cases, select an IEP with training in addressing health-sensitive environments.
› Ensure the selected professional is independent and not involved in the remediation work to avoid conflicts of interest.

❑ **Confirm Scope of Work:**

› Review the third-party assessor's proposed methods and standards to ensure they align with your specific needs.

Stage Five: Post-Remediation Reconstruction and Maintenance

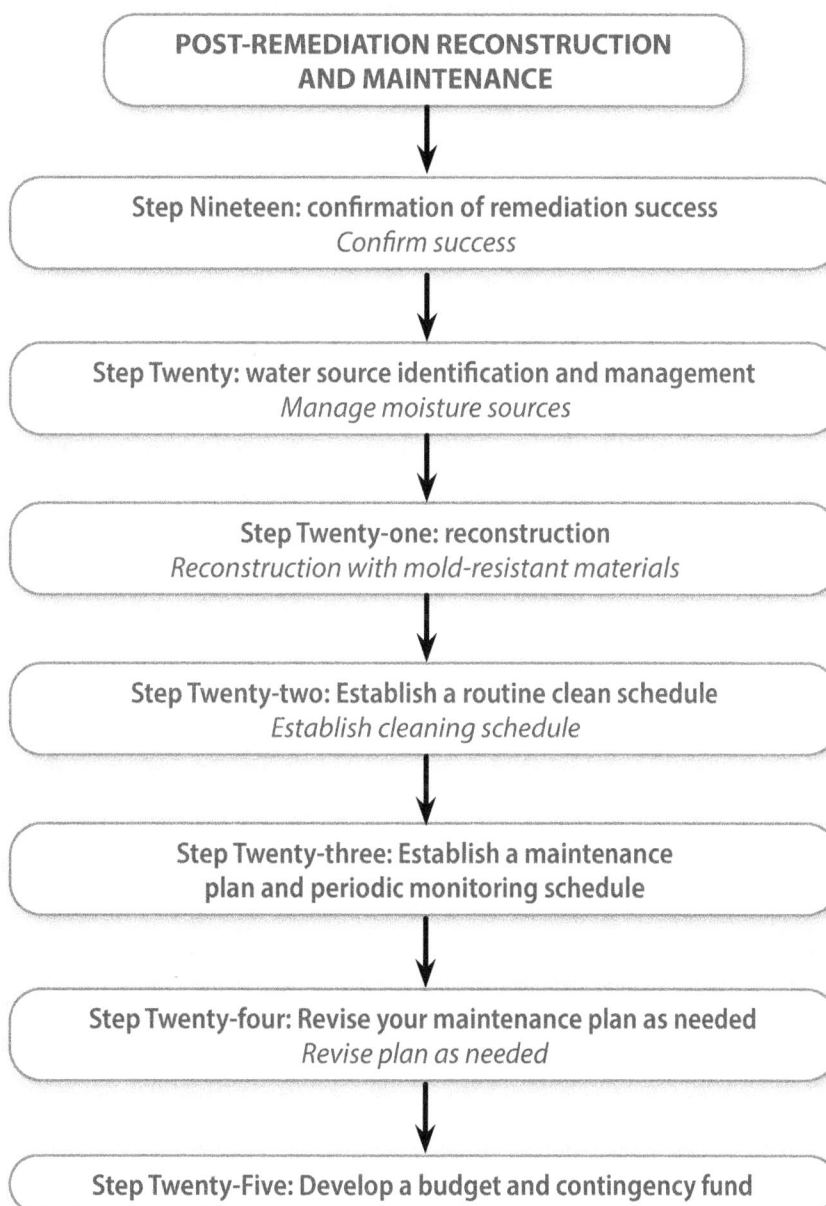

POST-REMEDIATION RECONSTRUCTION
AND MAINTENANCE

↓

Step Nineteen: confirmation of remediation success
Confirm success

↓

Step Twenty: water source identification and management
Manage moisture sources

↓

Step Twenty-one: reconstruction
Reconstruction with mold-resistant materials

↓

Step Twenty-two: Establish a routine clean schedule
Establish cleaning schedule

↓

**Step Twenty-three: Establish a maintenance
plan and periodic monitoring schedule**

↓

Step Twenty-four: Revise your maintenance plan as needed
Revise plan as needed

↓

Step Twenty-Five: Develop a budget and contingency fund

*Beyond Remediation: Cultivating a
Continuous Health-Conscious Habitat*

Stage Five focuses on ensuring the long-term success of mold remediation through Post-Remediation Reconstruction and Maintenance. This stage involves routine monitoring and sustainable practices to prevent future mold and water damage. It emphasizes the importance of managing the building's 'memory' of mold conditions, addressing the challenge of residues migrating from hard-to-reach areas into the living space over time. Reconstruction in this stage involves using mold-resistant materials, while maintenance includes establishing regular cleaning schedules and periodic checks. These practices are essential for those sensitive to mold and will enhance indoor environmental quality for those seeking a healthy living environment. The stage also advocates for a comprehensive budget and contingency fund for ongoing maintenance and unexpected issues. Stage Five is about solidifying the gains from remediation and ensuring a healthful, enhancing, mold-controlled environment. The philosophy moves away from the conventional 'kill the mold' strategy. Instead, it adopts a pacifist approach, recognizing that aggressive chemical treatments often lead to unintended, often detrimental, consequences. Dead mold retains harmful effects. Hence, the focus shifts to removing and rectifying conditions that facilitate mold growth. A 'healthy home' is more than just a mold-controlled space; it involves maintaining optimal air quality, balanced moisture levels, and a naturally balanced environment. This stage dives deeper into principles introduced in *Prescriptions for a Healthy House: A Practical Guide for Architects, Builders, and Homeowners, 4th edition,* I co-authored with Architect Paula-Baker Laporte, advocating for a living space that supports health and well-being.

Goals for Stage Five

By the time you have completed this stage, you should have the necessary information to be able to answer these questions:

❑ What strategies do you need to use to manage moisture sources, and what tools or professionals do you need to accomplish this purpose?

❑ How will mold-resistant materials and water management strategies contribute to your project's mold prevention and sustainability in reconstruction?

❑ How will Pathways™ Testing contribute to confirming the success of your mold remediation, and what additional purpose should it serve in ongoing maintenance?

❑ How will you implement a routine cleaning schedule to maintain a mold-controlled environment that is focused on the mold-sensitive individuals in your home?

❑ How often will you review and revise your home's maintenance plan and contingency fund?

Step 19: Confirmation of Remediation Success Before Reconstruction

Beyond the Remediation, Methods for Ensuring Success

Step 19 integrates multiple testing methods, including MSQPCR/HERTSMI-2, Pathways™ Testing, and Sequential Activation of Innate Immune Effects (SAIIE), to confirm the success of remediation before reconstruction begins. These methods provide nuanced insights into residual contamination, ensuring that remediation efforts have met the necessary standards for health and safety, particularly for sensitive individuals.

- **MSQPCR Testing and the HERTSMI-2 Score** provide detailed insights into mold types and quantities remaining in residual dust in different areas. Dust sampling from horizontal surfaces throughout the home helps determine the post-remediation contamination levels and guides decisions about additional cleaning or further remediation needs. (See Step 4)

- **Pathways™ Testing** screens for peptide bond and protein contamination, ensuring levels remain within normal background ranges. It also highlights surfaces showing increases, signaling residual conditions resulting from building memory, active growth, or hidden issues requiring further attention. (See Step 5)

- **SAIIE** offers a health-focused perspective by monitoring physiological responses to environmental challenges. It can detect biological changes in sensitive individuals before symptoms become apparent, serving as an early warning system to enable proactive action before reconstruction. *(See "Challenge Testing" on page 69)*

Together, these tools form a comprehensive evaluation framework, increasing the likelihood of identifying residual problems before reconstruction. This proactive approach safeguards the building and its occupants, ensuring a safe and healthful environment.

Exercise 19.1: MSQPCR and HERTSMI-2

❑ **Quantitative PCR (MSQPCR) and the HERTSMI-2 score** are valuable tools for evaluating mold contamination after remediation by analyzing dust samples to identify mold types and quantities. However, their effectiveness depends on proper timing, sufficient dust collection, and recognizing that visible dust may indicate deficiencies in cleaning. According to Step 16, post-remediation surfaces should be dust-free; visible dust on surfaces suggests that cleaning during remediation was inadequate. For MSQPCR to provide meaningful results, sufficient dust must naturally accumulate under normal living conditions following a thorough cleaning. Sampling too soon may fail to reflect the true environmental profile, and contamination from construction debris or gypsum can skew results. While waiting for appropriate dust accumulation is essential, combining MSQPCR/HERTSMI-2 with complementary methods like Pathways™ testing and SAIIE can accelerate the process. Pathways™ Testing provides immediate insights into biological residues, while SAIIE offers a structured health-centered evaluation, reducing delays and ensuring that remediation success is verified without stalling the project. Together, these tools form a comprehensive approach, confirming remediation effectiveness and maintaining progress toward a safe, clean environment.

› **Dust Quantity:** To obtain meaningful results from MSQPCR and HERTSMI-2 testing, an adequate amount of dust is collected from non-floor horizontal surfaces. Insufficient dust collection often indicates a recently cleaned environment, which is a desired outcome for effective cleaning. It also suggests that DNA testing is premature. Laboratories have the ability to perform analysis on as little as one milligram of dust, but such small quantities often lead to skewed results that fail to provide actionable insights. Rather than proceeding with minimal dust, which wastes resources and may offer misleading data, a delay in DNA testing until sufficient dust has naturally accumulated under normal living conditions isn't the only option. Pathways™ and SAIIE can proceed much more quickly.

› **Dust Composition:** If a significant amount of one kind of dust predominates, the composition may impact the MSQPCR/HERTSMI-2 results. If gypsum board dust dominates the sample, it often indicates inadequate cleaning. Gypsum dust, commonly present after remediation, often contains clay binders that inhibit DNA-based testing, resulting in unreliable outcomes for PCR testing. In such cases, the presence of significant visible gypsum dust already highlights the need for further cleaning, rendering analysis unnecessary at this stage. Prioritize additional cleaning to remove construction debris and ensure the collected dust represents the true environmental conditions before proceeding with any testing.

› **Timing for Dust Accumulation and Buildings to Forget:** The timing of dust collection is crucial for obtaining reliable MSQPCR and HERTSMI-2 results. Testing too soon after remediation often captures transient conditions rather than the true indoor environment, while waiting too long can delay reconstruction unnecessarily. Typically, a two-month waiting period allows dust levels to equilibrate, reflecting the actual indoor environment naturally. However, "building memory," the residual contamination from previous conditions, can persist and skew results. Thorough cleaning immediately after remediation helps "reset" the environment, removing historical contaminants and ensuring that subsequent dust represents ongoing conditions. Sequential sampling—collecting dust at intervals and cleaning between tests—balances the need for accurate data with timely reconstruction, providing meaningful insights into the success of remediation efforts.

› **Interpreting Results:** High-quality dust samples free from significant gypsum contamination can validate remediation success or reveal deficiencies in cleaning efforts. However, if substantial dust is present shortly after the remediation of the home is thought to be completed, it indicates a failure to meet visual cleanliness standards, making further testing unnecessary until thorough cleaning returns the environment to a dust-free state. MSQPCR testing should be used strategically to confirm the effectiveness of remediation or to pinpoint areas requiring additional attention, but visible dust must first be addressed, as its presence inherently signals inadequate cleaning.

Not Enough Dust?

The following strategy can be used over time for collection.

Sequential dust collection ensures enough representative dust is available for analysis while maintaining a clean environment. Follow these steps to maximize the effectiveness of MSQPCR testing:

Initial Sampling After Remediation:

- Immediately after remediation, collect a Swiffer® sample from non-floor horizontal surfaces within the remediated area. If there is insufficient dust to fill one side of the wipe completely, you will need to allow more dust to settle and collect more.

- Place the Swiffer in a double-sealable sandwich bag, label it, and store it.

Allow Dust to Accumulate:

- Wait one week to allow natural dust accumulation. Using the same wipe, collect additional dust along with the stored initial dust. If you still don't have sufficient dust, you will repeat the process as many times as necessary. You can proceed to clean your home after collecting the sample. This allows you to maintain a dust-controlled environment while continuing to collect it for analysis.

Repeat the Process as many times as necessary:

- Continue weekly sampling and cleaning cycles until a single Swiffer® wipe can collect sufficient dust (approximately 25–50 milligrams, enough to cover one side of the wipe completely).

- Focus on non-floor surfaces prone to natural dust settlement. Avoid collecting samples dominated by gypsum board dust or construction debris.

Analyze When Conditions Are Right:

- Only send a sample for analysis when sufficient dust has been collected and it is representative of the environment. Ensure the sample reflects ongoing conditions rather than transient post-cleaning states.

Exercise 19.2: Screen Surface Cleanliness Using Pathways™ Testing

❏ **Pathways™ Testing** measures peptide bonds and proteins on surfaces, which serve as an indicator of biological residues, such as mold fragments and other contaminants. This approach offers valuable insights into post-remediation surface cleanliness, particularly for households with sensitive occupants. Low levels of protein-based contamination indicate effective cleaning and a generally clean environment, while elevated readings may point to residual contamination or building memory that requires additional cleaning efforts. By integrating Pathways™ Testing into the post-remediation process, home surfaces can be objectively evaluated for residual surface conditions to ensure readiness for reconstruction. Pathways™ Testing was discussed in more detail in Step 5. The collection techniques are the same, and the remediated areas can be tested to ensure the peptide bond and protein levels indicate adequate cleaning. Additionally, Pathways™ Testing ensures that contaminated materials have been removed far enough to remove the visibly damaged materials and sub-visible contamination levels that cannot be visually observed. (for Pathways™ Testing instructions, see Step 5)

Pathways™ Testing offers a practical, actionable way to validate surface cleanliness and guide remediation adjustments. When used alongside MSQPCR testing, it forms a robust system for confirming remediation success and establishing a safe environment for reconstruction.

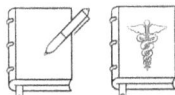

Exercise 19.3: Sequential Activation of Innate Immune Effects (SAIIE)

❏ **Sequential Activation of Innate Immune Effects (SAIIE)** provides a structured, health-focused framework for evaluating environmental exposures and their effects on sensitive individuals. Developed by Dr. Ritchie Shoemaker, this method integrates physiological monitoring during controlled re-exposure to determine if a remediated and cleaned environment is sufficiently free of contaminants to support healing. This approach is especially helpful for individuals who cannot reliably recognize contamination based on symptoms alone. When combined with Pathways™ Testing, SAIIE offers an evidence-based way to assess a property's suitability, cleaning frequency needs, and long-term livability.

Preparation: Work with your healthcare provider and provide informed consent. If the property has been recently cleaned, allow time for potential contaminants, such as mold fragments or microbial residues, to naturally settle before beginning the exposure trial. This is typically achieved by avoiding cleaning for a period equal to the expected interval between regular cleanings (e.g., two weeks). If time is limited, using negative air pressure to introduce particles from interior pathways can help accelerate the process. Pathways™ Testing conducted before the trial can provide additional insights into contamination levels by measuring peptide bonds and protein residues.

- Spend three or more days in a clean, safe, mold-controlled environment to reset your physiological baselines.

- Avoid exposure to any suspect-contaminated areas during this time.

- This "baseline reset" allows you to begin the trial with stabilized symptoms and lab markers, ensuring a reliable point of comparison for the re-exposure phase.

Entry Trial: Following this preparation, enter the property under controlled conditions for three successive days, spending a minimum of four to eight hours per day in the space. During the trial period, do not go anywhere; you might be exposed to contamination.

- During this time, track your symptoms closely in a journal, noting any changes in health, such as fatigue, brain fog, respiratory issues, or headaches.

- Conduct Visual Contrast Sensitivity (VCS) tests as your physician recommends to assess visual processing changes, and, if applicable, work with your healthcare provider to monitor biological markers like C4a, MMP9, or VEGF.

- If you experience significant adverse symptoms during the trial, stop immediately and consult your physician to determine the appropriate next steps.

After completing the re-exposure, evaluate the property's suitability based on the combined results of symptom tracking, VCS testing, and Pathways™ Testing. If symptoms remain minimal and Pathways™ Testing shows consistently low levels of contamination, this may indicate that the environment can be maintained with regular cleaning every two weeks. However, if symptoms worsen significantly or Pathways™ Testing reveals increasing levels of contamination, this suggests that the property may require more frequent or thorough cleaning, additional remediation, or even alternative housing.

Maintaining detailed records of your observations, test results, and environmental changes is essential throughout this process. A well-documented diary will help you and your healthcare provider make informed decisions and track progress.

For further information on SAIIE, its applications, and supporting research, visit SurvivingMold.com or consult resources such as "SAIIE Meets ERMI: Correlation of Indices of Human Health and Building Health." (Shoemaker R., 2008b).

||||||||||||||||||||||||||||||||||||||||||||||||||||||||||||||||||||||||||||||||||||||||||||||||||||||||||||||||||||||||||||||||||||||||||||||

The Role of Health Care Providers, IEPs, and Remediators in the SAIIE Process: A Collaborative Approach

Successfully implementing the Sequential Activation of Innate Immune Effects (SAIIE) process requires collaboration between healthcare providers, Indoor Environmental Professionals (IEPs), and remediation specialists. Each professional plays a distinct but complementary role in addressing mold-related health concerns and ensuring a safe living environment for individuals with sensitivities, such as Chronic Inflammatory Response Syndrome (CIRS).

Physician's Role

- **Medical Evaluation and Monitoring**: The physician helps evaluate and provide informed consent information, assesses the patient's health status, conducts diagnostic tests, and monitors symptoms before, during, and after controlled re-exposure in the SAIIE process. They determine the physiological impacts of environmental exposures and advise on whether the home environment is suitable for recovery.

- **Interpreting Health Data**: By analyzing biomarkers, symptom progression, and tools like Visual Contrast Sensitivity (VCS) testing, the physician provides crucial insights into the patient's response to environmental changes.

- **Guiding Health-Centric Decisions**: Based on medical data, the physician determines whether additional remediation or adjustments in cleaning frequency are necessary to meet the patient's health needs.

Indoor Environmental Professional's Role

- **Environmental Assessment**: The IEP evaluates the property to identify mold types, contamination levels, and hidden sources of moisture that may contribute to unresolved exposure. This includes conducting tests like MSQPCR or Pathways™ and providing actionable environmental data to complement the physician's findings.

- **Collaboration and Strategy Development**: The IEP collaborates with the physician and remediator to design a tailored remediation strategy that addresses health-centric concerns, focusing on reducing biological contaminants to support the patient's recovery.

- **Client Education**: The IEP educates the client about effective prevention strategies, such as controlling humidity, improving ventilation, and maintaining a routine cleaning schedule, empowering them to maintain a health-supportive environment.

Remediator's Role

- **Executing the Remediation Plan**: The remediator implements the strategies outlined by the IEP, ensuring that cleaning, containment, and removal efforts adhere to agreed-upon health-centric standards.

- **Ensuring Quality and Safety**: The remediator applies advanced techniques to achieve effective remediation, minimizing particle release and avoiding practices that could exacerbate contamination.

- **Feedback and Adjustments**: Collaborating with the IEP, the remediator provides updates on progress and incorporates adjustments as necessary to align with SAIIE findings.

A Holistic Approach to Patient Health and Home Environment

The SAIIE process emphasizes the integration of medical and environmental expertise. The physician's focus on the patient's health, the IEP's detailed environmental insights, and the remediator's practical implementation combine to create a robust framework for addressing mold-related challenges. Together, this team ensures that the home environment is not only clean but also supportive of long-term health and recovery for individuals with sensitivities. Regular follow-ups and ongoing communication among these professionals provide continuity and assurance, safeguarding both the patient and their living space.

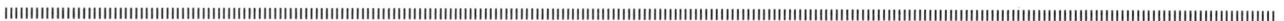

Step 20: Water Source Identification and Management

Thoroughly Assess and Address Moisture
Before Reconstruction Ensues

Identifying and managing moisture sources is essential to preventing future water damage and mold growth. This process involves thoroughly investigating moisture sources and implementing strategies to address them, such as repairing leaks or improving ventilation, before beginning reconstruction. Taking these steps ensures comprehensive repair and minimizes the risk of recurring mold issues.

In some cases, the source of water causing damage and microbial growth is evident from patterns of water staining or mold. However, the source must always be identified and addressed. Conducting leak testing after repairs and before reconstruction helps confirm the effectiveness of the repairs. This step helps ensure that the underlying issue has been resolved and reduces the likelihood of future problems.

Essay: Leak Testing for Windows, Doors, and other Penetrations
by Bill Weber

Where is that mysterious dripping sound coming from? How do I know if my window(s) and door(s) are leaking? How is the water getting into my basement or crawlspace? Leak detection is both an art and a science. It can be a difficult task for both the forensic building consultant and the property owner, sometimes taking a considerable amount of time, money, and energy. The good news is that even the most difficult and elusive leaks can be successfully traced to their origination point! If you get stumped and need help, look for a company with knowledge and experience in building science, construction techniques, and the right forensic tools and equipment; this should accelerate the process.

For leaks into crawlspaces and basements from the exterior, I recommend focusing on the waterproofing of the foundation and the groundwater management around the building. Although groundwater (natural springs) can sometimes be a problem, they are rarer than construction-related activities. Depending on the age of the house, waterproofing may not even exist around the foundation perimeter. Early *damp* proofing around basement walls generally consisted of a thin liquid applied asphaltic material. Over time, this material breaks down, allowing water to intrude. In newer buildings, typical waterproofing includes a liquid-applied membrane with a drain mat and dimple pad to allow water to flow to the French drain system. The French drain system should be installed at the lowest point of the foundation footing. Whenever possible, French drains should drain to daylight rather than relying

on sump pumps, which can fail due to mechanical issues or power outages—even with battery backup, which may still be insufficient during severe weather. Gravity, by contrast, doesn't fail. Tracer dyes used at the base of the basement walls can help define suspect areas. Tracer dye tablets are available in multiple colors that can best be seen with ultraviolet light.

If you are wondering if you have a leak in the supply plumbing, a check of your water meter (with no fixtures or appliances running for about an hour) can reveal whether or not there is a current leak. Leak detection companies use sonic listening devices to listen for leaks inside wall cavities and concrete slab foundations. The use of moisture meters and thermal imaging cameras can also help locate small and elusive supply plumbing leaks. Nondestructive moisture meters generally use impedance to determine density differences within a material. When using a moisture meter, be sure to compare material that is at "dry standard" with the suspect material. Thermal imaging measures the surface temperatures of materials; when conditions (temperature and relative humidity) are right, moisture will evaporate from surfaces, making a surface colder through evaporative cooling. Thermal imagers provide a visual picture of the evaporative cooling.

For doors, windows, light fixtures, and other penetrations into the building, there are guidelines for specific testing established by organizations, including the American Architectural Manufacturer's Association (AAMA) and ASTM

International. These standards are generally used for newly installed fenestrations and other architectural features. For older fenestrations, AAMA, in conjunction with the Fenestration and Glazing Industry Alliance, produced the *AAMA 511-22: Voluntary Guide for the Forensic Evaluation of Water Intrusion at Fenestration Products*. The purpose is to provide a guide for evaluating evident water penetration. If finding the leak can be less formal, applying water and mimicking rain with a garden nozzle may suffice. On the interior of the wall, removal of drywall and insulation at the tested fenestration is the best way to see where the water is coming in. Sometimes,

it is not the window or door but rather its installation or the water-resistive barrier (building paper) that is applied to the exterior of the building. If removing building materials is impossible, using moisture meters and thermal imaging devices, as noted previously, can be a viable option.

Regardless of the type of leak, it's crucial to dry building materials quickly, as mold can begin to grow within 24–72 hours under the right conditions. If the leak has been ongoing, mold remediation by a company experienced in medically important remediation is recommended.

Exercise 20.1: Verifying Repairs to Identified Issues

❏ Ensure that all previously identified moisture sources contributing to water damage and mold growth have been effectively repaired. This step focuses on confirming the success of repairs before reconstruction to minimize the risk of recurring problems.

- **Review Identified Issues:**
  › Compile a list of all recognized water intrusion sources, such as leaks, condensation, flooding, construction defects, or aging materials.

- **Inspect Repair Work:**
  › Visually examine all repaired areas to ensure the work appears complete and aligns with expected outcomes.
  › Check for remaining gaps, improper seals, or any visible signs of incomplete work.

- **Perform Leak Testing:**
  › Simulate potential water intrusion by spraying a garden hose on repaired areas such as windows, roofs, and exterior walls to identify leaks.
  › Observe open wall cavities and other areas during heavy rainfall if feasible. Look for signs of moisture ingress.

- **Document the Results:**
  › Record findings from the inspection and leak testing. Note any areas that require additional attention or follow-up.

- **Withhold Reconstruction Until Confident:**
  › Do not proceed with rebuilding until all sources of moisture have been conclusively addressed.

Keeping materials dry is the most effective and long-lasting solution for preventing mold growth and avoiding the potential pitfalls associated with chemical coatings. For those managing mold-sensitive environments, the focus must remain on controlling moisture, ensuring cleanliness, and choosing non-toxic methods to create a truly healthful living or working space. —IICRC, 2024

Exercise 20.2: Proactive Prevention for Other Potential Issues

Take a proactive approach to identifying and addressing areas of the home that may not yet have shown damage but are likely to fail in the future based on known patterns or conditions.

❏ **Evaluate Similar Risk Areas:**
- › If a window or other building component has failed, consider the likelihood that other windows or penetrations of the same age or condition will fail soon.
- › You've already considered whether any openings or penetrations, such as doors, ventilation openings, or drain lines penetrating the building envelope, may have allowed water entry. Now is the time to think about the future and anticipate future issues. It may be most straightforward to address these possibilities during the reconstruction process, but if that is not within your current budget, add these to your Step 23 Maintenance Plan and Step 25 Budget.

References

Office of Policy Development and Research, U.S. Department of Housing and Urban Development. (n.d.). *Moisture problems in manufactured homes*. HUD USER. Retrieved August 8, 2024, from https://www.huduser.gov/portal/publications/Moisture_Problems.html

Office of Policy Development and Research, U.S. Department of Housing and Urban Development. (n.d.). *Minimizing moisture problems in manufactured homes located in hot, humid climates*. https://www.huduser.gov/Publications/PDF/MoistureReportFinal.pdfS

Step 21: Reconstruction

Smart Moisture Strategies for Lasting Wellness.

Focus on using materials that inherently resist mold growth and don't trap moisture and implementing water management strategies during reconstruction. *Prescriptions* *for a Healthy House,* which I co-authored with Paula Baker-Laporte, offers insights into constructing and remodeling with health, sustainability, and mold prevention in mind, guiding safe and thoughtful rebuilding.

|||||||||||||||||||||||||||||||||||||||||||||||||||||||||||||||||||||||||||||||||||||||||||||||||||||||||||||||||||||||||||||||||||||||||||||||||||

Essay: Reconstructing a Healthy Home
by Paula Baker-Laporte FAIA-BBNC

Once a successful remediation has been completed, you are ready to rebuild. Reconstruction presents an opportunity to permanently fix any problems while making your home a healthier and more resilient environment in which to recover and thrive. The following are some essential points for you to consider when rebuilding a health-supporting environment. The 4th edition of *Prescriptions for a Healthy House (Prescriptions)*, a book coauthored by John Banta and me through 4 editions and over 25 years of collaboration, is the companion book that will walk you and your design/build professionals through the detailed information you need to help you achieve your goal.

Taking Care of the Cause of Moisture Damage

The first factor in a successful rebuild is understanding the cause of the moisture damage and assuring that it will never recur. Our building envelopes, consisting of the external walls, floors, and roofs, mediate between two complex and dynamic sets of conditions: the surrounding external climate and the occupants' activity within. Suppose your water damage problems were caused by moisture intrusion through the envelope, whether due to poor drainage, leaks, condensation, or wall or roof failure; the problem must be addressed at the core level to ensure that it never reoccurs. Rebuilding simply to meet the Building Code may not sufficiently address these problems. Moldy homes with built-to-code standards are, unfortunately, a common occurrence. *Prescriptions* can help you understand many of these conditions and how to address them; however, your situation may warrant consultation with a building envelope specialist familiar with how your local climate and built environments interact. He/she can help you to understand and find solutions for more complex envelope issues.

Rebuilding With Non-Nutritive Materials

Many standard building materials used in North America, as explained earlier in this book, are made of materials that are ready food for mold. OSB, standard drywall, plastic non-permeable finishes, etc., are all disasters waiting to happen. Just add moisture, and mold will quickly form. The good news is that more vapor-permeable, mold-resilient, nonnutritive materials exist for every application, and specifying them for your rebuild is worthwhile. *Prescriptions* can help you identify and find them.

Rebuilding With Healthier Materials

If you have been sensitized or made ill by mold exposure in your home, you may find that you or a member of your household has also become sensitive to chemicals that never bothered them in the past. *Prescriptions' major focus* is to help you reduce the chemical load in your rebuild, which is essential to creating the most conducive environment for regaining and maintaining health.

Even if you have never been sensitive to chemicals in the past, why introduce a chemical load into your home now? Unlike a decade ago, thanks to health emphasis by building related programs such as Declare, Safety Data reporting, Greengard, and LEED, the consumer can now learn more about the harmful chemicals commonly found in building products and access information regarding ingredients in individual products. Many material manufacturers have responded to increased market demand by creating healthier building products. It is now much easier to build back your home without harmful chemicals.

Unfortunately, this does not mean that every product advertised as "green" will be safe for you to use. It takes a bit of work to become an informed consumer when your goal is to use the healthiest materials. In *Prescriptions* we walk you through the process of vetting materials for health using a combination of available and free online resources. Throughout *Prescriptions*, we also provide several healthy options for each category of materials and have already done the research for you. Many listed products will be readily available at your local big box stores such as Home Depot. Others, although important to your health, must be specially ordered and require a little advanced planning. Note that if you have become severely chemically sensitive, then consider our listed materials as a good starting point. We recommend individual self-testing of all materials in some cases.

Rebuilding To Prevent Future Plumbing Water Events.
Whether or not your home was originally damaged due to a water loss event, you can take several simple steps while rebuilding to prevent or minimize future damage from leaks and flooding. A few of these include:

- Adding floor drains or catchment pans at laundry and mechanical room appliances.
- Selecting appliances with built-in flood control.
- Installing leak detection, alarm, and shut-off devices.
- Adding catch drains under sinks.
- Building removeable kicks at kitchens and bathroom cabinets.

In summary, construction renovation is a complex process, and the average homeowner has little experience with it. However, if your health is your priority and you have a willing and able design/build team on your side, this is an achievable and worthwhile goal.

Myth: Mold-Resistant Materials Prevent Mold Growth.
Fact: While mold-resistant materials can help reduce the risk of mold growth, they don't completely prevent it. If conditions are right, such as high humidity or water leaks, mold can still grow on these surfaces.

Exercise 21.1: Planning a Mold-Resilient Rebuild

❑ Develop a reconstruction plan that addresses the root causes of moisture damage and prioritizes mold-resistant materials and strategies for a health-supporting rebuild.

- **Understand the Cause of Damage:**
  › Review the identified causes of previous water damage (e.g., leaks, poor drainage, condensation).
  › Assess the building envelope (walls, floors, roof) to determine if structural changes are needed to prevent future moisture intrusion.

- **Consult Experts:**
  › If needed, consult a building envelope specialist to identify and address issues specific to your home's design and climate.
  › Record their recommendations for resolving complex moisture issues.

- **Choose Mold-Resistant Materials:**
  › Research and select materials that are non-nutritive to mold, such as paperless drywall, mineral-based plasters, and vapor-permeable finishes.

- **Plan for Vapor Management:**
  › Incorporate vapor-permeable materials and systems into your design to allow moisture to escape while preventing water intrusion.

- **Create an Actionable Rebuild Plan:**
  › Outline the steps required for reconstruction, focusing on preventing future mold growth.
  › Share the plan with your contractor or design/build team, ensuring alignment on health-supporting principles.

Exercise 21.2: Proactive Measures for Future Water Event Prevention

❑ Incorporate proactive strategies during reconstruction to prevent future water events and minimize potential damage from leaks and flooding.

- **Evaluate Vulnerable Areas:**
  › Identify areas of the home prone to water events, such as laundry rooms, kitchens, bathrooms, and mechanical spaces.
  › Document potential risks, such as old plumbing, appliances without flood control, or missing floor drains.

- **Plan for Preventative Features:**
  › Choose reconstruction features that mitigate water damage risks:
  › Floor drains or catchment pans in laundry and mechanical rooms.
  › Leak detection, alarm, and shut-off devices on appliances.

> Catch drains under sinks.

> Removable kick plates for kitchen and bathroom cabinets.

- **Upgrade Plumbing Systems:**

  > Specify high-quality plumbing materials designed to withstand wear and tear.

  > Install appliances with built-in flood control mechanisms.

- **Incorporate Design Solutions:**

  > Work with your contractor to integrate water management systems into the rebuild.

  > Ensure designs allow for easy monitoring and maintenance.

- **Test New Installations:**

  > After reconstruction, test installed systems (e.g., leak detectors, floor drains) to confirm they function as intended.

  > Create a maintenance schedule to ensure continued performance.

Step 22: Establish a Routine Effective Cleaning Schedule

Addressing Building Memory with Routine Effective Cleaning

Cleaning a dirty house can be particularly challenging for mold-sensitive individuals, as accumulated contaminants can exacerbate health issues. Establishing a routine cleaning schedule is crucial to interrupt the accumulation of "building memory" and the tendency of spaces to collect outdoor contaminants over time. Proactive cleaning prevents these contaminants from reaching levels that trigger symptoms, ensuring the environment remains healthy.

Mold-sensitive individuals often develop a heightened awareness of environmental changes, serving as an early warning system for potential problems. Subtle cues, such as unusual odors or increased dust, signal when contaminants may be accumulating. By paying attention to these changes, you can adjust your cleaning routine to address issues before they escalate, maintaining control over your living space.

A clean floor and horizontal surfaces are your home's best air purifiers. Every cleaning cycle acts like changing the filters in an air purifier, removing mold triggers, dust, and allergens that would build up to a point where they are released from the floor and begin to circulate in the air. Maintaining consistent cleanliness limits the "memory" effect of past contamination and reduces the burden on mechanical filtration systems, enhancing overall air quality.

Routine, thorough cleaning using effective methods and products ensures the physical removal of mold triggers while empowering individuals to take charge of their environment. This step is not just about maintaining a clean appearance—it's a proactive strategy to disrupt building memory, prevent mold recurrence, and foster long-term wellness. A well-maintained cleaning regimen tailored to the specific needs of your home and its occupants promotes confidence and ensures a healthy, mold-controlled living space.

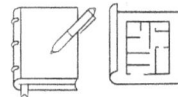

Exercise 22.1: Establishing a Proactive Cleaning Routine

❏ **Identify Key Cleaning Zones:** Begin by identifying areas of your home that are prone to contamination buildup. Focus on floors, horizontal surfaces, high-use zones like entryways, kitchens, living areas, and areas near windows, doors, and HVAC vents. Don't overlook "forgotten" spaces such as baseboards, behind furniture, and under appliances, as these areas can harbor dust and allergens if neglected.

❏ **Create a Cleaning Schedule:** Develop a cleaning schedule tailored to your home's and its occupants' needs. For high-use areas, include daily tasks to address the accumulation of clutter and ensure damp surfaces dry daily. If you have "hot spots" of contamination, you must address them as often as necessary before they get out of control. Establish weekly or every other week tasks, such as HEPA vacuuming, followed by effective cleaning of horizontal surfaces, as described throughout this book. Plan for monthly deep cleaning sessions on a rotational basis to tackle less frequently accessed spaces and surfaces, such as behind furniture, books stored on open shelving, personal possessions, and under appliances.

❏ **Choose Effective Cleaning Methods:** Use tools and products that effectively capture and remove contaminants. HEPA vacuums and disposable microfiber cloths are excellent for trapping fine particles without redistributing them. Use a damp microfiber mop with a safe detergent, like Branch Basics All Purpose, to remove biotoxin residues and allergens for hard floors. Avoid harsh cleaning chemicals that can leave behind irritating residues, especially for mold-sensitive individuals.

❏ **Adopt a Layered Cleaning Approach:** Employ a two-step cleaning process to maximize effectiveness. To remove loose particles, start with dry cleaning methods, such as HEPA vacuuming. Follow up with wet cleaning techniques, such as mopping or wiping with a damp microfiber cloth, to address residues and deeply embedded contaminants.

❏ **Prioritize High-Use Areas:** Pay special attention to high-traffic zones like entryways, kitchens, and living areas, which require more frequent cleaning to prevent the spread of contaminants. Additionally, focus on surfaces at or near breathing height, such as tables and countertops, where airborne particles are more likely to circulate and settle.

❏ **Treat Cleaning as Filter Replacement:** Approach each cleaning session with the mindset that *"a clean, hard-surface floor is better at controlling air quality than a room air purifier."* Just as an air purifier depends on clean filters to function effectively, your floors and horizontal surfaces act as natural air purifiers, capturing airborne contaminants and preventing them from circulating. Keeping these surfaces clean reduces dust, mold fragments, and allergens, significantly improving indoor air quality. Regular maintenance of hard-surface floors and horizontal surfaces ensures your home operates as a highly effective, self-sustaining air purification system.

❏ **Monitor and Adjust:** Pay close attention to subtle environmental cues, such as increased dust or unusual odors, as these may indicate the need for more frequent cleaning or adjustments to your methods. As you clean, monitor to see how dirty the wipe becomes. Aim for a cleaning schedule that adjusts to clean more frequently when the accumulated dust levels show up at a higher rate. Use a checklist to track completed tasks, ensuring consistency in your routine while allowing for flexibility as needed.

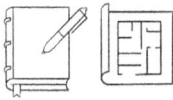

Exercise 22.2: Using Pathways™ Testing to Monitor and Guide Cleaning

Utilize Pathways™ Testing to monitor contaminant levels and refine your cleaning routine based on data-driven insights.

❏ **Conduct Follow-up Testing:** Periodically use Pathways™ Testing to evaluate protein-based contamination levels on floors, horizontal surfaces, personal possessions, and other key areas of your home.

❏ **Analyze Results and Refine Cleaning Strategies:** Compare protein levels from different locations to identify areas requiring more frequent or targeted cleaning. As the Pathways™ Testing results indicate, cleaning frequency should be increased in areas with higher contaminant levels. Damp disposable microfiber cleaning removes mold and bacterial contaminants more effectively from hard, smooth surfaces. If a persistently elevated level of proteins and peptide bonds emerges, this should be monitored closely and evaluated to see if a new area of concern or hot spot is developing.

❏ **Reassess Periodically:** Repeat Pathways™ Testing at regular intervals (e.g., quarterly) to monitor the effectiveness of your cleaning routine. Twenty Pathways™ tests per 1000 square feet targeting "areas of concern," but also collecting some from random surfaces can help adjust the schedule or methods as new trends or vulnerabilities emerge.

Step 23: Establish a Maintenance Plan and Periodic Monitoring Schedule

Proactive Maintenance: Setting the Stage for Long-Term Success

Establishing a maintenance plan and periodic monitoring schedule is essential for the early detection of new issues and the long-term health of your home. Regular inspections focus on areas prone to moisture and mold, enabling the prompt identification and resolution of any signs of water damage or mold growth. This proactive approach preserves the integrity of remediation work while minimizing the risk of future problems and associated expenses.

This step emphasizes the importance of systematic monitoring to detect potential issues before they escalate. By routinely checking areas susceptible to moisture accumulation and mold growth, you can address problems early and maintain a safe, healthy environment for your home's occupants.

A regular monitoring schedule reinforces the effectiveness of previous remediation efforts and prevents mold recurrence. This preventative strategy provides peace of mind and contributes to the overall well-being of your home. With routine inspections and proactive measures, you can safeguard your home against mold-related problems and maintain a healthy, mold-controlled living environment.

Exercise 23.1: Establishing a Maintenance Schedule and Monitoring Plan

❑ Create a general maintenance and monitoring plan to prevent moisture and mold issues, maintain a healthy home, and ensure the integrity of remediation work. For more detailed guidance, refer to the Maintenance chapter in *Prescriptions for a Healthy House*, which provides specific strategies tailored to health-focused home management.

› **Develop a General Maintenance Plan**: Identify key areas of your home prone to moisture or water damage, such as kitchens, bathrooms, laundry rooms, basements, crawl spaces, attics, and exterior elements like roofs and gutters. Create a list of regular tasks to address potential moisture issues, including cleaning gutters, checking for leaks, and

maintaining proper ventilation in high-risk areas. To ensure consistent, proactive maintenance, adjust the schedule for these tasks based on seasonal changes, such as increased vigilance during rainy seasons or in humid climates.

› **Establish a Monitoring Routine**: Conduct periodic inspections of moisture-prone areas, checking for early signs of water intrusion, mold growth, or system failures. Utilize tools like moisture meters or humidity sensors to detect hidden problems that may not be immediately visible. Document building-related observations in your project diary and health-related evaluations in your medical diary to create a clear record of patterns and progress. Address any issues promptly to prevent them from escalating into larger problems.

Exercise 23.2: Using SAIIE to Monitor Home Environment Changes

❑ Work with a qualified health provider to incorporate baseline parameters into your health maintenance and monitoring routine. The SAIIE framework can be used to detect and track subtle physiological responses to environmental conditions in your home over time. By comparing baseline data—collected when your home is a clean environment—with periodic health evaluations, you can monitor how changes in your living space may influence your health.

For example, if your health provider observes changes in biomarkers, symptoms, or visual contrast sensitivity (VCS) testing results, this may indicate a shift in the home environment, such as new moisture intrusion, hidden mold growth, or other contaminants. These changes could also be triggered by seasonal shifts, construction dust, building memory (residual contamination from prior issues), or lapses in routine cleaning. Changes in the frequency of cleaning, housekeeping staff, or cleaning methods can also influence the home's condition, potentially allowing contaminants to accumulate unnoticed.

To align SAIIE with your home maintenance routine:

• **Schedule periodic health assessments** to coincide with home inspections or seasonal maintenance tasks. This synchronization helps ensure your health and home environment are optimized together.

- **Use your project diary** to track environmental conditions (e.g., humidity levels, maintenance activities) and your medical diary to log health-related observations. Comparing the two helps identify potential correlations and ensures both aspects are effectively monitored.

Although SAIIE focuses on physiological responses, environmental monitoring tools like MSQPCR with HERTSMI-2 Score calculations and Pathways™ Testing can help detect contamination occurrences within the structure. Together, these methods provide a comprehensive approach to maintaining a mold-controlled environment and ensuring your living space remains optimized and conducive to healing and well-being.

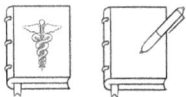

Exercise 23.3: Using SAIIE as an Early Warning System

This exercise helps you apply the Sequential Activation of Innate Immune Effects (SAIIE) protocol as an early warning system to monitor your health during emergencies or potentially lesser issues in your home. It can be used to monitor planned activities. It is also a way to monitor unplanned activities, emergencies, or accidents to detect changes in your body's response and uncover potential issues. Examples include when unrecognized contamination is released during routine remodeling, emergency water damage events are not dried quickly enough to prevent the amplification of organisms, or when adequate controls are not in place to prevent or recover from releasing unknown contaminants into your living space. By establishing baseline health parameters and performing timely monitoring, you can identify early signs that conditions are deteriorating. This allows you to assess whether emergency drying or temporary control measures are effective, if housing remains safe, and whether the level of personal protective equipment is sufficient when entering contaminated areas of the home.

It is important to recognize that this step relies on the heightened sensitivity of certain individuals to detect early signs that conditions in the home may be worsening. Their participation should always be voluntary, with informed consent, and only undertaken if their health condition allows such monitoring. This exercise is not intended for situations where a problematic area is entered unprotected or to test boundaries unnecessarily. Instead, it is designed for those unforeseen moments when an event, breach, or accident occurs.

- ❑ The Sequential Activation of Innate Immune Effects (SAIIE) protocol provides a structured method to assess whether the immediate measures taken are sufficient or if additional interventions are necessary to address the situation fully.

Relying on SAIIE for systematic evaluation rather than solely on perceptions or environmental testing ensures a timelier recognition of issues.

Establish Your Baseline SAIIE Parameters

- Work with your healthcare provider to determine and track the SAIIE parameters most relevant to your condition, such as:
  - › Biomarkers like C4a, MMP9, TGF beta 1, VEGF, or other inflammatory markers.
  - › Visual Contrast Sensitivity (VCS) scores.
  - › Symptom tracking tailored to your sensitivities.

Routine Monitoring

By consistently collecting and recording information at intervals in your Health Diary while living in a mold-controlled environment, you will establish baseline values that serve as a clear reference point for identifying changes in your health parameters if an issue arises.

Act Quickly After Water Damage or other emergencies to reestablish baseline parameters

If you discover water damage in your home, act quickly to evaluate its impact on you:

- Ideally, you should collect baseline SAIIE monitoring parameters the same day you discover the issue. This includes testing your biomarkers, repeating VCS tests, and noting any new or worsening symptoms.
- Record these results as your initial post-damage reference point.

Follow-Up Testing

Repeat SAIIE testing at logical intervals to track changes over time. After emergency drying measures are completed, conduct testing to assess their immediate impact on your health parameters. If remediation is needed, SAIIE tests and observations are performed to evaluate the effectiveness of each phase. Use these results to document whether your health parameters improve, stabilize, or worsen and to take appropriate actions to improve control measures or increase levels of effective cleaning.

Document Findings

Keep detailed records of all test results and observations throughout the process. These records can help you and your healthcare provider assess the impact and make informed decisions. These steps can.

- Provides objective evidence of whether water damage is affecting your health.
- Helps determine the success of drying and containment efforts.

- Guides you in deciding whether additional remediation is necessary.

- Offers valuable documentation for healthcare or legal purposes if needed.

Step 24: Revise your Maintenance Plan as Needed

Evolve Your Maintenance Strategy
Continually for a Healthy Home

As environmental conditions and home needs evolve, so should your maintenance strategy. Step 24 emphasizes the importance of regularly revisiting and updating your maintenance plan to respond to your home's specific characteristics, health, and broader changes in climate. Adopting a flexible and proactive approach will better anticipate humidity, moisture, and water damage concerns, ensuring a healthier living environment over time.

In a climate where global patterns are shifting and buildings are aging faster, adapting your plan with an eye to changing environmental conditions will help address potential risks before they become real. This includes using information from visual inspections, medical and building-related testing results, and awareness of how your home's unique features may react to new challenges over time. By continually refining your maintenance strategy, you can maintain a mold-resistant, safe, and resilient environment for years to come.

Exercise 24.1: Review the current maintenance plan

❑ **Evaluate** how your plan aligns with the home's changing needs and environmental conditions.

› **Inspect for Emerging Issues:** Conduct a visual inspection and note any new signs of moisture, wear, or mold. Pay special attention to high-risk areas like basements, crawlspaces, and attics.
› **Evaluate Seasonal Changes and Climate Impacts:** Look at how seasonal climate variations or recent extreme weather events may impact your home's needs.
› **Identify Areas Requiring Increased Attention:** Based on recent findings and testing results, mark areas that may require more frequent monitoring or maintenance.

Exercise 24.2: Adapt Maintenance Tasks for Climate Change

❑ **Modify or add tasks** in your plan to better address the effects of climate change, including increased humidity, higher temperatures, or changing precipitation patterns.

› **Increase Frequency of Key Inspections:** For example, increase checks for condensation and mold growth in enclosed spaces in areas with higher humidity.
› **Adjust Ventilation and Dehumidification Needs:** Revise settings or install additional dehumidifiers or ventilation solutions if humidity levels have risen.
› **Account for Temperature Extremes:** Evaluate the impact of recent heat waves or cold snaps on insulation, roofing, and weather seals, and adjust maintenance tasks accordingly.

Exercise 24.3: Update Long-Term Repairs and Replacement Schedule

❑ **Ensure your timeline** for significant repairs (roofing, HVAC, plumbing) reflects both climate conditions and materials' evolving durability.

› **Adjust Replacement Timelines:** Consider moving up the schedule for components exposed to harsher conditions, like roofing or siding in hurricane-prone areas.
› **Use Weather-Resilient Materials:** Plan to invest in durable, weather-resistant materials for future upgrades (e.g., moisture-resistant insulation or stormproof windows). Look for materials and systems that resist liquid entry but have permeability to allow water vapor to dry.
› **Create a Seasonal Checklist:** Develop a checklist of tasks to prepare your home for each season, reflecting local climate patterns and recent weather trends.

Exercise 24.4: Document and Monitor Adjustments

❑ **Be ready to adjust your plans.**

› *Log Adjustments and Observations:* Document each change made to the plan and note any improvements or challenges encountered.
› **Monitor Key Metrics:** Use tools like humidity sensors or energy usage monitors to evaluate how well adjustments meet your home's needs.
› **Review Annually or After Major Weather Events:** Set an annual or post-event review (after a significant storm) to evaluate the plan and identify further adaptations. For detailed recommendations on proactive care and long-term strategies, refer to the Maintenance chapter in *Prescriptions for a Healthy House*. This resource provides valuable guidance for refining your efforts and maintaining a healthy home environment.

Step 25: Develop a Budget and Contingency Fund

Prepare for Routine Upkeep and Unexpected Challenges

Develop a comprehensive budget and contingency fund for routine maintenance, unforeseen water damage, and mold expenses. With insurance policies increasingly limiting mold-related coverage, it's essential to anticipate and allocate funds for potential costs. Effective financial planning is key to the long-term health and stability of your property.

Follow these structured steps to create a budget that ensures you're financially prepared for regular maintenance and unexpected costs. Remember to account for your property's unique challenges, especially if it has confounding factors such as older construction, past water damage, or ventilation issues, which can increase ongoing maintenance costs. Additionally, plan for larger, long-term replacements, such as roofing, window, siding, and plumbing updates, which are critical to prevent mold and water damage over time.

Exercise 25.1: Assess Routine Maintenance Costs

❏ **Identify Regular Maintenance Needs**: List the routine maintenance tasks needed to maintain a mold-free environment. Everyday tasks include HVAC filter replacements, humidity monitoring, regular dehumidifier maintenance, gutter cleaning, and roof inspections.

❏ **Estimate Annual Costs:** Research the average costs of each maintenance item and compile a total for annual expenses.

Exercise 25.2: Evaluate Confounding Factors and Their Costs

❏ **Identify Property-Specific Challenges:** Review any confounding factors your property has, such as poor ventilation, previous water damage, or structural features that make maintenance more challenging.

❏ **Budget for Increased Maintenance Frequency:** For homes with issues like crawlspaces or older plumbing, expect to need more frequent inspections and maintenance, raising annual costs.

❏ **Account for Additional Repairs:** Properties with confounding factors often require unexpected repairs. Plan to allocate 10–20% of your yearly maintenance budget for these factors.

Exercise 25.3: Plan for Longevity Issues and Major Repairs

❏ **Budget for Long-Term Repairs:** Anticipate the need for significant repairs or replacements, such as a new roof, updated plumbing, or HVAC upgrades. These items are essential to prevent water intrusion and maintain air quality.

❏ **Roofing:** Depending on materials, estimate for replacement every 20–30 years.

❏ **Plumbing and Electrical Systems:** Plumbing pipes often need replacing every 20–50 years, especially if original materials are prone to leaks. Electrical system updates may also be required, particularly if mold exposure has affected wiring insulation.

❏ **Windows and Insulation:** Older or poorly installed windows or insulation can allow moisture intrusion, contributing to mold growth. If these are nearing the end of their life, include them in your budget.

❏ **Allocate a Major Repairs Fund**: Set aside a portion of your budget each year (5–10%) specifically for these larger expenses, even if they're not anticipated in the immediate future. This reserve will help spread costs over time rather than facing a large, unexpected outlay.

Exercise 25.4: Establish an Emergency Contingency Fund

❏ **Set Aside a Reserve for Unplanned Expenses:** An emergency fund is essential because water damage and mold issues can arise unexpectedly. Consider setting aside 10–15% of your property's annual maintenance budget.

❏ **Account for High-Impact Events:** If your property is in an area prone to heavy rainfall, hail, flooding, or humidity, budget extra for emergencies related to these conditions. This could include emergency water extraction, mold remediation, and temporary housing if areas of the home become uninhabitable.

❏ **Review and Adjust Annually:** Revisit the contingency fund each year, adjusting based on past maintenance costs and any new property conditions.

Exercise 25.5: Evaluate Insurance and Out-of-Pocket Costs

❏ **Review Insurance Coverage:** Understand the extent of mold and water damage coverage in your homeowner's insurance policy. Many policies now have caps or exclusions for mold-related claims.

❏ **Plan for Gaps in Coverage:** If your policy does not cover mold or has low limits, plan to cover a significant portion of potential remediation costs out of pocket. This may increase the amount you need to save in your contingency fund.

❏ **Explore Supplemental Insurance Options:** Some providers offer separate mold coverage; consider adding this if your property is especially vulnerable to water damage or mold growth.

Exercise 25.6: Track and Adjust the Budget Annually

❏ **Monitor Spending Against the Budget:** Track all maintenance and repair costs throughout the year to compare them to your initial budget. This data will help refine your estimates and ensure the budget meets actual needs.

❏ **Adjust Based on Property Condition and Changes:** If new issues arise or your property undergoes repairs that reduce risks, adjust your budget accordingly. Routine adjustments allow you to allocate resources effectively, ensuring sufficient funds for ongoing maintenance without over-reserving.

❏ **Include Inflation and Rising Costs:** As costs for labor and materials increase over time, adjust your budget annually by 3–5% to ensure it remains sufficient for future needs.

Part Three: Contents and Personal Possessions

ABOUT OUR THINGS

Our personal belongings fall into many categories. There are things we use to perform utility functions in our daily lives, including household appliances, entertainment equipment, tools for work, clothing, bedding, items we use for personal hygiene, and medical devices. Other things have a deeper meaning. Irreplaceable keepsakes remind us of good times, sad times, people and places we love, and memories or lessons we have learned. In most situations, our possessions in moldy, water-damaged buildings can be salvaged. Still, it depends on the amount of damage and the degree of personal sensitivity to mold.

The good news is that not everything has to be thrown away. Many things can be cleaned and returned to service. Even severely water-damaged items of value can often be preserved, stored, or displayed, for example, in an air-tight case or other ways that separate the affected person from the item.

When planning what to do with possessions, many hypersensitive people have bodies that overrespond. These extreme overresponses can be lessened or eliminated over time and with appropriate treatment. This is not to suggest that hypersensitive people will ever be able to expose themselves to contamination with impunity, but that, ultimately, the goal is to return mold levels and its by-products to normal background levels, which allow or facilitate the body to function.

Remediation, Restoration, and Preservation: Goals and Differences

Remediation involves physically removing mold and other contaminants from affected items or areas to ensure a safe and healthy environment. Just like with the building, the primary goal of remediation is to eliminate harmful substances by physically removing them rather than attempting to kill them. This process can include thoroughly cleaning by HEPA vacuuming and removing the particles and oils with microfiber cloths dampened with a detergent solution, provided the dampness will not damage the object. This is the first step toward restoration. The focus is on health and safety, ensuring that contaminants are effectively removed so the environment no longer poses a risk to the most sensitive person living in the home. Remediation removes contamination to render the item free of contaminants, but its appearance may still be damaged or stained. Repair restores function, while restoration returns function and appearance to their pre-damaged condition.

Restoration goes beyond remediation by repairing and restoring items or areas to their original or near-original condition. Restoration aims to address damage, making the items functional and aesthetically pleasing again. This process can involve repairing physical damage, refinishing surfaces, and replacing damaged components. Restoration aims to return the item or area to its pre-damaged condition in functionality and appearance, making it seem like the damage never happened.

Preservation, in contrast, focuses on maintaining the current state of an item or area to prevent further deterioration. The primary goal of conservation is to stabilize the environment and protect the item from future harm, often without making it suitable for active use. Preservation is used for personal possessions with sentimental or historical value that may no longer be suitable for regular use but desire to be kept intact. In some cases, when complete restoration is not possible, practical, or immediately necessary, preservation can be used to store the item to prevent further deterioration until restoration is deemed appropriate. The item may even be stored contaminated, but in a way where the contaminants will not be shed into the environment.

In summary, while remediation, restoration, and preservation all address damage and contamination, they have distinct goals and methods. Each approach is chosen based on the specific needs and circumstances of the items or areas in question, ensuring the most appropriate care and treatment.

CONTENTS OVERALL STRATEGY

Before discussing the specifics of content cleaning, it is helpful to understand the underlying philosophy and opinions regarding mold remediation of content. First, consider items with settled spores, particles, or fragments but no actual mold growth. Almost every item with settled spores and fragments can be returned to a healthy condition if enough time, effort, and money are spent.

- Many home items don't warrant wasting time, effort, and money because they can be replaced for far less than handling, cleaning, and storing.

- The degree of remediation needed should be based on the level of sensitivity of the most reactive person in the household.

- The most reactive person in the household is rarely the person who should be doing the cleaning but is frequently the most motivated to do a good job. Some sensitive people decide to do their own cleaning; while this is commendable, it often exacerbates symptoms. Personal protective equipment can help, but it is never 100%. If you are not accustomed to working with protective gear, you must be aware that it is often hot and uncomfortable and may not provide you with the level of protection or comfort you expect or need.

- The more significant the length of time a porous item such as an upholstered sofa has been exposed to spores and fragments, the greater the likelihood they have become "ground in" or "deeply penetrated," and the more difficult it will be to clean the item.

- Hard, non-porous objects like finished wood, glass, ceramic, metal, and plastic are significantly more straightforward to clean than soft, porous materials such as upholstered furniture.

- Thin, soft, porous materials such as shirts, blouses, pillowcases, towels, and other linens are much easier to clean by laundering than thicker, porous materials such as comforters and stuffed fabrics.

- Mattresses, pillows, and upholstered furnishings are among the most difficult or impossible to thoroughly clean. Barrier materials may be applied to the outside of these types of items to help protect them from contamination entering or exiting.

- Soft or porous materials with actual mold growth are rarely cost-effective to restore. In most cases, the growth can be identified visually by the staining, swelling, distortion, and musty odor present on the item.

IDENTIFYING POSSESSIONS WITH MOLD GROWTH

Just like our buildings, when our belongings grow moldy, it is always due to moisture. If items contain nutrients or dust with digestible ingredients and remain damp for a sufficient period, mold will grow. Wet/damp wood, paper, cardboard, natural fiber cloth, and stuffed upholstered furniture are nutrient-rich materials and will be invaded by root-like structures called hyphae if the item remains damp for a few days. The hyphae transport nutrients that support mold growth, much like plant roots absorb nutrients. Mold aids the digestion of nutrients by releasing acids and enzymes into the moisture layer, allowing the breakdown of the material. This process makes the nutrients soluble in the water, which nourishes growth. Digestion stops when the material dries out, causing the mold to go dormant, but it can begin again if the damp condition returns.

Mold growth on personal possessions can be caused by either liquid water or water vapor.

- Liquid Water: From rain, floods, pipe breaks, or other water damage emergencies can saturate personal belongings. These must be dried quickly and thoroughly to prevent mold from growing. Liquid water damage can also cause some belongings to crack, swell, buckle, cup, warp, and stain beyond repair long before mold growth can develop.

- Water Vapor: High levels of water vapor in the form of excess humidity can support mold growth without any liquid water being present. Sometimes, the dew point is reached, and condensation forms. A few types of mold can grow when the relative humidity at the surface of an item reaches 61%. Meanwhile, at 70% humidity, multiple types of mold readily grow on surfaces.

- Condensation: When condensation moisture forms and remains, it can initially produce a light layer of mold on the damp surface. If recognized and addressed early, restoring these items by drying and cleaning the surface before digestive enzymes cause permanent damage is often possible. However, if condensation repeatedly forms on surfaces or remains continuously damp, cumulative mold growth can cause permanent damage.

- Musty Odors: For books and papers, a musty odor from excess humidity may form long before visible damage. The odor is frequently the first sign that something has become too damp. Immediate drying can arrest further deterioration, and detailed cleaning can return the books or papers to a serviceable condition. Still, the items may not be worth the time and money necessary.

Hard plastic, glass, metals, stone, ceramics, and tile will only develop mold if there's a layer of nutrient-rich dirt or dust on them. These hard-surfaced items can almost always be cleaned to remove mold growth. However, if the moisture conditions that lead to mold growth remain uncorrected, the problem will reoccur.

Personal possessions damaged by mold growth should be evaluated case-by-case to determine if restoration, preservation, or remediation is appropriate. For example, preserving an original birth certificate or other legal documents may be necessary when only the certified original is considered valid. Storing each document page separately inside a clear, adequately sized, sealable plastic bag can allow the document to be examined from both sides through the bag.

Replacing inexpensive and readily available items may be the simplest and most cost-effective option. However, preservation, remediation, repair, and restoration might all be crucial for high-value items like a famous painting or work of art. Depending on the owner's choices, items with high sentimental value may be temporarily preserved until they can be remediated, repaired, or restored as necessary and desired. For valuable specialty items, it is a good idea to get the best expert advice you can. I will try to advise you on the general concepts for lesser items, but ultimately, you have to decide what is and isn't appropriate for your situation.

IDENTIFYING POSSESSIONS WITH SETTLED SPORES AND FRAGMENTS

Since mold and other microorganisms only grow in dampness or excess moisture, it is much more common for personal possessions to remain dry but become cross-contaminated when dust containing mold spores, fungal fragments, and other water damage-associated organisms become airborne, travels a distance from an area where the mold has developed and settles onto dry surfaces elsewhere in the home. This contamination not only affects the building but also settles onto our belongings.

Hard-surfaced items can be easily cleaned to remove this contaminated dust.

Cross-contamination spreads when items are moved from contaminated to clean areas. Proper cleaning of surface-contaminated items before moving them can return them to normal condition. However, cleaning without addressing sources of contamination allows new spores and fragments to spread and cause recontamination. This often results in the perception that the item was unsuccessfully cleaned when, in fact, the cleaning was successful, but cross-contamination was redeposited on the surfaces.

If you've spent time on discussion boards about mold and mold illness, you've likely seen advice suggesting that you throw away all your belongings and start over. While this scorched earth approach might initially seem compelling, I disagree. It has significant downsides, such as the unnecessary loss of valuable items, emotional distress, and financial strain. People who follow this approach often have more regret and harm than benefit. There are many things to consider, but when you are highly reactive, buying new things may not be the answer. Although brand-new furnishings and items are expected to be clean, this isn't always the case. Some manufacturing plants and storage facilities have mold contamination problems, which can transfer to new items during production or storage.

There are other ways that unanticipated mold can be introduced into indoor environments. For people who do not experience sensitivities, these may not present an obvious problem. However, more frequent, routine, effective cleaning may be a good choice for those with sensitivities to help prevent cross-contamination issues from developing.

Some other considerations include:

- Staged furnishings used in homes for sale have sometimes caused mold inspection failures, introducing mold into otherwise uncontaminated spaces and causing an otherwise acceptable space to be rejected.

- Secondhand stores are loaded with second-hand spores.

- Transporting contaminated items from one location to another without proper cleaning can spread microscopic spores and fragments, contaminating a clean home.

- Most people do not suffer notable effects and overlook the risk of cross-contamination, but mold-sensitive individuals can react severely. What triggers a reaction in one person may not affect another, and those with mold sensitivities can have varying responses. Authoritative sources agree that buildings should not cause occupant health complaints, and this principle should also extend to personal possessions. (ACGIH, 1999) (USEPA, 2008)

TRIAGING THE APPROACH TO ADDRESSING CONTAMINATED CONTENTS

When dealing with contaminated contents in your home, triaging your approach can significantly streamline the remediation process. Removing non-essential items from the house first helps facilitate building remediation by allowing for a more focused effort on addressing structural issues. Packaging and storing contaminated items is much faster than evaluating, cleaning, packaging, and storing them individually. This triage method prioritizes immediate removal over thorough cleaning, enabling quicker progress in restoring your living environment.

Unexpected complications may arise during the remediation process, potentially leading to cross-contamination. Packing personal possessions in boxes or wrapping them can help mitigate this risk. Protected items are far less likely to accumulate additional contamination. It's much easier to clean the outside of a box than to individually clean all the items stored inside. Storing these boxes offsite offers even more protection by ensuring that ongoing remediation efforts won't add further contamination to your belongings.

Some may argue that because everything in the home is already contaminated, boxing or wrapping items isn't necessary since they'll be cleaned eventually. However, my experience shows that upfront protection makes a significant difference. It can mean the difference between maintaining the expected level of cleaning versus undergoing multiple rounds to remove additional layers of contamination that might accumulate if things go wrong.

To implement an effective triage system, it's essential to have a clear, consistently used labeling process to avoid mixing up items. Color-coded labels are particularly useful for this purpose. The colors act as visual reminders when opening boxes, indicating the contamination status and whether the contents have been cleaned adequately. For example:

- **Red Labels**: Items that are heavily contaminated and have not been cleaned.
- **Orange Labels**: Items that are moderately contaminated and need further cleaning.
- **Yellow Labels**: Items that have been cleaned but may need additional cleaning or cautious handling.
- **Green Labels**: Items that have been thoroughly cleaned and are ready to return to the home after remediation and restoration are complete.

This color-coded system organizes and tracks contaminated items and ensures no confusion arises during remediation. When it's time to clean and restore these items, the labels will guide the necessary precautions and help prevent accidentally opening a box with contaminated contents.

Additionally, separating non-essential items and storing them temporarily helps maintain a clutter-free environment, making it easier to conduct thorough cleaning and remediation of the building. Once the structural remediation is under control, you can systematically address the stored items, ensuring they don't reintroduce contaminants into the cleaned environment.

When packing and protecting contaminated items, it's helpful to triage them according to the cleaning process they will undergo. For example, laundry should be packed together and sorted so that each box of items will be handled and cleaned the same way. Mixing items that need dry cleaning with those that can be washed in a machine would result in having to sort them again later. Grouping electronics, shoes, and non-washable accessories separately ensures each category is treated with the appropriate cleaning process, saving time and effort during remediation.

Additional ways to sort items can include:

- Breakable Dishes: Separate fragile dishes from resilient ones to prevent damage during storage and handling.
- Silverware, Pots, and Pans: Group easily cleaned kitchen items such as silverware, cutlery, pots, and pans.
- Artwork and Family Memorabilia: Keep valuable and sentimental items like artwork and family memorabilia separated from regularly used utility items.
- Books, CDs, and Record Albums: Sort media items by type to facilitate specific cleaning and restoration methods.
- Business Records: Group business records by topic, such as tax filing records, to keep them organized and accessible if needed. Keep one special box separate for things you are likely to need soon.
- Small Electrical Appliances: Pack small appliances like toasters and coffee makers separately from other items.
- Lamps and Lighting: Group lighting fixtures and lamps together.
- Stuffed Decorative Pillows: Keep soft furnishings like pillows or stuffed toys together.
- All Plastic toys should be separated from board games and other toys that have paper components.
- Musical Instruments: Store instruments separately, ensuring they are packed securely to avoid damage.

Some items might best be taken directly to a specialist for cleaning and safe storage. These high-value or specialty items include artwork, guns, jewelry, stamps, and coin collections. Items of significant value or requiring special care may even warrant storing in a safe deposit box or other secure storage facility for maximum security.

Consulting with professionals for these items can ensure they are properly cleaned and protected, avoiding potential damage and preserving their value.

Using a triage approach requires discipline and consistency in labeling and handling items. However, it can significantly reduce the stress and workload of dealing with mold-contaminated possessions, ultimately leading to a more efficient and successful remediation process. Later in the contents section, you will find an alphabetized list of different types of personal possessions, suggested cleaning methods, and other specialized handling and storage suggestions.

SORTING TO FACILITATE THE CLEANING PROCESS

Since no two situations will ever be the same, the process must be modified as necessary. Here is an example of one way to proceed.

Step One: Set Up a Priority Box

The priority box is for things you need to be available or do immediately, such as unpaid bills. This is also the place for Passports, driver's licenses, medications, and other possessions that must not get packed away where you can't find them. Set up a second box for necessary documents anytime in the next twelve months. This would include documentation for filling out your tax returns and other business or financial records that will need to be taken care of in a relatively short period over the next few days to a year. Mold remediation almost always takes longer than you anticipate. That's an unfortunate fact, but it is true—so don't fall into the trap of throwing everything together and allowing it to be mixed up. There's a good chance you'll have some delays. Also, prepare a bag with essentials that need immediate cleaning for the next few days, like preparing for a change of clean clothes.

Step Two: Trash the Trash

Now, walk through each room with an eye towards things that have no value, are trash or no longer wanted, and are going to be discarded. Get rid of them first. Have empty boxes or trash bags ready for things that will not be kept, such as assorted rags or clothing full of holes. If there's no chance you will use it again, then there's no reason to keep it. You don't need to catch everything, but the more unnecessary items that can be eliminated, the less that will be in the way.

Step Three: Document the Damage with Photos and Records

Taking photos or videos is one of the most effective ways to document the condition of your possessions. Be sure to include valuable items you may need to discard or donate. This documentation can be crucial for insurance claims and may be useful for tax purposes. Tax laws regarding casualty losses, medical expense deductions, and disability-related tax credits are complex. Consulting with a tax professional or accountant is essential to ensure you claim all eligible deductions and credits. They can also advise you on any necessary documentation, such as a doctor's prescription or declaration of medical necessity, which may be required to support your deductions.

This careful documentation and understanding of tax implications can help you manage the financial impact of water damage, mold contamination, or mold-related disabilities.

Step Four: Remember Your Plants and Pets

If you have house plants, they'll need some extra care. It is probably best to move them outside if it's that time of year when the weather permits them, and they won't suffer the consequences of being moved outdoors. Large-leafed plants are much easier to clean than small-leaf plants, but over time, even the finest of leaves can be cleaned by having them in an outdoor location where you can repeatedly spray them with a stream of water or air-wash them. But for now, get them outside if the weather permits. Realizing that your plants have died due to neglect or abandonment can be disheartening. Even more devastating is when a forgotten pet, like a turtle or fish, is remembered too late after it has passed away. Think about these things and how to approach them early on. Take dogs or cats to the groomer for a bath using a pet-safe soap or shampoo, followed by a thorough rinsing. It is not necessary and often dangerous to use toxic chemicals on pets or anything else. Be aware that although most internet advice is well-intentioned, some is malicious!

Step Five: Clean Items Twice

Plan on double-cleaning most things to create a contamination break. You can clean things by HEPA vacuuming and wiping with a dry microfiber cleaning cloth. Still, depending on whether the object can handle dampness, using a dampened microfiber cleaning cloth with a small amount of soap solution added to the water is better. Five drops of dish detergent to a quart of water spritzed from a spray bottle onto a disposable microfiber-type cloth is usually suitable for cleaning most items. If they are very greasy or have an oil film or polish, you may need to increase the amount of detergent. The trick is to use just enough detergent to emulsify the spores, fragments, and fat-soluble toxins so they can be wiped away without leaving soap residues behind. My first choice is always to use Branch Basics All Purpose Cleaner.

For fine wood furnishings, a detergent-based cleaner specially designed for wood furniture may be appropriate (for example, Bona, Murphy's, or Seventh Generation Wood Cleaner). Whatever you use, always test clean a hidden area first to be sure the cleaning agent and moisture won't damage the finish. Don't be fooled by advertising that promotes using biocides, antimicrobials, or other products to kill mold. In my opinion, these are unnecessary marketing tactics that frighten people into believing that mold spores or fragments that have settled onto surfaces require toxic options to be effective.

Items cleaned as they are placed into the packing box must be completely dry before packing. When arriving at their destination, they should be cleaned outdoors before being brought back after remediation or moving to a new place. Ideally, they come out of the box outside, and the packing material is discarded and never brought into your new home.

You may want to consider the benefits of keeping non-essentials boxed or wrapped in storage for a while and gradually cleaning the items as needed. Take time to clean them properly before moving them into the new place. Rushing the process may result in cross-contamination.

Step Six: How to Pack

Many cleaning aspects involve steps you would be doing during a regular move. Collect items and keep track of the rooms that they are in. Pack them so they don't get broken as they are boxed and transported. Fill boxes as much as they can reasonably hold and try to group similar things. Not filling boxes wastes storage space and increases the risk of breakage. Make sure that things are secure within the packaging. It's best to protect fragile contaminated items with clean packing paper. This is oftentimes available from packing stores in large rolls. You may also find it in rolls from companies that print newspapers. The idea is not to use newsprint because the ink may transfer onto your things. It's important not to trap moisture, so bubble wrap or plastic bags may not be advisable. Tyvek Building Wrap® can be used to wrap both large and small items and allows water vapor to diffuse through. This reduces the potential for trapped moisture, resulting in mold growth in items that have been stored before they are completely dry. It can also help allow condensation to dry before damage results.

Step Seven: Deciding to Sell, Donate or Gift

This is an individual decision you will need to make. Secondhand stores inadvertently and unknowingly accept many items contaminated with settled spores. Most people with hypersensitivity to mold intuitively know they can't shop at second-hand stores or their purchases must be adequately cleaned. If you decide to gift or donate items, a round of cleaning would be a kindness, but many people in need will be grateful to take a mold-contaminated item and clean it themselves.

Step Eight: Already Protected Items

Some of your things are already protected and packed, such as items in drawers, totes, boxes, or other protective covers. These items are frequently stored clean and don't need to be unpacked or repacked. Use a disposable microfiber cloth to clean the outside of the box container or enclosure. If the box is dirty, you may want to HEPA vacuum it first, then remove the items before disposing of the box. Items protected in clean drawers and cupboards are easy to seal into a clean box.

Step Nine: Label It

The trick to finding things later is ensuring your boxes are labeled accurately and clearly. Label sides, as well as the top. Labeling makes it easier to know what is in a box when stacked together. Label the boxes by the level of cleanliness, item category, and room. For example: "Not Cleaned," "Cleaned Once," "Unknown Cleanliness," Type of item—"Books," "Electronics," "Mixed Curios," "Ceramics"; Location—"Library," Kitchen," "Bathroom."

Step Ten: Sort by Item Type

Sort by type of item since similar items are cleaned in similar ways. Keep electronics together in the same box. Clothing, bedding, and linens that can be laundered should be sorted by type and packaged together. Separate dry-cleaning items from washable items. Keep books, records, audio tapes, videos, and CDs in separate boxes since each has its own way that needs to be cleaned. Also, it's much easier to clean things in batches or groupings where the same procedure will be used.

Step Eleven: Don't Overload Boxes

If they get too heavy, they'll be hard to move, and somebody may be injured. The smallest packing boxes are often referred to as book boxes. Since the number of books that can be stored in the box is fewer, there is less chance that the box will get too heavy.

Step Twelve: Use Packing Tape to Seal Seams

Use packing tape, not duct tape. It is easy to cut open and reseal the boxes. Sealing the seams will prevent contaminants such as spores, fragments, and dust from getting in or out.

Step Thirteen: Use Desiccant Packs

You may want to use silica gel packing packets to help absorb excess moisture. This is especially important if you are going to be using plastic bins, bubble wrap, or plastic bags, which can form condensation inside when temperatures fluctuate. Silica gel packets are designed for boxes and containers of different sizes. They should be big enough to protect your things by absorbing the excess moisture for as long as they are in storage or while being shipped. If you live in a humid area, it may be necessary to change the silica gel desiccant periodically. Some silica gel packets will change color when it is time to change them—but if you don't check often enough, it may be a problem. If items are being individually wrapped or stored in plastic bubble wrap or plastic bags, the silica gel must be inserted inside the plastic with the item to protect it. Items loosely packed in plastic bins need the silica gel packets in the bin. Silica gel packet sizes vary from the small packets used inside vitamin jars to protect the tablets from moisture to several pounds for large shipping cargo containers. Small packets are generally measured in grams. Larger packets are measured in ounces. There are approximately 30 grams to an ounce. A three-ounce packet is about right for helping protect a six cubic foot box that is 24" by 24" by 18". A one-ounce packet will generally be suitable for a small book box. These are general suggestions for the process, but every situation will be different, so it is necessary to use common sense and good judgment and modify these recommendations depending on the circumstances.

PREVENTION OF DETERIORATION DURING WATER DAMAGE EMERGENCIES

When contents are wet, the top priority is rapid drying. The faster an item dries, the lower the risk of mold development. Professional restoration companies often lift furniture off wet surfaces by placing rigid foam blocks under each leg to elevate the item and promote air circulation around its surfaces. Cardboard boxes on wet or damp floors should have their contents immediately transferred to a dry box, with wet items set aside for focused drying. The original box should be discarded to prevent further contamination.

It's often best not to wait for materials like linens and clothing to dry on-site. Sending them immediately to a professional laundry or dry cleaner can help prevent further damage. Items labeled "dry clean only" may shrink if not blocked or preserved in their original form. Specialty items such as jewelry, coin collections, musical instruments, firearms, and artwork should be promptly removed and taken to a specialist in the care and restoration of such items. Similarly, computers and electronic devices should be prioritized for backup and preservation to safeguard stored information.

Specialists are trained to preserve the maximum value and appearance of items, bringing them back to their best possible condition. They also know how to store specialty items to prevent further damage. For example, leaving a wine collection in an environment undergoing rapid drying with dehumidification could "bruise" the wine due to elevated temperatures. Additionally, the process might dry out the corks, increasing the risk of spoiling the wine.

PACKING CONTAMINATED ITEMS FOR A MOVE OR STORAGE

Regarding packing for cleaning contents, the primary goal should be maximum speed and efficiency and minimize inconvenience and cost. If you are hypersensitive to mold, it may not be appropriate for you to do this work yourself, yet you are probably the most motivated to have it done correctly. What follows are some things to consider as you go about the process.

If you are hypersensitive, get the work done by someone you trust. A well-positioned clear plastic window on the side of the containment can allow you to monitor workers' activities from a distance. A body cam worn by workers can also allow you to monitor and direct their activities at a distance.

Get rid of the perishable things that will spoil quickly and make no sense to put through a cleaning process.

Remember to empty the trash! Please remove perishables before they perish and develop mold in the trash can or compost bucket. The more disposable items you can eliminate by getting them out to the dumpster, the better and easier it will be for you to deal with the other things you want to save.

Avoid getting sentimental about the items you are cleaning or packing. If in doubt about a non-perishable item, don't waste time thinking or reminiscing—keep it and package it to store it. This way, you don't have to spend time cleaning it right away.

Don't feel like you must clean every item immediately to 100%. Many contaminated items can be stored for later processing and cleaning. Initially, focus your helpers on the things you will need right away. Give those the extra effort to clean them on the way out the door thoroughly and then do a second cleaning when they arrive at the new place before they are ever taken inside. Two rounds of cleaning are generally sufficient for hard-surfaced items. By breaking the cleaning into two separate rounds, with the last cleaning just before you bring items into the new place, you can help break the cross-contamination cycle. Clean outdoors whenever you can. This is much easier and less expensive than establishing and maintaining a containment with HEPA-filtered contamination control inside.

The contaminated items you're not so sure about needing or needing right away can be stored as is but preserved. Later, they must be cleaned before they are returned to use.

If you are hypersensitive to mold, you may want to talk with your medical practitioner about whether it's appropriate for you even to be a part of the cleaning process. Some people insist on being a part of the cleaning process no matter what! In that case, they must realize that even with personal protection, minor lapses in attention to detail may trigger their sensitivities and make them feel miserable. Unconsciously wiping the sweat off your forehead with the gloved hand you've been using to handle items with settled spores and fragments can result in significant exposure for a sensitive person. Such exposures may take extra time to recover or even be a further setback to medical treatment. Also, a person suffering from mold-induced "brain fog" may not make the best decisions or be very effective in their cleaning efforts.

CLEANING METHODS

Contents Remediation & Cleaning.

When a house is contaminated with mold or other micro-organisms related to water damage, it is usually necessary to remediate the home's structure and address personal possessions afterward. This is often referred to as content remediation or content cleaning. Factors that should be included in making decisions regarding contents cleaning include:

- history of water damage,
- physical damage to the item,
- value of the item,
- visual evidence of mold growth,
- musty odors,
- medical recommendations made by one's medical practitioner,
- laboratory results,
- the needs of the most hypersensitive person living in the household.

Due to the diverse materials used in manufacturing personal belongings, content remediation and cleaning often require more specific approaches than those used for a building's structure. Now, we focus on addressing various items, including evaluating the extent of contamination and employing preservation or remediation techniques when mold has developed. Additionally, we'll explore how to clean settled spores, fragments, and other particles from various materials and personal possessions. Remember, the

longer an item stays wet, the greater the risk of damage and mold growth. Keep things dry, and mold will never have the chance to thrive!

In many instances, the decision to keep or discard an item after water exposure hinges on the extent of the water damage, regardless of mold growth. Water absorption can cause a range of issues such as swelling, cracking, warping, buckling, cupping, staining, and pitting—often rendering an item irreparable before mold even has a chance to develop. Mold growth is just one of many consequences of prolonged water exposure. While some types of water damage and mold can be addressed, porous items that remain wet long enough for mold to establish itself are typically beyond restoration due to the physical deterioration caused by the water. Rapid drying is essential to arrest water damage before it becomes permanent, preserving the item's appearance and functionality and stopping mold from taking hold.

Even if possessions in a moldy house have remained dry, they may have settled spores, hyphae, and other mold and microorganism-related fragments that traveled on air currents around the home before settling onto the items.

- In general, spores and fragments can be removed from most surfaces by following the cleaning recommendations provided by the item's manufacturer. While these methods are often focused on maintaining appearance, a simple substitution—such as using a soft, damp microfiber wipe instead of a soft cloth—can significantly improve the cleaning of mold residues. The methods used to clean settled spores and fragments are often similar to those needed for cleaning dirt and grease from an item. Addressing the dirt and lipids or oils that accumulate on surfaces provides for effective cleaning.

- Hard, non-porous surfaces are easily cleaned using mild soap or detergent in water to dampen a microfiber cloth.

- Soft, porous items like clothing or linens can be successfully laundered or dry cleaned with laundry detergent.

- Cleaning thick, porous items like upholstered furnishings is challenging. The spores, fragments, and particles can be vacuumed from upholstered surfaces immediately after settling onto that surface. However, the longer the upholstered item is used in a contaminated environment, the deeper the particles are ground into the padding. It becomes a lot more work with less chance of success. Several minutes of daily HEPA vacuuming appears to reduce the contaminant level at the surface, which may provide temporary control. However, it is uncertain how long an increased level of cleaning will be necessary to return the items to normal.

- More specific suggestions for cleaning specialty items will follow later in this Chapter.

COMPLICATED ITEMS

Not every item falls neatly into the categories of porous or non-porous. Some, like leather, fall in between, and certain non-porous items, such as electronics, may be made of durable, waterproof materials but still have ventilation holes that make the interior vulnerable. Additionally, many objects are composed of different materials. For example, as I sit here, I'm looking at a ceramic drum with a leather skin stretched taut, secured by a metal ring held in place with braided macramé jute twine, decorated with fringes of string, yarn, beads, feathers, and felt-like materials. This drum includes various materials, ranging from completely non-porous to entirely porous. Contamination could be relatively simple to clean if contamination were limited to settled spores and fungal fragments. However, mold growth from prolonged moisture exposure would be a more significant challenge.

If the value of the drum lies in its sound quality, it could likely be restored to a usable condition by stripping and discarding the decorations. However, restoration becomes more complex if the value is in the decorations. Most items with mold growth can be restored to the point where they no longer pose a health hazard. However, they may not be suitable for hypersensitive individuals, and their appearance and functionality may remain compromised. Specialized experts can often restore severely damaged items, but restoration may not be cost-effective, depending on the item's value. For example, replacing a dime-store novel is far cheaper than restoring it. On the other hand, a first edition of *Tom Sawyer,* signed by Mark Twain, would merit professional preservation and restoration efforts.

PERSONAL PROTECTION

Anyone working to assist with cleaning mold from items should be protected. The level of protection needed depends on many factors, including the types and quantities of mold that will be encountered, the nature of the work activities, and where the work is going to be performed. Most people think of mold as only creating an airborne risk, but skin contact can result in skin and mucous membrane irritation, rashes, intense itching, and toxins absorption through the skin.

Personal protection goes beyond safeguarding the individual dealing with mold in their home. Inadequately protected support helpers can unknowingly carry mold contaminants back to their own homes, potentially exposing their families. While this may not pose an issue for most people, around one in four individuals have a genetic predisposition that makes them more sensitive to mold, potentially affecting them at much lower concentrations.

How Clean is "Clean Enough"?

The question of how clean items need to be is a highly individualized consideration, particularly for mold-sensitive individuals. For most people, the general goal is simply the absence of mold growth, with spores and fragments present in quantities and types similar to those typically found outdoors, along with an acceptable overall appearance. However, for those with heightened sensitivities, the required cleanliness levels may need to be much lower, making it difficult to predict how thoroughly personal possessions must be cleaned to avoid triggering a reaction.

Achieving a balance between cleanliness and immune health poses a unique challenge, especially in environments managed for mold-sensitive individuals. According to the hygiene hypothesis, overly sanitized environments may hinder the immune system's development by limiting exposure to everyday microbes that help "train" it. This theory suggests that asthma's prevalence in developed nations could be partly due to such hyper-clean conditions disrupting the immune response during critical postnatal stages. While it's essential to minimize mold exposure to prevent reactions, creating an excessively sterile environment could weaken immune resilience, ultimately requiring a nuanced approach to ensure cleanliness and immune support. (Bloomfield SF, 2006)

Cleaning Frequency and Surface Considerations

After remediation, maintaining appropriate cleanliness levels becomes an ongoing effort, especially for those who are hypersensitive. Repeated cleanings over time can help replace old contamination with newer, uncontaminated dust, gradually improving the acceptability of the environment. A study of randomly selected homes found that after detailed cleaning of carpeting, it takes approximately four weeks for the level of mold spores to return to pre-cleaning levels. (Anderson, n.d.)

Using a rule of thumb, if we estimate that 3% of mold contamination builds up daily on horizontal, hard, non-porous surfaces (e.g., tops of furniture, open shelves, and counters), cleaning once a week could keep the build-up at roughly 25% of the levels expected if cleaning were only performed monthly. Thus, a two-week cleaning cycle may be insufficient for sensitive individuals, but it is generally more than adequate for people without sensitivities. When an item has been allowed to accumulate mold residue for months, it may require multiple rounds of cleaning to remove the build-up adequately.

The type of surface also affects cleaning requirements and effectiveness:

- **Horizontal surfaces** like floors and tabletops accumulate the most dust, dirt, mold spores, and fragments.

- **Rough or textured surfaces** are more challenging to clean than smooth surfaces, as they trap more particles.
- **Personal possessions** left out in the open tend to collect dust quickly, adding to the cleaning burden.
- **Carpets** and area rugs can harbor significant dust and dirt, requiring more effort and time to clean than hard-surface floors.
- The **surface area of personal possessions** often exceeds the combined floor, wall, and ceiling surfaces in a home, making them a major contributor to overall contamination levels.
- **Spores and fragments** tend to settle downward. Large horizontal surfaces require more frequent attention than vertical surfaces or the undersides of objects. For example, a picture frame's top edge typically collects far more dust than its vertical surface.

Managing Clutter to Reduce Cleaning Efforts

The more cluttered an area is, the greater the cleaning effort required to maintain appropriate conditions. Items left out accumulate more dust and contamination, complicating the cleaning process and increasing the needed frequency. To reduce the cleaning burden, it is helpful to minimize clutter, especially in spaces that need to remain highly clean for hypersensitive individuals.

- **Reduce** the number of items displayed or stored out in the open.
- **Discard** what is no longer needed or useful.
- **Store items in enclosed containers** to limit the dust they can collect over time.

Decluttering simplifies cleaning and ensures that the remaining surfaces are easier to access, reducing the risk of hidden mold contamination and making regular cleaning more effective.

CLEANING AND PRESERVATION METHODS

The following are general methods that can be used to remove mold spores, fragments, and other types of contamination from surfaces. It is up to the user to use good judgment to determine if a certain method will be more effective for different items. Not all items can be cleaned effectively because the cleaning process may damage some things.

Air Washing: Air washing with compressed air works best for hard, rough surfaces like unfinished wood. It is used when damp or dry-wiping with microfiber cloths is impossible because the rough surface or the wood will snag the cloth. It also works well for irregular surfaces that are difficult to clean due to small nooks and crannies. Air

washing is labor intensive but does a good job of removing particles clinging to most items' surfaces and blowing them into the air. For this reason, air washing should be performed outdoors or in a cleaning chamber with filtered exhaust ventilation to prevent a buildup of contaminants.

Air washing is performed using compressed air blown at the material's surface to be cleaned. A fan-shaped air delivery tip can help spread and control the air stream to ensure maximum effectiveness. The compressed air velocity must be high enough to overcome the static or molecular forces that hold the dust on the surface but not so strong that it damages the surface or injures the cleaning person. According to OSHA29 CFR 1910.242 (b), The maximum safe air pressure velocity for air washing is 30 psi. Some air compressors develop much higher pressures, which are greater than necessary and can damage the surface being cleaned. Personal protection is essential. Care should be taken to be sure that the blast of air doesn't project the particles at high velocity, which can injure the hands, but also project large particles into the eyes. Hearing protection should be worn if the noise is loud enough to cause hearing damage. Special pressure-reducing nozzles are available at auto parts supply stores that automatically reduce the pressure to a proper safe level.

Air washing should first be performed on an inconspicuous surface to test and be sure it will not cause damage to the item. Examples of items that may be best cleaned by air washing would include concrete block or poured walls and floors, rough-cut wood with multiple splinters, the rough, unfinished backs of many types of cabinets or dressers, and inside stringed musical instruments like guitars, violins and cellos where the interior is accessible for air washing via a sound hole. A flexible tube-like nozzle tip may be helpful to direct the airflow into tight spaces, such as the interior of items with small or irregularly shaped openings.

Most accessible surfaces for an item that is going to be air-washed should be HEPA vacuumed first to remove the bulk of the dust, spores, and fragments without projecting them up into the air. This is followed by air washing, with a final microfiber cloth cleaning of the accessible surfaces of the item(s) that don't snag the cloth.

It is usually easiest to perform air washing outside, away from contamination. Blowing the spore and fragments off the item will put them into the air, quickly diluting them to normal background levels. If air washing is going to be performed indoors, it is usually necessary to construct a cleaning containment chamber with negative air around the surfaces that will attempt to be cleaned. This is very much like establishing a containment chamber for isolating and remediating mold growth, but in the case of a cleaning chamber, it is generally maintained as a clean area to protect the items that are being cleaned from cross-contamination with the rest of the home. Care must be taken to prevent the high-pressure air stream from the compressed air from overcoming the negative air pressure in the cleaning chamber containment and potentially spreading contaminants around or blowing them outside and into adjacent areas. Working in the capture zone of a HEPA-filtered air filtration device can act as a temporary moveable hood set up for local exhaust ventilation. It can be an excellent way of controlling the contaminants that blow off an object by the high-pressure air stream.

Damp Wiping: Damp wiping uses minimal water to clean a smooth or slightly rough, hard surface. Damp wiping is most effective when used in conjunction with a disposable microfiber-type cleaning cloth. The wipe is folded into a size that fits the hand for manual cleaning comfortably, or it can be installed onto a mopping system disposable cloth holder on a pole. For surfaces that can tolerate a small amount of moisture, the cloth is dampened with a couple of spritzes of water with about five drops of your favorite dish soap or detergent per quart of water. There is much more information about this cleaning method in the Stage Three, Step 14 on "Effective Cleaning" and "Microfiber Cleaning Cloths" in the 25 Steps Guide. The same techniques used for cleaning the walls, floors, and ceiling can be adapted for cleaning personal possessions. Damp wiping can only be used with items holding up to a small amount of moisture. Always test an inconspicuous surface to be sure it can tolerate wet wiping without causing damage.

Dry Wiping: Dry wiping is performed the same way as damp wiping, however no moisture is used. Dry wiping is primarily used when the item being cleaned is not able to get wet or damp. It can also be used as a final step after damp wiping. The dry disposable microfiber-type cleaning cloth can remove excess moisture left on surfaces and pick up minor residues left behind by the damp wiping method. The wipe is folded into a size that fits the hand for manual cleaning comfortably, or it can be installed onto a mopping system disposable cloth holder on a pole. Dry wiping is typically the final step in fine particulate cleaning, which removes microscopic particles from the air by precipitating them on the horizontal surfaces in the work area. When fine particle cleaning is performed, the personal possessions and contents should be removed from the work area or adequately protected.

Deionized Water: Deionized water has all the salts and minerals removed and doesn't conduct electricity. The dissolved salts and minerals in the water conduct the electricity that shorts out electrical and electronic equipment when it gets wet. Deionized water can be purchased by the gallon at the supermarket, but cleaning electronics or other electrical equipment with deionized water is not typically a do-it-yourself technique. However, it is frequently and effectively used by professionals with specialized cleaning equipment. Deionized water does not conduct electricity; cleaned items should always be unplugged. Residual salt or other conductive mineral or dust deposits may mix with the deionized water to become conductive. Internal electrical components such as capacitors may hold a charge that can result in severe shock or electrocution even when the equipment is turned off. Only qualified persons who understand how to service electrical equipment safely should attempt these procedures.

Items are cleaned using deionized water. Air washing can blow off the excess water and help dry the surfaces. Gentle heat, such as from a hair blow dryer, is often also used for drying small items. More extensive materials are commonly professionally cleaned with deionized water and dried using a special chamber designed explicitly for that purpose (See O'Dell Electronics Cleaning Station below).

Dishwashers: The dishwasher is an amazing tool that can clean contaminated dust containing mold spores and fragments off surfaces. Dishwashers can be used for more than just dishes, pots, pans, and flatware. As with all forms of cleaning, you must use judgment regarding items that can be successfully cleaned in a dishwasher. In general, anything that is waterproof and can withstand the high-pressure wash jets may be able to be cleaned in a dishwasher. Common sense should be used when determining what to clean this way.

It is important to realize that many dishwashers use room air during the drying cycle. The location of the vent that pulls the air into the dishwasher for heating and drying is not always apparent. This means that if a dishwasher is used in a mold-contaminated environment, cross-contamination may be brought into the dishwasher during the drying cycle and cause recontamination of freshly washed items.

Net-type dishwasher bags can be used to wash small waterproof items like small toy building blocks and other small toys and curios. The items are placed loosely in the bag and then run through the dishwasher on the rack. Some items may be able to be mechanically washed in the dishwasher but not tolerate high temperatures. It is important to evaluate the item to determine the appropriate water and drying temperature to prevent damaging the items.

Dry Cleaning is used primarily for relatively thin clothing, linens and fabrics that are listed by the manufacture as requiring dry cleaning. Dry cleaning uses a variety of non-water-based liquids for cleaning. For more information see the Chapter on Laundry and Dry Cleaning.

Freezing and Freeze Drying is a preservation technique that can slow or prevent further mold, bacteria and other biological contaminants from developing. If damage has already developed it will remain on the item, but further growth or damage may be arrested with varying degrees of success. Rapid or flash freezing at colder temperatures using commercial flash freezers or dry ice typically causes less damage to the item. Slower freezing, such as if you place a wet book in the freezer at home, may allow ice crystals to form, which can cause physical damage to the paper. Flash or rapid freezing creates less damage, but in an emergency, a home freezer may be better than nothing or can at least start the chilling process while a flash freezer is located to finish the process. Rapid action by freezing items such as valuable books or documents during the first 24 hours after they get wet can frequently halt further deterioration and allow the item to be restored to almost as good a condition as before it was wetted.

Once frozen, a freeze-drying process similar to that used in food preparation to make instant coffee and dehydrated survival foods can remove the water and prevent additional microorganisms from growing. The drying part happens when the frozen item is placed in a chamber that keeps the item at freezing temperatures but at the same time depressurizes to a point where the ice sublimates. This means the ice turns directly into water vapor without passing through a liquid phase. The water vapor is continuously exhausted from the depressurized chamber as it forms—hence the drying. Once the excess water is removed to a point where mold or bacteria cannot grow, the item can be removed from the chamber to restore it to its original condition. Not all types of books and papers freeze well. Some types of water-based printing inks will run, and some pages will melt together, making them impossible to salvage. Carefully placing sheets of wax paper between the pages before freezing is a technique art conservators may use to help limit the damage. Some specialty water damage restoration contractors have semi-truck-size freezer units and large commercial freeze-dry chambers that can be used when catastrophic events like floods or hurricanes damage libraries with large quantities of irreplaceable literature. Some taxidermists have small freeze-dry chambers that can dry a few frozen items at a time. Meat lockers for specialty butchers that cater to hunters and small farms and ranches will usually be able to flash freeze boxes filled with books to preserve them until arrangements can be made for drying in a freeze-drying chamber.

HEPA Vacuuming is essential for removing large quantities of contaminated dust and dirt from the surface. In general, a vacuum cleaner creates suction between the head or nozzle of the vacuum and the surface being cleaned. The nozzle should have spacers to position it slightly above the surface, allowing air to flow across the area being cleaned for more effective vacuuming. The loose materials become aerosolized into the air stream and pulled into the vacuum cleaner, where a series of filters remove the debris, dust, and particles before the air is exhausted back into the room. To clean, the vacuum cleaner must have enough suction or lift to capture and pick up the various forms of dirt and particulate. When working to clean up contaminants generated by water damage, the vacuum must also have sufficient filtration capacity to collect and contain the tiny particles that are sucked into it, so they aren't released by the vacuum cleaner back into the room air. To adequately filter the air before it is released back into the room, the vacuum cleaner should have an adequately sized HEPA filter so that it doesn't restrict the airflow leaving the vacuum cleaner. As the filter becomes clogged, the airflow reduces, and the suction or particle lifting ability declines, so the vacuum cleaner no longer cleans effectively.

Since mold spores and fragments are mixed right in with the dust and dirt, HEPA vacuuming helps remove loose contaminants while simultaneously cleaning. HEPA vacuuming is generally the first step in cleaning a surface contaminated with by-products from water damage, such as mold and bacteria. Professionals in the mold remediation industry were incorrectly taught for decades that cleaning should always begin and end with a round of HEPA vacuuming. This was called a "HEPA Sandwich". We know today that the second round of HEPA vacuuming is useless and may reintroduce new contamination particles. It also creates a static charge on the vacuumed surface, causing a thin layer of dirt and contamination to become stuck to the surface. HEPA vacuuming is best used as a first step to remove large quantities of dust and debris and not blow contaminants back into the air. It is typically followed by effective cleaning techniques such as Laundering and Damp or Dry Wiping using microfiber or electrostatic cloths. The HEPA vacuuming removes the largest amount of debris, dirt, spores, and fragments, so the Laundering or Wiping can pick up the last bits of mold particulate and remove the other residues.

Just because a vacuum cleaner advertises it has a HEPA filter does not mean it will always work. One study of HEPA-type vacuum cleaners found that about half were not functioning up to standard and were spewing mold and other water-damaged organisms and fragments back into the air every time they were used to vacuum carpets. (Brandys, 2012)

A Laser Particle Counter can check HEPA vacuum cleaners to ensure the HEPA filter functions. Air from the unit's exhaust is drawn into the particle counter past a laser beam focused on a light-sensing surface. Each particle causes the light to scatter onto a different part of the sensor. The equipment then interprets the sensor information so the size and quantities of the particles can be determined and reported.

Laundering is used primarily for relatively thin clothing, linens, and fabrics, except for those items that cannot be laundered.

Microfiber Type Cloths (disposable): Examples of disposable microfiber-type cleaning cloths for use in cleaning up fine particles such as mold spores and fragments include unscented Swiffer Wipes, Rubbermaid Hygen® Wipes, and others. The finely divided fibers are less effective than a new reusable microfiber cloth. Still, they are better for use on highly contaminated surfaces since they can be discarded. I am not a big fan of loading our landfills with discarded items, but when dealing with mold contamination from settled spores, I would rather discard a disposable microfiber-type cloth than the item itself.

The difference between the cleaning ability of a disposable microfiber-type cloth and a paper towel is amazing. Microfibers pick up and retain more contamination, whereas paper towels quickly load and smear the contamination around instead of removing it.

Microfiber Cloths (reusable): Microfibers pick up and retain contamination, whereas regular cloth towels quickly load and smear the contamination around instead of removing it. Unfortunately, microfiber cloths need special cleaning measures, so they are rarely cared for properly. This means they are not generally doing the best possible job. To be adequately cleaned, reusable microfiber cloths must be cleaned with special detergents and held at temperatures between 165° and 185° Fahrenheit for multiple cycles of washing, typically requiring almost an hour. They can not be laundered with other items or exposed to chlorine bleach or other harsh chemicals. The higher temperatures during this cleaning process allow the microfibers to relax and release dirt and contaminants. If the specialized laundering processes are not used, substantial amounts of contaminants remain in the wipe and can potentially re-contaminate surfaces instead of cleaning them.

Pressure Washing: Pressure washing should only be used to clean durable or waterproof items. Pressure washing is often used as a first round of cleaning waterproof items instead of HEPA vacuuming. If you have oily or greasy items or spilled dried liquids, then pressure washing may be an excellent first step for cleaning. Portable pressure washing systems can also be used outside to clean items. As with every cleaning method discussed, it is important to test clean items to be sure they will not be destroyed or damaged by the high-pressure wash stream. As with all wet cleaning processes, wet items should be rapidly and thoroughly dried before being brought inside to avoid contributing to mold growth on more sensitive surfaces with moisture or humidity transfer.

Ultrasonic Cleaning: Ultrasonic cleaning uses high-frequency vibration to clean waterproof items that can fit in the ultrasonic cleaning tank. These machines range in size from those for small items such as jewelry cleaning to large, long tanks used for cleaning Venetian blinds and other more oversized items with intricate surfaces. The equipment used for ultrasonic cleaning is expensive, so it is not typically a do-it-yourself method. Still, compared to the time necessary to effectively hand clean an intricate surface like a Venetian blind, it can be worth transporting the item to a professional facility specializing in ultrasonic cleaning. It is important that the facility changes the cleaning solution between batches and that the items be rinsed well after being removed from the tank to remove the residues.

Ultrasonic cleaning using deionized water has been effectively used to clean electronic circuit boards, computer system interiors, and other electronic and electrical equipment. This specialized equipment is usually only available from specialty cleaning professionals.

Odell Electronics Cleaning Station: The Odell Electronics Cleaning Station specializes in cleaning electronics and electrical components. It's a high-end piece of equipment that professionals use rather than DIY enthusiasts. One of its standout features is deionized water, which doesn't conduct electricity, making it safe for cleaning delicate electronic parts that would otherwise be damaged by tap or stormwater due to their mineral content. This system ensures that circuit boards, computer components, and other electronic items can be thoroughly cleaned with a reduced risk of electrical shorts or damage.

The Odell machine also has a built-in drying chamber, which prevents moisture from lingering in the equipment after cleaning. Thorough drying is critical because any remaining dampness could lead to mold regrowth or further damage. This integrated cleaning and drying process ensures that items like dehumidifiers or other sensitive electronics are restored to a safe, functional condition.

The Odell system is ideal for severe cases of insufficient standard cleaning methods. The machine maintains a controlled environment by utilizing a negative air exhaust to prevent dust and debris from escaping during cleaning. This professional-level cleaning process is highly effective for removing mold spores, dirt, and contaminants from complex electronic devices, providing care that is difficult to achieve with manual cleaning methods. Professional cleaning services using systems like the Odell can help recover electronics that might otherwise be deemed unsalvageable. Their advanced cleaning technology ensures that even severely contaminated items can be restored to functionality, prolonging their useful life and contributing to healthier indoor environments.

GENERAL PROCEDURES FOR CLEANING PERSONAL POSSESSIONS

The following methods outline the general procedures for cleaning various types of surfaces. Since personal possessions can be made of a wide range of materials and combinations, applying common sense and adjusting these recommendations to suit the specific item and situation is important.

These procedures assume that the materials being cleaned are dry. If wet or damp items are found, cleaning alone will not prevent further damage. Deterioration will continue until the items are properly dried. The cleaning methods should always be selected based on the type of material and its condition.

Mold Growth on Natural Fabrics (Natural—Wool, Cotton, Silk, Hemp)

Natural fabrics such as wool, cotton, silk, and hemp can support mold growth if they become wet and remain damp for an extended period. When mold grows on these fabrics, it digests and weakens the fibers, often resulting in discoloration or staining. This damage typically makes restoring the item impractical and not cost-effective. However, it may be possible to preserve and, in some cases, restore historical or sentimental fabrics that have sustained mold damage. The success of such efforts depends on factors such as the degree of saturation, how long the item remained damp, the temperature during that period, and the nutrients available for mold growth.

The acids and enzymes produced by mold can severely compromise the structural integrity of the fabric, preventing it from being returned to a usable condition. However, the item's damaged appearance may still be preserved to avoid further deterioration, but the priority must be drying the item to stop any additional growth. Restoration of significantly mold-damaged, high-value materials can be expensive and may require expert assistance at the curator level. Preservation, which aims to halt further deterioration, is usually less costly but will still need expert advice beyond the scope of this book. Preservation may involve neutralizing or removing the acids and enzymes in the fabric and packing the item in an airtight, desiccated container or display.

In most cases, natural fabric items with actual mold growth are unlikely to be restored for regular use, particularly for individuals with mold sensitivities.

Settled Mold Spores and Fragments on Natural Fabrics

Natural fabrics that have settled mold spores or fragments without mold growth can typically be cleaned using the laundering or dry-cleaning methods recommended by the manufacturer. However, these fabrics generally do not function well as barriers and often allow the penetration of mold spores and fragments, depending on the tightness of the weave. One exception is tightly woven silk barrier covers for mattresses and pillows, which can encase items and prevent the penetration of mold spores and larger fragments. More research is needed to understand why silk works effectively as a barrier in these cases.

Most thin natural fabric items, such as comforters, quilts, and jackets (less than half an inch thick), can be successfully cleaned of settled spores and fragments through laundering or dry cleaning. Thicker items may require a case-by-case assessment to determine their salvageability. In general, two rounds of laundering with soap or laundry detergent is sufficient to remove most mold spores and fragments. However, individuals with mold sensitivities may benefit from a third cleaning round, especially if the "sticky" organism *Chaetomium globosum* is present, to help maximize thorough decontamination.

Mold Growth on Synthetic Fabrics

Synthetic fabrics themselves do not support mold growth when they become wet. However, a layer of dust, dirt, or skin cells can provide the nutrients necessary for mold to colonize the synthetic material and grow on or around the fibers. Once mold begins to grow in synthetic fabrics, the extent of the damage depends on the fabric's stability when exposed to the acids and enzymes released by the mold as it digests the dirt and other nutrients present on the surface. Many fabrics are blends that include synthetic and natural fibers, and these mixed fabrics are less likely to be successfully restored once mold growth occurs.

In many cases, laundering synthetic materials can remove mold growth and the dirt or nutrients deposited on the fabric. The process typically begins with HEPA vacuuming to remove a substantial amount of dirt, spores, and fragments. This is followed by one or two rounds of laundering or dry cleaning, depending on the sensitivity of the individual using the item, the type of mold contamination, and the effectiveness of the cleaning method. Each round of cleaning should include the use of laundry detergent to ensure thorough removal of contaminants.

Settled Mold Spores and Fragments on Synthetic Fabrics

Settled mold spores and fragments can be easily removed from synthetic fabrics through laundering or dry cleaning *(refer to "Laundering" on page 323, "Dry Cleaning" on page 321)*. Some synthetic fabrics are also effective barriers, preventing the penetration of mold spores and fragments. For woven synthetics, the tightness of the weave plays a significant role in determining their effectiveness as a barrier. At the same time, non-woven fabrics like Tyvek are particularly good at blocking tiny spores and fragments. This means that certain padded or stuffed synthetic fabric items, such as jackets and winter wear, may only need surface cleaning—such as HEPA vacuuming—followed by laundering or dry cleaning to remove dirt, dust, and contaminants from the fabric surface.

Mold Growth on Leather Suede or Vinyl

Leather and suede can support mold growth if they remain wet for a sufficient period, as the organic nature of these materials provides nutrients for mold. In contrast, vinyl does not support mold growth directly, but an accumulation of dirt and dust on its surface can provide the organic nutrients needed for mold to grow. Once mold growth begins on these materials, the extent of the damage depends on the material's stability when exposed to the acids and enzymes released as the mold digests the dirt and other nutrients present on the surface.

Settled Spores on Leather Suede or Vinyl

Settled mold spores and fragments can be easily removed from leather, suede, and vinyl surfaces by using a HEPA vacuum and cleaning with microfiber cloths. Specialty soaps, detergents, or surfactant-based cleaners are available for hand-cleaning these materials and can typically be used with disposable microfiber cloths. Testing an inconspicuous area first ensures the material is colorfast and can be cleaned without damage. Leather, suede, and vinyl generally act as practical barriers against the penetration of mold spores and fragments, making it possible to clean padded or stuffed jackets and winter wear by removing surface dirt, dust, and contaminants with HEPA vacuuming, followed by the manufacturer-recommended cleaning method.

However, some leather, suede, or vinyl materials have small perforations that penetrate through the material. It may be necessary to examine the material closely with a strong magnifying lens or microscope to determine if these holes go all the way through. If they do, mold spores and fragments may pass in and out of the items during use, creating potential reservoirs of contamination. While the surface of the leather can be cleaned, items with penetrations may still be unsuitable for individuals with mold sensitivities due to the risk of spores and fragments being released from the padding.

METAL, GLASS, CERAMIC
Mold Growth on Metal, Glass and Ceramic

- Metal, glass, and ceramic are hard, non-porous materials with smooth surfaces that do not provide the nutrients needed to support mold growth. However, these materials can still become contaminated by settled spores or fragments present in dust. If the surface becomes damp, a film of organic material or biofilm can develop, providing the nutrients necessary for mold growth. Cleaning mold growth from these surfaces should focus on removing the nutrient layer or biofilm. In cases of actual mold growth, more aggressive mechanical cleaning methods may be required, such as using a dishwasher, ultrasonic cleaner, or pressure washer.

- Typically, a soap, detergent, or surfactant cleaner is sufficient to remove surface films. It is important to use low-suds detergent when using mechanical cleaning equipment according to the manufacturer's instructions. If high moisture levels have caused rust or corrosion on metal surfaces, addressing the corrosion may require professional evaluation and restoration, as it goes beyond the scope of this book.

- If the metal component is part of an electrical system, there may be an increased risk of fire, shock, or electrocution due to the damage. In such cases, professional evaluation is necessary to ensure that the function and safety of the item have not been compromised.

MOLD GROWTH ON STONE OR CONCRETE

Remediation for stone and concrete is similar to metal, glass, and ceramic; however, stone and concrete often have rougher surfaces. Like metal, glass, and ceramic, these are hard, non-porous materials that do not contain nutrients to support mold growth but may become contaminated by settled spores or fragments in dust. The rough or pitted surfaces of stone and concrete can make them more challenging to clean. A nutrient-rich film can develop on the surface if the material is damp, supporting mold growth. Therefore, cleaning efforts should focus on removing this nutrient or biofilm.

When mold grows on stone or concrete, aggressive mechanical cleaning methods such as a pressure washer, ultrasonic cleaner, or dishwasher may be necessary. In most cases, a soap, detergent, or surfactant cleaner will effectively remove the surface film. It is crucial to use a low-suds detergent and follow the manufacturer's instructions when using mechanical cleaning equipment.

Settled Mold Spores and Fragments on Stone and Concrete

Cleaning settled mold spores and fragments from stone and concrete surfaces is similar to cleaning mold growth. For surfaces with heavy dust or debris, it is best to begin by using a HEPA vacuum to remove the bulk of contaminants. Spores and fragments can often be easily wiped away using microfiber cloths for smooth-surfaced stone or concrete.

For rough-surfaced stone or concrete, mechanical cleaning methods such as a dishwasher, ultrasonic cleaner, or pressure washer can save significant time and effort compared to detailed hand-cleaning, provided the items fit in the equipment. When dealing with large horizontal surfaces, the recommended method is to start with HEPA vacuuming, followed by using a truck-mounted extraction cleaner. This cleaning removes contaminants into a wet collection tank, with the contaminated air exhausted outdoors. Ideally, the exhaust should be HEPA filtered, but in most cases, exhausting the air several feet above the truck and away from buildings or obstructions is sufficient. Using a low-suds detergent surfactant in the cleaning solution helps contain the mold particles and fragments, allowing them to be safely flushed down the sanitary sewer system.

Mold Growth on Paper or Cardboard

Books, documents, and other items made of paper or cardboard that get wet must be rapidly dried to prevent mold growth. Blowing dry air from fans can effectively dry items that can be spread out, such as individual pages of documents or photographs. This method may leave the items wrinkled, but gently ironing them with clean linen or pressing them in a paper press can often help remove the wrinkles and return them to an acceptable condition. If an item cannot be completely dried within 24 to 48 hours, the risk of mold growth increases significantly. Flash freezing is another option, preventing mold growth from starting or arresting it in its early stages. This method allows the item to be preserved for later freeze-drying. Freeze-drying requires sophisticated and expensive equipment, typically reserved for high-value, irreplaceable books and documents. The drying process involves depressurizing the chamber to create a vacuum, allowing the frozen water to sublimate directly into vapor, which is then exhausted from the chamber. Some meat packing plants that cater to hunters offer flash freezing and storage services while arrangements are made to send documents and books to a freeze-drying chamber. Rapid freezing helps minimize the size of ice crystals that form, reducing physical damage. Some taxidermists have the equipment for smaller quantities of books to perform this process. Specialty water damage restoration companies may also provide these services.

It is unlikely that paper or cardboard with established mold growth can be fully restored. In most cases, discarding and replacing the item is more cost-effective. However, when the information must be preserved but is unlikely to be used again, moldy items may be dried and packaged for storage without mold remediation. After the necessary retention period, documents that were never needed can be incinerated. Workers can retrieve the item from storage using appropriate personal protective equipment and photograph or copy it if the information is required. For example, some tax records must be kept for seven or more years but may never be needed. In such cases, the moldy items can be dried and stored without remediating the mold. Materials with information known to be required again can be copied or photographed for future retrieval.

Settled Mold Spores and Fragments on Paper or Cardboard

Papers, photographs, books, and other paper or cardboard-based memorabilia that only have settled spores or fragments and never got wet can be cleaned to remove the surface contamination. Generally, cleaning with a dry disposable microfiber cloth is required for settled contamination. Items that have been wrapped, boxed, or placed in albums with protective sleeves may be able to be removed from the contaminated outer covering, which is discarded, without needing to clean the recovered items.

Book and Paper Storage

It is common for books and papers to develop musty odors without visible growth in storage. This occurs in the beginning stages of mold contamination. If musty items remain damp, the development will worsen until the item can no longer be restored. Rapid drying and cleaning of the musty item may restore the item to an acceptable condition. However, silica gel desiccant packets are far better to keep these materials dry and prevent growth issues.

Mold Growth on Plastics

Plastics do not inherently support mold or other biological growth. However, accumulating surface dirt and dust can provide the organic nutrients that allow mold growth. Once mold growth begins on plastic surfaces, the extent of the damage depends on the material's stability when exposed to the acids and enzymes released by the mold as it digests the dirt and other nutrients present on the surface.

Settled Mold Spores and Fragments on Plastics

Heavy accumulated settled spores, fragments, and dust can be easily removed from plastic surfaces by HEPA vacuuming. However, the electrostatic charge on many plastics often leaves a fine contamination layer. This residue can be effectively removed by wiping with microfiber cleaning cloths dampened with soapy water, detergent, or surfactant-based cleaners. Depending on the item, solid plastics can also be effectively cleaned using pressure washing or running them through a dishwasher, using low-suds soap or detergent in water.

Mold Growth on Wood

Cleaning and restoring finished wood with water damage or mold growth depends on the type of wood, the finish, and the nature of the moisture exposure, as these factors influence the types and quantities of organisms that can grow. Surface mold on wood finishes or polishes is common in humid, damp environments. Mold can grow on the oil, wax, or polish applied over the finish, appearing as a fuzzy layer of dust on the surface. In such cases, the wood remains in good condition but requires cleaning to remove the mold and the nutrient layer of polish. The cleaning approach should be based on how deeply the mold hyphae have penetrated the wood. Sometimes, wiping the surface with a microfiber cloth dampened with a furniture soap, followed by a fresh coat of polish, is sufficient. However, suppose the mold growth has penetrated the wax or polish, affecting the varnish or wood itself. In that case, the item will need to be evaluated on a case-by-case basis to determine whether it is worth attempting restoration.

Mold growth on unfinished softwood can lead to swelling, cracking, warping, or staining caused by water damage. If the physical damage is not too severe, surface mold growth may be removed and cleaned to a condition where it no longer triggers reactions in hypersensitive individuals. Sanding while simultaneously using a HEPA vacuum is the typical method for effectively removing mold from softwood. This is followed by dry or damp wiping with a microfiber cloth to remove any remaining fine dust.

Some specialty woods may naturally display various colors due to mold stains that develop while the tree grows. These stains are dyes that have entered the wood cells and do not contain mold spores or fragments. Mold-related staining that develops in trees has not been reported to pose a problem for sensitive individuals. Any decayed parts are removed and discarded at the lumber mill. Mold-stained woods typically have a protective coating to preserve the wood and enhance the natural colors.

Restoration is generally unlikely in cases of mold growth on unfinished composite woods, such as oriented strand board (OSB), particle board, and medium-density fiberboard. If composite wood has been exposed to moisture long enough for mold growth, the water damage will typically have caused swelling and structural weakening, making the material unrestorable. An exception occurs when high humidity causes light surface mold growth without direct liquid contact. The wood may be cleaned using the same techniques for cleaning settled spores, as discussed in the next section.

Settled Mold Spores and Fragments on Wood Surfaces

Settled mold spores, fragments, dust, and debris can accumulate on wood surfaces. When visible dirt, dust, or loose debris is present, the first step is to use a HEPA vacuum to thoroughly clean the surface until no more loose material can be removed. After vacuuming, the surface should be wiped down with a clean microfiber cloth, either damp or dry, until no more dust or dirt can be removed.

Next, inspect the surface under strong lighting, viewing it from different angles or using a magnification lens to check for any remaining dirt, grease, or grime. If the surface still appears dirty and can tolerate some moisture, it may require damp cleaning. Damp cleaning is performed with a mild, unscented soap or detergent solution, such as five drops of dish detergent mixed into a quart of water in a spray bottle or a specialty wood cleaner like Bona or Murphy's. Instead of spraying the item directly, lightly spritz the microfiber cloth (two spritzes should suffice) and use it to clean the surface.

The goal is to clean the item until it is free of visible dust or dirt. A second dry wipe should then be used to confirm cleanliness. For example, a single wipe should be able to clean the top, underside, and legs of a 48 by 48-inch table, with the second wipe coming back clean and free of any visible dust or dirt.

Settled Mold Spores and Fragments on Rough or Irregular Wood Surfaces

When cleaning rough or irregular wood surfaces with intricate designs, grooves, nooks, and crannies, additional attention is required to effectively clean hard-to-reach areas. After HEPA vacuuming, evaluate the surface to determine if rough areas cannot be effectively cleaned with a reusable or disposable microfiber cloth due to snagging. If the item has intricate carvings or areas that are difficult to access, air washing may be the most effective method for removing settled spores and debris.

An unscented disposable Swiffer wipe can be cut into 0.5 by 1.5-inch strips and wrapped around a cotton-tipped swab to detail smaller areas. Dip the swab into a mild, soapy cleaning solution, squeeze it as dry as possible, and use it to clean the intricate details and grooves. Discard the swab when it becomes visibly dirty and continue with a fresh one. Repeat this process until no more dirt or debris is picked up by the Swiffer-covered swab.

Use reasonable judgment to determine the level of cleaning needed for rough surfaces that snag cleaning cloths. Air washing will remove the bulk of the item's dust, mold spores, and fragments. Since rough-surfaced items are unlikely to come into frequent close contact with people, the dry vacuuming and air-washing process may be sufficient to clean the item. A few remaining particles stuck to the surface are unlikely to cause problems for a hypersensitive individual, as they will not quickly become airborne or transfer through handling.

SPECIFIC CONSIDERATIONS FOR CLEANING PERSONAL POSSESSIONS

The following provides general guidance for cleaning specific types of items. If you are mold-sensitive, unsure how to clean an item, or unable or unwilling to do so yourself, this information can help you communicate with a knowledgeable individual who can evaluate the item. Together, you can decide whether the item is salvageable and determine the appropriate cleaning methods for removing mold and fragments associated with water damage. Given the wide range of items and circumstances, providing detailed instructions for every situation is impossible. This guide assumes you already have a basic understanding of the item you want to clean and know how to handle it safely without risking harm or damage to the item. For instance, this section assumes you know never to introduce moisture into the interior of electrical equipment and that handling or cleaning internal components of an electrical device—while it's plugged in or operating—is dangerous. While most items can be effectively cleaned, consider whether the cost of cleaning exceeds the item's value.

Air Purifiers

Cleaning air purification units should be performed following the manufacturer's instructions. Generally, the exteriors are made up of hard surfaces that can be cleaned like any hard-surfaced small appliance. The outside is typically cleaned with a disposable microfiber cloth dampened with a few spritzes of a non-toxic soap or detergent cleaning spray, as described earlier. If the interior needs cleaning, the disposable filters and gas-absorbing media are generally unable to be reused and should be removed and discarded. Protective screens or covers may provide access to the motor/fan assembly. In some cases, it may be

possible to use compressed air to clean interior surfaces without having to access them directly. If it can be done safely, the inside may be air-washed through the vent openings while the air purifier operates outdoors (without filters) as designed to be used. This allows the machine to help clean itself. New replacement filters can then be installed before use.

Appliances: Large (see the specific appliance)

Appliances should be maintained in accordance with the manufacturer's maintenance and safety instructions. In general, the outsides of large appliances are easy to clean using HEPA vacuuming followed by damp wiping. The horizontal surfaces accumulate more spore—and fragment-contaminated dust than the vertical surfaces. Large appliances should be pulled out once or twice a year to allow cleaning of their backs and sides, especially the condensation pan underneath. While they are out, it is an excellent time to clean the floors and walls that are otherwise inaccessible.

Cleaning the motors, pullies, belts, compressors, and other internal components that may be present in large appliances generally requires the assistance of a repair technician. Unfortunately, few are familiar with cleaning settled mold spores and fragments from the equipment they service, but many are willing to assist with their hourly service fee. By combining the information in this book with their knowledge of the appliance, they can effectively clean the internal components of these appliances. Generally, a HEPA vacuum cleaner and microfiber cleaning cloths can access most of the components. This can usually be performed with the appliance pulled out to access the top, bottom, back, and sides. If air washing is needed to blow out internal components, the appliance would typically need to be moved outside to prevent blowing contaminants into the house. Or it may be cleaned within a specially constructed cleaning chamber.

Appliances: Small

Most small appliances are kept put away where they are protected from settled dust. The outsides should be cleaned and maintained in accordance with the manufacturer's instructions. Generally, the outside can be cleaned with a disposable microfiber cloth dampened with a couple spritzes of a non-toxic soap or detergent cleaning spray. If the small appliance, such as a blender, food processor, or toaster has vent holes that lead to the interior, it may be able to be adequately cleaned by using compressed air to blow contaminants out of the interior through the vent openings (see "Air Washing" page 306). If it can be done safely, small appliances with a motor inside may be able to be air-washed through the vent openings while they are operating normally in the way they are designed to be used. A repair technician may also be able to open the appliance and use a combination of HEPA vacuuming, air washing and microfiber cleaning cloth to effectively clean the interior of the device.

Area Rugs
(See "Carpets and Area Rugs" on page 316)

Artwork

The nature and value of artwork influence how artwork is cleaned. Art can be made of various materials that may require different cleaning methods to prevent additional damage. The decisions and cleaning methods for art go well beyond the scope of this book and should be made with the assistance of a professional art curator experienced in the media that is being evaluated. The Conservation Center in Chicago is a well-established company that provides evaluation, stabilization, and restoration services. theconservationcenter.com

||||||||||||||||||||||||||||||||||||||||||||||||||||||||||||||||||||||||||||||||||||||||||||||||||||||||||||||||||||||||||||||||||||

Essay: Restoring Valuables After Water Damage
by Ramona Gallahger

Following water or moisture events, you may find yourself in the challenging position of needing to have your valuable, sentimental, and irreplaceable items cleaned or restored. The stress of deciding what to keep and what to discard can feel overwhelming, especially as your stress level during this time may be at an all-time high. Fortunately, many high-value antiques and fine decorative arts can retain their worth if properly conserved. Acting quickly to prevent further damage is crucial.

What to Do First
Stay Calm: It's important not to panic. You will navigate through this situation successfully.

Separate Items: The first step is distinguishing between damaged and undamaged items. Place anything that is dry and does not require mitigation in a clean, dry area away from wet, damp items to minimize further damage and cross-contamination. Remember, the key to success is preventing further damage.

Handling High-Value Antiques
Furniture: High-end antique wood furniture can be stripped and refinished. Upholstered items may be renewed, and new fabrics and cushioning can be replaced. Wet or damp furniture should be elevated on blocks to facilitate drying and airflow until a furniture restorer can assess the damaged item for restoration. It is essential to find a reputable furniture restorer specializing in valuable furniture who can address the perseveration of the patina. This fine layer builds up over time and enhances the appearance. Unknowingly removing it could permanently devalue the highly prized antique. When restored correctly, little or no value is lost.

Fine Art: Fine art—including oil paintings, watercolors, mixed media, and works on paper—can also be conserved. A key factor in minimizing further damage is the handling (or not handling) of the damaged fine art. Keep artwork hanging until a professional can safely remove it to a safe and healthy environment. Moisture or water damage can occur to frames; moving them can damage the gold leaf or gesso, the decorative edge of elaborate gold frames. Damage to the frames can be expensive and time-consuming to repair. Improper handling can also offset the corners or stretcher that binds the painting in place. If unable to keep artwork hanging in place, wet or moist paintings can be carefully laid out on a flat surface with the painted side up and with a protective barrier between the painting and the flat surface. This is usually done on blocks or a screening that allows airflow. Do not attempt to remove works on paper from their frames if the artwork is stuck to the glass.

Caring for Decorative Arts Sculptures and Ceramics: Non-porous decorative items that don't absorb moisture, such as metals, glass, and other non-permeating surfaces, can be gently cleaned with a damp cloth.

Decorative porous or semi-porous items should be staged to allow airflow to begin the drying process. A specialized expert should perform cleaning. Intricate pieces or those with areas that are difficult to access surfaces may require professional cleaning using controlled steam or air pressure.

Oriental Rugs
High-value oriental rugs are hand-knotted and usually made in the Middle East or Asia. Antique rugs are made from vegetable dyes and are susceptible to color runs and dye bleeds. When wet carpets become saturated with water, they are difficult to move. Never hang or fold a wet oriental rug, as it can easily damage the rug's foundation and might trigger additional color runs or bleeds. A rug cleaning expert should process valuable rugs.

Preserving Documents and Textiles
Documents and Books: If the water or moisture damage is minimal, and an environmentally safe and healthy area is available, then individual papers can be placed flat on a clean surface and air dried before conservation. Valuable documents, papers, and books can be freeze-dried to minimize the effects

of water or moisture damage. Specialized experts offer freeze-drying services. Freeze drying is an expensive process and is typically used when the value of the damaged item is greater than the cost of the service. The wet or damaged documents, paper, or books should be carefully packed with a dry barrier between the wet or damp layers. Wet or damp paper items should be shipped to a commercial freeze-drying facility immediately upon packing to prevent further contamination. If papers are stuck together, do not attempt to pull them apart. Once the damaged documents are dried or freeze-dried, they can be transported to the conservator for further evaluation and conservation.

Clothing and Textiles: Articles of clothing with direct water damage may show signs of color runs and dye bleeds and may not warrant salvaging. If clothing items are of high sentimental, historical, or other value where professional conservation or preservation is desired, then cotton, nylons, and polyesters can be washed according to the manufacturer's specifications at the correct water temperature to avoid shrinkage. Wools, cashmere, leathers, and expensive or designer fabrics should be processed according to the manufacturer's specifications. Wet clothing can be hung or laid out to be air-dried to

prevent further deterioration. At the same time, a decision is made to determine what will be necessary for cleaning and preservation. Dry cleaning items should go to a dry cleaner for proper cleaning. Most dry cleaners offer a laundry service where clothing can be washed and folded onsite. If you have an entire house or an apartment of textiles to clean, it is usually easier to call a specialized expert as soon as possible to remove these items. It is very time-consuming and would take several full days to wash and dry all the clothing in most average-sized houses.

The Importance of Professional Help

It is generally beneficial to call a specialized expert as soon as possible in the event of water or moisture damage to begin restoring, conserving, and preserving valuable, sentimental, and irreplaceable items. The specialized expert would be able to best guide you in the proper procedures and triage for the individual pieces or categories of items. They will also correctly pack the items for transport, saving you valuable time and emotional stress. If it is not possible to retain a specialized expert right away, then caution must be taken as items can easily be further damaged due to improper handling or care.

||||||||||||||||||||||||||||||||||||||||||||||||||||||||||||||||||||||||||||||||||||||||||||||||||||||||||||||||||||||||||||||||||||||||||||||||||||||

Automobiles, Cars, Vehicles

(See "Vehicles" on page 331)

Battery-Operated Electronics and Toys

Most battery-operated electronics and toys can be cleaned with damp wiping and air washing nooks and crannies in accordance with the manufacturer's instructions. Generally, the outside can be cleaned with a disposable microfiber cloth dampened with a couple of spritzes of a non-toxic soap or detergent cleaning spray, with air washing being used for cracks and difficult-to-access parts. *(See "Air Washing" on page 306).*

Books, Magazines, Journals, Bound Ledgers

(See "Mold Growth on Paper or Cardboard" on page 312)

Carpets and Area Rugs

Most wall-to-wall carpets in the United States are sold with synthetic backing material, less prone to mold growth than jute backing, which was commonly used in the US before the availability of plastics. Jute-backed rugs that remain chronically wet are a common source of nutrients supporting *Stachybotrys* growth in the carpet. This is also the case with paper seaming tape for joining wall-to-wall carpet, where it transitions from one room to the next, and when it is used to seam together smaller pieces of carpet, they fit a large room. Even 100% synthetic carpets that get

chronically wet can support mold growth in the dust and dirt they accumulate.

In most cases, the amount of moisture required for *Stachybotrys* to grow is too great for growth to happen in carpeting unless it is sitting on a chronically wet slab, such as in a damp basement or garage. *Penicillium* and *Aspergillus* organisms don't require as much moisture and will thrive on the various nutrients found in house dust.

When water flows into the carpet, there is a limited amount of time before it begins to fester and allow microorganisms to grow. The amount of dirt and house dust found in carpets provides nutrients so that when moisture is added, the spores begin to soak and prepare for germination. People who are not hypersensitive to mold may have up to 24 hours to discover and start the drying process. Still, families with hypersensitive individuals may only have a fraction of that amount of time before the carpet begins to support the growth of a variety of bacterial organisms, many of which can start multiplying much more rapidly than mold. (Holland, 2012) (IICRC, 2024) Since rapid drying involves air movement, it may be best to remove wet carpet from the home for drying or disposal. Since the carpet pad is made of sponge-like materials that hold large amounts of water—if drying is delayed, it is best if it is removed and discarded. (IICRC, 2021) For homes occupied by people with sensitivities to organisms associated with water damage. In most cases, they shouldn't even have wall-to-wall carpet. (CIRSx Institute, 2024)

Some companies performing professional water damage restoration want to lead by spraying wet carpets with an antimicrobial or a deodorizer. Unfortunately, this practice does not help much and frequently worsens matters. Chemical treatments such as antimicrobials or biocides are quickly broken down by organic materials such as the dirt that has built up in carpeting. Even when the treatments are considered safe, they may react with other substances in the soil to form more harmful by-products. People hypersensitive to organisms that develop during water damage are often sensitive not only to mold and microorganisms but also to antimicrobials, biocides, enzyme treatments, and fragrances or deodorizers they contain.

If a rapid drying response involving double extraction of the water, followed by cleaning and rapid drying, is impossible, the carpet should be removed and discarded. High-value area rugs may be able to be salvaged. Still, they should typically be removed and sent for specialized cleaning in a vat where they can be submerged, cleaned, and extracted under water multiple times until all the soils have been removed before beginning the drying process. This is a time-critical process that needs to start within 24 hours for the greatest success, ideally. Once mold has grown in carpets, they can rarely be salvaged cost-effectively.

The biggest problem with carpets is that they require a greater level of ongoing maintenance and cleaning than most people are willing to provide to remain healthy. In most water-damaged buildings, the carpet will have elevated mold spores and fragments deeply ground into the material. These contaminants have not grown in the carpet but were floating in the air and settled onto the carpet. The contamination is on the carpet's surface and can easily be removed. The longer the contamination is allowed to sit on the carpet, the more deeply it becomes ground in and engrained. Daily thorough HEPA vacuuming of carpet in a home with contamination being released from another area can remove the surface contamination before it has a chance to become deeply embedded. The longer settled mold contamination is allowed to remain on carpeting, the more labor-intensive it will be to get it under control.

Area rugs vary dramatically in the types of materials used for their manufacture. But, just like wall-to-wall carpet, all area rugs will develop mold growth in the soils they contain if they get wet and stay wet for a long enough time. Since area rugs are more accessible to remove for cleaning, they are generally easier to maintain than wall-to-wall carpets.

One study cited by the Carpet and Rug Institute showed that homes with adequately maintained carpets can have better indoor air quality than homes with bare, surfaced floors. (Buttner, 2002) The caveat is the carpet must be properly maintained by effective routine cleaning. At low contamination levels, carpets tend to trap and hold the dirt and particles. However, I have experienced that very few people routinely vacuum their carpets sufficiently to be considered adequately maintained. In addition, regular vacuum cleaners do not trap mold contamination. A HEPA-type vacuum cleaner is needed to remove the small mold-sized spores and fragments of mold effectively.

Cleaning mold-contaminated carpets involves repeated HEPA vacuuming using a properly functioning vacuum to clean the carpet from multiple directions until no more dust or dirt can be removed. Using a vacuuming pattern from all directions is important since the carpet fibers do not fully release the soil they contain when only using a back-and-forth motion. Thorough initial cleaning should be performed dry to remove as much soil as possible. Beginning the cleaning process with water will cause mud to form with the deeply embedded soils, making it more difficult or impossible to get them out. HEPA vacuuming multiple times at a rate of 2 minutes per square yard has been found to be often necessary to reduce mold contamination to normal levels. For example, a 12 by 12-foot carpeted room typically needs about 30 minutes of continuous HEPA vacuuming on three sequential days to sufficiently clean from mold contamination buildup. During the third day of vacuuming, no fine dust should be able to be collected. If three days of intensive HEPA vacuuming does not sufficiently reduce the build-up of dirt, there is a good chance that a dirt reservoir has migrated through the carpet and pad to the floor below. In one instance, I collected three pounds of dirt from the floor under a ten-year-old carpet in an apartment. The accumulated dirt was tested to determine what mold and bacteria were present at different levels. We found that the carpet and pad did not stop the penetration of mold and bacteria. The contamination levels under the carpet and pad were as high under the carpet as on top. (Holland, 2012) For people with mold sensitivities, cleaning and maintaining 1600 square feet of carpeting in a 2,000 square foot moldy home would require 6 hours to perform a weekly cleaning of just the carpet. For this reason, hard-surfaced flooring is preferable and can be cleaned and maintained much more quickly and effectively.

Cassette Tapes

Most cassette tapes are kept put away in a case where they are protected from settled dust. The outside case should be cleaned and maintained by dry wiping with a microfiber cloth. If needed, the interior cassette can also be cleaned the same way. Gentle air washing may also help blow out the internal parts of a cassette tape left out of its case. Cassette tapes should be kept protected from moisture. If they get wet, they are probably ruined and must be replaced. Irreplaceable content may be transferred to a CD or other electronic media by contractors specializing in recovering electronic and audio content from damaged media.

Compact Disks – CDs (DVDs)

Most Compact Disks are stored in a case that protects them from settled dust. The outside of the case should be cleaned and maintained by dry or damp wiping with a microfiber cloth. If needed, the interior disk can be cleaned using a disk cleaning kit available at electronics supply stores.

Cell phones

(See "Battery-Operated Electronics and Toys" on page 316)

Clothing

(See "Laundering" on page 323)

Clothes Dryers

When appropriately used, clothes dryers play a vital role in preventing mold growth by effectively removing excess moisture from freshly laundered clothing and linens. Built from materials that do not typically support mold growth, dryers can maintain a mold-free environment when correctly installed and maintained. However, improper installation, maintenance, or dryer use can introduce mold problems within the unit, exhaust ductwork, or the home. Even well-maintained dryers can exacerbate mold issues by depressurizing the home, pulling mold spores from wall cavities, and redistributing them into the air or onto clean clothing.

Conventional vented clothes dryers, commonly used in the U.S., must vent to the outside to expel moisture and, in the case of gas dryers, harmful combustion gases like carbon monoxide. When venting or airflow is compromised, such as when dryer lint clogs the vent duct, moisture can build up, leading to mold growth and cross-contamination of laundry. If the duct develops leaks or comes loose, damp lint and moisture-laden air can accumulate in hidden spaces, resulting in mold growth. Proper installation, regular maintenance, and venting to the outside are essential to prevent mold issues and ensure the dryer operates effectively and safely.

Essentials: Vented Clothes Dryers

Clothes dryers can cross-contaminate cleaned clothing when used in a building with a mold problem by depositing spores and mold fragments.

1. Clothes dryers must always be installed and operated according to the current code and the manufacturer's instructions. If you are unsure, consult a qualified installation and repair technician.

2. Clean the lint screen every time you use the clothes dryer. A clogged lint filter can accumulate enough to prevent clothes from drying and allow moisture to build up.

3. Have the dryer duct and exhaust vents inspected and cleaned at least every year to remove excess lint and ensure proper function.

4. Clothes dryers should only be used in clean areas free of mold contamination. Vented clothes dryers pull large quantities of room air into the machine, which can immediately cross-contaminate freshly laundered items when operated in a contaminated building.

5. Open a window in the laundry room while using the clothes dryer. This will help reduce the risk of potential contamination being pulled from wall cavities and other hidden spaces.

6. Use a clothesline to dry clothing temporarily until your home has been successfully remediated.

7. Ensure the dryer duct exhausts to the outside and does not blow damp, hot air into a wall cavity, attic, or crawlspace. Damp air can result in mold growth.

8. Unvented clothes dryers are top-rated in Europe but not very common in the US. A growing number of brands are becoming available.

   › They remove moisture from clothing by condensation instead of heat,
   › Are more energy efficient and less likely to cause a house fire or leak moisture-laden air into the building.
   › Establish normal pressurization levels with fresh outdoor air—so they don't pull mold contamination out of building wall cavities. This reduces the risk of recontamination of freshly laundered linens.

Collectibles

There are so many types of collectibles that each needs to be considered individually, depending on the materials used for their construction. If they get wet, immediate action may save them, but this depends on the item. A wet coin collection may be easily cleaned and dried, whereas wet baseball cards will deteriorate quickly, require specialty restoration, or may not be restorable. In many cases, collectibles are stored in boxes where they do an adequate job of preventing contamination from penetrating. This means only the outside box or case requires cleaning or replacement.

Computer (Desktop)

Unless you are experienced and comfortable opening and accessing the interior of your computer, this is probably best left to a repair technician or someone with experience. Generally, the outside can be cleaned with a disposable microfiber cloth dampened with a couple of spritzes of a non-toxic soap or detergent cleaning spray. A computer repair technician should be able to open the desktop computer and use air washing to effectively clean the device's interior. Some parts inside a laptop are sensitive to static discharge and may be damaged by some cleaning processes. HEPA vacuuming without properly grounding the components, the computer, the person cleaning the machine, and the vacuum cleaner may result in damage from static discharge. Blowing compressed air at too high a velocity may damage the internal fans if they can spin too quickly.

Computers (Laptops)

All the comments about desktop computers apply to laptops. Another consideration about laptops is that they are smaller and have less space to dissipate heat. The more compact design means they are often more challenging to access the interior. Unless you have special skills, they would require a professional computer technician for cleaning and restoration.

Computer (Monitors)

In most cases, an experienced person should only open computer monitors for cleaning. This is especially true for monitors that have capacitors inside them. Capacitors can hold a solid electrical charge for days after the monitor is unplugged, sufficient to cause a severe shock. The outsides of most monitors can be cleaned just like any other piece of hard-surfaced furniture. Still, the interiors should probably be air-washed with compressed air—used outdoors or in a filtered negative air pressure cleaning chamber.

Computer backup Disks and USB Drives

For backup Disks, see Compact Disks—CDs, DVDs. For USB and external hard drives, see Electronics (also see Battery-Operated Electronics and Toys)

Couches

(See "Furniture (Upholstered)" on page 322)

Curios

There are so many different types of curios that each would need to be evaluated separately to determine their material composition and if and how they should be restored. Durable waterproof curios may be cleaned using an acceptable automatic dishwashing detergent. Small curio items may be able to be placed into net bags to keep them from falling to the bottom of the dishwasher during the cleaning process. Delicate waterproof curios may be less likely to be damaged by high-pressure water streams if cleaned in an ultrasonic cleaner, but this is not always true. Sometimes, the sound waves may cause certain delicate items to fracture. Professionals who perform ultrasonic cleaning should be able to advise on the suitability of this cleaning method. Hand washing and damp wiping are more labor-intensive methods that can be used for various curios. Porous curios would need to be evaluated item-by-item to determine effective cleaning. A baseball signed by a famous sports personality may be gently cleaned using a dry microfiber cloth. Still, in some cases, it might already be protected in a glass or plexiglass display case to protect it from additional settled dust getting in and to prevent settled spores and fragments from getting out.

Dehumidifiers

Whole-house dehumidifiers are often expensive and difficult to maintain, rarely meeting specific moisture control needs. These systems are fixed, making it hard to manage different areas requiring dehumidification. Mold frequently develops inside whole-house units, particularly in hard-to-clean regions, even with UV lights. For most homes, portable dehumidifiers offer a more practical and flexible solution, providing better control over specific areas and easier maintenance and monitoring to see how well the moisture levels in the home are being maintained. Initially, they collect larger amounts of water, which reduces with drying.

The levels should then drop, signifying that the excess moisture load is controlled. If it doesn't fall or you see a sudden spike, it may signal an unresolved moisture issue in the home.

While useful, portable dehumidifiers require regular upkeep. The water collection bucket should be emptied daily to prevent mold growth. When traveling, a helpful option is setting up the dehumidifier inside a bathtub or shower with a hose leading directly into the drain. This allows the unit to operate continuously and reduces the risk of overflow, especially when you're away.

Encourage the unit to dry out daily by removing and emptying the collection tank from the unit and using a portable fan to blow moisture through the dehumidifier assembly and collection tank to completely dry the interior of the equipment daily.

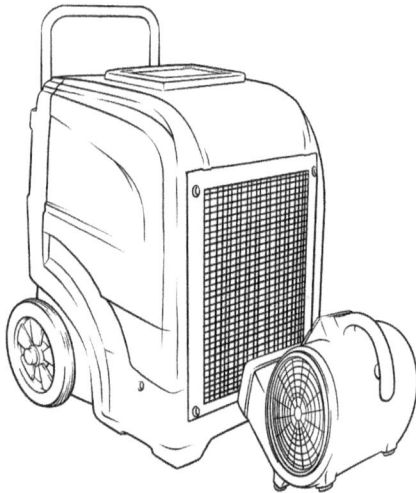

Figure 6-1: Using an air mover to dry dehumidifiers daily will help interrupt the growth cycle and prevent internal hidden mold growth.

If mold develops inside a dehumidifier, immediate attention is necessary. In severe cases, replacement may be the best option. Professional cleaning using non-conductive soap and deionized water is recommended for less severe mold growth, ensuring the unit is completely dry afterward. This is generally not a do-it-yourself project since most dehumidifiers have an internal capacitor that can hold its charge for some time after the unit is unplugged. Accidental discharge of the capacitor during cleaning or accessing the internal components can result in a massive discharge of electricity into the person working on the unit. For professional-grade cleaning, the Odell Electronics Cleaning System can be particularly effective. This system uses deionized water and controls drying to safely clean and restore electronic components, including dehumidifiers, ensuring the unit remains functional and reducing the risk of future mold problems. Regular maintenance with such systems can extend the lifespan of the dehumidifier and help maintain a healthful indoor environment.

Dishes, Pots and Pans, Utensils

Run them through a dishwasher using a non-toxic detergent designed for automatic dishwashers. An automatic dishwasher can remove caked-on eggs and other dried foods, so its ability to remove mold spores and fragments is excellent. Items can also be hand-washed and dried.

Dishwashers

When appropriately used, dishwashers will do a good job of cleaning their interiors and the items they are used to clean. However, this means that all but the smallest of food scraps should be scrapped from the dishes before they are placed in the machine. Grease should be wiped from plates, put into the trash, and not flushed down the drain. If you find that a greasy film is building up in your dishwasher, you are either not using sufficient automatic dish detergent or are leaving too much grease and food scraps on the dishware you are washing. Soap or detergent formulas must be low-sudsing, or you will find gobs of soap bubbles filling the dishwasher and spilling out onto the floor. You also can't use vinegar, baking soda, borax, or other pseudo-cleaners often promoted for non-toxic cleaning. They will not work.

It is important to read the owner's manual, remove and clean the filter screens, and perform other routine maintenance recommended by the manufacturer. Even with proper maintenance, calcium or mineral deposits can build over time. About once a month, I like to run an empty load on the highest temperature and maximum water setting using a packet of LemiShine® Cleaner for automatic dishwashers to help remove the excess buildup before it impairs the ability of the dishwasher to clean effectively. When you first begin this type of maintenance, it may be necessary to perform the LemiShine® cleaning more than once to overcome the buildup.

Settled mold spores and fragments can be removed from the outside of the dishwasher by cleaning it and maintaining it following the manufacturer's instructions. Typically, a disposable microfiber cloth dampened with the 5-drop detergent in a quart of water works well for this purpose. Cleaning the motors, pullies belts, and other internal components in a dishwasher generally requires the assistance of a repair technician. Unfortunately, few are familiar with cleaning settled mold spores and fragments from the equipment they service, but many are willing to assist with their hourly service fee. By combining the information in this book with their knowledge of the appliance, they can effectively clean the internal components of these appliances. Generally, a HEPA vacuum cleaner and microfiber cleaning cloths can access most of the components. This can usually be performed with the dishwasher pulled out to access the top, bottom, back, and sides. If air washing is needed to blow out internal components, the dishwasher must be moved outside or cleaned in a containment to prevent contaminants from blowing into the house. Also, see the section in this chapter on large appliances.

Draperies & Curtains

Draperies with mold growth usually indicate condensation moisture forming on cold walls or windows. The home is also being maintained at a relatively high humidity level. Usually, draperies with visible mold growth will not be able to be returned to a normal appearance. They can be cleaned first by HEPA vacuuming to remove most mold contaminants, followed by laundering or dry cleaning appropriate for the material (see "Laundering" on page 323, "Dry Cleaning" below). Although the mold is gone, this is unlikely to remove the staining and return it to an acceptable appearance. The source of the elevated moisture levels needs to be determined and controlled to prevent a reoccurrence. Some draperies impede air circulation and prevent the moisture from drying quickly. If this is the case, a different drapery may be considered to allow better ventilation between it and the wall. Another option is to ensure the areas can dry completely every day by removing the drapes, wiping up excess moisture, and promoting air circulation. Laundering or dry cleaning is appropriate to effectively clean settled spores and mold fragments from draperies and curtains.

Dry Cleaning

Despite the name, dry cleaning involves wet cleaning with solvents to remove dirt, grease, and particulates from items like clothing that might be damaged by water. About 90% of dry cleaners use perchloroethylene (perc), a solvent that may not be well-tolerated by individuals with chemical sensitivities. Many dry cleaners do not continuously distill their cleaning fluids but rely on filtration. This allows submicron contaminants, such as mold spores, fragments, and biotoxins, to remain in the cleaning fluids until properly distilled.

A 2016 study found bacterial contamination in two of fourteen dry-cleaning facilities, likely due to mixing highly contaminated items with uncontaminated ones. This issue can also occur with mold, as filtration systems commonly used in dry cleaning are ineffective at removing microscopic mold spores and mycotoxins. Continuous distillation, rather than filtration alone, is essential to eliminate these contaminants properly.

A "funky" or chemical odor after cleaning indicates that the cleaning fluids were likely not properly distilled. Heavily contaminated items may require two cleaning rounds, but ensure the fluids are distilled between each round to prevent redepositing contaminants. Cross-contamination between customers' items is possible, so whenever possible, request that your items be cleaned separately with freshly distilled solutions.

In some cases, detergents are added to dry-cleaning fluids to help remove fats, oils, and mycotoxins. These should only be used during the initial cleaning cycle, followed by a rinse with freshly distilled solvent. However, laundering is generally better than dry cleaning, especially for chemically sensitive individuals. Laundering with detergent effectively removes both fat-soluble and water-soluble toxins and avoids the potential contamination risks associated with reused dry-cleaning fluids.

Electronics

(See "Battery-Operated Electronics and Toys" on page 316)

Freezers

(See "Refrigerators & Freezers" on page 328)

Furniture with Growth (Hard Surfaced)

Wood furniture saturated with water is usually ruined by the water long before mold grows. The wet wood can swell, crack, buckle, warp, cup, and stain. These types of physical damage can rarely be fixed cost-effectively to return the item to an acceptable condition. There may be specialty situations where restoration of "special" items may be warranted. These will usually require the services of specially trained woodworkers and refinishers. Mold grows on the surface of wooden items and can sometimes be removed by surface cleaning. This is most likely successful if the mold is limited to the surface and the hyphae have not yet penetrated the wood. Many furniture polishes are made with organic materials such as beeswax and carnauba wax. The cleaning and restoration of the item may be as simple as following the following steps:

1. HEPA vacuum all furniture surfaces outside or in a negatively pressurized cleaning chamber with a nozzle attachment designed for vacuuming hard surfaces.

2. Examine the surfaces closely with a magnifying glass to see if the mold is limited to the surface or if it penetrated the finish into the wood.

3. Strip or remove the wax finish or polish and re-examine the surface to determine if any areas were missed.

4. If the mold growth has penetrated the shellac, varnish, or other top coating but not damaged the underlying wood, it may be necessary to have the furniture stripped for refinishing.

5. Clean the furniture thoroughly inside and out using a wood furniture cleaner designed to clean wood without damaging the surface. Bona® wood floor cleaner or Murphy's® Oil Soap typically have good results. Spot

tests an inconspicuous area first to be sure the cleaner will not cause additional damage.

6. Testing items after cleaning can help determine if the mold has truly been cleaned to a level appropriate for you. Pathways™ Testing discussed in Steps 2, 17, and 19 in the 25 Step program may be helpful in determining if the contents have been adequately cleaned. Professional testing may also be worth considering.

7. Once you are satisfied that the item has been cleaned to an acceptable level, a new coat of wax or polish should be applied to protect the finish further and spruce up its appearance.

Furniture with Settled Spores and Fragments (Hard Surfaced)

Wood furniture with settled spores and fragments can usually be cleaned by HEPA vacuuming, followed by cleaning the surfaces with a disposable microfiber cloth and an appropriate wood furniture cleaner. It is not necessary or recommended that you use expensive products that claim they are specially designed for cleaning or killing mold. The purpose of cleaning is to remove the spores, fragments, and residues, and this can be done quite well with regular dish detergent in water, as described in the Sections on Effective Cleaning and Effective Cleaning Products. However, you should always spot-test whatever product you decide to use to be sure it will not damage the finish. Intricately carved or grooved wood surfaces may be best cleaned by air-washing or cutting microfiber cloths into strips that can be used on the tip of a cotton swab to get into the small spaces as described in the Section of this Chapter on Wood—under General Procedures for Cleaning Personal Items. That section also applies if you have furniture of different types of materials, for example, hardwood drawers and cabinet fronts with a particle board back and plywood shelves.

Furniture (Outdoor)

Most outdoor furniture is designed and constructed to withstand some moisture, such as dew and rain. Over time, outdoor molds may grow on these materials. Some people may be individually hypersensitive to the usual types of outdoor molds. These are hard to avoid—since they are everywhere. The Section of this Chapter on General Procedures for Cleaning Personal Items should contain information to help you evaluate and determine the methods for removing mold from outdoor furniture. In many cases, it will not be cost-effective—so it is better to prevent mold on such items by either taking them in when not in use to keep them dry or choosing materials like metal, glass, cement, ceramic, and plastic so they don't deteriorate and become mold infested in the first place. Wicker is a poor choice for outdoor furniture and, if used outdoors, will require frequent replacement.

Furniture (Upholstered)

Upholstered furniture is one of the most challenging things to restore when affected by mold growth. The padding or stuffing is frequently made up of various types of foam, feathers, and batting materials such as polyester, cotton, wool, or other very porous materials. Over time, skin cells and other organic dust will settle on the surfaces of these furnishings. If mold spores and fragments are present, they will settle with the dust. We push out some air as we sit or lie on the item. When we get up or move around, the air is sucked back into the item and carries the particles into the material. Over time, the dust and accumulated mold spores and fragments move deeply into the materials. If the item is in a typical environment, it collects normal levels and types of dust and mold. If the item is in a water-damaged environment with elevated levels of problem types of mold present, some contaminants will be sucked into the matrix with each movement, while others will be ejected back out.

In addition, it is common for heavy cardboard to be used inside upholstered furniture as shims and to help round the corners over the internal wood frame. On a few occasions I have tracked down mold contamination in upholstered furnishings to cardboard used in the construction that was contaminated with mold growth. In one case, the furniture was brand new, with no evidence of ever being wet. It was apparent that moldy cardboard had been used to construct the sofa. Upholstered furnishings left outside in the rain or dew are practically guaranteed to develop mold internally. The bulky cushioning acts as a sponge to hold the moisture, and the internal components of cellulose have the nutrients for growth to develop.

Glassware

Most glassware can be cleaned in an automatic dishwasher using soap or detergent designed for use in automatic dishwashers. Delicate or high-value glassware may need to be hand-washed using dish soap. Glassware should be thoroughly dried before packing for storage.

Humidifiers and Vaporizers

Humidifiers add moisture to the air. They are frequently used in sick rooms for congested patients to help ease their breathing under dry conditions. It is recommended that whole-house humidification systems be avoided. They are expensive, difficult to maintain, and rarely meet expectations. In addition, the damp or wet components will frequently develop mold and bacteria contamination if they aren't kept scrupulously clean. Whole-house humidifiers are often difficult to access and can't be moved around or easily adjusted to facilitate specific humidification needs. Some units have had UV lights added to help prevent growth from developing inside the humidifier, but this rarely works. UV can only prevent growth on surfaces that are exposed to the light. The internal components create shadows that the light cannot reach, and those surfaces will frequently support growth. They require almost constant maintenance and upkeep, including frequent cleaning, to remain sanitary and effective.

Thirty to fifty percent relative humidity is generally considered an ideal comfort range. I have encountered several cases where clients have complained of the air feeling dry and wanted to install humidification when, in fact, the humidity levels were already well above the typical comfort level. In most of these cases, the perception of dryness was more likely irritation of the mucus membranes in the nose and eyes from exposure to elevated mold levels. The last thing these houses needed was humidification.

Portable humidifiers generally have a water reservoir that is kept full of water to be vaporized into the room air. If a humidifier is necessary, it is best to fill the unit with only the amount of water needed each day. The reservoir should be cleaned and inspected daily, along with the rest of the unit, for signs of growth. Choosing a unit with components that can be accessed for inspection, cleaning, and drying can help prevent mold growth inside the unit. The manufacturer's information should be consulted for cleaning instructions. Using chemical water treatments to prevent mold and algae growth is usually unacceptable for people with hypersensitivities. Humidifiers that add moisture by atomizing the water by vibrations to produce droplets are more prone to aerosolization mold than steam-based humidifiers. The atomization process will frequently atomize the contaminants in the water, whereas A steam base humidifier is less likely to vaporize the contaminants.

If humidification is needed to treat medical conditions, it is preferable to have the humidity produced and delivered directly in the vicinity of the patient allowing the rest of the house to remain dry. If more than a couple of days of humidification is needed, the humidifier should be turned off, cleaned, and dried before refilling and continuing to use. This is especially important before storage.

Jewelry

There is a wide variety of materials used for jewelry. Each piece would need to be evaluated separately to determine its potential for developing mold. Metal and gemstones do not support mold growth, but if dirty, the dirt may provide the nutrients necessary for growth if elevated moisture is present. The string used for stringing necklaces or bracelets is one material that can frequently support mold growth when it gets damp. A jeweler should be able to replace these moldy materials by restring them. Most jewelers have ultrasonic cleaners that do a good job of removing mold spores and contaminants.

It is more common for jewelry to have mold that transfers onto it from either being in contact with moldy materials or settled spores. The container or box used for storing jewelry should be kept clean and dry. If jewelry does become contaminated, it can usually be easily cleaned using a microfiber cloth or other soft cloth available from jewelry suppliers.

Laundering

Laundry is about more than removing dirt—it's key to keeping garments, bedding, and linens sanitary and healthful. Machine washing is highly effective in removing mold spores and residues from most fabrics. (Schrantz, n.d.)

Most clothing with settled spores but no growth can be successfully cleaned of mold and biotoxins using two laundering cycles with additional detergent added between cycles. Since *Chaetomium globosum* tends to affix itself more firmly to linens than other types of mold—use three cycles instead of two when it is present. Use quality, non-toxic, well-tolerated detergents like Branch Basics All Purpose Cleaner supplemented with their laundry booster. Despite internet advice, avoid using supplements like vinegar, baking soda, borax, antimicrobials, or essential oils, as they may neutralize or adversely affect the results.

Washing machines can leak or flood, causing mold growth in our homes. Leaving wet clothing in a washer can cause the clothing to grow mold.

1. Washers must always be installed and operated according to the current code and the manufacturer's instructions. Have your washer installed by a qualified installer or repair technician.

2. If you must locate your laundry room in an area subject to water damage, a catch pan that drains outside or can hold a whole load of water and a power shut-off may also help prevent widespread water damage.

3. Respond immediately to spills, leaks, and any water intrusion.

4. While waiting to accumulate a load of laundry, allow wet or damp linens to dry by hanging them so they have air circulation on all sides.

5. After washing the load, remove wet linens and clothing and put them on a clothesline, drying rack, or clothes dryer. Leaving them bunched in the washer can cause mold growth and musty odors to develop if you accidentally forget a load in the washer. Please don't remove the laundry; add more detergent, rewash it, then remove it to the outside to line dry. This will allow you to evaluate if the recleaning was successful outdoors. If

you notice any remaining mustiness, then it is likely that significant growth occurred, and the items should be discarded.

6. Perform a monthly maintenance cleaning following manufacturer recommendations.

7. Run a cleaning cycle using the hottest water and largest load settings with an enzyme-based powdered laundry detergent designed to dissolve sludge buildup in washers. (i.e., Lemi Shine washing machine cleaner)

8. Front-load washers are especially prone to mold growth due to the door gasket trapping moisture, leading to musty odors that can affect sensitive individuals. Hand drying the gasket after you finish the loads for the day, keeping the door open, and having a fan circulate the air inside the drum area can help, but top-load washers are generally easier to maintain. Top-load models may still develop mold in detergent and other inaccessible compartments, but these are typically easier to clean and prevent with air movement from a fan.

9. Keep the Door open when the washer is not in use to allow it to air dry. If the interior is not drying quickly, a portable fan aimed at the inside of the unit may provide extra drying power to keep your washer from becoming a problem.

Mattresses

To maintain a healthy sleeping environment, prevent mold growth and accumulation in mattresses. While no method is 100% effective, long-term cleaning measures can significantly reduce settled mold spores, fragments, and allergens. A 2012 Taiwanese study demonstrated that daily HEPA vacuuming of mattresses could reduce fungal contaminants by 85%, providing foundational insights into keeping mattresses cleaner and safer. 11 (Banta J. , 2017)

In 2017, I tried replicating part of the Taiwanese study, explicitly focusing on mold removal from mattresses by HEPA vacuuming. I used Mold Specific Quantitative Polymerase Chain Reaction (MSQPCR), a DNA analysis method for mold evaluation. A moldy mattress donated by a client was cleaned daily over eight weeks in a containment chamber built by Anderson Group International, a mold remediation contractor. The cleaning process and laboratory analyses were crowd-funded by 40 supporters, with additional contributions allowing us to test various dust mite covers and materials for their ability to block mold spores and fragments. The study verified the Taiwanese study results. While cleaning can be effective, it's crucial to incorporate protective strategies for long-term mold control in mattresses. (Wu, 2012)

I also tried HEPA vacuuming nonstop for two hours on another donated contaminated mattress and found a similar reduction in fungal load. Based on the Taiwanese

study, the elevated mold levels are expected to build to the original level approximately six weeks after stopping the daily vacuuming.

In another study, I found that wrapping a mattress with Tyvek soft wrap could halt virtually 100% of contaminants from passing through the barrier. Here are the instructions for wrapping a mattress:

Protecting Your Mattress

Wrapping your mattress in an effective barrier is essential to protect it from further mold exposure. The following graphic illustrates the best practices for wrapping a mattress, including selecting materials that block mold spores and prevent moisture buildup. This strategy complements cleaning efforts and provides additional protection for those concerned with mold sensitivities and long-term mattress health.

Materials Needed:
Soft Tyvek #1443R
Tyvek Tape
MERV 11 furnace filter
Mattress

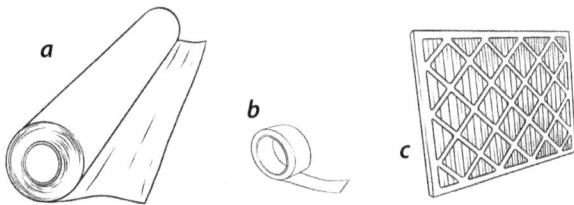

*Figure 6-2, 3, 4: You'll need Tyvek® Soft Wrap 1443R (**a**), Tyvek Tape® (**b**), and a MERV 11 or 13 furnace filter (**c**).*

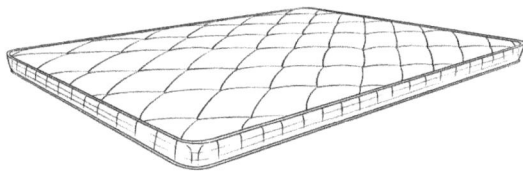

Figure 6-5: Measure your mattress.

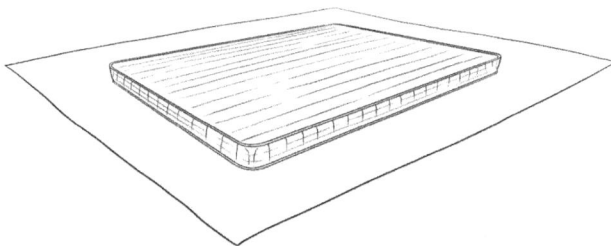

Figure 6-6: Flip the mattress top side down onto a sheet of Soft Tyvek #1443R that has been appropriately sized

to be large enough to wrap the mattress like you would a package. You may need to join two sheets together with Tyvek Tape so the mattress cover will be big enough.

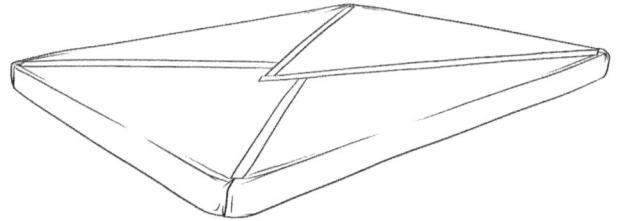

Figure 6-7: Fold and tape the seams.

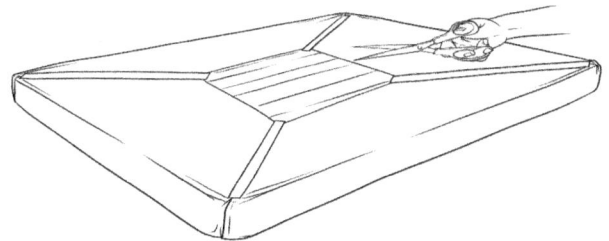

Figure 6-8: Cut a hole a few inches smaller than the furnace filter. The filter will act as a pressure release valve, letting filtered air in and out of the mattress.

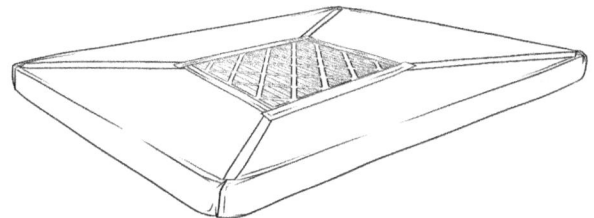

Figure 6-9: Tape the filter securely in place. Flip the mattress right side up, and it is ready to add a washable top pad, sheets, and bedding.

Microwave Ovens

Microwave ovens should be cleaned and maintained in accordance with the manufacturer's maintenance and safety instructions. In general, the accessible outsides and cooking chamber are easy to clean regularly by using damp wiping. Built-in microwaves would need to be pulled out to allow cleaning of their backs and sides and underneath and the otherwise inaccessible walls.

Cleaning the internal components should only be performed by an experienced, trained microwave repair technician since improper assembly can cause dangerous leaks of microwave energy. Unfortunately, few microwave service technicians are familiar with cleaning settled mold spores and fragments from their equipment. Still, many are willing to assist for their hourly service fee. Combining the information in this book with their knowledge of the appliance, they should be able to clean the internal components effectively. Generally, using a combination of HEPA vacuum cleaning, air washing, and microfiber cleaning cloths will effectively clean most of the components. Microwave ovens are frequently used in kitchens where grease, fats, and oils can accumulate. Damp wiping with an appropriate mixture of soap, detergent surfactant, and water (as described in the Damp Wiping section of this chapter) may be able to be effectively used for most of the internal components but will require the experience and judgment of your repair technician. This is usually best performed with the microwave oven enclosed in a small cleaning chamber with a HEPA vacuum cleaner, which assists with controlling any internal spores and fragments containing dust that may be present. If air washing is needed to blow out internal components, the microwave must be moved outside or into a chamber to prevent blowing contaminants around the house.

Mirrors

Since mirrors are usually mounted vertically, they accumulate less dust and fewer spores and fragments. Mirrors are easily cleaned using your favorite window glass cleaner with a microfiber-type cloth.

Musical Instruments

There are a wide variety of musical instruments. Some hold up well to short-term moisture, such as flutes, trumpets, and woodwinds. These musical instruments must be made of moisture-resistant materials because saliva and humid breath continuously pass through them. These instruments fare best when cleaned and thoroughly dried after each use. Even when the materials with which they are made are resistant to mold and bacteria growth, a biofilm can build up inside the instrument, which can provide nutrients and lead to the amplification of a variety of microorganisms that have been associated with hypersensitivity pneumonitis, asthma attacks and exacerbation of respiratory symptoms. Most music repair technicians who work on these types of instruments have access to various equipment that can flush out debris and dissolve away the biofilm that has built up inside. Ultrasonic cleaning tanks are also commonly used. Routine at-home cleaning can help prevent problems from developing. Still, annual or as-needed professional service and cleaning may be necessary for people with sensitivities who want to continue practicing their art.

Since multiple chemical sensitivities are frequently shared in people with sensitivities to water damage-related organisms, it is necessary to discuss the use of any chemicals with your repair technician to be sure they will not create a post-cleaning problem for the user.

Musical instrument cases also have a higher risk of developing mold inside the case. This is especially true for brass horns, woodwinds, and other instruments when moisture from saliva and the breath is deposited. Instruments should be stored in cases with silica gel desiccant packets to control excess humidity. It is recommended that the packets used should have color change indicators that will tell when they can no longer adsorb the moisture. The packets should be changed with fresh ones or reactivated following the manufacturer's instructions. Almost all can be reactivated in an oven; some are designed to be dried and reactivated quickly in a microwave oven. The reactivation instructions must be followed carefully; otherwise, the packets or the microwave oven may be damaged.

Musical instruments in a water-damaged home are vulnerable to moisture and the drying processes used to restore the property. Aggressive drying techniques often applied in water-damaged homes can harm delicate instruments, which may need to be removed when extensive drying is required. Percussion, electronic, and string instruments, in particular, may need special care when wet. Improper drying can lead to issues such as warping, swelling, buckling, or cupping of materials if under-dried, while over-drying can cause excessive shrinkage, cracking, and loosening of joints. If pianos, organs, or other delicate instruments are in the affected area. In that case, it's often best to relocate them to a different part of the home where extra controls and monitoring can help prevent further damage. Ideally, they should be moved to a controlled environment for drying, cleaning, and storage until the home is restored to a safe condition.

Electronic instruments that get wet require special care for the computer boards and electrical circuits in addition to the instrument's needs. When in doubt, it is best to consult with an experienced repair technician. They can advise and often offer their facilities and experience.

Musical Instruments and Settled Spores, Particles and Fragments

Cleaning musical instruments of settled spores can range from easy to complicated, depending on the instrument. In most cases, a disposable microfiber cloth dampened with a mild detergent solution (5 drops of detergent to a quart of water) will work great. If the instrument has sound holes, such as a guitar or violin, it may be necessary to use compressed air outdoors or in a cleaning chamber to blow the contaminants out. Pianos and organs can be tricky and will usually require the assistance of a piano repair technician. The piano should have a containment with negative air controls built around it or be moved outside. Depending on the level and locations of contamination, the piano may need to be partially disassembled to reach the inner works. The keyboard often accumulates dust under the keys, and dust may work its way in behind the soundboard. A combination of HEPA vacuuming, compressed air, and damp wiping will generally restore the piano to a clean condition before it is reassembled.

Ovens and Stovetops

The most challenging thing about cleaning an oven is being able to access it from all sides. Stovetops and Ovens are made to be easy to clean. The construction materials are hard and non-porous and, therefore, easy to maintain in a sanitary condition. Generally, a HEPA vacuum cleaner and microfiber cleaning cloths can access most of the components when the unit is pulled out to access the top, bottom, back, and sides. There are typically no internal fans or hidden components that are difficult to access. When air washing is used, the oven should ideally be moved outside to prevent contaminants from blowing into the house.

Papers and Documents

(See "Mold Growth on Paper or Cardboard" on page 312)

Photographs

Depending on their age, type, extent of damage, and historical value, photographs may be able to be cleaned of settled spores and particles associated with water damage by cleaning them with a dry or slightly dampened Swiffer wipe. Always spot-test first to be sure that the photos can withstand moisture and abrasion. Older photographs were usually developed with a wet development process. However, with age, the paper may become brittle and unable to withstand the cleaning method. Often, the photographs will need to be pressed flat to eliminate curling. Historical or high-value photographs or photos of other water damage and mold growth should be sent to an art conservatory for cleaning *(See "Artwork" on page 315)*.

Pillows

Pillows are rarely able to be cost-effectively cleaned when mold growth has occurred on them or they have been exposed to high levels of settled spores and fragments from water damage. The longer the item has been exposed and the greater the use, the greater the likelihood that the contaminants will have worked deeply into the stuffing materials. If the pillow cover has value, it is usually possible to open a seam along one edge of the pillow for removing and discarding the stuffing. The outside cover is then laundered or dry cleaned as appropriate before re-stuffing the pillow with clean new materials.

Plants (Indoor)

Indoor plants with visible mold growth are unlikely to be successfully restored. You may be able to prune away the bad parts. Mold growth associated with indoor water damage is unlikely to occur on indoor plants. It is more likely that the visible mold growth is mildew, a group of molds that grows on living plants. Regardless, the plant should probably be discarded.

You may be able to clean settled spores' dust and particles from plants by taking them outdoors and gently spraying them multiple times. If the weather is good and will not kill the plant, it is likely best to clean it multiple times over several days.

If mold grows on the soil of potted plants, it can usually be controlled by taking the plant outside and gently scraping off about an inch of soil. The soil is discarded and then replaced with a new layer of potting soil.

Watering house plants from the top can increase the risk of mold growth on the soil. To help prevent this, consider using a root watering system. Often made from plastic, glass, or clay, these systems use a hollow tube inserted into the soil to deliver water directly to the roots.

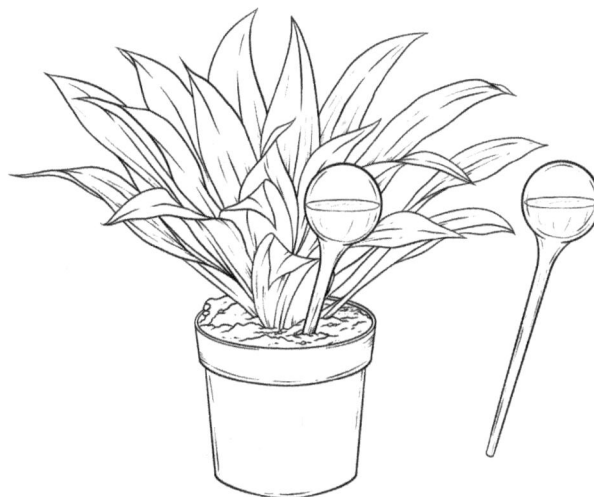

Figure 6-10: A plant root watering system keeps the soil surface drier, helping prevent mold from growing on soil surface.

Plants (Artificial)

The ability to successfully clean artificial plants often depends on the materials used for their construction. Plastic plants can often be hand washed, and some can be put in a net bag and run through a dishwasher with the drying cycle turned off since the high drying temperatures may melt the plastic. Silk and paper are difficult to clean successfully without causing damage. In most cases where hand cleaning or special handling is necessary, the amount of time or cost of having the work done will far exceed the value of the artificial plant.

Purses

Purses that develop mold or are water-damaged are rarely able to be restored and will generally need to be discarded. They should be stored in dry places to protect them if they need to be preserved. A one-ounce silica gel desiccant packet inside the purse will generally help control moisture. Keeping the purse interior dry will help prevent mold from growing inside. Closed-top purses do a good job of preventing settled spores and contaminant fragments from collecting inside. A thorough HEPA vacuuming is usually sufficient to remove any extraneous contaminated dust that may have gotten inside. Cleaning the exterior would need to be evaluated on a case-by-case basis, but it would generally include HEPA vacuuming and possibly air washing or damp wiping.

Record Albums

Records are generally kept in an album cover case, protected from settled dust. The album cover should be cleaned and maintained by dry wiping with a microfiber cloth. The interior of the album cover may be cleaned with gentle air washing. If needed, the interior record can be cleaned using a record cleaning kit available at electronics supply stores.

Refrigerators & Freezers

Refrigerators and freezers are typically not cost-effectively reparable after a significant flooding event that wets the interior mechanical components. If they have been in a moldy or water-damaged environment but did not get wet, they should be cleaned and maintained in accordance with the guidance in the appliance section of this chapter. The exterior and interior refrigeration and freezer compartments are typically designed to make cleaning easy.

In contrast, the interior of the mechanical section of refrigerators and freezers can be challenging to clean and is prone to a rarely addressed issue with the condensation defrost cycle collection pan. The purpose of this pan is to collect the liquid that drains from the refrigerator during the self-defrosting cycle or from the condensation moisture that forms on the cooling coils. The pan is often set close to the compressor, condenser, and heat distribution coils. This is because the heat generated by the refrigeration process can dry the pan by evaporating the excess moisture into the room air. In theory, the heat dries the pan, so the moisture never sits there long enough to form mold and other organisms to grow in the water. This may be true as long as the pan stays clean. Over time, house dust can build up in the pan to a point where the heat can no longer evaporate the moisture from the pan. The dust buildup acts like a sponge to hold the moisture, and house dust is a perfect nutrient for some molds and microorganisms. It is common for *Auerobasidium pullulans* to grow at high levels in the condensation pan. Fortunately, this contamination does not usually require remediation of the building to get it under control. Refrigerator cleaning and maintenance can keep it under control. Older refrigeration units were designed with the collection pan toward the front and easily accessible for removal and cleaning. Most newer refrigerator units now have the condensation collection pan bolted into the interior areas in ways that make it difficult to access for routine cleaning.

Cleaning the internal mechanical components and the condensation pan in a refrigerator generally requires the assistance of a repair technician. Unfortunately, few of them are familiar with cleaning settled mold spores and fragments from the equipment and usually don't have a HEPA vacuum to assist with the cleaning. This can result in high levels of mold that grew in the condensation pan being released into the kitchen and then migrating into other areas of the home.

Many refrigerator repair persons are willing to assist with the cleaning for their hourly service fee. By combining the information in this book with their knowledge of the appliance, they can effectively clean the internal components. Generally, using a HEPA vacuum cleaner and microfiber cleaning cloths dampened with soapy water can clean most of the components. If air washing is needed to blow out internal components, the refrigerator must be moved outside or a containment chamber constructed to prevent blowing contaminants into the house.

Safes

Many safes are designed to protect the contents from fire, water intrusion, and theft. The exterior of the safe is made of a hard, non-porous material that does not support mold growth. Various mold spores and other contaminants associated with water damage can settle on the outside of the safe, but these should be easily cleaned using a dampened disposable microfiber cleaning cloth.

It is common for mold to grow on the contents inside safes when condensation forms due to a drop in temperature that results in the interior of the safe reaching dew point temperature. It is inexpensive insurance to keep a silica gel desiccant packet in the safe's interior to protect against excess moisture resulting in condensation. The silica gel should be replaced or recharged annually or as needed.

Stove Tops
(See "Ovens and Stovetops" on page 327)

Suitcases and Luggage

Ideally, suitcases and luggage will be kept dry and stored in areas that do not have mold problems. Their purpose is to transport and protect the contents inside. Unfortunately, this means they are subjected to exposure to the weather. I have on many occasions looked out airport windows down at the tarmac, watching as passengers' luggage is loaded in the rain into the hold of an airplane, and thought about whether I would arrive quickly enough at my destination so I could thoroughly dry my baggage before mold growth would set in. Once luggage has developed mold, it can rarely be successfully cleaned of the growth. Canvas or soft-shell luggage is prone to absorbing the moisture that gets on the surface. To prevent mold growth, it should be emptied and wholly dried every day of your trip. When dried daily, mold spores will not have a chance to germinate and begin growing.

Hard-shell luggage generally does a better job of preventing growth on the outside of the case. It is usually made of leather or synthetic materials that shed liquid water and avoid an exchange of water vapor into the clothing and items stored inside. This may seem like hard-shell luggage is the best choice, but they are more prone to condensation moisture developing inside. Earlier in this chapter, I told the story of a client who had massive amounts of mold growing on her things in a shipping container due to condensation moisture trapped inside the container. The same thing can happen on a smaller scale with hard-shell suitcases. As the temperature drops, any dampness from water vapor trapped inside the hard-shell luggage can condense inside, forming enough water activity to allow mold spores to germinate and begin growing inside the contents of the luggage. It is common for the temperatures inside the baggage hold of an airplane to get quite chilly at 30,000 feet, resulting in condensation and moisture forming. In most cases, the moisture is released. It can dry adequately overnight, but sometimes, with long trips or delays and especially with travel in tropical countries, mold growth develops inside the case. One clue that this has happened is if you open the suitcase and get hit with a blast of musty odor. Silica gel desiccant packets can help prevent condensation moisture problems from developing. A one-ounce packet should be adequate for protecting a standard-size suitcase while you travel. Hard-shelled luggage stored in a garage or unconditioned shed is also prone to developing interior mold, which can be prevented with a dry silica gel packet inside. The packets should be changed to dry at least once a year or as needed.

Soft-shell luggage is generally less likely to develop mold from trapped condensation moisture but more likely from wetting the outside from rain or heavy dew. The greater the amount of wetting and the longer the duration, the greater the likelihood that the interior contents will also be affected. Keeping a desiccant packet inside soft-shelled suitcases can provide additional protection for the contents inside. Still, it will not prevent mold from growing on the outside of the bag, so it is important to dry these items as much as possible during travels and before storing them. Unloading a wet case and placing it in front of the air stream coming off a hotel's in-wall heater/AC or in the bathroom with the exhaust fan running can assist in more rapid drying.

Soft-shell luggage contaminated with settled spores can be effectively cleaned by HEPA vacuuming. Hard-shell cases can be wiped with disposable microfiber cloths to clean settled spores effectively and fragments from the surfaces.

Televisions

In most cases, television sets should only be opened for cleaning by an experienced person. Televisions have capacitors inside them. Capacitors can hold a strong electrical charge for days after the monitor is unplugged, sufficient to cause a severe shock. The outsides of most monitors can be cleaned just like any other piece of hard-surfaced furniture in accordance with the manufacturer's instructions. Still, the interiors should probably be air-washed with compressed air—used outdoors or in a negative air pressure-filtered cleaning chamber.

Tools: Electrical

The outsides should be cleaned and maintained in accordance with the manufacturer's instructions. Generally, the outside can be cleaned with a disposable microfiber cloth dampened with a couple of spritzes of a non-toxic soap or detergent cleaning spray. When tools such as drills, electrical saws, routers, and planers have vent holes leading to the interior, they may be adequately cleaned by using compressed air to blow contaminants out of the interior through the vent openings. If it can be done safely, electrical tools with a motor inside may be able to be air-washed through the vent openings while they are operating normally in the way they are designed to be used. A repair technician may also be able to open the tool and use a combination of HEPA vacuuming, air washing, and microfiber cleaning cloth to clean the device's interior effectively.

Tools: Hand

Each tool needs to be evaluated individually to determine the most effective techniques. Most hand tools are made of durable, hard, non-porous materials and are easily cleaned. Many can be easily cleaned by running them through a dishwasher with detergent and then dried. Small parts like sockets for use with socket wrenches can be placed in net bags to keep the small parts from getting lost inside the dishwasher. The internal ratcheting mechanism for a socket wrench may not tolerate the moisture. It may need hand cleaning by damp wiping with a microfiber cleaning cloth. Hand tools with moving parts, like a pair of pliers, may require a small amount of lubricant added to the pivot point after cleaning to keep the moving parts functioning smoothly.

Toys

Toys come in so many different types that judgment needs to be used to determine if and how they will be restored and cleaned. The toy's cost is often insignificant compared to the time and effort spent cleaning. In these cases, replacing the item may be far more expedient and cost-effective. Many items, however, are easy to clean. Electronic toys are handled like other electronic items *(see "Electronics" on page 321)*. They would be cleaned like clothing for thin cloth or material and laundered or dry cleaned. Air washing, HEPA vacuuming, and Damp or dry microfiber cleaning cloths are the most common methods, but ultrasonic cleaners and dishwashers may also be used. Wooden toys would be handled the same way as wooden furniture.

Toys (small) Lego's and Other Small Toys

Mesh bags are available for enclosing small items, including toys, that can go through a dishwasher. After washing, the most important thing is ensuring the items are thoroughly and rapidly dried. Hand drying may be needed. A fan may be used to help accelerate the drying of these items. Air washing with compressed air can help blow excess moisture from hard-to-reach areas.

Toys (Stuffed)

Stuffed toys with mold growth or water damage are unlikely to be successfully restored. However, a small child rarely cares about appearance. Heroic measures may be unnecessary depending on the degree of water damage and growth. The toy may be able to have a seam cut, the stuffing removed and discarded, and the fabric exterior laundered or professionally dry cleaned to return it to a sanitary condition. This may require multiple launderings (typically, two rounds are sufficient). A peroxide-based cleaner may also help remove some of the discoloration. Since the child may be in intimate contact with the toy, post-cleaning testing may be helpful for peace of mind. Once the exterior material has been adequately cleaned, the toy will be re-stuffed with clean new material, and the seam will be re-stitched.

Settled spores that land on stuffed toys that are displayed but not handled may be successfully cleaned using HEPA vacuuming. If the contamination has been worked into the fabric and stuffing, the method described above for removing the stuffing, cleaning the outside, and re-stuffing with new, clean fill can be used.

Trash Compactors

Trash compactors often develop mold problems. The internal components are complex to access and keep clean, and wet garbage contributes moisture that can result in mold growth inside the unit. Some trash compactors have a place for deodorizer packets inside the unit. As you have likely gathered from other parts of this book, I do not endorse covering up problems with air fresheners or other scents-releasing products. I recommend eliminating trash compactors and replacing them with a trash receptacle that can be easily removed for routine cleaning outside.

Utensils

Any non-porous utensils such as metal, plastic, or glass that can be run through a dishwasher can be effectively cleaned of spores and growth. Wooden spoons and other wooden utensils with growth are unlikely to be restored and should be discarded. Settled spores can also be cleaned from these and more delicate items by hand washing. Always use an appropriate soap or detergent for the item that is being cleaned.

Vacuum Cleaners

Vacuum cleaners are used to clean but must also be cleaned and properly maintained. Some people shun bagless vacuum cleaners because they mistakenly believe the bag will protect from contaminants being released back into the room. In fact, opening the vacuum cleaner to change the bag typically releases a cloud of invisible dust particles back into the room you have been working to clean. The bag is unable to contain microscopic contaminants. The space inside the vacuum cleaner after the airflow leaves the bag contains massive amounts of small particles and microscopic pollutants. Whether the vacuum cleaner has a bag or is bagless, emptying the vacuum cleaner should always be done outdoors. Professional mold remediators may change the bag inside the containment within the capture zone of the HEPA-filtered air filtration device to create a negative air pressure during the remediation.

- Emptying the vacuum cleaner should typically be done by someone not hypersensitive to the contaminants cleaned up by vacuuming.

- Take the vacuum cleaner outside before opening it.

- When possible, remain upwind from the vacuum cleaner while you open, empty, and clean the interior of the vacuum cleaner.

- The debris or full bag should be removed directly into another bag that can be sealed before placing it into the trash receptacle.

- There is a good chance that changing the bag or emptying a bagless vacuum cleaner has resulted in some level of contamination depositing on the outside of the equipment. The outside of the vacuum cleaner can be cleaned before bringing it back into the home by wiping it with a damp disposable microfiber cleaning cloth. Repeat the damp wiping as many times as necessary so that the final wiping does not reveal any visible dust or dirt from the outside of the equipment.

- HEPA and other vacuum cleaner filters should be changed when there is a noticeable reduction in suction or airflow.

- The vacuum cleaner should be taken outside.

- The bag (if present) or collection canister should be emptied as described above.

- The HEPA and other filters should be removed and discarded according to the owner's manual and manufacturer's instructions.

- I am not a fan of attempting to clean the HEPA filter. It is too easy to damage it during attempts at cleaning.

- The interior of the vacuum cleaner should be cleaned using a disposable microfiber cloth as described above.

- If it can be done safely, I like to temporarily reassemble the vacuum cleaner without filters or bag, then plug it in and turn it on to flush internal components that cannot be reached for manual cleaning. Flushing with air for 2 to 5 minutes should be adequate.

- The air flushing is followed by a second interior and exterior cleaning using a disposable microfiber cloth, and then new filters and a bag are installed for use.

Venetian Blinds

Venetian Blinds made of vinyl or aluminum can typically be cleaned of mold growth and settled spores and fragments by sending them out for ultrasonic cleaning. Wood and material-covered blinds are seldom effectively restored from mold growth but can be easily cleaned of settled spores using a combination of HEPA vacuuming, microfiber cleaning cloths, and air washing.

Vehicles

Vehicles like cars, trucks, and motorhomes pose unique challenges in maintaining a healthful environment. While vehicle interiors are generally not mold-friendly, transported items such as cardboard, food, and dirt can create mold-friendly wet conditions. Cross-contamination from contaminated items can also introduce mold spores, and vehicles stored in unconditioned areas are prone to condensation. Many issues can be avoided by choosing vehicles designed for easy maintenance, such as those with non-porous floor mats, leather or vinyl seats, efficient cabin air filters, and properly draining, easily accessible air conditioning systems.

Cleaning Vehicles to Reduce Settled Spores and Fragments

Though creating a mold-free vehicle is impossible, you can significantly reduce spores and contaminants to maintain a healthful environment. Air washing, HEPA vacuuming, and microfiber wiping effectively control these particulates. Cleaning should be done outdoors for fresh air dilution and to prevent the spreading of contaminants in your garage. Routine cleanings can help avoid the buildup of mold over time.

1. **Remove Loose Items:** Remove anything not attached, like mats and personal belongings, and clean them separately.

2. **Initial HEPA Vacuuming:** Lightly vacuum to remove loose dirt before detailed cleaning.

3. **Use HEPA or Central Vacuums:** HEPA vacuums collect small particles. Choose central vacuums for car washes so you can park away from the discharge point.

4. **Air Washing:** Use compressed air (no more than 30 psi) to dislodge particles from hard-to-reach areas like seat rails and under consoles.

5. **HEPA Collection:** Simultaneous vacuuming while air washing can help capture dislodged particles and reduce cross-contamination.

6. **Repeated HEPA Vacuuming:** Vacuum repeatedly to remove lingering particulates, especially from carpets and upholstery.

7. **Damp Wiping:** Spray a disposable microfiber wipe with five drops to a quart of water detergent to clean surfaces like dashboards and seats. Follow with a dry wipe to remove moisture.

8. **Routine Maintenance:** Regular cleaning controls mold levels and prevents the need for deeper remediation.

Mold Growth in Vehicles

To prevent mold in vehicles, keeping the interior dry is essential. Moisture can enter through wet shoes, spills, leaks, or the air we exhale. The waterproof exterior then traps this moisture inside. Dirt, skin cells, or food provide nutrients for mold, so cleaning and drying any moisture that accumulates ideally within 24 hours is best. Condensation or clogged AC drains can also cause dampness, and storing vehicles in unconditioned spaces may lead to condensation moisture buildup. Parking in a conditioned space and using dehumidifiers if needed can help, especially in humid regions. Using the car's heater to warm the interior and rolling windows down to exhaust damp air can assist with temporary moisture control. Using silica gel packets can help protect against minor moisture, but larger spills may require fans and dehumidifiers.

Remediating Mold in Vehicles

Once mold develops in porous materials like seats or carpets, they often need replacing. Minor issues from limited moisture can sometimes be resolved with rapid drying, but trapped moisture under mats or carpets increases mold risk. Minor mold issues may be fixed by removing the source and thoroughly cleaning, but products claiming to kill mold often worsen conditions for sensitive individuals. Extensive water damage, such as from flooding, usually renders a vehicle unsalvageable, especially for people with mold sensitivities. Flooded cars often suffer from mechanical and electrical damage as well.

Avoid Purchasing Flooded Vehicles

Insurance companies often declare flooded vehicles a total loss, but they may still be resold. Disclosure is required but may appear in fine print. The car's title may be marked "Flood" or "Salvage" to indicate it had past flooding, but some states use a code that is hard to decipher. Using a service like Carfax can help make it more straightforward. Repairs and restoration may only address function and cosmetics while masking mold with deodorizers. Signs of flooding include musty odors, air fresheners, stained upholstery, rust, mud in hidden areas, and corrosion in electrical components.

Cabin Air Filter Replacement

A musty odor when the air conditioner is turned on often indicates mold growth from condensation moisture in a vehicle's air conditioning system. Filtered air flowing through the system helps prevent dirt from accumulating as a nutrient for mold. Most vehicles today have a cabin air filter to help filter outdoor and recirculate air as a first line of defense against mold. The filter should be replaced annually, or every 15,000 miles, but more frequent changes may be necessary if driving in dusty conditions or wildfire smoke.

The filter is usually located behind the glovebox and can be changed by following instructions in the owner's manual or online videos. Ensure the new filter fits snugly to avoid air bypassing it. While the filter is out, carefully clean the surrounding area with a HEPA vacuum or microfiber cloth to prevent debris from entering the system. If the AC air smells musty, the filter may have damp debris causing mold. Replacing it may solve the problem. However, if mold grows on the coils or condensation pan, thorough cleaning or costly disassembly will be required, as deodorizers only mask odors and don't eliminate mold. Keeping the system dry when not in use also helps prevent mold growth.

Keeping a Vehicle's AC System Dry When Not in Use

Mold can grow in the AC system if excess moisture accumulates and doesn't dry completely. Silica gel packets won't address this moisture, so ensuring the condensation pan drains entirely each time the air conditioner is used is essential. To determine the best AC drainage position, turn off the AC with the car aimed uphill, downhill, and on level ground to see which position tilts the vehicle to allow the maximum water flow from the condensation pan. This will help you identify which position allows the most complete drainage. We have a hill a few minutes from our home. By turning off the AC but leaving the fan running on high and driving up the hill, the car's condensation pan empties entirely, and the fan helps dry the cooling coils and residual moisture in the system. This results in the system being dry when we get home and shut off the car. This prevents standing residual water from remaining, which promotes mold growth.

Video Games
(See the appropriate media in this section, and "Electronics" on page 321)

Video Tapes

Most videotapes are kept in a case that is protected from settled dust. The outside case should be cleaned and maintained by dry wiping with a microfiber cloth. If needed, the interior cassette can also be cleaned the same way. Gentle air washing may also help blow out the internal parts of the cassette that have been left out of its case. Video Tapes should be kept protected from moisture. If they get wet, they are probably ruined and must be replaced if desired. Irreplaceable content may be transferred to a DVD or other electronic media by contractors specializing in recovering electronic and audio content from damaged media.

Washers
(See "Laundering" on page 323)

References

American Conference of Governmental Industrial Hygienists (ACGIH). (1999). *Bioaerosols: Assessment and control.* American Conference of Governmental Industrial Hygienists.

U.S. Environmental Protection Agency. (2008). *Mold remediation in schools and commercial buildings* (EPA 402-K-01-001). Retrieved from www.epa.gov/mold

Bloomfield, S. F., Stanwell-Smith, R., Crevel, R. W., & Pickup, J. (2006). Too clean, or not too clean: The hygiene hypothesis and home hygiene. *Clinical & Experimental Allergy, 36*(4), 402–425. https://doi.org/10.1111/j.1365-2222.2006.02463.x

Anderson, R. L. (1969). Biological evaluation of carpeting. *Applied Microbiology, 18*(2), 182–187.

Brandys, R. C., & Brandys, G. M. (2012). *In-field test methods and reference standards for portable high-efficiency particulate air filtration (PHEAF) equipment.* OEHCS Publications.

Holland, J., Banta, J., Cole, G., & Passmore, B. (2012). Bacterial amplification and in-place carpet drying: Implications for category 1 water intrusion restoration. *Journal of Environmental Health, 74*(9), 8–14.

Institute of Inspection, Cleaning, and Restoration Certification (IICRC). (2015). *ANSI/IICRC S520: Standard and reference guide for professional mold remediation.* IICRC.

Institute of Inspection, Cleaning, and Restoration Certification (IICRC). (2015). *ANSI/IICRC S500: Standard and reference guide for professional water damage restoration* (3rd ed.). IICRC.

Buttner, M. P., & Cruz-Perez, P. (2002). Measurement of airborne fungal spore dispersal from three types of flooring materials. *Aerobiologia, 18*(1), 1–11.

Schrantz, M. (Host). (n.d.). *IEP Radio #19: Contents cleaning with Ralph E. Moon, PhD—A review of "mold-contaminated" fabrics* [Audio podcast episode]. IEP Radio. Retrieved from https://clmmag.theclm.org/home/author

Banta, J. (2017). *Mattress contamination study* [Unpublished study].

Wu, F. F., Wu, M. W., Pierse, N., Crane, J., & Siebers, R. (2012). Daily vacuuming of mattresses significantly reduces house dust mite allergens, bacterial endotoxin, and fungal β-glucan. *Journal of Asthma, 49*(2), 139–143. https://doi.org/10.3109/02770903.2011.648297

OTHER RESOURCES

Dry & Dry Silica Gel Desiccant dryndry.com

Other Silica Gel Desiccant sources: Amazon.com

Part Four: Epilog

Each of us is shaped by the sum of our experiences, a collection of moments that leave indelible marks on who we are and how we see the world. As a child growing up in Southern California, I vividly remember the immense power of earthquakes. They didn't frighten me, but they were fascinating. Later, at the age of ten, my mother and I took a trip to visit family in Indiana, arriving in South Bend shortly after the Great Tornado of 1965 had left its mark. Driving through the heart of the damaged areas, I can still picture a brick manufacturing facility on the outskirts of town. The two side walls stood untouched, framing a channel of destruction that ran straight through its center. A stark juxtaposition of stability and chaos. A reminder of both nature's fury and the fragile boundaries that define safety.

There have been many additional events throughout my life that have shaped my healthy home philosophy. The first 15 years after I married my wife, Trisha, I treated our home with bug bombs and applied the termiticide Chlordane to combat termites, a chemical banned shortly after I used it. When Trish was nine months pregnant with our first daughter, heavy rains and poor community drainage led to our home flooding with half an inch of water. I naively cleaned it with a rented carpet shampooer from the local supermarket, failing to address the water damage properly. Then our home was crop-dusted—twice—with the fungicide Benomyl, a widely used product at the time, later linked to carcinogenicity and DNA damage concerns. Its extensive use in paint also contributed to developing fungicide resistance in molds, creating "super-strains" that have rendered other antimicrobial products less effective and led to widespread challenges in agricultural and environmental settings. The pilot responsible for spraying our home later sprayed four school children in the schoolyard on the other side of the orchard and was grounded by the agricultural commissioner for two weeks—a slap on the wrist,

essentially an enforced vacation. These risks ultimately led to Benomyl's removal from the market and delisting by the EPA approximately 20 years later, in 2001.

In 1982, I inadvertently poisoned my family with lead-based paint while sanding and stripping it from the exterior of our home. At that time, I was less aware of the dangers of lead exposure and the importance of proper precautions. Later, we rented a house that had been used as a clandestine drug lab, with hazardous materials—including a leaking tank of hydrogen chloride gas—discarded in the crawlspace. I made that discovery three days after moving in, which led to the property being declared eligible for Superfund restoration funds. Over time, these repeated exposures took a toll, and Trish became seriously ill.

By her mid-thirties, Trish's health had declined significantly, and we were struggling to find answers. At the time, little information was available to guide us. Doctors were baffled by her symptoms, and when her condition didn't align with their knowledge base, they often dismissed her suffering as psychosomatic or labeled her as "crazy." But I knew better. Over the years, our family continued camping every summer, and we noticed something remarkable. In the fresh mountain air, Trish's health would steadily improve. The first few days of each trip were challenging, with her symptoms as severe as they were at home, but by the end of the first week, she experienced a dramatic recovery, feeling as well as she had during our first 15 years together. Unfortunately, the relief was fleeting. Within minutes of returning home, her symptoms would reappear, and by the next day, it was as if we had never left.

On some level, it feels as though I was destined to become an environmental consultant—a path forged as a survival mechanism against these experiences. While I may have been slow to learn, each challenge became a stepping stone, shaping my career and mission. I now focus on educating others and helping the public understand that safer alternatives exist. The risky behaviors of manufacturers, distributors, marketers, and salespeople—practices I once unknowingly supported—are not only unnecessary but have caused profound harm.

SLAPP Suits

Strategic Lawsuits Against Public Participation (SLAPP suits) are legal actions designed to intimidate or silence individuals or organizations who speak out on public interest issues, often by burdening them with costly and time-consuming litigation. Several of my colleagues in the environmental field have faced these types of legal challenges while striving to communicate inconvenient truths. A prominent example is the lawsuit filed by Sharper Image against *Consumer Reports* after the magazine published a critical review of Sharper Image's portable ozone generators. The suit backfired, as *Consumer Reports* successfully defended its findings, and the court awarded $50,000 in damages to the magazine. This legal loss, coupled with increasing awareness of the dangers of ozone generators, contributed to Sharper Image's decline; the company is no longer in business.

Another tactic I have personally experienced involves the use of confidentiality agreements. Early in my career, I signed such an agreement several times while conducting research funded by companies interested in evaluating their products or applications. These companies assured me they wanted an honest understanding of their product's capabilities and limitations. However, when my research revealed significant limitations. I found myself threatened with legal action if I discussed the problematic findings, which, unfortunately, became classified as their trade secrets. These agreements effectively silenced me, restricting my ability to share critical insights that could have prevented harm or misapplication.

While writing this book, I have been careful not to breach these agreements or divulge proprietary information. However, I remain unreserved in citing independent, peer-reviewed university or other research that has identified similar issues. This highlights the importance of transparency and independent investigation, as confidentiality agreements can be weaponized to suppress truth rather than foster improvement.

Portable ozone generators, which Sharper Image once promoted heavily, have since been outlawed for consumer sale in California due to health risks. However, a legal loophole permits their installation in HVAC systems, creating an ongoing problem. I have personally encountered several cases where these systems worsened indoor environmental quality, exacerbating health issues rather than improving them. These situations highlight the importance of truthful, science-based communication and the need for legal protections to shield professionals and organizations from retaliatory lawsuits when they speak out to protect public health and safety. Anti-SLAPP laws serve as a critical countermeasure, often allowing defendants to recover costs and, in some jurisdictions, imposing significant penalties on those who misuse the legal system for intimidation.

When Trish developed her chronic illness, it became the final impetus not just to survive but to advocate for healthful, informed choices that protect both people and their homes.

There is much more to that story, but in short, it set me on the path to becoming a home environmental consultant specializing in building health, long before it was widely recognized as a critical issue. I've been doing this work for over 35 years, and about 27 years ago, Trish used her ability to sense mold issues to find the first home where she could truly begin to heal. Guided by her internal sense of whether an environment felt good, she called my attention to the house. When I saw it, I was able to confirm that her instincts were right—it was naturally healthful. By that time, I had already begun studying Baubiologie and had the privilege of meeting architect Paula Baker-LaPorte and medical doctor Erica Elliott. Together, we co-authored *Prescriptions for a Healthy House: A Practical Guide for Architects, Builders, and Homeowners*. What started as a collaboration has endured for 25 years, culminating in the fourth edition of that book being released shortly before I developed my own health crisis.

Early in my career, I recognized that mold made people, including Trish, sick in their homes. After more than a decade of illness, Trish had developed an internal early warning system, or the ability to sense when indoor conditions weren't healthful for her.

By 2017, I had come to realize the need for a book specifically about mold, one that could help the general population—and particularly those affected by mold illness and their families—understand the complexities of mold and water damage. While *Prescriptions for a Healthy House* was in its third edition, I increasingly felt compelled to write a book devoted entirely to mold. As I began outlining and drafting chapters, I saw there were still gaps in knowledge that needed to be filled. Determined to address these gaps, I launched an Indiegogo crowdfunding campaign, raising over $15,000—primarily through $25 contributions—to support my research.

The research was successful, and as a perk, I promised all contributors an electronic copy of the book upon its completion. Along the way, I shared 15 chapters of information with my supporters. I originally planned to finish the book in 2020, but like so many others, my plans were disrupted by the COVID pandemic. Although delayed, the challenges only strengthened my resolve to complete the work and provide the guidance many desperately need.

Like many, COVID-19 affected our lives and my work in unforeseen ways. At the pandemic's start, my consulting career with RestCon grew beyond capacity, with 12-hour days becoming the norm. When the virus hit, my in-person appointments quickly evaporated. People with biotoxin illness were more afraid of COVID-19 than their mold problems. However, by shifting to online consultations, my schedule quickly filled again, and I could continue working remotely. Concerned about the potential for a housing market collapse, my wife, Trish, and I sold our California home and moved to Prescott, Arizona, where we hoped to use our equity to buy a house debt-free. After months of searching, we abandoned our original plan and purchased a home with visible mold at a reduced price, with the plan to remediate it myself to ensure it was safe for us.

During the COVID-19 crisis, remediation proved incredibly difficult. Supplies like respirator cartridges were in short supply, and I only had a limited stock on hand. Based on my years of experience working with mold, I believed I was immune and that exposure wouldn't harm me. However, I didn't realize then that I, too, was genetically predisposed to mold sensitivities. My ability to detox nightly in the safe homes we had created for Trisha had likely protected me for years, but that was about to change.

While Trisha went to live with our youngest daughter, I began the remediation work on our newly purchased fixer-upper in Arizona. Protective gear was scarce, and I had only three respirator cartridges to complete the project. These cartridges were supposed to be replaced daily, but without replacements available, I stretched each one to last two weeks. This meant that during the six weeks it took to remediate the home successfully, there were times when I was inadequately protected.

In hindsight, I began experiencing slight tremors and cognitive decline within weeks of finishing the work. At the time, I chalked it up to aging—I was in my mid-60s, and minor changes in memory, multitasking, and organization seemed like typical signs of growing older. Despite these challenges, I successfully remediated the home, and it turned out to be a good place for us. Any adverse symptoms from my safety shortcuts didn't seem significant and were easy to ignore. This home was where I first began developing the Pathways™ Testing methodology, using the home as a field experiment and the primary method of detecting where hidden problems were located and testing for cleanliness in the home. The home allowed me to try firsthand the methods that my research suggested were very helpful in achieving the necessary cleanliness for a home occupied by someone with sensitivities. Pathways™

Testing has become an essential tool in my work. We lived in that home successfully for about three years.

Eventually, we sold the Arizona home and moved to Virginia to be closer to family. During the cross-country move, I became seriously ill with an infection that was incapacitating and caused a complete loss of hearing in both ears. Over the next eight weeks, my hearing was partially restored through treatment with antibiotics and steroids. Still, this treatment destroyed my microflora and triggered a Candida infection, further complicating my recovery. I could still consult with clients via Zoom, but my writing ability suffered greatly. I could not organize my thoughts or write coherent sentences, which stalled my progress in writing this book.

It wasn't until Dr. Eric Dorninger of Roots and Branches intervened that I began to understand the full extent of my health decline. Eric and his colleagues Dana Bjerke and Genevieve Lamancusa had been referring patients to me for years, and we often collaborated on cases. One day, after a consultation, he pointed out that he had noticed tremors developing during our conversations. His observation was a wake-up call. I realized how much my health had deteriorated, and it became clear why I had been struggling with the completion of this book. The cognitive decline and tremors were no longer something I could dismiss—they were symptoms of something far more serious.

I am happy to share that after several months of diagnostics and treatment following the Shoemaker protocol, my health and writing ability have been restored, allowing me to complete this book. This journey has been humbling and enlightening, teaching me resilience and reinforcing the value of persistence in uncertainty. What began as a professional effort to share knowledge and empower others has taken on a deeper personal significance. Finishing this book is a professional achievement and a testament to recovery and the profound lessons it brings. It has shaped my practice philosophy, reminding me of the importance of empathy, informed decision-making, and the strength to emerge from challenges.

If you or someone you care about is grappling with mold illness, this is your moment to take action. Mold-related health challenges can feel overwhelming, but knowledge and proactive steps can make all the difference. Understanding the connection between water-damaged environments and health is not just critical for recovery—it's essential for prevention. The tools and insights in this book are meant to empower you to take control, seek appropriate solutions, and advocate for better awareness and care.

The rising prevalence of mold-related illnesses is not an isolated issue; it reflects deeper systemic problems in how buildings are constructed, maintained, and remediated.

A lack of accountability, inadequate education within the restoration and medical industries, and widespread misinformation have left many to suffer unnecessarily. By addressing these root causes and demanding better practices, we can create safer, healthier environments for everyone.

How Bad It Is: Inadequate Remediation Practices

Inadequate remediation practices lie at the heart of the mold crisis. While much attention is given to killing mold or cosmetically addressing it, the real issue often lies in hidden contamination and the superficial measures used to address it. Effective remediation requires the physical removal of affected materials, particularly porous ones, where mold can penetrate deeply and thrive. Unfortunately, many remediation efforts rely on chemicals such as antifungals, biocides, or agents that bleach discoloration, which may make surfaces appear clean but leave the underlying problems unresolved. Moisture intrusion and nutrient-rich materials, like paper-faced gypsum, remain unaddressed, allowing mold to persist.

The widespread use of chemicals and biocides in remediation is particularly concerning. These products are often marketed as quick fixes that "kill mold" or prevent its return but can create more problems than they solve. Toxigenic molds, for example, produce biotoxins as a defense mechanism and may respond to biocides by producing even higher levels of these toxins, making the environment more hazardous for sensitive individuals. Similarly, bleaching agents may remove visible mold discoloration but fail to resolve the structural and environmental conditions that promote its growth. This approach leads to a cycle of superficial fixes and recurring contamination, leaving occupants at ongoing risk and perpetuating the mold crisis.

The Anderson v. Allstate Case: A Catalyst for Change

The late 1990s marked a turning point for the mold crisis in the insurance industry, epitomized by the landmark case of *Anderson v. Allstate*. This case resulted in an $18.5 million jury verdict against Allstate Insurance, one of the largest mold-related judgments. The case centered on Mr. Anderson, a man in his nineties, who experienced significant property damage due to burst frozen pipes resulting in water damage and mold contamination. His home became uninhabitable, and Allstate refused to cover the full cost of remediation, which was estimated at approximately $132,000.

Jurors in the initial trial expressed frustration with what they perceived as Allstate's deliberate legal maneuvers to delay proceedings, seemingly in the hope that Mr. Anderson would pass away before the case went to trial.

When the case finally reached a verdict, the jury awarded $18.5 million in damages, a sum intended not only to compensate Mr. Anderson but also to send a message about the insurance company's conduct. However, Allstate appealed the verdict and succeeded in reducing the award to $500,000—a sum substantially higher than the original remediation estimate but far from the resounding victory initially declared.

Mr. Anderson, never received the original multi-million dollar sum, but the case became a watershed moment for the insurance industry. The staggering potential for mold-related payouts sent shockwaves through the sector, prompting insurers to take aggressive steps to limit their exposure. This included the introduction of mold caps and exclusions in homeowner policies, effectively transferring the financial burden of remediation onto homeowners. These measures signaled a shift in priorities, focusing on short-term cost containment rather than addressing the underlying causes of mold and water damage.

The PLRB Conference and Missed Opportunities

In the wake of the Anderson case, I was invited to speak at a Property and Liability Resource Bureau (PLRB) conference to address the growing mold crisis. The industry was in a state of panic, searching for ways to mitigate the financial risks posed by mold claims. I was asked to give a presentation at the conference. In it I suggested that the insurance industry's response to the crisis should not mirror its reaction to Anderson—limiting coverage and shifting responsibility to policyholders—but should instead draw inspiration from its handling of the electrical fire crisis in the early 20th century.

Back then, insurers faced a similar existential threat due to widespread electrical fires caused by faulty wiring and substandard materials. Rather than capping payouts, the insurance industry provided seed money to establish organizations like Underwriters Laboratories (UL) and the National Fire Protection Association (NFPA) to develop safer standards, materials, and practices. This proactive approach drastically reduced fire-related losses while preserving the industry's viability. I urged the insurance sector to adopt a similar model for mold, advocating for investments in research, better building practices, and the adoption of moisture-resistant materials like DensArmor Plus, a paperless form of gypsum.

Manufacturing Failures: The Rats-Can-Fly Approach

Unfortunately, the insurance industry and manufacturers took a different path. Instead of focusing on moisture control and less nutrient-rich building materials, manufacturers attempted to treat the paper-facing of gypsum board with biocides. This approach reflected a "rats-can-fly" mentality where a rat is thrown off the top of a building and it fly's to the ground. If you stop the study before the collision of the rat with the soil, the rat flew! What was learned was that the addition of chemicals could slow mold growth under ideal conditions, but it failed to address real-world complexities. Research showed that while biocides in paper-facing did initially slow mold growth, it did eventually catch up with the ultimate result of also triggering toxigenic molds to produce significantly higher levels of biotoxins when mold eventually developed. This reaction made the environment more hazardous than if the materials had simply been left untreated and dried quickly.

This reliance on chemical additives has mirrored the broader industry's overdependence on short-term solutions. Instead of addressing the core issue—moisture management—this approach created a cycle of reactive, ineffective measures that often-worsened conditions for sensitive individuals. The rats-can-fly analogy highlights the inherent flaw in stopping studies before observing the inevitable outcome: the biocides may delay mold growth, but when it occurs, the result is even more toxic than before. (Chakravarty, 2012)

The Promise of MSQPCR and the Barriers to Its Adoption

Mold-Specific Quantitative Polymerase Chain Reaction (MSQPCR) represents one of the most promising advancements in the field of mold and environmental health. This DNA-based methodology enables precise identification and quantification of mold species, offering unparalleled clarity compared to traditional techniques like spore traps or bulk sampling. By accurately measuring mold levels in a given environment, MSQPCR provides actionable insights, empowering remediation professionals to target contamination effectively and protecting vulnerable populations from prolonged exposure.

A Revolutionary Tool for Mold Investigation

Developed by the Environmental Protection Agency (EPA) over two decades ago, MSQPCR was designed to address critical gaps in mold detection. Unlike older methods that relied on culturing or visual inspection, MSQPCR provided the ability to identify a wide range of mold species quickly and precisely. It was heralded as a tool that could revolutionize how professionals evaluated mold contamination, helping to standardize the industry and improve public health outcomes.

The technology's applications extended beyond simple detection. MSQPCR allowed professionals to assess the effectiveness of remediation efforts, evaluate the severity of contamination, and correlate mold levels with health outcomes. For individuals with mold sensitivities, such

as those with Chronic Inflammatory Response Syndrome (CIRS), this level of specificity was transformative. For the first time, there was a reliable tool that could uncover hidden issues and validate whether environments were truly healthful.

Attempts to Suppress Its Impact

Despite its promise, MSQPCR faced significant resistance. Early on, misconceptions about its reliability and practicality delayed its adoption. The industry's resistance stemmed partly from its association with the Environmental Relative Moldiness Index (ERMI), a statistical research tool also developed by the EPA using MSQPCR data. While ERMI was designed for epidemiological studies, not individual diagnostics, its limitations were unfairly conflated with the underlying MSQPCR methodology.

The ERMI controversy provided ammunition for critics, many of whom were aligned with industries that stood to lose from widespread adoption of MSQPCR. Opponents argued that the technology was too complex, expensive, or unnecessary, dismissing its value without fully understanding its capabilities. This narrative was bolstered by a lack of education among professionals, who were often unaware of how MSQPCR could enhance their work.

Industry Pushback and Strategic Suppression

The pushback against MSQPCR was not limited to criticism. Attempts were made to squelch its influence through strategic suppression. Some industry players questioned the technology's validity in court, sowing doubt about its admissibility as evidence. Others promoted outdated methods as simpler and more cost-effective, even when those methods failed to provide the same level of accuracy or insight.

Moreover, the widespread marketing of ineffective biocides and "quick-fix" solutions further sidelined MSQPCR. By emphasizing surface-level cleaning and superficial remediation techniques, manufacturers and service providers avoided addressing the deeper issues that MSQPCR could reveal. The industry's reluctance to invest in long-term solutions perpetuated the cycle of inadequate remediation and ongoing health risks.

The EPA's Evolving Stance

The EPA's own communications about MSQPCR and ERMI added to the confusion. In a 2006 bulletin, the agency stated that ERMI was intended for research purposes and not validated for general use. This message was repeated in subsequent updates, including a strongly worded 2013 bulletin ordered by the EPA's Office of Inspector General. While these statements clarified ERMI's limitations, they were often misinterpreted as a rejection of MSQPCR itself.

In 2021, the EPA clarified its position further, acknowledging that MSQPCR was a valuable tool for quantifying mold contamination. The bulletin emphasized that the technology was developed in response to recommendations from the Institute of Medicine, which had called for more precise methods to assess mold exposure. Despite this endorsement, the lingering stigma around ERMI continued to overshadow MSQPCR's potential. (USEPA, 2021)

Another Missed Opportunity

Had MSQPCR been embraced earlier, it could have transformed the industry. By providing a robust scientific foundation for mold investigations, the technology could have mitigated many of the issues that persist today, from inadequate remediation practices to disputes over contamination levels. Instead, misinformation and resistance have slowed its adoption, leaving vulnerable populations without the full benefit of this groundbreaking tool.

A Call for Hope: Advancing Solutions and Inspiring Progress

The challenges posed by mold and water damage are daunting, but the tools, knowledge, and expertise to address them are already emerging. At the heart of the solution is a growing collaboration among healthcare professionals, Indoor Environmental Professionals (IEPs), remediators, educators, and policymakers. Together, these experts are working to create healthier environments and advance our understanding of mold's impact on health and buildings. Through their combined efforts, we can turn the tide and build a future where homes and workplaces foster well-being.

The Essential Role of Healthcare Professionals

Healthcare professionals are at the forefront of this transformation. As awareness of conditions like Chronic Inflammatory Response Syndrome (CIRS) grows, more physicians are recognizing the link between environmental exposures and complex health conditions. By identifying mold-related illnesses, guiding patients toward appropriate treatments, and collaborating with environmental experts, physicians play a pivotal role in bridging medical care with environmental science.

Organizations like CIRSx are leading the charge by providing education and resources for healthcare providers. They offer training to help physicians better understand mold-related illnesses and equip them with the tools to address these challenges in their patients. This growing engagement among healthcare professionals is critical,

as it ensures that individuals affected by mold and water damage are no longer dismissed but instead receive the care and attention they need to recover.

Physicians also work closely with Indoor Environmental Professionals (IEPs) and remediators to align medical treatment with environmental interventions. By ensuring that patients' living and working environments are healthful, healthcare providers are driving a more holistic approach to recovery—one that addresses both the individual and their surroundings.

The Vital Work of Indoor Environmental Professionals (IEPs)

IEPs serve as the investigative arm of the mold and water damage response. These experts perform thorough assessments to uncover hidden contamination, identify sources of moisture, and evaluate the full scope of microbial hazards, including mold, Actinobacteria, and gram-negative bacteria that produce harmful endotoxins. IEPs provide independent, science-based recommendations to guide remediation efforts, ensuring that actions taken are effective and health-focused.

IEPs are indispensable as third-party advocates who verify that remediation efforts are thorough and align with medical needs. Their objective evaluations protect clients from superficial fixes and hold remediators accountable for delivering quality results.

Remediators: The Hands-On Problem Solvers

Remediators are the practitioners responsible for addressing contamination identified by IEPs. Their work involves more than cleaning visible mold; it requires physically removing contaminated materials, addressing moisture problems, and implementing solutions to prevent future growth. For individuals with hypersensitivities, including those with CIRS, remediators must follow stringent protocols to ensure healthful results.

Unfortunately, the widespread use of antifungals, biocides, and other chemical treatments often creates more problems than it solves. These substances may bleach discoloration or superficially clean surfaces but leave contamination and harmful residues behind. Remediators must instead prioritize physical removal, thorough cleaning, and moisture control as the gold standard for health-focused remediation.

The Comprehensive Nature of Water-Damage Organisms

Mold is only part of the problem. Water-damaged environments can host a variety of harmful microorganisms, including Actinobacteria and gram-negative bacteria. These organisms produce exotoxins and endotoxins, which can trigger severe inflammatory responses, respiratory issues, and immune dysfunction. A complete approach to water damage must address all these hazards, ensuring that spaces are safe and healthful for occupants.

Avoiding the Pitfalls of Toxic Chemicals

The reliance on chemical treatments to solve mold problems is a pervasive issue. Biocides, antifungals, and other treatments may seem like quick fixes, but they often exacerbate the situation. For example, toxigenic molds can produce even greater quantities of biotoxins when exposed to these chemicals, creating environments more harmful than before.

Effective solutions prioritize physical removal and cleaning over chemical shortcuts. By addressing moisture problems and eliminating contamination at its source, we can create truly healthful environments without introducing new risks.

Empowering Change Through Education and Collaboration

Organizations like **CIRSx** and **IICRC** are paving the way for progress. CIRSx focuses on educating healthcare professionals, IEPs, and remediators about the complexities of mold-related illnesses, fostering a more informed and collaborative approach. Meanwhile, IICRC provides the industry with clear, actionable standards for mold remediation and water damage restoration, emphasizing prevention, physical removal, and thorough verification.

These organizations represent a model for how collaboration and education can drive meaningful change. Their work ensures that healthcare providers, environmental professionals, and remediators have the knowledge and resources needed to address mold challenges effectively.

A Call for Leadership

When I began my career as an environmental consultant, formaldehyde was a significant concern due to its widespread use in building materials and its associated health risks. The Environmental Protection Agency (EPA) addressed this issue under the Clean Air Act (CAA), which grants the agency authority to regulate hazardous air pollutants, including formaldehyde. Through stringent regulations and emission standards, the EPA effectively reduced formaldehyde levels in indoor environments, leading to a substantial decline in related health issues.

This success story underscores the importance of empowering the EPA with clear mandates to tackle environmental health challenges. Just as the agency mitigated formaldehyde exposure through its regulatory authority, a similar approach could be applied to mold and other indoor air quality concerns. By granting the EPA the

necessary authority and resources, we can develop comprehensive strategies to address these issues, ensuring healthier environments for all.

The formaldehyde case exemplifies how coordinated efforts between regulatory agencies, industry stakeholders, and the public can lead to significant improvements in environmental health. It serves as a model for addressing current challenges, such as mold contamination, by highlighting the effectiveness of regulation, research, and public awareness in mitigating health risks.

In conclusion, the progress made in reducing formaldehyde exposure demonstrates the potential for success when the EPA is empowered to act decisively. By applying similar strategies to mold and other indoor pollutants, we can create safer, healthier living and working environments for everyone.

To truly turn the tide, the Environmental Protection Agency (EPA) must be empowered with a federal mandate to address mold and water-damage issues comprehensively. With its scientific expertise and experience in setting environmental standards, the EPA is uniquely positioned to lead this effort. A mandate would enable the EPA to:

1. **Fund Research**: Support studies on mold-related illnesses, the genetic predispositions that make some individuals more vulnerable, and effective prevention strategies. Develop advanced detection methods like MSQPCR to improve accuracy and accessibility.

2. **Establish Standards**: Create enforceable guidelines for mold inspection, remediation, and prevention that prioritize health and safety.

3. **Promote Public Education**: Raise awareness about mold's health impacts, signs of water damage, and best practices for prevention. Empower individuals to make informed decisions about their environments.

4. **Coordinate Efforts**: Partner with organizations like IICRC and CIRSx to align standards and education across industries, fostering a unified approach to mold management.

The mold crisis is a challenge, but it is not an insurmountable one. Through collaboration, education, and a commitment to science-based practices, we can create a future where homes and workplaces are safe and healthful. By empowering the EPA, supporting the invaluable contributions of healthcare providers, IEPs, and remediators, and embracing advanced methodologies like MSQPCR, we can transform the way we approach mold and water damage.

Let us seize this opportunity for progress. Together, we can protect public health, support vulnerable populations, and build environments that nurture well-being for generations to come. This is our call to action—and our chance to make a lasting impact.

References

Chakravarty, P. (2012). Evaluation of five antifungal agents used in remediation practices against six common indoor fungal species. *Journal of Occupational and Environmental Hygiene, 9*(2), 81–92. https://www.epa.gov/system/files/documents/2021-09/updated-fact-sheet.ermi-_9.9.21.final_new-template_508-compliant_0.pdf

U.S. Environmental Protection Agency (EPA). (2021, September). *The Environmental Relative Moldiness Index (ERMI): Updated fact sheet.* Retrieved from https://www.epa.gov/system/files/documents/2021-09/updated-fact-sheet.ermi-_9.9.21.final_new-template_508-compliant_0.pdf

About the Author

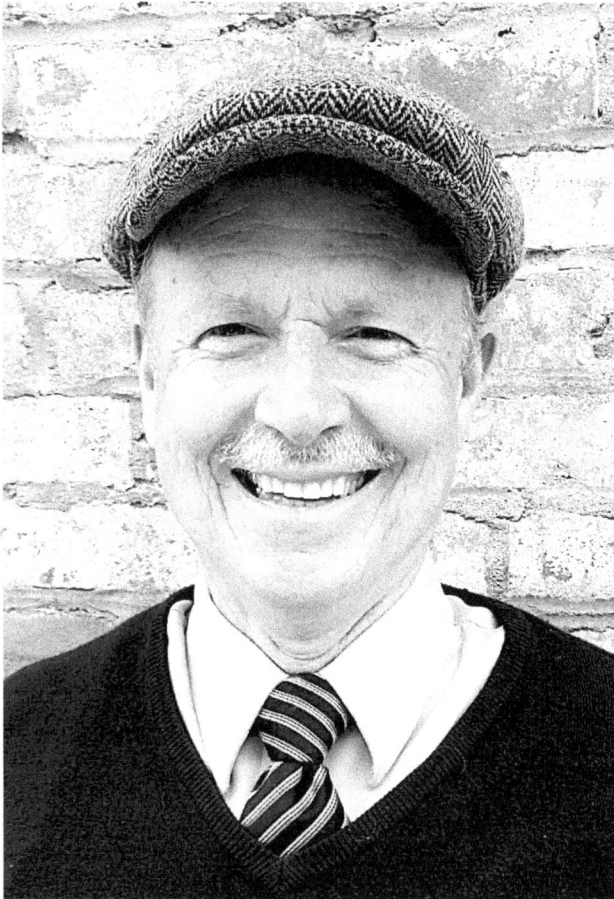

JOHN BANTA has spent over 37 years specializing in indoor environmental quality, with a focus on Medically Important Remediation for individuals sensitive to mold and water-damaged buildings. A retired Certified Industrial Hygienist and one of the first Baubiologists in the United States, he has consulted on thousands of cases, working closely with physicians, building professionals, and individuals with hypersensitivities. As the co-author of *Prescriptions for a Healthy House,* John has dedicated his career to developing science-based, non-toxic solutions for creating healthful indoor environments.

John has lived in multiple regions across the United States, giving him firsthand experience with how different climates, construction styles, and environmental factors influence mold and water damage. His work has taken him from humid coastal areas to arid desert regions, helping clients navigate the unique challenges of each setting.

For the past 27 years, John has provided consulting services through RestCon Environmental info@restconenviro.com. He specializes in Medically Important Remediation, helping individuals with complex health conditions create and maintain mold-controlled living environments.

When he's not consulting, teaching, conducting research or writing, John enjoys traveling and exploring nature with his wife, daughters, and grandchildren, embracing the outdoors as an extension of his passion for healthy living.

Contributors

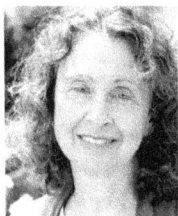

PAULA BAKER-LAPORTE, FAIA
Paula Baker-Laporte is the founding principal of EcoNest Architecture in Ashland, Oregon. A Fellow of the American Institute of Architects and a Building Biologist, Paula specializes in creating environmentally sound, health-enhancing homes. Her clients range from individuals with severe health challenges to those seeking optimal, eco-conscious living environments.

Over the past 30 years, she has focused on alternative mass wall building systems that integrate health and ecological performance. Her firm also consults internationally on the health impacts of the built environment, collaborating with owners, architects, and construction teams.

Her dedication to health in architecture was inspired by her own recovery from living in an unhealthy home. Paula's published works include the 4th edition of *Prescriptions for a Healthy House* (2022) and two natural building books co-authored with her husband, Robert Laporte: *EcoNest: Creating Sustainable Sanctuaries of Clay and Timber* (2007) and *The EcoNest Home* (2015).

Contact: info@econestarchitecture.com

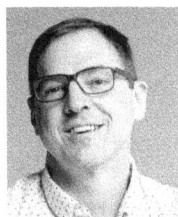

ERIC DORNINGER, ND, LAc
Dr. Eric Dorninger completed his Doctor of Naturopathic Medicine and Master of Science in Acupuncture at Bastyr University in 2003, followed by a two-year residency in Naturopathic Primary Care. In 2005, he founded Roots and Branches Integrative Healthcare, a clinic dedicated to solving "mystery illnesses" by uncovering the root causes of chronic, unrelenting health conditions. Dr. Dorninger focuses on "why you have it" rather than just "what you have," guiding his practice with the principle of "removing obstacles to cure."

Dr. Dorninger is a co-founder of CIRSx (CIRSx.com), an organization dedicated to "leading the way in treating, educating, and serving those with Chronic Inflammatory Response Syndrome."

Learn more at drdorninger.com
Photograph by Caleb Henry (Wild Inc.)

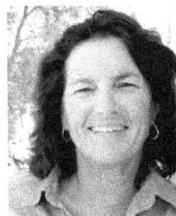

CINDY EDWARDS, General Building Contractor
Cindy Edwards is a general building contractor with over 40 years of experience in the field. She is also a certified building analyst with extensive expertise in home performance contracting. Cindy has studied and mastered the specialized knowledge required to assess and remediate buildings for CIRS patients. After observing many failed attempts by other mold experts, she developed her own successful approach to addressing these complex challenges. Cindy now teaches these skills to others, offering practical solutions and renewed hope to families dealing with CIRS. A beacon of hope for patients seeking recovery, she co-authored the MIR (Medically Important Remediation) 101 training through the CIRSx Institute. Cindy is also the co-author of *Mold Illness: Surviving and Thriving*.

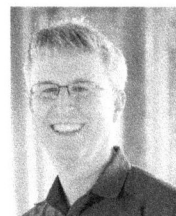

SCOTT FORSGREN, FDN-P
Scott Forsgren, FDN-P is a health coach, blogger, podcaster, health writer, and advocate. He is the editor and founder of BetterHealthGuy.com, where he shares his 28-year journey through the world of Lyme disease, mold illness, and the myriad of factors that chronic illness often entails.

His podcast *BetterHealthGuy Blogcasts* interviews many of the leaders in the field and is available on his web site, BetterHealthGuy.com, and on Apple Podcasts, Spotify, Amazon Music, YouTube, and Odysee. He has been interviewed on numerous podcasts and has lectured on his recovery from chronic illness at conferences and on several online summits. He has written for the *Townsend Letter* and other publications.

He is the co-founder of The Forum for Integrative Medicine which hosts an annual conference bringing together some of the top integrative practitioners to share practical tools for treating complex, chronic illness. He serves on the Board of Directors of LymeLight Foundation which provides treatment grants to children and young adults recovering from Lyme disease.

Today, Scott is grateful for his current state of health and all that he has learned on this life-changing journey.

Editor and Founder, BetterHealthGuy.com
Host of *BettherHealthGuy Blogcasts* Podcast

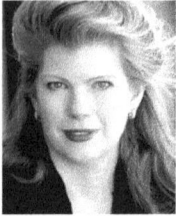

RAMONA GALLAGHER, Personal Property Expert

Ramona Gallagher graduated from the University of Massachusetts, Amherst, with a degree in Retail Management. Her career in inventories began in the 1980s while interning with Bloomingdale's, later overseeing inventories for companies like G. Fox, Filene's, and August Max. For over 25 years, she has specialized in insurance loss inventories, including seven years as Senior Project Manager at Comprehensive Inventory Services, managing high-value personal property losses. In 2006, Ramona founded Great Estates Inventory, LLC, serving businesses, individuals, and professionals. She holds a Certificate in Appraisal Studies in Fine and Decorative Arts from the Rhode Island School of Design and is trained in Uniform Standards of Professional Appraisal Practice (USPAP). Certified as a Property Insurance Appraiser (CPIA) since 2016, she is also a Registered Third-Party Evaluator (RTPE) and a voting member of the IICRC S320 Standards Committee. Licensed as a public adjuster in multiple states, Ramona is a member of several professional associations and is pursuing the Contents Loss Specialist (CLS) designation. She is the proud mother of two, Ashley and Rylan.

greatestatesinventory.com
Email: info@greatestatesinventory.com

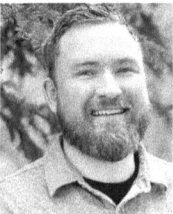

RYAN HOLSAPPLE, PH.D

Dr. Ryan Holsapple, holding a Ph.D. in Depth Psychology from Pacifica Graduate Institute, is Co-owner and Co-Director of the Center for Creative Choice alongside Karen Johnson. Founded in 1973 by Dr. Roger Strachan, a lifelong psychologist and therapist, the Center is home to the Self Soul Spirit model, a profound approach to psychology. Dr. Strachan mentored Dr. Holsapple for over a decade, training him in client work, genetic psychology, neurophysiology, gestalt therapy, and applied philosophy. After years of rigorous preparation, Dr. Strachan entrusted Dr. Holsapple with the continuation of the Center and the Self Soul Spirit model. Dr. Holsapple integrates scientific principles with soulful and spiritual approaches, drawing inspiration from Carl Jung and James Hillman. His unique perspective supports clients and groups in self-discovery, healing, and authenticity. Passionate about empowering others, he facilitates transformative experiences and offers educational training to ensure the Self Soul Spirit model's legacy. Dr. Holsapple is dedicated to helping people access their innate wisdom and live with greater empowerment and purpose.

Dr. Holsapple is currently taking clients and families dealing with CIRS and other chronic illnesses.

centerforcreativechoice.com
ryan@centerforcreativechoice.com

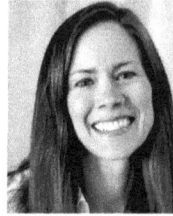

JENNY JOHNSON, MSPT, FMCHC, NBC-HWC

Jenny is a licensed Physical Therapist, National Board-Certified Functional Medicine Health Coach, and CIRS Coach & Consultant. Jenny holds a Bachelor's in Biology from Duke University and a Master's in Physical Therapy from the University of Colorado. She is certified in Functional Nutrition for Chronic Pain, Professional Life Coaching, HeartMath™, the Safe and Sound Protocol, the Bredesen Protocol, and the Shoemaker Protocol, among others. A Surviving Mold Proficiency Partner since 2019, Jenny draws from personal experiences with Lyme Disease, CIRS, Autism, MCAS, POTS, and Alzheimer's. As founder of Simplified Wellness Designs, LLC, Jenny supports clients virtually as a coach, consultant, and educator. Her compassionate approach fosters personal growth, equips clients to enhance health, and guides them in making choices for lasting well-being. She is a faculty member of the CIRSx Institute, and co-authored the CIRSx Coach and Consultant Course for allied health professionals.

Jenny's signature programs and offerings include:

CIRS Healing Collective: educational support network

Equipped to Overcome CIRS: group coaching program and online course for CIRS patients

Salugenex™ for CIRS: group wellness program for individuals overcoming CIRS

Private Coaching & Consulting: individuals seeking personal support navigating environmental illness.

jenny@simplifiedwellnessdesigns.com
simplifiedwellnessdesigns.com

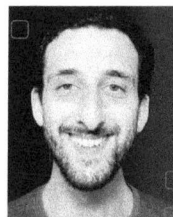

ALEX KESSLER

Alex Kessler is a translational scientist in precision medicine and the founder of the YouTube channel *Healthy Home Guide*. After experiencing severe chronic illness caused by toxic mold exposure, Alex dedicated his life to empowering others with actionable, evidence-based solutions for improving indoor air quality. Combining scientific expertise with personal experience, he creates budget-friendly, DIY protocols that are practical and effective, even for renters. Alex's mission is to make healthy homes accessible for everyone. His work focuses on transforming science into real-world strategies to help people create living spaces that promote healing and long-term well-being.

healthyhomeguide.com
YouTube: Healthy Home Guide
Email: alex@healthyhomeguide.com

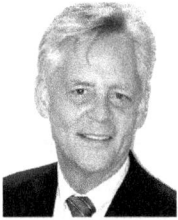

KEN LARSEN, CR®, WLS®, FLS®, CLS®, ERS®, CMP®, CSDS
Ken Larsen, has been in the restoration industry since 1978. Recipient of the 32nd RIA Martin L. King Award for his many contributions and sincere dedication to the Restoration Industry, his career includes 18 years as an independent property restoration contractor, consultant to restorative drying during catastrophes and large loss drying coordination, expert witness, and now the author of one of the industry's leading technical resource book on the subject of structural restorative drying—Leadership in Restorative Drying. He is currently an IICRC Approved instructor of WRT, ASD and CDS certificate courses. Larsen is also an RIA instructor of the restoration industry's advanced certification credentials: Water Loss Specialist (WLS®), Fire Loss Specialist (FLS®), Contents Loss Specialist (CLS®), and Certified Restorer (CR®). He serves as Chairman for RIA approved Instructors, Trainers and Subject Matter Experts, a sub-committee of RIA's Education Committee. He is also a Registered Third Party Evaluator® (RTPE). Ken lives in Clearwater area in Florida.

ken@drystandard.org

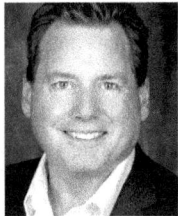

SCOTT W. McMAHON, MD
Dr. Scott W. McMahon earned his Bachelor of Science in Chemistry in 1985 and his Medical Degree in 1989, both from Creighton University. He completed his pediatric residency at Duke University Medical Center in 1992 and has been a board-certified pediatrician practicing in Roswell, New Mexico, for over 26 years. His journey into Chronic Inflammatory Response Syndrome (CIRS) began in 2009 when a local family sought help for their daughter's illness linked to a water-damaged school.

Inspired by his visits to Dr. Ritchie Shoemaker's office, Dr. McMahon established a practice focused on diagnosing and treating CIRS. He became the first physician worldwide to complete Dr. Shoemaker's CIRS Certification Program.

Dr. McMahon has authored two books, co-authored three consensus statements, and frequently speaks at medical conferences. He continues to serve CIRS patients at his Roswell clinic.

wholeworldhealthcare.com
wwhcinfo@wholeworldhealthcare.com

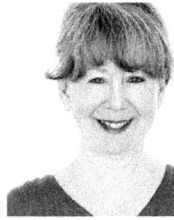

MARILEE NELSON
Marilee is a Board-Certified Nutritionist, Certified Building Biologist, and building materials specialist. She is also on the advisory board for Documenting Hope. For 33 years, she has worked with the chronically ill, children with disabilities, and mold and chemically injured. She lives in the Texas Hill Country with her husband and is the Founder of Branch Basics. Her family's story about how and why Branch Basics was Formulated and Developed is on page 92: The Making of a Healthy Cleaning Line in *Prescriptions for Healthy House*.

BranchBasics.com

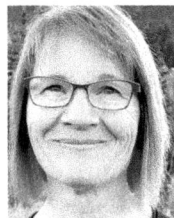

JANE PRESCOT, FMCHC
Trained as a Registered Nurse and Certified Midwife prior to emigrating to Canada, Jane worked in a variety of acute care and community nursing specialties before pivoting, as a result of her own health journey, to focus on Environmentally Acquired Illness / Biotoxin Illness (Chronic Inflammatory Response Syndrome). Jane became a Functional Medicine Certified Health Coach (FMCHC) in 2019 and Shoemaker CIRS Proficiency Partner in 2020. She was a founding member of the International Society for Environmentally Acquired Illness (ISEAI). Jane has received training in the Biology of Trauma and Medically Important Remediation. She is a faculty member of the CIRSx Institute and co-authored the CIRSx Coach and Consultant Course for allied health professionals

Jane's human rights complaint against her employer has set a precedent in Canada for ERMI / HERTSMI-2 testing for environmentally sensitive individuals in the workplace.

Flourish Clinic fatiguetoflourish.com
getmymoldylifeback.com

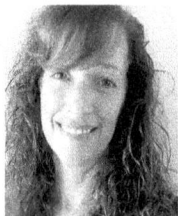

LAURIE ROSSI, RN
Laurie Rossi is a Registered Nurse with 40 years of experience specializing in oncology, integrative medicine, and patient education. As a CIRS patient, Laurie worked closely with Dr. Shoemaker to achieve her recovery and now dedicates her efforts to helping others navigate their journey to health. Since 2010, she has been deeply involved in educating and supporting CIRS patients, medical practices, and environmental professionals, fostering collaboration among compassionate individuals to meet the unique needs of this community. Laurie is the co-author of *Mold Illness: Surviving and Thriving*.

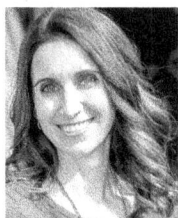

JENNIFER SCHRANTZ, REALTOR®, ABR®, GREEN
Jennifer Schrantz has been a REALTOR® in Arizona since 2013 and became the Designated Broker of OMNI Homes International in 2022. She is passionate about guiding clients through the home buying and selling process, ensuring their needs are met every step of the way. Jennifer specializes in working with clients affected by Chronic Inflammatory Response Syndrome (CIRS). Drawing from her collaboration with her husband, Michael Schrantz, an IEP and owner of Environmental Analytics, Jennifer tailors her approach to address environmental exposures, such as water damage and mold. Her expertise has helped many CIRS patients find homes that serve as safe sanctuaries. Outside of real estate, Jennifer is a pilot and flight instructor. She and her husband, Mike, have two boys and enjoy spending time outdoors hiking, swimming, and playing games as a family.

OMNI Homes International
Office Email: Broker@ohisupport.com
Personal Email: Jennifer.M.Schrantz@gmail.com

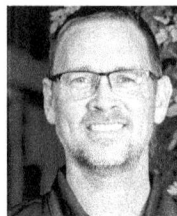

MICHAEL SCHRANTZ, CIEC, CMI
Michael Schrantz is the founder of Environmental Analytics LLC, a leading indoor environmental quality consulting firm. With over 27 years of expertise and involvement in more than 6,800 projects globally, he specializes in identifying contaminants, developing remediation protocols, and educating the public on indoor air quality. Michael is a board member of ISEAI and ACAC, a published author (publications and coursework), and a frequent speaker at conferences. Passionate about creating healthier living environments, he also hosts the educational platform IEP Radio, providing invaluable insights into building science and indoor environmental quality.

Podcast: *IEP Radio* on YouTube & SoundCloud
mike@environmentalanalytics.net

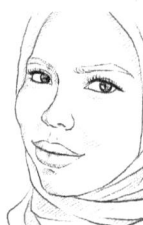

ATIK SUGIWARA
Atik Sugiwara is an artist and graphic designer with a background in traditional fine art and over five years of experience in digital illustration. Her work reflects a unique blend of freehand digital drawing and meticulous detail, offering vibrant, high-resolution Illustrations tailored to each project. Atik specializes in botanical, digital watercolors, and object illustrations, bringing a fresh, captivating perspective to each piece. She values clear communication, ensuring her clients are informed at every step of the creative process. Passionate about bringing ideas to life, Atik delivers quality, professionalism, and a collaborative spirit that makes her work stand out.

Atik created the illustrations in this book.

fiverr.com/atiksugiwara
instagram.com/atik.sugiwara

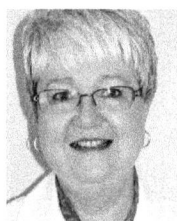

PAULA VETTER
Paula Vetter is a Holistic Family Nurse Practitioner with over 40 years of experience in both traditional and functional medicine. She served as a critical care instructor at the renowned Cleveland Clinic for more than a decade and has taught at colleges in Ohio. Paula also maintained a private practice in Central California, where she was a Shoemaker Certified CIRS Practitioner until her recent retirement. Passionate about empowering individuals and families, she is dedicated to helping others take charge of their health and transform their lives. Paula is the co-author of *Mold Illness: Surviving and Thriving*.

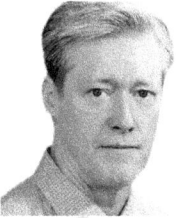

GREG WEATHERMAN, CMC
Since 1997, Greg Weatherman has specialized in addressing mold and bacteria, beginning as a Virginia Class A contractor with expertise in asbestos abatement. He has worked with Dr. Shoemaker's patients since 2001 and is now based in the southeastern U.S., operating as a licensed Florida Mold Assessor. Greg's company, Surviving Remediation, focuses on testing mold and bacteria in water-damaged indoor environments. Recently, he served on two IICRC standards committees: the S520 Standard for Professional Mold Remediation and the S700 Standard for Professional Fire and Smoke Damage Restoration. Greg is also a co-founder of CIRSx.com and one of the inventors and principals of Aerobiological Solutions, creators of the patented air-cleaning product AeroSolver. He offers both on-site and virtual inspections worldwide.

SurvivingRemediation.com
AeroSolver.com
gw@aerosolver.com

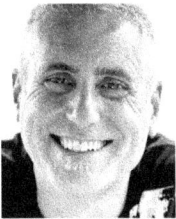

BILL WEBER, G.C., CR, CIEC, CMRS
Bill Weber is a Principal Consultant for AVELAR, a Northern California firm specializing in the forensic analysis, design, and repair of commercial properties and residential buildings. A founding member of the Building Science Institute and active in ISEAI and CIRSx, he holds prestigious certifications including Certified Restorer (RIA), Board-Certified Indoor Environmental Consultant (CIEC), and Board-Certified Microbial Remediation Supervisor (CMRS). He is also a Certified Building Science Thermographer (CBST) and a California licensed general contractor, serving as a Subject Matter Expert for the Contractors State License Board.

Bill has over 27 years of experience in remediation, mitigation, investigation, and repair of construction defects and smoke, fire, and water-damaged structures. He has contributed to the IICRC S500 and S520 standards, the *Surviving Mold Remediation Consensus Document*, and *Prescriptions for a Healthy House*. A recognized speaker, Bill has presented at training sessions, insurance panels, and environmental workshops nationwide.

Contact Bill Weber at bweber@avelar.com
AVELAR@avelar.net

Index

odors, musty: 18, 51, 59, 138, 139, 147, 167, 175, 180, 184, 185, 191, 205, 218, 226, 236, 253, 298, 299, 312, 323, 324

odors, chemical: 13, 131, 321, 330

outdoor dust sampling: 52, 203, 205

outdoor mold: 24, 38, 52, 55, 57

outdoor mold ecology: 45, 55

over-drying: 101, 115

ozone: 232, 253, 336

Paecilomyces variotii: 87

Pain: 21, 173

Pain, Abdominal: 22, 24, 173

Pain, Facial: 23, 173

Pain, Joint: 173

painted surfaces: 48, 138, 180–181, 315

paper-faced gypsum board: 12, 26–27, 52, 54–55, 60, 72, 73, 114–116, 122, 123, 126, 145, 148, 178, 179, 182–185, 188–189, 191, 196, 209, 250–251, 271–272, 338

paperless gypsum board: 143, 178, 286, 338

Parkinsons disease: XX, XXI

particle behavior: 9, 38, 43, 46, 47, 49, 51, 55, 57, 58, 62, 64–65

particle cleaning: 62–69

pathways: 21–22, 48, 51, 62, 66, 146, 178, 209, 215, 269, 273

Pathways™ Testing: 62, 137, 157–158, 203–206, 211–224, 214–216, 225, 227, 237, 253, 257, 260, 268, 270–273, 337

Pathways™ Testing post-cleaning: 69, 71, 121, 279–282, 289, 291, 322

Paula Baker-Laporte: 5–6, 28, 140, 186, 278, 285, 336

Paula Vetter: 30, 348

PCR (polymerase chain reaction): 10, 68, 199, 200, 205, 279

Penicillium brevicompactum: 74, 80

Penicillium chrysogenum: 80

Penicillium corylophilum: 80

Penicillium crustosum: 80

Penicillium spinulosum: 80

Penicillium variable: 81

PCO (photocatalytic oxidation): 232, 253–254

peptide bond residues: 15, 69, 157, 206, 211

personal diary: 166–168

personal possessions: 122, 297–332

pest inspections: 143

pet safety: 10, 113, 301

photographic documentation: 98, 102–103, 111, 126, 135, 200, 202, 235

physical removal: 10–11, 25–27, 32, 38, 52, 72, 116–117, 121, 158, 232, 234, 250–252, 254, 265, 288, 338, 340–341

plumbing, frozen: 149, 194

plumbing, leaks: 150, 187, 283

plumbing, traps (u-traps, p-traps): 148, 187

plumbing, vent stacks: 148

plumbing, AAV (Air Admittance Valve): 26, 148

polystyrene insulation: 144

pool, indoor: 179

portable air purifiers: 254

post-remediation assessment: 69, 121, 123, 232, 270, 275, 280

post-remediation: 9, 66, 69, 162, 229, 250,268, 271, 277

post-remediation verification: 3, 108, 121, 240

post-remediation reconstruction: 158–159, 277, 279

PPE, personal protective equipment: 65, 95–97, 103, 122–123, 180, 235, 252, 259

predatory practices: 104, 197

pre-existing conditions: 104, 125, 139

pre-loss conditions: 11, 125–126

Prescriptions for a Healthy House: 5–6, 140–148, 158, 185, 278, 285, 286, 293, 336

preservation: 43, 77, 116, 176, 226, 297–299, 303–307, 310

preservation (e.g., artwork, collectibles): 315–316

preventative measures: 105, 130, 141, 143, 150, 158, 169, 176, 266, 284, 285–286, 303

prevention: 105, 137, 141, 143, 158, 183, 266, 282, 284–286, 303, 341

Primal Trust: 36, 37

protein residues: 15, 69, 157, 206, 211

psychological impact: 28–30, 37–41, 376

psychrometry: 119

public records: 132

qualifications: 31, 104, 107, 199

quality control: 200, 202, 235, 240, 268, 273

Ramona Gallagher: 315, 346

rapid drying: 100, 116, 119–120, 150, 177, 303–304, 312, 316–317, 329, 332

rapid response: 98, 101, 150, 177

Rash: 17, 22, 28, 173, 305

REAC, (HUD Real Estate Assessment Center): 139

re-aerosolization: 58, 66

real estate transactions: 31–32, 130–132,137

real estate resources: 132–135, 175, 197, 268

reasonable accommodations: 48, 137, 139–140, 163

recontamination: 50, 62, 67, 69, 124, 156, 162, 205, 217, 242, 269, 279–280, 288, 290, 299, 307

Red Eyes: 21, 173

red flag: 132, 135, 137–138, 140, 175

refrigerator/freezers: 321, 328

regulations: 139, 160–161, 176, 228, 231, 233–234, 250, 276

remediation: 32–33, 66–69, 108, 117, 149, 170, 228–239

remediation plan implementation: 240–267

remediation quality control: 268–276

rental, inspections: 138

Reservation of Rights Letters: 127–128

reverse stack effect: 192, 260

Rhizopus stolonifer: 86–87

RIA (Restoration Industry Association): 102

rodent damage: 25–26, 147–148, 157, 179, 213–214, 259–260, 262

roof: 178–179, 188, 194, 260, 283, 285, 290, 293, 294

Ryan J. Holsapple, PhD: 14, 38, 346

ventilation: 28–29, 55, 58, 146, 148, 152, 155, 179, 259, 260
ventilation, local exhaust: 158,239, 242, 244–247, 250, 252
ventilation, moisture control: 5, 71, 103, 142, 158, 180–185, 266–267
Vertigo: 22, 173
vinegar: 67
visible damage: 11, 59, 63, 110, 147, 299
VOCs (volatile organic compounds): 12–14, 17, 28, 255

Wallemia sebi: 89–90
wallpaper: 62, 191
Water Activity (Aw): 60–61, 73
Water alarms: 102
water shutoff valves: 110
Water stains: 55, 118, 138, 175, 188, 226, 241, 252
water table, elevated: 177
water vapor: 58–60, 180, 298, 302
water-damage organisms
water-resilient materials
Weakness: 21, 173
wear and tear: 136, 144, 147, 175
weep holes: 146–148
weep screed: 146–147
window, condensation: 181–182
window, insulation: 182
wine: 43, 44, 116, 303
wine room: 179, 221,
Word Finding Difficulty: 22, 173
WRT, Water Damage Restoration Technician: 104, 106, 115

Stay Connected and Informed

Mold Controlled marks a milestone in addressing the challenges of mold and water damage, but the journey doesn't stop here. As new information emerges and innovative solutions develop, staying informed is essential.

Subscribe to **JohnCBanta.com** to receive intermittent updates directly in your inbox. Here's what you can expect:

- **Exclusive Book Updates:** Expanded content and related insights from Mold Controlled and Prescriptions for a Healthy House.

- **Research Highlights:** The latest studies on mold and water damage.

- **Product and Service Evaluations:** Updated reviews and recommendations to help guide your decisions.

- **Pertinent News:** Industry developments, regulatory updates, and more.

- **Calls to Action:** Opportunities to make a difference and support meaningful change.

- **Ask the Expert:** Submit your questions about mold, water damage, and environmental health. If I don't know the answer, I probably know someone who does! And if there's no currently known answer, it may be added to a research needs list.

Take the next step in creating a safer, healthier indoor environment.

Subscribe today at:

JohnCBanta.com

www.ingramcontent.com/pod-product-compliance
Lightning Source LLC
Chambersburg PA
CBHW081143020426
42333CB00021B/2644